In Vitro Methods in Toxicology

edited by

G. JOLLES
Rhône-Poulenc Rorer
Antony
France

and

A. CORDIER
Rhône-Poulenc Rorer
Vitry-sur-Seine
France

ACADEMIC PRESS
Harcourt Brace Jovanovich, Publishers
London San Diego New York
Boston Sydney Tokyo Toronto

ACADEMIC PRESS LIMITED
24/28 Oval Road,
London NW1 7DX

United States Edition published by
ACADEMIC PRESS INC.
San Diego, CA 92101

This book is printed on acid-free paper

A catalogue record for this book is
available from the British Library

ISBN 0-12-388175-7

Based on the Proceedings of the Sixth International Round Table of the
Rhône-Poulenc Rorer Foundation, Les Pensières 1990

Typeset by Photo graphics, Honiton, Devon
and printed in Great Britain by
The University Printing House, Cambridge

Contributors

Acosta, D. The University of Texas at Austin, Department of Pharmacology and Toxicology, College of Pharmacy, Austin, TX 78712, USA.

Aran, J.M. Laboratoire d'Audiologie Expérimentale, INSERM U-229, Université de Bordeaux II, Hôpital Pellegrin, 33076 Bordeaux, France.

Atterwill, C.K. The CellTox Center, Division of Biosciences, Hatfield Polytechnic, College Lane, Hatfield, Herts, UK.

Bach, P.H. Polytechnic of East London, School of Science, Romford Road, London E15 4LZ, UK.

Balls, M. FRAME, 34 Stoney Street, Nottingham NG1 1NB, UK.

Berger, A.E. Cell Biology Research Unit, The Upjohn Company, Kalamazoo, MI 49001, USA.

Bergmark, E. Department of Environmental Health, SC-34 University of Washington, Seattle, WA 98195, USA.

Bkaily, G. Department of Physiology and Biophysics, Faculty of Medicine, University of Sherbrooke, Sherbrooke, Quebec J1H 5N4, Canada.

Boyer, J.L. Liver Center and Department of Medicine, 333 Cedar St., Yale University School of Medicine, New Haven, CT 06510, USA.

Branstetter, D.G. Investigative Toxicology Unit, The Upjohn Company, Kalamazoo, MI 49001, USA.

Brodie, C. Departments of Psychiatry and Pharmacology, University of Colorado School of Medicine, Denver, CO 80262, USA.

Bruinink, A. Institute of Toxicology, ETH & University Zurich, CH-8603 Schwerzenbach, Switzerland.

Brun, P-H. Unité d'Endocrinotoxicologie, Institut de Recherche sur la Sécurité du Médicament, Rhône-Poulenc Rorer SA, 20, Quai de la Révolution, 94140 Alfortville, France.

Cailliau, E. Laboratoire de Biochimie Toxicologique et Cancérologique, Université Catholique de Louvain, UCL 7369, Avenue Mounier 73, 1200 Bruxelles, Belgium.

Calleman, C.J. Department of Environmental Health, SC-34 University of Washington, Seattle, WA 98195, USA.

Chang, C.C. Department of Pediatrics/Human Development, Center for Environmental Toxicology, Michigan State University, East Lansing, MI 48824, USA.

Claude, J.R. Laboratoire de Toxicologie, Faculté de Pharmacie, 4, Avenue de l'Observatoire, 75006 Paris, France.

Cordier, A.C. Institut de Recherche sur la Sécurité du Médicament, Rhône-Poulenc Rorer, 20, Quai de la Révolution, 94140 Alfortville, France.

Costa, L.G. Department of Environmental Health, SC-34 University of Washington, Seattle, WA 98195, USA.

Courjault, F. Unité de Néphrotoxicologie, Institut de Recherche sur la Sécurité du

Médicament, Rhône-Poulenc Rorer SA, 20, Quai de la Révolution, 94140 Alfortville, France.

Cramer, C.T.   Investigative Toxicology Unit, The Upjohn Company, Kalamazoo, MI 49001, USA.

Davies, D.   Departments of Psychiatry and Pharmacology, University of Colorado School of Medicine, Denver, CO 80262, USA.

Davila, J.   The University of Texas at Austin, Department of Pharmacology and Toxicology, College of Pharmacy, Austin, TX 78712, USA.

Deboyser, D.   Laboratoire de Biochimie Toxicologique et Cancérologique, Université Catholique de Louvain, UCL 7369, Avenue Mounier 73, 1200 Bruxelles, Belgium.

Dulon, D.   Laboratoire d'Audiologie Expérimentale, INSERM U-229, Université de Bordeaux II, Hôpital Pellegrin, 33076 Bordeaux, France.

Dunkel, V.C.   U.S. Food and Drug Administration, 200 C Street, S.W. Washington, DC 20204, USA.

Dupont, E.   Department of Pediatrics/Human Development, Center for Environmental Toxicology, Michigan State University, East Lansing, MI 48824, USA.

Ekblad-Sekund, G.   Unit of Neurochemistry and Neurotoxicology, Stockholm University, S-106 91 Stockholm, Sweden.

Fitzgerald, D.J.   The Flinders University of South Australia, School of Biological Sciences, Bedford Park, S.A. 5042, Australia.

Frazier, J.M.   The Johns Hopkins University, 615 North Wolfe Street, Baltimore, MD 21205, USA.

Goethals, F.   Laboratoire de Biochimie Toxicologique et Cancérologique, Université Catholique de Louvain, UCL 7369, Avenue Mounier 73, 1200 Bruxelles, Belgium.

Guguen-Guillouzo, C.   INSERM U49, Unité de Recherches Hépatologiques, Hôpital Pontchaillou, 35033 Rennes, Cedex, France.

Guillouzo, A.   INSERM U49, Unité de Recherches Hépatologiques, Hôpital Pontchaillou, 35033 Rennes, Cedex, France.

Heuillet, E.   Institut de Recherche sur la Sécurité du Médicament, Rhône-Poulenc Rorer, 20, Quai de le Révolution, 94140 Alfortville, France.

Hiel, H.   Laboratoire d'Audiologie Expérimentale, INSERM U-229, Université de Bordeaux II, Hôpital Pellegrin, 33076 Bordeaux, France.

Ivanov, M.A.   Institut de Recherche sur la Sécurité du Médicament, Rhône-Poulenc Rorer, 20, Quai de la Révolution, 94140 Alfortville, France.

Johnston, H.   The CellTox Center, Division of Biosciences, Hatfield Polytechnic, College Lane, Hatfield, Herts, UK.

Kalimi, G.   Department of Pediatrics/Human Development, Center for Environmental Toxicology, Michigan State University, East Lansing, MI 48824, USA.

Kentroti, S.   Departments of Psychiatry and Pharmacology, University of Colorado School of Medicine, Denver, CO 80262, USA.

Krutovskikh, V.   International Agency for Research on Cancer, 150 Cours Albert Thomas, 69372 Lyon Cedex 08, France.

Madhukar, B.V.   Department of Pediatrics/Human Development, Center for Environmental Toxicology, Michigan State University, East Lansing, MI 48824, USA.

Mahouy, G.   INSERM, Institut d'Hématologie, Hôpital Saint-Louis, 75010 Paris, France.

Mangoura, D.   Departments of Psychiatry and Pharmacology, University of Colorado School of Medicine, Denver, CO 80262, USA.

Mather, J.   Genentech Inc., South San Francisco, CA, USA.

Melcion, C.   Institut de Recherche sur la Sécurité du Médicament, Rhône-Poulenc Rorer, 20, Quai de la Révolution, 94140 Alfortville, France.

Nakazawa, H.   International Agency for Research on Cancer, 150 Cours Albert Thomas, 69372 Lyon Cedex 08, France.

New, D.A.T.   Physiological Laboratory, University of Cambridge, Cambridge CB2 3EG, UK.

Nilsson, M.   Unit of Neurochemistry and Neurotoxicology, Stockholm University, S-106 91 Stockholm, Sweden.

Odland, L.   Unit of Neurochemistry and Neurotoxicology, Stockholm University, S-106 91 Stockholm, Sweden.

Oyamada, M.   Department of Pathology, Sapporo Medical College, Sapporo 060, Japan.

Paine, A.J.   DH Department of Toxicology, St. Bartholomew's Hospital Medical College, University of London, Dominion House, 59 Bartholomew Close, London EC1 7ED, UK.

Petrella, D.K.   Drug Development Toxicology Unit, The Upjohn Company, Kalamazoo, MI 49001, USA.

Puddington, L.   Cell Biology Research Unit, The Upjohn Company, Kalamazoo, MI 49001, USA.

Purchase, I.F.K.   ICI Central Toxicology Laboratory, Alderley Park, Macclesfield, Cheshire SK10 4TJ, UK.

Ramos, K.   The University of Texas at Austin, Department of Pharmacology and Toxicology, College of Pharmacy, Austin, TX 78712, USA.

Renault, J.-Y.   Institut de Recherche sur la Sécurité du Médicament, Rhône-Poulenc Rorer SA, 20, Quai de la Révolution, 94140 Alfortville, France.

Roberfroid, M.   Laboratoire de Biochimie Toxicologique et Cancérologique, Université Catholique de Louvain, UCL 7369, Avenue Mounier 73, 1200 Bruxelles, Belgium.

Romert, L.   Department of Genetic and Cellular Toxicology, Stockholm University, S-106 91 Stockholm, Sweden.

Saito, T.   Laboratoire d'Audiologie Expérimentale, INSERM U-229, Université de Bordeaux II, Hôpital Pellegrin, 33076 Bordeaux, France.

Sakellaridis, N.   Departments of Psychiatry and Pharmacology, University of Colorado School of Medicine, Denver, CO 80262, USA.

Smith, M.A.   The University of Texas at Austin, Department of Pharmacology and Toxicology, College of Pharmacy, Austin TX 78712, USA.

Smyrniotis, T.   Commission of the European Communities, Directorate General for the Environment, Nuclear Safety and Civil Protection.

Sun, E.   Investigative Toxicology Unit, The Upjohn Company, Kalamazoo, MI 49001, USA.

Swann, J.   The University of Texas at Austin, Department of Pharmacology and Toxicology, College of Pharmacy, Austin, TX 78712, USA.

Toutain, H.   Unité de Néphrotoxicologie, Institut de Recherche sur la Sécurité du Médicament, Rhône-Poulenc Rorer SA, 20, Quai de la Révolution, 94140 Alfortville, France.

Trosko, J.E.   Department of Pediatrics/Human Development, Center for Environmental Toxicology, Michigan State University, East Lansing, MI 48824, USA.

Ulrich, R.G.   Investigative Toxicology Unit, The Upjohn Company, Kalamazoo, MI 49001, USA.

Vernadakis, A.   Departments of Psychiatry and Pharmacology, University of Colorado School of Medicine, Denver, CO 80262, USA.

Vintezou, P.   Institut de Recherche sur la Sécurité du Médicament, Rhône-Poulenc Rorer, 20, Quai de la Révolution, 94140 Alfortville, France.

Walum, E.   Unit of Neurochemistry and Neurotoxicology, Stockholm University, S-106 91 Stockholm, Sweden.

Wilks, M.F.   ICI Central Toxicology Laboratory, Alderley Park, Macclesfield, Cheshire SK10, UK.

Yamasaki, H.   International Agency for Research on Cancer, 150 Cours Albert Thomas, 69372 Lyon Cedex 08, France.

Zbinden, G.   Institute of Toxicology, Swiss Federal Institute of Technology and University of Zurich, Schwerzenbach, Switzerland.

Participants

Adolphe, M. Société de Pharmaco-Toxicologie Cellulaire, 15, Rue de l'École de Médecine, 75006 Paris, France.

Amiel, C. UER Xavier Bichat, INSERM U 251, 16, Rue Henri-Huchard, 75018 Paris, France.

Ballet, F. Rhône-Poulenc Rorer, Institut de Recherche, sur la Sécurité du Médicament, 20, Quai de la Révolution, 94140 Alfortville, France.

Baron, H. Rhône-Poulenc Rorer, Institut de Recherche, sur la Sécurité du Médicament, 20, Quai de la Révolution, 94140 Alfortville, France.

Bazin, H. Commission des Communautés, Européennes, Direction Générale de la Science de la Recherche et du Développement, Centre Commun de Recherche, Rue de la Loi 200, B-1049 Bruxelles, Belgium.

Beaune, P. Faculté de Médecine Necker - Enfants Malades, Biochimie Pharmacologique et Métabolique, 156, Rue de Vaugirard, 75730 Paris Cedex 15, France.

Bertrand, M. École Nationale Vétérinaire de Lyon, 1, Avenue Bourgelat, B.P. 83, 69280 Marcy-l'Etoile, France.

Bonnod, J. IFFA-CREDO, Centre de Recherche et d'Élevage du Domaine des Oncins, B.P. 109, 69210 l'Arbresle, France.

Bost, P.E. Rhône-Poulenc Rorer, Direction Recherche et Développement, 20, Avenue Raymond Aron, 92165 Antony Cedex, France.

Brown, N. MRC Experimental Embryology and Teratology Unit, St. George's Hospital Medical School, Cranmer Terrace, London SW17 0RE, United Kingdom.

Bruggmann, A. Pharma Information, Birsigstrasse 4, CH-4054 Basel, Switzerland.

Burnol, F. Institut Curie, 26, Rue d'Ulm, 75231 Paris Cedex 05, France.

Caillard, L. Rhône-Poulenc Interservices, Direction Qualité Sécurité Environnement, Service Toxicologie, Les Miroirs, 18, Avenue d'Alsace, 92097 Paris La Défense, France.

Cano, J.P. Sanofi Recherche, Centre de Montpellier, Direction Scientifique, 371, Rue du Professeur Blayac, 34082 Montpellier Cedex 2, France.

Carmichael, N. Rhône-Poulenc Secteur Agro Toxicologie, 14-20, Rue Pierre Baizet, B.P. 9163, 69263 Lyon Cedex 09, France.

Carvallo, D. IFFA CREDO, Centre de Recherche et d'Élevage du Domaine des Oncins, B.P. 109, l'Arbresle, France.

Catinot, R. Rhône-Poulenc Rorer, Institut de Recherche sur la Sécurité du Médicament, 20, Quai de la Révolution, 94140 Alfortville, France.

Deregnaucourt, J. Rhône-Poulenc Rorer, Direction Projets, 20, Avenue Raymond Aron, 92165 Antony Cedex, France.

Detaille, J. Y. Rhône-Poulenc Secteur Agro, Centre de Recherche, 355, Rue Dostoievski, Sophia-Antipolis, 06561 Valbonne, France.

Douzou, P. INRA, 147, Rue de l'Université, 75341 Paris Cedex 07, France.

Fetter, A.W. Rhône-Poulenc Rorer, Central Reseach, 800 Business Centre Drive, Horsham, Pennsylvania 19044, USA.

Firth, M.   49 Woodstock Avenue, London NW11 9RG, United Kingdom.

Foster, P.M.   ICI, Central Toxicology Laboratory, Alderley Park, Macclesfield, Cheshire SK10 4TJ, United Kingdom.

Fournier, E.   Rhône-Poulenc Rorer, Institut de Recherche sur la Sécurité du Médicament, 20, Quai de la Révolution, 94140 Alfortville, France.

Fumero, S.   Istituto di Ricerche Biomediche, "Antoine Marxer" RBM SpA, Via Ribes, 1, 10010 Colleretto Giacosa (TO), Italy.

Gautheron, P.   Laboratories Merck Sharp & Dohme - Chibre, Route de Marsat, B.P. 134, 63203 RIOM Cedex, France.

Ghosh, M.   Rhône-Poulenc Rorer, Institut de Recherche sur la Sécurité du Médicament, 20, Quai de la Révolution, 94140 Alfortville, France.

Gopinath, C.   Huntingdon Research Centre Ltd, P.O. Box 2, Huntingdon, Cambridge PE18 6ES, United Kingdom.

Granier Bompard, C.   P.A.EX.A., 10, Place Léon Blum, 75011 Paris, France.

Grosse, M.   Biologie Servier, Laboratoire de Toxicologie Génétique, 905, Route de Saran, Gidy, 45403 Fleury-Les-Aubrais Cedex, France.

Guillot, R.   Faculté de Médecine de Paris Ouest, Laboratoire d'Histoembryologie, 45, Rue des Saints-Pèris, 75270 Paris Cedex 06, France.

Hillaire, S.   Rhône-Poulenc Rorer, Institut de Recherche sur la Sécurité du Médicament, 20, Quai de la Révolution, 94140 Alfortville, France.

Jegou, B.   Université de Rennes 1, Laboratoire de Biologie de la Reproduction, CNRS UA 256, Campus Universitaire de Beaulieu, 35042 Rennes Cedex, France.

Jolles, G.   Rhône-Poulenc Rorer, Direction Scientifique, 20, Avenue Raymond Aron, 92165 Antony Cedex, France.

Kelley, M.   Rhône-Poulenc Rorer, Central Research, 800 Business Center Drive, Horsham, Pennsylvania 19044, USA.

Kramer, P.   E. Merck, Institut für Toxikologie, Frankfurter Strasse 250, Postfach 4119, 6100 Darmstadt 1, Germany.

Laduron, P.   Rhône-Poulenc Rorer, Centre de Recherche de Vitry-Alfortville, 13, Quai Jules Guesde, 94403 Vitry-sur-Seine Cedex, France.

Le Bail, R.   Rhône-Poulenc Rorer, Institut de Recherche sur la Sécurité du Médicament, 20, Quai de la Révolution, 94140 Alfortville, France.

Mansuy, D.   Laboratoire de Chimie et Biochimie, Pharmacologiques et Toxicologiques, 45, Rue des Saints-Pères, 75270 Paris Cedex 06, France.

Marano, F.   Université de Paris VII, Laboratoire de Cytophysiologie et de Toxicologie Cellulaire, 2, Place Jussieu, 75251 Paris Cedex 05, France.

Marguerie de Rotrou, G.   Centre d'Études Nucléaires 85X, DBMF/Laboratoire d'Hématologie, INSERM U 217, 38041 Grenoble Cedex, France.

Massingham, R.   Riom Laboratoires-CERM, Route de Marsat, B.P. 140, 63203 RIOM Cedex, France.

Mazuret, A.   Rhône-Poulenc Rorer, Institut de Recherche sur la Sécurité du Médicament, 20, Quai de la Révolution, 94140 Alfortville, France.

Melcion, C.   Rhône-Poulenc Rorer, Institut de Recherche sur la Sécurité du Médicament, 20, Quai de la Révolution, 94140 Alfortville, France.

Merieux, C.   Fondation Mérieux, 17, Rue Bourgelat, B.P. 2021, 69227 Lyon Cedex 02, France.

Moonen, G.   Université de Liège, Faculté de Médecine, Institut Léon Frédericq, Service de Physiologie Humaine et Physiopathologie, 17, Place Delcour, B-4020 Liège, Belgium

Morin, J.P.   Centre International de Toxicologie, Miserey, B.P. 563, 27005 Evreux Cedex, France.

Osborne, B.   Southern Research Institute, Frederick Research Center, Toxicology Operations, 7470-C Technology Way, Frederick, MD 21701, USA.

Picard, J.J.   Université Catholique de Louvain, Laboratoire de Génétique du Développement, Place Croix-du-Sud 5, Bte 3, B-1348 Louvain-La-Neuve, Belgium.

Pierre, R   OPAL, 63, Boulevard des Invalides, 75007 Paris, France.

Pouradier Duteil, X. Imedex, Zone Industrielle des Troques, B.P. 38, 69630 Chaponost, France.

Printz, P. Ministère de la Recherche et de la Technologie, 1, Rue Descartes, 75231 Paris Cedex 05, France.

Puiseux Dao, S. Université Paris VII, Laboratoire de Cytophysiologie et de Toxicologie Cellulaire, 2, Place Jussieu, 75251 Paris Cedex 05, France.

Robin, J.L. Rhône-Poulenc S.A., Direction Scientifique, 25, Quai Paul Doumer, 92408 Courbevoie Cedex, France.

Rogiers, V. Vrije Universiteit Brussel, Faculteit Geneeskunde en Farmacie, Laarbeeklaan 103, B-1090 Brussel, Belgium.

Roquet, F. Rhône-Poulenc Rorer, Institut de Recherche sur la Sécurité du Médicament, 20, Quai de la Révolution, 94140 Alfortville, France.

Roux, C. Faculté de Médecine Saint-Antoine, Laboratoire d'Embryologie, 27, Rue de Chaligny, 75571 Paris Cedex 12, France.

Rouzioux, J.M. Pasteur Mérieux, 1541, Avenue Marcel Mérieux, 69280 Marcy l'Étoile, France.

Sanders, J. Rhône-Poulenc Rorer, Central Research, 800 Business Center Drive, Horsham, Pennsylvania 19044, USA.

Schlütter, G. Bayer A.G., Pharma Forschungszentrum, Institut für Toxikologie Pharma, Postfach 101709, D-5600 Wuppertal 1, Germany.

Silice, C. Rhône-Poulenc Secteur Agro Toxicologie, 14-20, Rue Pierre Baizet, B.P. 9163, 69263 Lyon Cedex 09, France.

Sommet, M. Rhône-Poulenc Rorer, Direction Scientifique, 20, Avenue Raymond Aron, 92165 Antony Cedex, France.

Thibault, N. Rhône-Poulenc Rorer, Institut de Recherche sur la Securité du Médicament, 20, Quai de la Révolution, 94140 Alfortville, France.

Thybaud, V. Rhône-Poulenc Rorer, Institut de Recherche sur la Sécurité du Médicament, 20, Quai de la Révolution, 94140 Alfortville, France.

Tocque, B. Rhône-Poulenc Rorer, Institut de Biotechnologie, 13, Quai Jules Guesde, 94403 Vitry-sur-Seine Cedex, France.

Tulkens, P. Université Catholique de Louvain, Faculté de Médecine, Laboratoire de Chimie Physiologique, UCL 7549, Avenue Hippocrate, 75, B-1200 Bruxelles, Belgium.

Valette, L. Fondation Mérieux, 17, Rue Bourgelat, B.P. 2021, 69227 Lyon Cedex 02, France.

Vandenberghe, Y. Searle European Development Centre, Parc Scientifique de Louvain-la-Neuve, Rue Granbompré 11, B-1348 Mont-Saint-Guibert, Belgium.

Van Der Venne, M.T. Commission of the European Communities, Directorate-General Employment, Industrial Relations and Social Affairs, Health and Safety Directorate, Bâtiment Jean Monnet, L-2920 Luxembourg, Luxembourg.

Van Looy, H. OCDE, Direction de l'Environnement, 15, Boulevard de l'Amiral Bruix, 75016 Paris, France.

Van Maele-Fabry, G. Université Catholique de Louvain, Laboratoire de Génétique du Développement, Place Croix-de-Sud 5, Bte 3, B-1348 Louvaine-La-Neuve, Belgium.

Vannier, B. Roussel Uclaf, Direction du Développement Préclinique Santé, Département de Toxicologie, 102, Route de Noisy, B.P. No 9, 93230 Romainville, France.

Vintezou, P. Rhône-Poulenc Rorer, Institut de Recherche sur la Sécurité du Médicament, 20, Quai de la Révolution, 94140 Alfortville, France.

Weill, N. Société Hazleton, B.P. 0118, 69593 l'Arbresle Cedex, France.

Woolley, A. Life Science Research, EYE, Suffolk IP28 7PX, United Kingdom.

Zucco, F. Consiglio Nazionale delle Ricerche, Istituto Tecnologie Biomediche, Via G.B. Morgagni 30/E, 00161 Roma, Italy.

Preface

In the field of drug research, toxicologists face a paradox: how can they guarantee consumer safety through implementing the increasingly stringent standards of the regulatory authorities and yet, at the same time, drastically reduce animal experimentation, even though these tests are currently considered to be the methods which provide the best prediction of possible adverse effects in Man?

In vitro toxicology emerges as a possible solution to this dilemma; but what is the real status of this approach at the beginning of the 90s? Does it actually offer an alternative to the more conventional methods?

The present volume is an attempt to answer some of these questions. It is published in the wake of an International Round Table attended by about one hundred experts from eleven different countries. However, it is not simply the Proceedings of that meeting, but rather a monograph compiled especially to report the reviews which were presented and the discussion which took place. It has been designed to provide a rational assessment of the current potential of the alternatives to animal experimentation.

The first part of the book constitutes an introduction to general aspects of the question. The reader will then find a second part, which presents a pragmatic summary of the existing techniques and methods currently used in *in vitro* toxicology and relating to the most important target organs such as the kidneys, liver, central nervous system, heart, eyes and ears. The ability of the methods to assess reproductive toxicity and carcinogenicity is also thoroughly discussed. The various chapters are intended to provide a precise statement and discussion of the existing knowledge. Extensive bibliographies give access to the very numerous studies which have been published in the literature.

The final section considers questions of principle. How are the various parties involved in drug research reacting to the use of *in vitro* technologies? Is there a consensus regarding their validity and their potential contribution to the assessment of drug safety? In the successive statements and the discussions which followed, opinions were heard from representatives of the legislators, drug manufacturers and animal protectors, as well as academic and research institutes. This review should enable readers to grasp the complexity of the problem and reassess their own positions with a view to future action.

This book therefore has a dual purpose: to provide a technical overview of the current state of the art and to suggest a more theoretical definition of the border between what is already possible and what remains a goal to be achieved.

It is also hoped that this book may help to show that the search for methods to replace animal tests is of permanent concern to all involved in drug research and manufacture. Huge progress has already been achieved, thanks to the tireless efforts of a large number of research teams, amongst which we are proud to count many from the pharmaceutical industry.

G. Jolles and A. Cordier

Acknowledgements

Our warmest thanks go to all the speakers and participants who attended the International Round Table on "*In Vitro* Toxicology: An Alternative to Animal Testing?". Despite the topic, which frequently raises hot and even fierce debate, active cooperation and free discussion in a friendly atmosphere clearly marked this conference. We are extremely grateful to the chairmen of the sessions for their effectiveness, and would like to make special mention of the outstanding contribution of Dr M. Balls, from the Fund for the Replacement of Animals in Medical Experiments (FRAME), who acted as the moderator of the Panel Discussion: his firm but fair chairmanship combined with his talent in formulating accurately the questions from the audience and for stimulating the discussions, largely ensured the success of this very interactive and lively part of the meeting and enabled its presentation in this volume. We are further very grateful to Dr G. Zbinden from the Swiss Federal Polytechnic School (ETH) in Zurich for his generous advice during the preparation of the Round Table.

We are particularly indebted to Mrs M. Sommet and Mrs M.Ghosh from the Scientific Directorate of Rhône-Poulenc Rorer; Mrs Sommet assisted us most diligently in the organization of the meeting and afterwards patiently and efficiently finalized the manuscripts received from the contributors. Mrs Ghosh carefully reviewed all the articles, with special emphasis on the linguistic aspects: without their efforts, the publication of this volume would never have been possible.

We express our gratitude to the managements of the Rhône-Poulenc Rorer Foundation and of the Fondation Universitaire des Sciences et Techniques du Vivant, who jointly and very generously sponsored the conference; the hospitality of Dr Charles Mérieux in the beautiful estate of Les Pensières beside Lake Annecy and the assistance of the local organizing committee under the leadership of Dr L. Valette were very much appreciated.

Transcription of tapes of the discussion was performed by Dr Mary Firth and we wish to acknowledge thankfully her skill and competence.

Finally we wish to thank Dr Carey Chapman and the staff of Academic Press Ltd (London) for their expert and kind assistance in producing this volume.

G. Jolles and A. Cordier

Contents

Part I

General Aspects of *In Vitro* Testing

Development of *In Vitro* Toxicology

G. ZBINDEN

Institute of Toxicology, Swiss Federal Institute of Technology and University of Zurich, Schwerzenbach, Switzerland

Toxicology Under Indictment

The controversy about the ethical justification of animal experimentation has gathered momentum in recent years. Toxicologists find themselves right in the middle of the quarrel. It is not because their research methods are more cruel than those of other biomedical scientists, or that they use the largest number of animals. As a matter of fact, only about 10 to 15% of the laboratory animals required for biomedical research are used for safety studies. However, chemical pollution of the environment, accumulation of waste products, hazards from drugs and consumer goods, and pesticide residues in food are subjects that are very high on the general public's list of worries. They evoke fear and aggressive feelings against science and technology in general. Toxicology is intimately involved in the management of these problems, and is thus pronounced guilty by association. In addition, a minor toxicological procedure, the assessment of irritant properties of chemicals on skin and mucous membranes, the so called Draize test, has caught the attention of animal rights advocates, and has now become the focal point of their agitation against experimental toxicology as a whole.

Before dealing with the subject of *in vitro* methodology in toxicology,

IN VITRO METHODS IN TOXICOLOGY
ISBN 0-12-388175-7

it must be pointed out that the failure to conduct appropriate safety studies in animals has been the cause of many serious accidents in the past. Moreover, from personal experience and that of many colleagues, I can state unequivocally that much human misery has been prevented because toxicological studies have identified untoward effects of new chemicals that were then never introduced into the human environment (Zbinden, 1990a). It is for these reasons that society has charged toxicologists with the duty of detecting and assessing the toxic properties of chemical substances, old and new, and to determine safe levels of exposure. As long as toxicologists are asked to carry this responsibility, they must be permitted to use the research methods they consider to be adequate. Thus, the question is not whether we should replace experiments done in live animals with *in vitro* tests, but rather how and when *in vitro* procedures can contribute to the overall safety assessment required for chemical substances.

Alternatives to Animal Experimentation

The approach to obtain useful scientific information through investigations with *in vitro* model systems has been used successfully in biomedical research for many years. As an alternative to animal experimentation, it has much appeal for those educated laymen who basically support the view that research is needed for the benefit of all living beings, and to assure the survival of future generations, but are unable to accept that live animals must be sacrificed to achieve these goals. Scientists known that *in vitro* research represents a different dimension, providing information that is often useful, but rarely equivalent to that obtained from animal experiments. As a consequence, reasonable people in both camps have come to agree on a definition of alternative research that can be formulated as follows:

> Alternative methods in the strict sense of the word are procedures in which living animals are replaced by systems that feel no pain and anxiety, and provide information that is equivalent to that obtained in animal experiments (replacement).

> Included are research methods that use no living animals, but yield only part of the information obtainable in animal experiments, or provide data of a different quality (partial replacement).

> Alternative methods in the wider sense of the word are procedures that result in a reduction of the number of animals, and permit

a lessening of pain and anxiety. This includes a change-over to phylogenetically and neuropsychologically less developed animal species (reduction, refinement).

In vitro methods are widely used whenever a specific type of information is needed. This is evident from the contents of presentations (posters and oral communications) given at biomedical congresses. The examples given in Table 1.1 show that at least half of the research communications presented by fundamental biomedical scientists are based on data obtained in *in vitro* models (Zbinden, 1990b). In toxicology, represented by the 1990 meeting of the Society of Toxicology, only about a third of the studies reported were conducted with the help of *in vitro* procedures (Zbinden, 1990a). Moreover, if one considers that much of the work of toxicologists deals with routine *in vivo* safety studies which are rarely reported at scientific meetings, one comes to the conclusion that the actual percentage of *in vitro* work done in experimental toxicology is much lower.

Applications of *In Vitro* Methods in Toxicology

Replacement

In the basic biomedical sciences, *in vitro* methods are used whenever a specific question needs to be answered ("experiments done to know").

Table 1.1

Phylogenetically highest *in vivo* or *in vitro* system used in scientific communications

			Methods used (% of total research)				
Society*	Year	Communications (total)	Large laboratory and farm animals	Rabbits and small rodents	*In vitro* procedures	Humans	Others incl. insects, computers
USGEB	1974	171	2	26	66	2	4
USGEB	1984	373	1	19	62	4	14
FASEB	1989	6649	10.1	29.2	48.0	7.9	4.8
SOT	1990	1235	4.2	59.3	29.1	2.3	5.2

*USEGEB: Union of Swiss Societies for Experimental Biology; FASEB: Federation of American Societies of Experimental Biology; SOT: Society of Toxicology.
Note: In the SOT figures 101 presentations reporting theoretical concepts or retrospective surveys are not included.

This is also true for toxicology. For example, in the field of mutagenicity testing, *in vitro* models were favoured right from the beginning. It is a clear-cut case where specific biological qualities, i.e. the ability of a substance or its metabolites to induce point mutations, to break chromosomes or to disturb mitosis, are investigated.

However, in many cases, the goals of toxicologists are different. Experiments are done to exclude the presence of adverse effects in whole organisms ("safety studies"), or, quite often, to determine the spectrum of toxicity over a broad dose range. Thus, a typical toxicological experiment aims at detecting a great variety of toxic effects that manifest themselves not only by disturbance of selected biochemical processes at the cellular and subcellular level (for which *in vitro* tests could be very useful), but by complex dysfunctions and structural damage of many organ systems that cannot be modelled with isolated organs, tissues, cells, and cell fractions.

For a small number of toxicological procedures, a direct (1:1) replacement by an *in vitro* method seems possible. Examples are the Limulus Amoebocyte Lysate test as a replacement of the pyrogen assay in rabbits, and a high-performance liquid chromatography (HPLC) procedure for the control of insulin production batches which can be done instead of the bioassay with mice (Fisher and Smith, 1986). However, for the majority of toxicity studies performed with chemical substances, a direct replacement by an *in vitro* model appears to be out of the question.

Partial Replacement

General remarks

The most promising development is the use of *in vitro* methods as supplementary measures to enhance the efficacy of standard safety studies and to detect undesirable properties of new chemicals at an early stage. A survey of the applications of *in vitro* procedures reported at the 1990 annual meeting of the Society of Toxicology (SOT) shows in which direction these developments are moving (Table 1.2).

From the table it is evident that *in vitro* methods are most often used to assess cytotoxic properties of chemicals, and these studies are usually performed for screening purposes. It is also seen that organotypic cell cultures are used more and more frequently, replacing, to a certain extent, unpretentious cell lines such as HeLa cells and the robust but plain fibroblast cultures.

A rapidly developing field of activity is also the use of *in vitro* methods

Table 1.2

Toxicological in vitro models used in 307 posters and short communications at the SOT 1990 annual meeting

Organ	n	Toxic effects and screening	Mechanisms	Metabolism
Liver	97	25	24	48
Nervous system	37	20	13	4
Miscellaneous cells	30	17	12	1
Kidney	30	19	8	3
Skin	24	12	3	9
Lymphoreticular system	21	15	4	2
Lung	16	9	0	7
Heart	13	10	2	1
Whole organisms	9	8	0	1
Bone	7	4	3	0
Blood vessels	7	3	2	2
Female sex organs	6	2	3	1
Connective tissue	5	3	1	1
Male sex organs	5	3	1	1

for the elucidation of toxicological mechanisms. It is still mainly limited to investigations of hepatotoxicity, but a few researchers are expanding into biomechanistic studies with cells or cell fractions of other organs. Another active area of scientific exploration is the use of tissue slices, cell cultures and tissue fractions for the assessment of the metabolism of foreign chemicals. Understandably, it is still preferentially done with liver tissue and cells. A particularly promising development here is the increasing use of human tissues which permits early detection of important species differences that could become a problem for the extrapolation of animal toxicity findings to man. Finally, it should be mentioned that *in vitro* techniques often provide the most accurate information on the critical toxic concentrations at the relevant target sites. Together with pharmacokinetic and metabolic data, these findings play a pivotal role in risk assessment.

Cytotoxicity and toxicological screening

Historically, *in vitro* toxicology has mainly been concerned with detecting cytotoxicity. For the assessment of adverse properties of chemicals that are due to direct contact with living tissue, this approach is certainly justified. It has been used widely and with some success for the development of *in vitro* tests to screen chemicals for their irritant and corrosive properties on the skin and mucous membranes.

Human ingenuity to devise techniques that permit (semi)quantitative evaluation of toxic cell damage and cell death is almost limitless. But most experimental approaches that have been developed fall within one of the five basic classes summarized in Table 1.3, which lists the principal end points used as indicators for cell injury.

Cytotoxicity and cell death are also logical targets if one wants to study cell damage induced by metabolites formed under the influence of u.v. radiation. Relatively simple procedures in which cytotoxicity of chemicals is compared in the presence and absence of u.v. radiation are, therefore, very useful to identify phototoxic chemicals (Beijersbergen van Henegouwen, 1988).

If we deal with direct cell injury induced by chemicals, the type of cells used as indicator systems is of relatively little importance. It is acknowledged that there are differences between various cell types with regard to sensitivity against cytotoxic injury, but, in general, the ranking order of cytotoxicity obtained with a series of chemicals in different cell preparations is very similar. An exception to this empirical rule are the toxins that need to be formed from inert precursors through the action of metabolizing enzymes. Such chemicals are often considerably more cytotoxic in hepatocytes which are better endowed with metabolizing enzymes than other cell types (Ekwall and Acosta, 1982).

In recent years, the interest of toxicologists has expanded into assessment of selected cellular responses other than cell death. This development was greatly aided by improvements of cell culture techniques which permit satisfactory maintenance and propagation of many cell types. In addition, morphological, biochemical and immunochemical assay procedures have been developed that permit quantitative determinations of many specific cellular elements such as enzymes, components of the cytoskeleton, receptor proteins, etc. As an example, the large variety of biochemical properties that can be studied individually in the NG 108-15

Table 1.3
Variables measured in cytotoxicity tests

---

1. Active exclusion of substances (Trypan Blue)
2. Active uptake of substances (Neutral Red)
3. Loss of cell constituents (lactate dehydrogenase (LDH))
4. Loss of activity of intracellular enzymes (MTT dehydrogenase)*
5. Reduced synthetic activity (albumin)

---

*MTT, 3-(4,5-dimethyl-2-thiazolyl)-2,5-dimethyl-2H-tetrazolium bromide.

mouse neuroblastoma–rat glioma hybrid (Singer and Tiemcyer, 1985) is mentioned (Table 1.4). Another illustration is a technique capable of assessing cell–cell communication by ways of tight junctions. It is based on the observation of transportation of a fluorescent dye from one cell to an adjacent one in which fluorescence was abolished by photobleaching (Bombick, 1990). Both systems can be used for toxicological screening, the first one for the detection of specific neurotoxic agents, the second one for chemicals that inhibit intercellular communications and, thus, possess an activity that is characteristic of tumour promoters.

Elucidation of toxicological mechanisms

For the evaluation of toxicological findings and for risk assessment, the understanding of biological mechanisms has become of great importance. This is particularly true in the area of carcinogenicity, since an increase in tumour incidence in a lifetime bioassay in rodents can be the consequence of a variety of biological mechanisms. Without the knowledge of the underlying biological processes, risk assessment for man remains a futile statistical exercise.

Table 1.4

NG 108-15 mouse neuroblastoma – rat glioma hybrid variables measured (Singer and Tiemeyer, 1985)

Growth and metabolic activity
    Cell count, total protein
    Lactate dehydrogenase
    α- and β- Galactosidase
    α- and β- Glucosidase

Synthetic enzymes
    Choline acetyltransferase
    Tyrosine hydroxylase
    Glutamic acid decarboxylase

Neurotransmitter uptake
    [^{3}H] Choline
    Mazindol binding (dopamine)
    Imipramine binding (5-hydroxytryptamine)

Receptor binding
    Quinuclidinicyl benzilate (cholinergic)
    Muscimol (γ-aminobutyrate)
    Cyanopindolol (β-adrenergic)
    Cholecystokinin

A good understanding of how a toxic reaction comes about is also important for many other fields of toxicology. Cell culture methods are very useful for providing pertinent data, e.g. on the enzymes affected by a toxic substance, the generation of free radicals, the interaction with specific cell constituents such as tubulin, or cell organelles, e.g. lysosomes or mitochondria. From such biomechanistic studies, it is sometimes possible to develop new screening tests that can then be employed to assess the toxicological characteristic of newly synthesized substances. An example is the *in vitro* assay for peroxisome-inducing properties in hepatocyte cultures (Gray *et al.*, 1983).

Foreign substance metabolism and risk assessment

The importance of metabolites as the ultimate toxic species is now well recognized. The investigation of metabolic pathways in the microsomal fraction of liver, in liver slices and liver cell cultures has proven to be a very useful technique for a rapid identification of the breakdown products formed by metabolizing enzymes. It is particularly appropriate, since it permits comparisons across several laboratory animal species with relatively low expenditure of time and money. In addition, data obtained in liver tissue of animals can be compared with those gained from comparable preparations from human liver.

In recent years, efforts have also been made to study not only the qualitative aspects of hepatic metabolism, but also to investigate the kinetics. From a comparison of the *in vitro* kinetics observed in appropriate liver preparations with *in vivo* data in one animal species, conversion factors can be obtained that can also be applied to the *in vitro* data of other species including man. This then permits reasonably realistic predictions of the *in vivo* kinetics of the metabolic processes in the other species (Green and Provan, 1990).

It is obvious that the detection of species differences gives invaluable information for extrapolation of animal toxicity data to man. Moreover, *in vitro* studies can also provide information on the critical concentration of a chemical or its metabolites that are necessary to induce an adverse effect in the principal target organs. Pharmacokinetic and metabolic studies designed to determine whether or not this minimal toxic concentration can be reached under specific exposure conditions in man can provide a realistic assessment of risk that is much more relevant than a comparison of the tolerated dose (no-adverse-effect dose) in an animal model and the dose administered to man under realistic conditions of use. An example is the risk assessment procedure for insoluble bismuth salts. In this process the determination of the minimal toxic bismuth concentration in brain cell cultures was a significant piece of information without which realistic predictions for human risk could not have been made (Zbinden *et al.*, 1990).

Conclusions

The use of *in vitro* techniques in toxicological research is on the increase. The most important application of many *in vitro* procedures is as tools in toxicological screening. Here, simple assessment of cytotoxicity is a widely used technique for the evaluation of local tissue injury and for a general indication of the intrinsic toxic potential of test chemicals. But more and more, organotypic cell and tissue culture preparations are used not only to demonstrate non-specific tissue injury and cell death, but also for the detection and quantitative assessment of specific functional, biochemical and structural defects that do not inevitably lead to cell death. A particularly promising application is the toxicological screening of chemicals for embryotoxic and teratogenic effects for which several *in vitro* models are already in common use.

Unfortunately, the attitude of many regulatory agencies towards incorporation of *in vitro* tests into standard toxicological procedures is not encouraging. For example, it has been known for many years that cytotoxicity tests can predict and exclude irritant and corrosive properties of chemicals with high probability. It is acknowledged that these tests are not totally accurate. However, the proposal of the British Toxicology Society (Fielder *et al.*, 1987) to accept *in vitro* data for skin and eye irritation when they indicate cytotoxicity, and to proceed with *in vivo* testing in a single animal only when the result of the *in vitro* test was negative, has not yet been endorsed by any national or international regulatory body. Such an act would greatly advance the development towards partial replacement of the Draize test, an *in vivo* procedure whose scientific value and ethical justification is increasingly questioned by a large percentage of toxicological experts.

The prospects for a replacement of most of the other standard toxicological tests are, unfortunately, even less favourable. Current regulations demand that toxicological studies be performed to gain data on the whole spectrum of toxic effects over a very broad dose range. It is unrealistic to expect that *in vitro* models can be found that would provide comparable information. Even more unrealistic are the expectations that *in vitro* tests could be used to determine "safety", i.e. the absence of toxicity. For this purpose, it is still necessary to rely on *in vivo* studies with large numbers of animals. On the other hand, *in vitro* techniques have found an increasing acceptance for the evaluation of biomechanisms of toxicity. Since biomechanistic investigations are becoming an integral part of every toxicological assessment of new chemicals, it can be predicted that the use of *in vitro* techniques for this purpose will greatly expand in many areas of toxicology. Ultimately, such investigations will become much more important than the standard safety studies done today.

Finally, it must also be recognized that the selection of species for toxicological studies, and risk assessment for man on the basis of such investigations, are only possible if one takes into consideration the toxicokinetic characteristics and the metabolic pathways of the test substances. The progress made in the last 10 years towards obtaining much of the relevant information in *in vitro* systems, and the possibility to expand these investigations into human cells and tissues, are further reasons to believe that *in vitro* research techniques will continue their progress and will become an unquestioned part not only of scientific research in toxicology, but also of routine studies performed in industrial laboratories.

References

Beijersbergen van Henegouwen, G.M.J. (1988). *Arch. Toxicol., Suppl.* **12**, 3–9.
Bombick, D.W. (1990). *In Vitro Toxicol.* **3**, 27–39.
Ekwall, B. and Acosta, D. (1982). *Drug Chem. Toxicol.* **5**, 219–231.
Fielder, R.J., Gaunt, I.F., Rhodes, C., Sullivan, F.M. and Swanston, D.W. (1987). *Hum. Toxicol.* **6**, 269–278.
Fisher, B.V. and Smith, D. (1986). *J. Pharmacol. Biomed. Anal.* **4**, 377–387.
Gray, T.J.B., Lake, B.G., Beamand, J.A., Foster, J.R. and Gangolli, S.D. (1983). *Toxicology* **28**, 167–169.
Green, T. and Provan, M.W. (1990). *In* "Basic Science in Toxicology" (G.N. Volans, J. Sims, F.M. Sullivan and P. Turner, eds), pp. 69–78. Taylor & Francis, London.
Singer, H.S. and Tiemeyer, M. (1985). *In* "In Vitro Toxicology. A Progress Report from the Johns Hopkins Center for Alternatives to Animal Testing" (A.M. Goldberg, ed.), pp. 266–291. Mary N. Lieber Inc., New York.
Zbinden, G. (1990a). *Regulat. Pharmacol. Toxicol.* **14**, 167–177.
Zbinden, G. (1990b). *TIPS* **11**, 104–107.
Zbinden, G., Bruinink, A. and Mitchell, D.B. (1990). *Proc. 1990 Eur. Meet. Toxicol. Forum*, in press.

Discussion

E. Walum

Prof. Zbinden said that our main responsibility as toxicologists is to man, and he talked about replacement. Could he please comment on the possibility that part of *in vitro* toxicology is concerned with developing methods which do not replace anything but are in the frontier, if you like, of toxicology – new methods in areas like immunotoxicology and neurotoxicology, where we are not replacing any animals but developing *the* method from the beginning in *in vitro* systems?

G. Zbinden

I hope I did not say that the only obligation of toxicologists is to man. Our obligations are to man, animals and the whole living environment. I have not mentioned the great contribution that *in vitro* toxicology is already making routinely to ecotoxicology, where there are alternative targets like fish, shrimps, fish eggs and so on. *In vitro* techniques to protect the environment are already used widely because they are the natural techniques to use.

I certainly agree that the *in vitro* studies can be right from the beginning. We are increasingly interested in biomechanistic studies. If we have identified, or even only speculated about, a mechanism that could become a target of toxicity, this is quite possible. If we say, for example, that free radical generation, denaturation of cell proteins or activation of peptidases in the cell is an important aspect of ageing, if we think that chemical exposure for a long time, particularly in the presence of an oxidizing drug, can activate this system, I think we could start immediately by developing the *in vitro* model, based on either established or speculated mechanisms.

J.R. Claude

Prof. Zbinden said it was not possible to obtain an agreement with the regulatory agencies for the alternative procedure proposed for the Draize test. As a member both of the European Economic Community Safety Group for Drug Evaluation in Brussels and of the French Regulatory Agency, I have to defend a little the position of the regulatory toxicologists.

First, there is the validation problem, a formal problem. It is very difficult to consider many of the alternative methods as validated. Secondly, the impression given to the consumers. We are worried in the agencies about having problems with consumers if there were large, or not so large, accidents with a new drug and if the risk assessment had been performed only in a control system or not sufficiently in whole animals. This very big question is also under discussion in the Food & Drug Administration. I think these two reasons explain why it is so difficult to include the alternative methods in the regulatory assessment.

I hope very much that it will be possible to include some techniques within a few months or within a few years in other cases. For instance, in the case of chemicals, not drugs, I think the comparative studies performed for the Draize test by the group led by Mrs van der Venne is a good example of the efforts being made by the regulatory authorities to include alternative methods in the near future.

G. Zbinden

I appreciate the problems of the regulators and their insistence that the new methods should be validated. It is worth mentioning that of course the old methods were never validated. There was not a single validation study, for example, for the long-term carcinogenicity study. If there had been, that model would never have been accepted because a model with more than 50% false positives and quite a number of false negatives would never have got through a scientific review. This is just a historical remark.

It is clear that much of what is done in toxicology is to reassure ourselves and to protect the regulators, ourselves and the manufacturers against unfair claims from people. If we can say that 10 000 animals have been killed and nothing has happened, then something that happened to someone cannot be due to our chemical.

However, I think we have to get away from that. By insisting on partial replacement, I provide the regulators with a way out of their dilemma. I tell them that so far the only assay we want to *replace* is the insulin assay; there is no question that high-performance liquid chromatography is vastly superior to what is done with animals and there is no reason for not approving it.

In all other areas we want partial replacement. I almost cannot talk about the Draize test any more. It is clear to me that if a compound in an *in vitro* system kills cells at a relatively low concentration, that compound will be a risk for people if they get it in the eye. If a compound is identified as a cytotoxic agent, it can be labelled as a risk for humans.

We also admit that there are a very few compounds which are not cytotoxic but are still a risk for people when they get in their eyes. For that, the British Toxicology Society (BTS) wants to sacrifice one rabbit. We experience extreme frustration when talking to people at the Environmental Protection Agency (EPA) because they will not listen. They say that is fine – but they want six animals, full dose, 100%. What are we going to do in this situation? We do not want to replace the Draize test, but just want to make it scientifically right. Not one scientist has brought a valid objection against the BTS proposal – but we are still waiting for approval. The problem lies with the EPA, not with the Europeans.

P. Tulkens

I liked Prof. Zbinden's statistics of the number of communications dealing with tissue or other *in vitro* models. I am slightly puzzled about another kind of statistics dealing with the rate of success or failure of such approaches in the evaluation of compounds. By failure, I mean situations in which misuse of the *in vitro* model has led to the wrong conclusions. I am not talking only about toxicology but I can identify a few cases where *in vitro* models clearly led to wrong conclusions and to the development of compounds which were later proven to be either inefficacious or toxic.

A refinement of the statistical analysis that may be needed would be to find out how much these systems have demonstrated success or usefulness.

G. Zbinden

That is a very good point. If there is a scientific question, it is important to say that what is found with an *in vitro* model is true for that particular circumstance. It is our fault if we make a poor extrapolation from it. The classic example of a wrong prediction, of course, is the Ames test. Bruce Ames led us to believe that if in an *in vitro* system combining S9 fraction and manipulating *Salmonella typhimurium*, a point mutation is found, this indicates a human carcinogen. The Ames test is a 100% valid model for defining chemicals that in the circumstance of a particular *in vitro* model generate toxic metabolites capable of interfering with DNA.

It depends upon what is made of the findings. Dr Tulkens points out that people have made wrong predictions. There is nothing wrong with the model; the model is true only for the situation for which it is designed. The same applies *in vivo*. If a study is done in the rat, the result is valid and true only for the rat and nothing else. In extrapolating this result to other species including man, there has to be a tremendously complex input, which is where mistakes can be made – but that is not the fault of either the rat or the *in vitro* model.

J. Frazier

Once we get past the issues of gross toxicology we immediately focus on target organ toxicity, to which basically two factors contribute:

1) The particular sensitivity of a tissue because it has an enzyme that is sensitive, it lacks a detoxification mechanism and so on.
2) The kinetic factors targeting a particular tissue because the chemical will concentrate in that particular tissue.

What does Prof. Zbinden see for the future for *in vitro* approaches for predicting the toxicokinetics of compounds?

G. Zbinden

Toxicokinetics is a key issue, but one major advantage of the *in vitro* model is that it gives the local concentration that is affecting that particular target organ. It is very difficult to predict how much of a given compound will go to the liver in man, but progress is being made. I showed one example where the blood kinetics of methylene chloride (not its organ kinetics) could be modelled very well by looking at the *in vitro* kinetics in the liver (the major target of metabolism) and scaling it up with one *in vivo* model in which the mouse was used.

Many other things can be used to predict kinetics in humans. Lipid solubility can be included as a factor in our computer model, the water/octanol partition, the pK_A and so on. With the *in vivo* kinetics, some reasonable suggestions can be made. It is obvious that this is only partial prediction and that we will often have to use a whole animal or human model, but there is a possibility that models can be found.

The reason I am so excited about this is because in the old days when I was in the drug industry when we had a new compound and wanted to go into humans, we gave $1/10$ LD_{50} as the first dose. To my surprise, this "caveman" procedure is still used by some modern pharmaceutical companies who take the first dose as $1/10$ LD_{50} in the mouse, or something slightly more elaborate.

In my opinion, the only way to select the dose is to ask the pharmacologist what is the active concentration, and then to ask the toxicologist what is the toxic concentration at the target organ. For this, probably *in vitro* models would be very useful. Then we should tell the pharmacokineticist the structure of the compound and its lipid solubility, and ask him to make an educated guess how this would be handled – because he will have worked with similar compounds – and to say what is the dose that will be below the toxic concentration but in the pharmacological range. This is the progress which will be made.

Here again, *in vitro* models play only a partial, but very important, role and the better we are at doing this the more elaborate we become. Newer techniques are now also being developed on membrane permeability of compounds using *in vitro* models; for example, passive diffusion uptake into cells can be modelled into the kinetic models and then used. I see great progress in this area.

H. Baron

Does Prof. Zbinden not feel that we might also consider among the so-called alternative methods perhaps more carefully conceived and improved conduct of animal studies? So often toxicology studies are conceived to determine toxicity at a very high dose. Does he not feel that for mechanistic reasons we could learn a lot from very carefully conceived experimental procedures, timed sacrifices, advanced fixation and morphological techniques? This could give us a lot of information about lesion kinetics and complement the information obtained from the *in vitro* methods.

G. Zbinden

I definitely agree. It is included in the alternatives in the wider sense of the word which I have not discussed. It is my absolute conviction that with the modification of the standard technology which Dr Baron mentioned chemicals can be detected. For example, we have developed a nephrotoxicity screen which has so far been validated with about six animals per drug with 16 compounds, covering a very broad range from almost non-nephrotoxic to very seriously nephrotoxic. This screen picks up nephrotoxicity if a compound is nephrotoxic; if it is not nephrotoxic, nephrotoxicity is not found. There is no question that toxic effects can be detected by applying techniques, again mainly in the area of toxicological screening.

When we have identified a compound as the one we want to continue with, and it is the best from all the *in vitro* and *in vivo* work, there is still an obligation to society, as Dr Claude pointed out, first, to admit that we do not know everything, there may be something we have missed in our models and, secondly, to prove the absence of toxicity. There is no scientific way to demonstrate lack of toxicity, so some insurance type of experiment has to be done, in which a number of animals are loaded with a relatively high dose – and if nothing happens we feel better.

This is nothing to do with science; it is purely admitting that we may have missed something in our models – which happens, it happens to me quite often – and that we have an obligation to lean over backwards to do more for safety than has been done in the past. How much more is a matter of debate. I think much too much is done in many areas, particularly in carcinogenicity testing. In time perhaps it will be possible to reduce it. Unfortunately, every time a regulation comes out there is more of the same, rather than less. We will have to work on this a little more.

D. Acosta

With regard to the problem of validation, the regulatory agencies are waiting to see how some of these *in vitro* techniques work out. There has to be a source of funding for this work. Federal agencies and private industry are two possible sources. With Prof. Zbinden's background in this area, how does he see that much of this type of work can be supported if regulatory agencies claim they do not have a lot of funds to support it? Federal agencies claim they would rather support basic research as opposed to applied research which would involve a lot of screening, etc. Private industry may be doing some of this work in-house, but they are reluctant to release some of the information obtained within their own particular company.

Does Prof. Zbinden see a problem in terms of worldwide funding of this type of effort, and how can this be coordinated if funding becomes – or is – difficult?

G. Zbinden

Validation is probably the most boring and scientifically unchallenging activity in the life of a scientist. I have just come from a meeting in Johannesburg where, for about the 10 000th time, somebody demonstrated that acetaminophen is hepatotoxic in liver cells. The whole approach goes back to taking standard compounds, developing these techniques with them and proving repeatedly that they are toxic. In my opinion, this is not the right thing to do.

Funding is very difficult to obtain in Europe too because this work is very costly. The German Ministry of Research and Technology has given a large amount of money for the Draize test and for the LD_{50}. We will probably hear from Dr Balls about the validation study, but the results coming out of it show that, for cytotoxicity, these models, more or less whatever cell type is used, give the same rank order of toxicity.

My hope is that in the future validation will be forward looking. When chemical and pharmaceutical companies have a compound and their primary purpose is to get it on the market, I would like to see them doing what the regulators require, but also using the *in vitro* models that are available now. When the chemists who are making new compounds talk to the people doing *in vitro* toxicology and not to those doing *in vivo* toxicology 5 months later, that to me is the way to establish validation. When the chemist asks them to tell him what a compound does in *this* cell type because he wants to modify and improve it, then we have achieved our aim.

I know some companies already do this, for example, ICI and I think Rhône-Poulenc. They have to do the standard techniques now, but I hope they will also do additional methods. I have not talked about teratogenicity testing, but there are several good tests to measure potential teratogenicity. I see no reason why materials cannot be put into a hydra and a post-implantation embryo culture side by side. I predict that in some cases the *in vitro* studies will show something that the *in vivo* studies missed.

A classic case has recently been published by Diether Neubert, that of acyclovir, a compound that causes a wrong base incorporation into virus DNA. Because of its biochemical action, acyclovir should be a teratogenic, but it was not teratogenic in the standard animal test. Neubert then used a post-implantation embryo culture, and not only identified acyclovir as a potent teratogen but also was able to identify the teratogenic concentration *in vitro*. He said that if that particular concentration is reached *in vivo*, then acyclovir must be teratogenic, so the standard assay was modified and two doses were given on one day only. The predicted concentration was found, and sure enough, the *in vivo* test was positive. Finally, he found that the concentration that caused teratogenicity in the *in vitro* system was exactly the same as that which caused it *in vivo*. This was about 10 times higher than the peak concentration in women, so the risk assessment was made that acyclovir is potentially teratogenic but that this is of no concern to either women or children.

If this is done on a routine basis it will sometimes give better information. I admit frankly that it can lead us in the wrong direction, but how many times have we been misled by the animal experiments? The animal experiments have often led us astray.

H. Brun

What does Prof. Zbinden think about extrapolating the MIC_{50} results from an *in vitro* model to the plasma concentration found *in vivo* after drug administration in order to validate a culture model in terms of the *in vivo* findings?

G. Zbinden

The use of the plasma concentration as a fixed point to compare *in vitro* and *in vivo* is very important. I am not anxious to have an ED_{50}, because the ED_{50} is selected. I think the minimum toxic concentration is much more relevant.

Groups in Sweden and East Germany have been comparing ED_{50} values or toxic concentrations in *in vitro* systems with lethal concentrations of the same chemicals in humans. If the concentrations of a chemical that kill a human are compared with the concentrations that kill cells, surprisingly, but truly, they are almost identical. The predictability can be greatly improved if, say, active concentrations in the plasma are compared instead of using dose or some kind of extraneous factor. Plasma has to be used, because target organ concentrations cannot be obtained.

2

In Vitro Strategy for the Safety Assessment of Drugs

A.C. CORDIER

Institut de Recherche sur la Sécurité du Médicament, Rhône Poulenc Rorer, 20, Quai de la Révolution, 94140 Alfortville, France

Introduction

Experimental toxicology is the first and necessary step in assessing the safety of a new drug. It corresponds to both ethical and regulatory requirements. The pharmaceutical industry has an ethical duty to offer the highest possible guarantee of the safety of candidate drugs when these are first administered to healthy volunteers or to patients. On the same ethical grounds, the regulatory authorities also require experimental toxicology tests before clinical trials can begin or a product licence is granted.

A large number of widely varied tests are included in the battery of regulatory toxicology studies. These tests involve animals of various species: rat, mouse, rabbit, guinea-pig, dog and monkey. Five main areas of investigation can be defined: (1) general toxicity studies, which range from acute, single administration to repeated administration over periods of up to one year; (2) reproductive toxicity studies, which test more specifically for the possibility of a toxic impact on fertility, embryo development or perinatal psychomotor development; (3) mutagenicity tests, which are carried out essentially *in vitro*, and usually investigate

IN VITRO METHODS IN TOXICOLOGY
ISBN 0-12-388175-7

the impact on three end points: gene mutations, chromosome aberrations and primary DNA damage; (4) carcinogenicity studies, which are carried out in rodents and involve treatment lasting throughout most of the animals' lifespan; (5) various other special tests, such as hypersensitivity, phototoxicity and skin reactions.

The studies should provide answers to the following questions:

> 1) Which organs/tissues or cells are the targets for any toxic impact, and which physiological functions are affected by the pharmacological activity or adverse effects of the drug?
> 2) What are the highest doses which can be administered safely and what is the safety margin?
> 3) What is the risk of causing genetic damage, congenital abnormalities or neoplastic changes?

Toxicological assessment is therefore complex, since all organs and all physiological systems are potential targets. It is multidisciplinary and calls for clinical observation, haematological and biochemical tests, gross pathological and histopathological examinations as well as multigeneration behavioural studies. The findings of all these studies have to be interpreted in the light of kinetic data concerning the absorption and metabolism of the drug in the various experimental species and in man.

This rapid overview of the experimental toxicology of drugs makes it abundantly clear that we cannot hope to replace all experimental studies in animals by *in vitro* tests. The complexity of the living organism cannot be reduced to a range of cell types which can then be tested individually *in vitro*.

Reasons for the Development of *In Vitro* Toxicology

Progress in cellular and molecular biology, improvement of cell culture techniques and the establishment of differentiated cell lines have permitted the rapid development of *in vitro* toxicology. The application of this new and rapidly expanding scientific discipline to the evaluation of drug safety is an ethical, scientific and economic necessity.

More and more people are increasingly concerned about the welfare of animals used in laboratory research, and various institutions and laboratories now publish detailed ethical guidelines concerning the care and protection of laboratory animals. The number of animals used in biomedical research has fallen substantially and steadily over the past decade; however, a considerable number of animals is still required for the exhaustive evaluation of the toxicological potential of a new drug. There is, therefore, an ethical necessity to develop and apply alternative methods, to refine animal testing, to reduce the numbers of animals used, and in a few cases to replace animal tests.

It is difficult to predict the effects of a new drug in man, because it involves extrapolating experimental data obtained in one species to another species. Experience has shown that only 50% (or, if we exclude subjective effects, 70%) of the side effects observed in man will have been detected in animal tests. Conversely, fortunately only 20–30% of the effects found in animals will also occur in man. There is therefore a scientific need to improve the predictive accuracy of toxicological studies through better understanding of the toxic mechanisms involved. The use of cell cultures provides a method not only of investigating toxicity mechanism in detail, but also of avoiding extrapolation problems related to species specificity by using human cells whenever possible.

The usual research and development costs of a new drug can be estimated to be 150 million US dollars. The process is highly selective, and for each drug on the market place, 4000–5000 compounds have to be synthesized. Toxicology constitutes a very considerable hurdle and plays a major role in this process of selection. The proportion of molecules eliminated on toxicological grounds ranges from 20 to 50%, depending on the stage reached. Out of 44 compounds which drop out of the race at some point during the emergence of a new drug, 29 will be brought down by toxicological data.

There are therefore economic reasons for the pharmaceutical industry to develop methods which can eliminate molecules with prohibitive toxicity and identify the least toxic ones as early as possible.

Ethical, economic and scientific reasons, backed up by the introduction of cellular and molecular biology into toxicology, have all contributed to the development of alternative or complementary methods in toxicology which are essentially *in vitro* methods.

Areas of Application of *In Vitro* Toxicology

The development of *in vitro* methods makes it possible to develop three new sectors outside the area of regulatory toxicology: screening toxicology, selective toxicology and explanatory toxicology.

Screening Toxicology

The rationale for *in vitro* screening is that the degree of exposure to a given hazard determines the risk incurred. *In vitro* tests are able to determine the toxic potential which constitutes the "hazard". If this potential were to be zero, then the risk would be zero.

In vitro screening tests must be quick, they must use only small quantities of test substances (which may be in short supply at this early stage) and must be able to handle large numbers of molecules.

In validating these tests, particular attention must be paid to specificity in order to avoid discarding potentially valuable drugs as a result of false positive results. At this stage, the sensitivity of the tests is less important, because these preliminary screening tests will inevitably be followed by conventional tests, which can be relied on to pick up any false negatives that occur.

The potential effects targeted must be restricted to those that would prohibit, or severely restrict, the use of the drug, e.g. mutagenicity or teratogenicity.

It is important to realize that between 20 and 25% of molecules are positive in Ames tests, that 30–35% of molecules show *in vitro* clastogenic activity and that 10–15% are positive in certain teratogenicity tests. Since the overlap of these effects is only partial, it follows that at least 30% of the molecules synthesized will have to be weeded out by these tests. If this is done at an early stage, resources can be focused on molecules with a genuine therapeutic potential, thus avoiding the fruitless use of animals in testing molecules that will inevitably be eliminated later.

Toxicological screening should take place as soon as a range of molecules with interesting pharmacological activity has been identified. In this new approach, pharmacological and toxicological screening are simultaneous and the findings can be fed back to guide chemical synthesis before any animal tests have to be carried out.

Selective Toxicology

As Paracelsus pointed out over 400 years ago, all chemicals are toxic above a certain dose level. The best drug is not therefore the most potent, but the one which offers the best activity/safety ratio.

Primary selection of the least toxic compounds using a wide battery of *in vitro* organ-specific methods composed of cells from different origins (heart, liver, lungs, kidneys, etc.) is hardly realistic in view of the vast number of possible sites of impact. To assess organ-specific toxicity, general parameters reflecting cytotoxicity, such as the release of LDH, are meaningless, since they are not specific and so give little information, as virtually the same result would be obtained regardless of whether fibroblasts, hepatocytes or renal tubular cells were used.

In fact there are two possible approaches. If one is dealing with drugs which belong to a category with well-defined toxicity, such as the anthracyclines or the aminoglycosides, an *in vitro* target organ toxicity test can be used which is appropriate to the specific organ and type of toxicity being tested for. However, more frequently one is faced with new chemical entities, and in this case, given the vast range of possible targets, it would be illusory to attempt to use *in vitro* toxicity methods until whole animal studies have identified the target organs or cells and, if possible, given some indication of the probable mechanism.

The identification of the target organ and the integration of the global toxicological data, notably including pharmacokinetic and metabolic data, must be used to establish an appropriate *in vitro* model to select the best candidate for drug development. This approach should involve the use of human cells whenever possible.

Correct use of *in vitro* methods to evaluate organ toxicity is based on several principles.

1) Cytotoxicity indicators are not good parameters for detecting organ toxicity; they must be used simultaneously with specific indicators in order to distinguish between specific effects and those caused by general toxicity. For example, triglyceride accumulation in hepatocytes occurring *in vitro* at concentrations much lower than that at which the hepatocyte is killed is indicative of steatogenic potential. Similarly, reduced synthesis of testosterone at a concentration that is not toxic toward Leydig cells *in vitro* is an indication of specific impairment of secretory function.

2) Models involving isolated cells are very useful for the investigation of a specific response, but more complex models involving multicellular interactions are more appropriate as a representation of the *in vivo* situation. Such models include co-cultures, three-dimensional cultures and perfused organs, slices, etc.

3) The fact that human cells can be used is one of the major advantages of *in vitro* methods or of investigating organ-specific toxicity. There are, of course, ethical problems relating to their supply and use, but the results can be directly extrapolated to man.

The basic principle – and the most important one – in handling *in vitro* methods is to recognize the exact limits of the models used and to pinpoint the exact question which they can answer. In general, each specific problem requires an appropriate model to be defined.

There is no universal *in vitro* model which can replace the whole animal. Simple tests give simple answers, whereas living organisms are in fact complex.

Explanatory Toxicology

All the principles underlying *in vitro* organ toxicology can also be applied to the field of explanatory toxicology. An understanding of the mechanisms of toxicity is fundamental to good safety assessment. In this respect, the implications for human risk assessment of a testicular injury found in animal tests is not the same if the injury is irreversible damage of germ cells as if it consists of an impairment of spermatogenesis caused by a temporary inhibition of the synthesis of testosterone in Leydig cells. Use of an *in vitro* model involving Leydig cells and of a Sertoli/germ cell co-culture offers a valuable tool with which to clarify this type of problem.

Acquiring an understanding of the toxic mechanism may be a lengthy and costly process. It necessitates the use of a large number of methods and specialist teams as well as fundamental research. Even though cell cultures can make a major contribution in the area of explanatory toxicology, this is only one of the large number of tools required to obtain an understanding of the complex mechanisms of toxicity as it occurs in the whole animal or in man.

A Progressive Strategy

The usefulness of *in vitro* methods in screening and in the elucidation of toxic mechanisms is now beyond dispute. However, with the exception of the very specific field of genetic toxicology, no tests or batteries of tests have yet been validated and approved as alternatives to whole animal tests in regulatory toxicology. As stressed earlier, in view of the complexity of the living body it is impossible to envisage the systematic replacement of *in vivo* by *in vitro* tests. However, we must consider whether in certain specific fields we should not envisage a new approach, involving an *in vitro/in vivo* mix of tests in which the *in vitro* tests are not intended to eliminate whole animal tests, but to reduce their number.

In 1987 the British Toxicology Society proposed a progressive approach to the evaluation of ocular irritation. They suggested that preliminary evaluation should be carried out by means of investigation of the physicochemical properties of a substance and *in vitro* tests. Only if these tests are negative is there any need to go on to carry out a skin irritation test and only if this is negative is an ocular irritation test carried out in a single rabbit. If this test is negative, then a full-scale conventional ocular irritation test is required. This approach not only reduces considerably the number of animals undergoing ocular irritation tests, but also reduces the suffering to which they are subjected.

A similar progressive strategy can perhaps be envisaged towards the evaluation of teratogenicity. The first stage would involve a battery of *in vitro* cellular tests with differing and complementary end points, such as the micromass assay. If the findings are negative, the next step could be the performance of *in vitro* whole embryo tests, which could be performed with metabolic activation by rat, rabbit or human hepatocytes. If the findings here are also negative, then final confirmation *in vivo* could be carried out in a single species.

In adopting such an approach, it is important to find out whether a teratogen could escape detection and, as a corollary, whether the use of a second species *in vivo* is indispensable. A scientific answer must be provided to this question before the requirement for tests in a second species can be eliminated.

A similar progressive approach is possible in the evaluation of carcinogenic potential. The first step would be a battery of regulatory mutagenicity tests, designed to detect genotoxic carcinogens, and the second step, a battery of promotion tests, which remains to be designed and validated. This battery would include, for example, tests of cell cooperation, cell proliferation and possibly a test of oncogene activation. If these batteries were also negative, then a second step would be required, during which the findings of chronic toxicity studies would be evaluated in order to identify any warning signs of a precancerous state, such as hypertrophy or hyperplasia, particularly of endocrine glands, abnormal mitoses and chronic inflammation. If all findings were negative, then a carcinogenicity study in a single species, probably the rat, should suffice to confirm the absence of any carcinogenic potential.

Conclusion

In vitro toxicology has a key role in the exclusion of candidate molecules with prohibitive toxicity and in the selection of the least toxic molecules from within promising chemical families. It is now making a major contribution to the rapid development of a scientific and rational approach to toxicology by increasing the reliability of risk assessment. A considerable amount of work remains to be done in the area of validation and in developing new and specific models as well as in devising innovative approaches which combine *in vitro* and *in vivo* studies.

Discussion

M. Adolphe
Dr Cordier talked about co-culture and multicellular cooperation. I agree with him, but does he think that such a complex battery of models and

tests is too great a problem for industry to carry out, also in terms of economics?

A. Cordier

I agree. When we start doing *in vitro* toxicology we use very few, simple models and simple parameters, such as cytotoxicity. When we go deeper into it, more precise and more reliable parameters are needed. Also, to answer many specific questions more sophisticated models like co-culture have to be used to determine the interaction of the cells for a specific toxicity. This is why I think *in vitro* methods are not cheap; they cost both time and money and become increasingly difficult as we go into more detail in this field.

A. Vernadakis

The discussion so far has not addressed fetal toxicology. I am not referring to teratology or perinatal toxicity, but fetal toxicity. How do we and the pharmaceutical industry approach the problem of fetal toxicity, of the fetus being exposed to potential toxic compounds through the mother? I noticed that the whole embryo was mentioned as a model.

A. Cordier

That is not for the fetus but for the embryo. The problem of the fetus is complicated because the impact of a drug on the fetus occurs after all the organs are formed. The main toxic effect is on later brain and psychomotor development. The usefulness of the *in vitro* approach is perhaps limited here. It is also more difficult than in other fields like teratology.

A. Vernadakis

(*interrupting*) I think it is too late when we are studying teratology because we are then studying an end point. I am asking how *not* to reach that end point.

E. Walum

The possibility occurs to me that psychomotor lesions are usually produced by selective destruction or selective inhibition of correct development of certain populations of neurons. This can of course be assayed in an *in vitro* system, provided that there is a central nervous system culture representative of the organ in its composition. There might be such cultures, for example, reaggregate or micromass cultures.

Prof. Zbinden gave a very good example of the use of chick brain cells in a quantitative risk assessment and its extrapolation to man. Dr Cordier strongly stressed the need to use human cells. This is what we feel, but is there substantial evidence that human cells will provide better results than animal cells in culture?

A. Cordier
Not for all the end points but for several. We have results in hepatotoxicity in one species, the rat, but not in dogs. To determine the risk for man, we can compare the toxicity with the same end point using rat, dog and human hepatocytes and can see the relationship between toxicity in rat and human hepatocytes. If toxicity is seen neither in dog nor human hepatocytes it can perhaps be expected that toxicity will not be found in man. This is one example, but I agree there are others where human cells are not so useful. For some kinds of toxicity, some specificity, say, in kidney cells or in specific functions, human cells might be more appropriate than other cell types.

J. Boyer
As a hepatologist, I am very pleased to hear Dr Cordier emphasize the need to use human hepatocytes. Now that liver transplantation is being performed it will become increasingly possible to obtain human tissue. Human tissue may not be needed for cytotoxic problems, but human culture systems should be very useful for the idiosyncratic reactions that are dependent upon metabolism.

P. Laduron
Dr Cordier said that when we are faced with new chemical series it is important to determine the target organ, but does he think that the target organ is in fact determined by the pharmacological profile?

A. Cordier
The target organ is not usually known with a new chemical entity and its toxicity is not necessarily determined by its pharmacological profile. It is too time consuming to always use a large battery composed of many different cell types using several end points. So if we want to select the least toxic compound, we must first have some idea about the target *in vivo*.

J.J. Picard
I was interested that Dr Cordier suggested that his teratology scheme would be carried out in three steps, each of which would predict in some way what could happen in the next step – admittedly with some errors. The first steps he suggested for teratology were the micromass test, cell attachment and metabolic cooperation. Do those tests really have

something to do with the next step, which would be the embryo? If three other steps were chosen that would not be suggested as being related to embryology, such as hepatotoxicity, Ames and neurotoxic tests, would there not be about the same results, the same errors and the same predictability as with *in vitro* test on the whole embryo culture?

A. Cordier

It depends upon how the tests are performed. We have modified the limb-bud micromass assay in order to decrease its sensitivity but to increase the specificity of the first screening towards 100% (it is now perhaps 95%). This means that only real teratogens are picked up by this test – but we lose a lot. We have taken the same approach with the cell attachment method, modifying the original technique in order to decrease its sensitivity, so that it does not pick up all the compounds but only those which act with this end point. When these two tests are combined there is very good specificity and the sensitivity is also increased.

If we take another end point, for example, clastogenicity, (since a compound that is clastogenic can also induce malformation), if we add such a test in the first screening it will also provide some information on that.

The problem about the first step is that many compounds have to be tested, and 1000 compounds a year cannot be handled with the whole-embryo culture. With the limb-bud micromass assay, however, 1000 or 2000 a year can be handled very easily because we have miniaturized and computerized tests. The first screening will not eliminate all the compounds but, since the specificity (not the sensitivity) is very high, when there is a positive result it means that the compound is a real teratogen and thus can be eliminated.

We use this screen, but I agree it is only a proposal. With the three end points we can perhaps use clastogenicity in place of cell cooperation or cell attachment.

P. Kramer

With regard to finding the appropriate cell type for *in vitro* testing, Dr Cordier said that it is necessary to identify the target organ in a preliminary short-term toxicity assay. What is meant by "short-term", because a lot of target organs will not be identified after a short time?

A. Cordier

I agree. Some target organs will be identified after perhaps 3- or 6-months' treatment, for which the same strategy cannot be applied. *In vitro* toxicology does not answer all the questions, but in a very short time – for example, we use an 8-day treatment in rats – it is possible to identify a likely target organ for a new chemical entity. Using the appropriate *in vitro* method we can then select compounds with activity and which are devoid of the specific toxicity for this family – and only this family. We have been successful with two or three chemical families, identifying specific cell types on specific target organs, specific mechanisms, and have developed a totally new *in vitro* approach which can be applied in the particular family. It cannot of course be applied to all the problems, but it can in some specific cases.

N.G. Carmichael
Prof. Zbinden identified a problem with compounds with low water solubility. One of the unifying factors of pesticides, in fact, is that almost all of them have low water solubility. How big a problem will this be in practice to have a good *in vitro* system for screening pesticides?

A. Cordier
Water solubility is one of the major problems in *in vitro* tests and we are always having to deal with it.

B. Bkaily
In talking about embryology, the use of embryo, fetal human or whatever, we must be careful about the age of the embryo. The pharmacology of any organ in an embryo, whether chick or fetal human, at certain ages will be completely different from that in an adult embryo. If we want to use culture cells we must be very careful about the way the cell may return to some embryonic state or the receptor and pharmacology may be completely different from the adult. We must be very careful about using embryonic cells or organs.

A. Cordier
I agree. It is why I emphasized the need to know exactly the limitation of a test, exactly what questions it can answer. This is the most important problem.

J.R. Claude
First, Dr Cordier's references to extrapolation to man came from a period when pharmacokinetic and metabolic studies were not so well performed as they are now. One way of making a better extrapolation from animals to man is through the great progress and the increasing role of safety in pharmacokinetics. This is very important. Toxicokinetics are described in the Appendix to the 1983 European Economic Community (EEC) recommendations.

Secondly, related to the schedule of the investigation concerning teratogenicity and the special case of the rabbit, it is true that the rabbit is probably a good model if the studies are performed on only one species, but in many cases there are few pharmacokinetic and metabolic data on the rabbit. Also, the rabbit is probably not a good species in terms of the pharmacokinetic data compared with man.

Thirdly, I agree absolutely that the use of two species, especially the use of mice, is completely irrelevant in carcinogenicity studies. I think Dr Cordier's data have underlined that the use of the rat alone is quite sufficient to perform the assay for carcinogenicity. Some European agencies are promoting the idea that carcinogenicity studies in one species, the rat, are sufficient to evaluate correctly the carcinogenicity of a new product.

A. Cordier

First, I agree that in recent years we have increasingly used pharmacokinetic data to make more accurate extrapolation from animals to man. This certainly increases the predictivity of toxicological study in animals.

With regard to the problem of teratology and the choice of species, the rabbit has of course been used because of the problem of thalidomide, but I do not know whether it is more accurate than to use the rat. If we have only the rat teratogenicity, I do not know whether that is sufficient, or what is the "plus" of the rabbit for all compounds, except in the case of thalidomide, where we had a very specific effect.

I am pleased to hear Dr Claude and Prof. Zbinden's comments about carcinogenicity studies. It reminds me of the paper by Tennant in *Science* (1987) in which he compared the results of and the accuracy between four *in vitro* tests with those of rodent carcinogenicity tests for 73 compounds tested in the national toxicological programme in the USA. The accuracy, in terms of the combined sensitivity and specificity, for all the four tests, Ames, sister chromatin exchange, mouse lymphoma and chromosome aberration, is 60–62%. The accuracy with the same 73 compounds between rat and mouse carcinogenicity studies is 66%: it is not known between rodent and man. Several mechanisms are involved in carcinogenicity, of which genotoxicity is only one: there are non-genotoxic and genotoxic carcinogens. An accuracy of 60–62% between *in vitro* tests and rodent carcinogenicity studies is certainly better than that 66% between rat and mouse *in vivo*.

J. Frazier

I believe this discussion raises the issue of which databases are appropriate for validating methodologies.

3

In Vitro Toxicology: An Alternative to Animal Testing in Safety Evaluation?

A.J. PAINE

DH Department of Toxicology, St Bartholomew's Hospital Medical College, University of London, Dominion House, 59 Bartholomew Close, London EC1 7ED, UK

Introduction

Determining the safety of a chemical requires a fine balance between the risk of its toxicity and the benefit of its use. In reality, "safety" as a lack of harm can only be demonstrated retrospectively by continued health or well-being despite exposure to some circumstance or preparation. To be useful, however, protection against harm, which involves predicting "safety", requires forecasting absence or minimization of risk in the future on the basis of present evidence. Important elements underlying safety evaluation are therefore knowledge of the hazard linked to an understanding of potential exposure.

Toxic hazard is usually determined by established test methods, the majority of which use animals and the results of which are credited internationally (OECD, 1981). Against this established background there is a well supported move to reduce the use of living animals for evaluation of toxicity (Balls *et al.*, 1992; this volume). It is important, however, to realize that the ethical, scientific and practical issues involved do not

IN VITRO METHODS IN TOXICOLOGY
ISBN 0-12-388175-7

apply specifically to toxicology but pertain equally to all aspects of medical research.

Types of Toxicity

A range of toxicity tests will be done in the development of a new chemical entity (Paine, 1991) and a variety of adverse effects may result (Table 3.1). These may be manifested as functional disturbances, evidenced by changes in behaviour or increased incidence of infection because a chemical is suppressing the immune system, and range to newer aspects of the subject, such as effects on the endocrine system and all of its consequences. For example, pathological changes produced in the pituitary, thyroid, ovary, breast or pancreas are all due to a common action on prolactin levels via the hypothalamus. Accordingly, in view of the diversity of toxic effects, current consensus is that the best chance of detecting the large range of adverse effects many of which depend on integrated body systems is by using the appropriate animal model.

Countervailing Strengths of *In Vivo* and *In Vitro* Models

Toxicologists have a wide range of systems available to them for toxicity testing (Table 3.2) but, in general, as the complexity of these decreases

Table 3.1
Types of toxicity

(1)	Functional:	based on clinical observation, e.g. behavioural toxicology, immunotoxicity
(2)	Biochemical:	mechanisms underlying dysfunction, absorption, distribution, metabolism and excretion of toxins
(3)	Structural:	pathology based at the levels of organs/tissues including carcinogenesis
(4)	Environmental:	accumulation/transformation in soil, water, air, animals (including ruminants), birds, insects, fishes and plants
(5)	Newer aspects:	irritancy, endocrine toxicology, genetic toxicology, reproductive toxicology (including fertility, teratology, postnatal development)

Table 3.2
Systems available for toxicity testing

COMPLEXITY	Advantages for basic research		COMPLEXITY	Advantages for testing
		Intact organism		
		Perfused organs		
		Organ culture/tissue slices		
		Primary cell cultures		
		Established cell lines		
		Tissue homogenates		
		Subcellular fractions/prokaryotes		
		Purified enzymes		

so does the advantage for identifying chemical hazard because simple techniques cannot be expected to detect the broad array of toxic effects that result from disturbances in integrated body functions. In addition, activation to a toxic metabolite may occur in one organ with the end effect occurring at a remote site, e.g. the metabolism of aromatic amines to proximate carcinogens in the liver that only act in the bladder. Vital body systems have evolved to respond homoeostatically to adverse stimuli, e.g. the controls over water and electrolyte metabolism via the kidneys and endocrine glands, the interrelated neural and paracrine regulators of cardiac function and blood pressure and the entire humoral, cellular and innate immune systems. Toxic effects on these multilevel systems can only be investigated at first by *in vivo* studies because otherwise there would be no indication of which target organ or mechanism to examine (Table 3.3). In contrast, however, as the complexity of the test system decreases so the advantage for determining precise mechanisms of toxicity and their extrapolation to man may increase. Thus, *in vitro* systems have played an important role in safety evaluation by demonstrating instances of rodent-specific toxicity which may be unimportant in relation to human risk assessment (Lock *et al.*, 1989; Green, 1990). Thus, the validity of *in vitro* tests as predictive tools and the degree to which they can be useful depends entirely on the sorts of questions being asked as well as the answers being sought (Table 3.4).

In contrast with whole animal studies, no one *in vitro* system can, therefore, be expected to detect the whole array of toxic effects or for that matter the wide range of target organs of toxicity. Thus, knowledge of the mechanism of toxic action is the surest foundation for the success of an *in vitro* model, but even here pharmacodynamic influences may diminish the performance of an *in vitro* model (Paine and Hockin, 1982; Goldberg and Frazier, 1989). Even if we can show a toxic effect *in vitro*, we may be faced with the problem of an extra tier in the extrapolation

Table 3.3
In vitro systems in toxicology

System	No toxicity	Toxicity
Perfused organs ⎫ Organ culture ⎪ Tissue slices ⎬ Cell cultures ⎭	Wrong target organ?	How to extrapolate to animal data base and compare ED_{50} with LD_{50}? How to get NOEL and ADI?
Tissue homogenates ⎫ Subcellular fractions ⎬ Purified enzymes ⎭	Wrong target organ? Missing co-factor/ mediator?	What does end point mean? Could it have been repaired *in vivo*?
Prokaryotes	Antibacterial? Epigenetic carcinogen?	Mutagen but what will be *in vivo* response?

Abbrevations: NOEL, no-observable effect level; ADI, acceptable daily intake.

Table 3.4
In vitro – in vivo extrapolations

Question	Answer
Is a chemical which is mutagenic *in vitro* a potential risk for man?	Yes!
Are chemicals which cause cell transformation *in vitro* potential carcinogens for man?	Yes!
Are inhibitors of cell proliferation *in vitro* potential poisons for man?	Yes, because of the ubiquitous nature of cell cycle events and mitosis
Can these responses be anticipated *in vivo*?	No, the chemical's disposition may be different

to man (Fig. 3.1). For example, how do we relate the median effective dose (ED_{50}) determined *in vitro* to the *in vivo* toxicity database (Fry *et al.*, 1988)? Then how do we relate the end point measured *in vitro* to derive a no-observable effect level (NOEL) and hence an acceptable daily intake (ADI) to protect the consumer of residue-containing foodstuffs? Although these parameters are considered by some to be pragmatic at best, they must also be considered successful on the basis

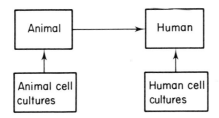

Fig. 3.1 *In vitro–in vivo* extrapolations.

of published statistics on poisonings, accidents and even pensions for industrial injuries, which indicate that harm to man is rare unless there is a breach of current safety standards.

Conclusions

A dilemma faced by toxicologists is that public concern about the use of experimental animals in testing for toxicity is increasing in tandem with public demand for improvements in product and drug safety. In general, toxicity tests *in vivo* have been capable of predicting most risks and even of overpredicting some when it has been possible to compare findings in man and animals (Lumley and Walker, 1987). Past errors and tragedies arose for fundamental and practical reasons. For instance, when the animals used in experiments have physiological and metabolic responses that diverge from man or the statistical power of experiments with a limited number of animals meant that idiosyncratic reactions could not be detected. Although methods are being improved and the number of animals employed in toxicity testing reduced by the introduction of the "fixed dose procedure" (Van den Heuvel *et al.*, 1987) and the British Toxicology Society's approach for testing for irritancy (Fielder *et al.*, 1987), animal studies are likely to remain the mainstay of toxicity testing methods for the foreseeable future. This is because only with *in vivo* studies can the full range of direct and indirect effects and disturbed physiological mechanisms be studied in a way that will support extrapolation to man and other species. Even though notable advances are being made in the development of alternatives, the adoption of such tests faces more than just the technical barrier of validating a new technology. Testing is an integral part of many regulatory schemes as well as product liability law and hence validation ultimately rests on acceptance by all members of the community including the general public themselves. Thus "safety" is more than just the prediction of damage, it is the societal decision that something or some activity is acceptable because it is worth more overall than the harm it may cause!

Acknowledgement

I am grateful to Professor Anthony Dayan for stimulating discussion and many of the ideas presented in this paper.

References

Balls, M., Botham, P., Cordier, A., Fumero, S., Kayser, D., Koeter, H., Koundakjian, P., Gunnary Lindquist, N., Meyer, O., Pioda, L., Reinhardt, C., Rozemond, H., Smyrniotis, T., Spielmann, H., Van Looy, H., Van der Venner, M.T. and Walum, E. (1992). *ATLA* **18**, in press.

Fielder, R.J., Gaunt, I.F., Rhodes, C., Sullivan, F.M. and Swanston, D.W. (1987). *Hum. Toxicol.* **6**, 269–278.

Fry, J.R., Garle, M.J. and Hammond, A.H. (1988). *ATLA* **16**, 175–179.

Goldberg, A.M. and Frazier, J.M. (1989). *Sci. Am.* **261**, 16–22.

Green, T. (1990). *Annu. Rev. Pharmacol. Toxicol.* **30**, 73–89.

Lock, E.A., Mitchell, A.M. and Elcombe, C.R. (1989). *Annu. Rev. Pharmacol. Toxicol.* **29**, 145–163.

Lumley, C.E. and Walker, S.R. (1987). *Arch. Toxicol.* **S11**, 295–304.

OECD (1981). "Guidelines for Testing of Chemicals", Paris, France.

Paine, A.J. (1991). *In* "General and Applied Toxicology" (P. Turner, T. Marrs and B. Ballantyne, eds), chapter 13. Macmillan, London, in press.

Paine, A.J. and Hockin, L.J. (1982). *Toxicology* **25**, 41–45.

Van den Heuvel, M.J., Dayan, A.D. and Shillaker, R.O. (1987). *Hum. Toxicol.* **6**, 279–291.

Part II

Target Organ Toxicity

A. General Aspects

4

An *In Vitro* Approach to the Study of Target Organ Toxicity

D. ACOSTA, K. RAMOS, M.A. SMITH, J. SWANN, and J. DAVILA

The University of Texas at Austin, Department of Pharmacology and Toxicology, College of Pharmacy, Austin, TX 78712, USA

Introduction

Exposure to drugs and chemicals often results in toxicity to living organisms. We have come to appreciate the fact that not all compounds are equally toxic to all parts of the living system, because the toxic actions of many compounds are manifested in specific organs. These organs are known as target organs of toxicity. This concept has developed into the evaluation of toxicants via their target organ specificity.

Several factors determine the susceptibility of a particular organ to toxicity. These factors include the pharmacokinetics of the compound, the metabolic fate of the chemical and the organ's ability to respond to the toxic insult. The liver, kidneys and lungs are capable of metabolizing chemicals to toxic reactive intermediates. The *in situ* metabolic activation of chemicals results in selective toxicity. These reactive intermediates can initiate toxicity via covalent binding to cellular macromolecules, generation of reactive oxygen species or peroxidative injury.

IN VITRO METHODS IN TOXICOLOGY
ISBN 0-12-388175-7

The application of *in vitro* model systems to evaluate the toxicity of xenobiotics has significantly enhanced our understanding of drug- and chemical-induced target organ toxicity. From a scientific perspective, the popularity of *in vitro* model systems has been justified for several reasons (Acosta *et al.*, 1985). From the public perspective, *in vitro* model systems enjoy increasing popularity because their application in toxicity testing may allow a reduction in the number of live animals employed. *In vitro* models commonly used in target organ toxicity testing include: perfused organ preparations, isolated tissue preparations, single cell suspensions and tissue culture systems. Because these models are used as predictors of the human response, when applicable, all preparations should be derived from species which respond with fidelity to the toxic challenge.

The expression of target organ toxicity ranges from subtle abnormalities of cellular organelles to permanent loss of organ function. Because each organ system is characterized by a large degree of structural and functional heterogeneity, the assessment of toxicity *in vivo* is often complicated. In this regard, *in vitro* model systems can be used to define general mechanisms of toxicity or to screen potentially toxic drugs and other chemicals. An essential consideration in attempting to validate *in vitro* systems is that data obtained *in vitro* should always be correlated to observations made *in vivo*.

A major goal of our laboratory has been the development of primary culture systems that retain differentiated functions and responses characteristic of intact tissues *in vivo*. Specifically, we have developed cellular models of primary cultures of heart, nerve, skin, cornea, liver and kidney cells to explore the mechanisms by which drugs or chemicals may be toxic to key organs of the body and to develop new techniques by which xenobiotics may be evaluated or identified as potential toxicants to living systems. The objective of this paper is to provide a brief overview of our approach to the study of target organ toxicology with *in vitro* cellular systems: liver, kidneys and central nervous system (CNS) have been selected as representative examples for our discussion of models.

Model of Liver Toxicity with Primary Culture System of Rat Hepatocytes

Drug metabolism and chemical hepatic injury can be studied by *in vivo* and *in vitro* models. *In vivo* models provide information about the major parameters of drug disposition including absorption, distribution, Phase I and II metabolism and elimination. *In vivo* models are used for studies of overall metabolism and metabolite(s) production, as well as for pharmacokinetic studies. These models are important for the demonstration that drugs or chemicals have a truly adverse effect on the liver in a setting of physiological significance. In addition, urine, bile and blood samples can be collected to study drugs or other chemicals with unknown drug disposition. However, *in vivo* systems have some disadvantages. For example, they are very complex systems and sometimes are not suitable for studying specific reactions involved in the metabolism of a drug or for studying the mechanism of a particular reaction. Similarly, there are problems with other variables such as age, sex, nutrition, pregnancy and genetic predisposition. Furthermore, qualitative and quantitative differences exist between the reactions of various animal species to chemicals. Not only do pharmacological and toxicological assessments with animals suffer from these limitations, they are also very costly and time consuming.

In contrast, *in vitro* models may be used to elucidate specific aspects of metabolism or cell injury. An important application of *in vitro* systems is the preliminary screening of xenobiotics for potential systemic effects (Grisham, 1979; Acosta *et al.*, 1987). Some of the advantages and disadvantages of *in vitro* models will be explained below.

Primary cultures of rat hepatocytes offer a suitable experimental model for studying the chemical biotransformation, cytotoxicity and genotoxicity of drugs and xenobiotics. They are useful tools for studying and evaluating potential toxic chemicals, and for studying the mechanism(s) by which chemicals and other xenobiotics may be screened or identified as potential toxicants to living organisms. Primary cultures of rat hepatocytes offer several potential advantages over whole animals when used as a model for drug biotransformation, detection of toxic chemicals, toxicity assessments and for evaluating their cellular mechanism of toxicity.

Some of these advantages are: (1) blood flow, heterogeneity of cell type and nervous and humoral factors are eliminated; (2) better control is obtained of nutritional and hormonal status, oxygen supply and concentration and time exposure to xenobiotics; (3) the morphology of individual cells can be easily observed under the microscope and direct contact between the compounds and the target is assured; and (4) the mechanism of the resulting toxicity can be examined and determined.

Liver cell cultures also offer several advantages when compared with other *in vitro* systems, such as liver cell suspensions. For example: (1) cells have time to recover from trauma sustained during the isolation procedure; (2) monolayer cultures initially consist of viable cells and can be maintained for long periods of time; and (3) monolayer cultures permit the study of the effects of toxicants on functions requiring organization of cells.

Historically, the major drawback of cultured liver cells is the decline of their cytochrome *P*-450 content, which makes the results of biotransformation studies difficult to interpret. Furthermore, cellular structural integrity and intercellular relationships are disrupted after dissociation of the tissue. However, it has been demonstrated that this culture system maintains several liver-specific differentiated functions, characteristic of normal parenchymal cells (Acosta *et al.*, 1978; Nelson *et al.*, 1982). Examples include: sulphobromophthalein (BSP) uptake and conjugation with glutathione; retention of activity of the L-isozyme of pyruvate kinase for over 20 days in culture; maintenance of glutathione levels; ability to synthesize urea; maintenance of a normal lactate to pyruvate ratio; and the retention of high levels of cytochrome *P*-450 activity for a long period of time. Of particular value is the ability of this *in vitro* system to reproduce conditions which are similar to those occurring *in vivo* but without the restraints imposed by the whole animal or the limitations which occur during the use of other *in vitro* systems.

Over the past several years, we have been able to demonstrate that a primary culture system of rat hepatocytes is a useful experimental model for studying the metabolism and potential cytotoxicity of various toxicants (Anuforo *et al.*, 1978; Acosta *et al.*, 1980; Davila *et al.*, 1989). We have shown that drugs and xenobiotics which produce liver injury in man may also be toxic to cultured hepatocytes, and that such toxicity may be evident after treatment with directly acting hepatotoxins or with indirectly acting agents, which produce allergic reactions within the liver. In previous studies, we have suggested that indirectly acting hepatotoxins, which typically produce hypersensitivity reactions by an idiosyncratic mechanism in man, may also be toxic to the liver *in vitro* (Davila *et al.*, 1990). This is true, for example, of papaverine hydrochloride, which has been shown to have an intrinsic effect on liver cells leading to hepatic injury.

Thus, primary monolayers of liver cell cultures can be used to investigate metabolism-mediated cytotoxicity of hepatotoxic drugs or xenobiotics; furthermore, they are useful systems for predicting toxicological responses to xenobiotics anticipated *in vivo*.

Model of Kidney Toxicity with Primary Culture System of Rat Proximal Tubule Epithelial Cells

The kidneys are dynamic organs involved in body homeostasis. Although they comprise less than 1% of total body mass, they receive approximately 20% of the total cardiac output. The nature of renal structure and function renders the kidneys susceptible to toxic insult by xenobiotics.

The high rate of renal perfusion allows compounds to reach high concentrations within the kidneys. The ion transport systems and renal concentrating mechanisms can also increase the exposure of the kidneys to foreign compounds. These factors, along with their inherent metabolic capabilities, make the kidneys very vulnerable to xenobiotic-induced toxicity.

Renal function can be analysed through the use of several *in vitro* techniques. These methods include the isolated perfused kidney, renal slices, isolated tubules and renal cell culture. Some of these methods have been applied to toxicity evaluation (Hirsch, 1976). Isolated kidney cells and renal tubule fragments have also been used in drug metabolism studies (Jones *et al.*, 1979). *In vitro* systems are easily manipulated and allow direct observation of changes in renal function. The use of *in vitro* techniques can help clarify the information gathered from *in vivo* studies. For example, renal transport can be studied *in vivo* through the use of *p*-aminohippurate and inulin clearance. These parameters can be monitored *in vitro* without the influence of changes in glomerular function. In this way, tubular functions can be studied independently of glomerular function.

Cell culture systems have become accepted as useful tools for toxicology studies. Primary cell cultures, cell lines and cell strains have all been used to evaluate the toxicity of various xenobiotics. Aside from simple gross observations of toxicity, cultured cells have been used to determine the mechanisms of toxicity.

Cultured cells facilitate the study of cellular injury that results from toxic insult. Valuable information can be obtained through the correlation of biochemical alterations with changes in cell morphology. These correlations can provide insight into the mechanisms of toxicity. Culture systems are a reliable, reproducible and inexpensive way to assess toxicity at the cellular level.

Primary cultures of renal cortical epithelial cells have been widely used in investigations of drug toxicity (Smith and Acosta, 1986; Smith *et al.*, 1987; Ambudkar *et al.*, 1988). Primary cultures have also been passaged for use in drug toxicity studies (Trifillis and Kahng, 1988). All cell culture techniques offer the advantage of rigorous control of the extracellular environment, and simplified manipulation of the cells.

Cell culture also excludes uncontrolled nervous, endocrine or haemodynamic influences. In addition, the use of cell culture permits prolonged exposures to xenobiotics, which is a distinct advantage over the isolated perfused kidney preparation, renal slices, renal tubule suspensions and renal cell suspensions.

Primary renal cortical epithelial cultures offer many advantages over other *in vitro* preparations in the study of xenobiotic toxicity. These cultures are relatively homogeneous; care is taken to separate epithelial cells from other cell types and to suppress the growth of fibroblasts. Because very little time elapses between the isolation of the tissue from the intact animal and the use of the culture in cytotoxicity studies, primary cultures offer the advantage of maintained differentiated functions. Cell lines, on the other hand, may have been in culture for decades (since 1958 for the MDCK line), and thus have undergone dedifferentiation (Sakhrani and Fine, 1983).

In addition, cell lines have been shown to possess features that are not characteristic of their presumed cell type of origin. This may result in an altered cellular response to toxicants. Indeed, the exact origin of cell lines cannot be determined in many cases, since they were obtained from renal homogenates which are very heterogeneous. In addition, the validity of toxicological studies performed on essentially transformed cells may be questionable.

Primary cultures are not without disadvantages. Because the kidney is a very heterogeneous organ, knowledge of the exact origin of cells grown in culture is limited. Studies of compounds that must be metabolized to cause toxicity may be hindered by the decline over time of drug-metabolizing enzyme activities *in vitro*. Considerable effort is required to limit contamination of the culture by fibroblasts.

Before cells in culture can be used for toxicity testing, it must be demonstrated that the cells have retained some of their differentiated functions. The metabolic capabilities of the kidneys have been well documented (Anders, 1980). Because it is thought that renal metabolism may be involved in the toxicities of various compounds, it is important that the metabolic status of the kidney cells be maintained in culture. Renal cytochrome *P*-450 has been implicated in the formation of reactive intermediates which cause tissue damage. The presence of marker enzymes, alkaline phosphatase and maltase, indicate proximal tubular brush border function. The kidney tubules are responsible for the transport of many organic anions and cations. Since some nephrotoxic agents can have an effect on renal transport systems, it is necessary that cultured kidney cells maintain this function. Cultured kidney cells which maintain their drug-metabolizing capacity, brush border functions and transport properties are more valid indicators of *in vivo* function. Alterations in these parameters can then be used to monitor xenobiotic-induced renal cell injury.

The primary culture system of rat kidney cortical epithelial cells used in our laboratory has been demonstrated to retain several differentiated kidney functions (Smith and Acosta, 1986). It has been demonstrated that primary cultures of rat renal epithelium maintained adequate activities of brush border enzymes (alkaline phosphatase and maltase) for at least 3 days in culture. Moreover, relatively stable levels of cytochrome *P*-450 and cellular glutathione were demonstrated, consistent with values previously reported for cells in culture.

Cytokeratin is an intermediate filament of the cytoskeleton found only in epithelial cells (Darnell *et al.*, 1986). The presence of these filaments was demonstrated in our culture system by indirect immunofluorescence. Transmission electron microscopy revealed the presence of junctional complexes, which are also characteristic solely of epithelial cells. Scanning electron microscopy revealed the presence of endocytic pits and of apical microvilli, demonstrating that normal cell polarization is maintained in culture.

Once the functionality of the cell culture system has been established, it is then possible to use the system to evaluate nephrotoxins. The cellular response to toxicity can be monitored via alterations in the normal cellular functions. Changes in renal transport, metabolism and enzyme function can serve as indicators of nephrotoxicity. The time–response and dose–response effects of a compound on these functional parameters can provide information about its toxic mechanisms.

In addition to organ-specific functions, biochemical markers common to all cell types can be used to monitor toxicity. Our laboratory has used the leakage of cytoplasmic lactate dehydrogenase (LDH) and cellular potassium content as indicators of plasma membrane integrity. The activity of mitochondrial succinate dehydrogenase (SDH) and cellular adenosine triphosphate (ATP) content serve as indicators of mitochondrial function. Other useful indicators of cellular organelle function include lysosomal acid phosphatase activity and microsomal glucose-6-phosphatase activity. The changes in cell membrane integrity and organelle function that occur after toxic insult can serve as an aid in localizing the cellular sites of toxicity. When combined with studies of renal-specific function, these parameters can help delineate the progress of xenobiotic-induced renal injury.

To establish the validity of primary renal cell cultures as a toxicological tool, it is necessary to evaluate several compounds known to be nephrotoxic *in vivo*. Heavy metals, analgesics and antibiotics have been shown to cause nephrotoxicity *in vivo*. The evaluation of known nephrotoxic agents in a cell culture system establishes guidelines for determining toxicity. Criteria delineated by changes in organ-specific functions, cellular organelle functions and cell-morphology can then be applied to the evaluation of potential nephrotoxins *in vitro*.

In our laboratory, we have evaluated the cytotoxicity of several well-known nephrotoxic agents in a primary culture system of rat kidney cortical epithelial cells. We have shown that mercuric chloride, cadmium chloride, acetaminophen, cephaloridine and gentamicin produced toxicity similar to that demonstrated in *in vivo* models (Smith and Acosta, 1986; Smith *et al.*, 1987; Swann *et al.*, 1990; Swann and Acosta, 1990).

Model of Neuronal Toxicity with Primary Culture System of Rat Hippocampal, Cerebellar and Astrocyte Cell Cultures

Complex biochemical phenomena can be satisfactorily studied with CNS neural tissue *in vitro*. Several techniques currently used are: slices, organotypic cell cultures, cell lines and primary cell cultures. Primary neuronal cell cultures are obtained by culturing (for more than 24 h) dispersed cells from neural tissue taken directly from the animal (Federoff, 1966; Stammati *et al.*, 1981). The brain tissue of the animal at an optimal embryological or postnatal stage of brain development is chosen for culturing specific cell types from various brain regions. Primary cell cultures of the mammalian CNS offer certain advantages over other tissue culture systems used for studying neurotoxicity. First, differentiation of neuronal properties is more fully expressed in primary cell cultures than in cell lines. Second, the extracellular environment can be more precisely controlled than in organotypic cell cultures. The main disadvantage of working with primary neuronal cell cultures is the presence of a "contaminating" non-neuronal cell population which can interfere in the interpretation of specific neurotoxic effects on neuronal function by a toxin. A separate and parallel primary culture of non-neuronal cells treated with the same neurotoxin should resolve the specific and non-specific toxic effect(s) on neuronal function.

In our laboratory, primary cultures of rat hippocampal pyramidal cells (primarily GABAergic), cerebellar granule cells (glutaminergic) and cerebral astrocytes were used as models to examine the selectivity and sensitivity of aluminium neurotoxicity in the CNS. This model offers several advantages over *in vivo* testing. First, neurotoxic effects which occur shortly after exposure to aluminium can be easily determined. Second, a comparison can be easily made between different parameters of cytoxicity so that the most sensitive indicators of aluminium neurotoxicity can be determined. Third, with the use of a relatively homogeneous cell population, the investigator can examine the cell-specific toxicity of aluminium.

With the increased use and consumption of aluminium-containing products, there is now a greater need to understand the biological fate of aluminium in humans. Most of the previous studies were concerned primarily with characterizing the pathological effects resulting from elevated brain aluminium levels. Only a few studies have been conducted that were aimed specifically at determining the molecular mechanisms of aluminium neurotoxicity. In addition, none of the studies to date have determined the selective vulnerability of the hippocampus, out of all other brain regions, to the neurotoxicity of aluminium. Part of the reason may be the inability of investigators to characterize fully the toxicity of aluminium among the various cell types of the hippocampus. The present study was designed specifically to determine the selective neurotoxicity of aluminium among three hippocampal cell types and to detect any differences in sensitivity of cellular function to aluminium toxicity.

Our results showed that aluminium neurotoxicity was expressed differently in the three cell types examined. Differences were found in membrane permeability, aluminium distribution and the activity of neurotransmitter-related enzymes following exposure of the cell cultures to toxic concentrations of aluminium.

Cultures of hippocampal pyramidal cells, cerebellar granule cells and cerebral astrocytes (a non-neuronal cell type) were previously shown to exhibit differences in cellular morphology, lactate dehydrogenase (LDH) activity, K^+ content and protein content following aluminium treatment (Kisby and Acosta, 1985, 1987). In the general toxicity studies, we saw significant decreases in cerebellar LDH activity (total), hippocampal total cellular K^+ and both astrocyte LDH activity (total) and total cellular K^+ following treatment of cultures with aluminium chloride. We report here that differences may also exist for glutamate dehydrogenase (GLDH) and glutamic acid decarboxylase (GAD) activity in these neuronal and non-neuronal cell cultures.

The mechanism of aluminium neurotoxicity is not well understood. In the present study, we have used *in vitro* models as an approach to understanding the specific neurotoxic mechanism(s) of aluminium and its selectivity in the CNS. We have found that three different cell types from the rat CNS differ in their response to toxic concentrations of aluminium *in vitro*. We have shown that aluminium interferes with the membrane permeability to ions and the activity of the cytoplasmic enzyme, LDH. Although studies in the past demonstrated that aluminium interferes with a number of neuronal properties, our studies indicate that these effects caused by aluminium may be cell specific. We found that the three cell types were different in their permeability to K^+ and similar in their prevention of LDH release after aluminium exposure. Changes in the permeability characteristics of the synaptic membrane to ions could lead to increased intracellular concentrations of neurotoxic metal ions (e.g. Al^{3+}). In the aluminium distributional studies, we demonstrated that differences do exist in the cellular aluminium content among hippocampal, cerebellar and astrocyte cultures. The results of these findings indicate that the higher aluminium levels in one cell type may be a reflection of its membrane properties. In addition, the higher concentrations of aluminium in a specific cell type (glutaminergic cerebellar granule cells) suggest that the distribution of aluminium in certain brain regions of experimental animals with aluminium-induced encephalopathies is probably related to alterations in the membrane characteristics of specific cell types. Our findings also indicate that certain cell types within brain regions may be more vulnerable to the toxic effects of aluminium.

The aluminium toxicity studies with the intracellular enzymes (e.g. LDH, GLDH and GAD) indicate that the toxic effects of aluminium on cytoplasmic and neurotransmitter-related enzymes differ depending on the cell culture (or type). Hippocampal LDH activity was unaffected by aluminium whereas cerebellar and astrocyte LDH activity was significantly reduced. We found that GAD activity (a marker for GABAergic neurons) in hippocampal cultures was unaffected by aluminium treatment, while GLDH (a marker for glutaminergic neurons) was signficantly reduced. In addition, we found that aluminium treatment of cerebellar granule cell cultures, a relatively pure population of glutaminergic neurons, produced significant decreases in GLDH activity after treatments of 12 h–10 days with 10 μM or 0.2 mM. Together, these results suggest that aluminium neurotoxicity in the hippocampus may be selective, although its role in dementia is still unclear.

From the results, it appears that hippocampal glutaminergic neurons may be especially sensitive to the neurotoxic effects of aluminium. However, further comparative research between aluminium and the different CNS cell types and their neurotransmitters is needed to understand the underlying mechanisms of aluminium neurotoxicity in the CNS. A key to determining the selectivity of aluminium for a specific cell type in the hippocampus will be the study of the effects of aluminium on aspartergic neurons. However, research in this area is particularly difficult since the metabolism and catabolism of aspartate is so closely related to glutamate. Assuming improvements in amino acid analysis, the results from these aluminium–aspartergic studies will, however, provide critical information on the selective neurotoxicity of aluminium to a particular cell type in the hippocampus.

Conclusions

The successful application of *in vitro* model systems to the evaluation of the target organ toxicity of xenobiotics has evolved from many years of coordinated research efforts. Future research should be directed towards the refinement of existing methodology and the development of new alternatives. As the level of technological sophistication advances, an increasing number of toxic drugs and chemicals are likely to be identified. Aggressive strategies must be designed to generate the database required to successfully manage potential toxicities. Although *in vitro* model systems are now recognized as powerful tools in toxicity testing, their full potential remains largely unexplored.

An important element in the development of *in vitro* systems for toxicity testing is the appropriate use of cytotoxicity assays for the evaluation of potential toxicity of xenobiotics. These assays should be sensitive measures for detecting toxicity, relatively inexpensive to use and highly reproducible between different experiments and laboratories. In addition, toxicity assessment should not be limited to a simple cytotoxicity test. There has been too much emphasis by some scientists in promoting the use of one test over another in evaluating the cytotoxic effects of chemicals in *in vitro* systems. For example, the promotion of viability tests (e.g. neutral red, MTT reduction, etc.) as ultimate indicators of cytotoxicity does not really contribute to a better understanding of a chemical's toxicity. Measurement of the loss of cell viability should in fact be used in conjunction with other tests which assess cell function and integrity. In our laboratory, we advocate the use of a battery of tests for evaluating the potential cytotoxicity of a test chemical. For liver cell culture systems, we evaluate specific hepatocyte functions (e.g. urea synthesis, cytochrome *P*-450 activity, sulphobromophthalein uptake, lactate/pyruvate ratios, etc.), as well as cell viability by neutral red uptake, enzyme leakage, and MTT reduction. Thus, we obtain an overall assessment of target organ toxicity of a specific compound.

Target organ toxicology has become an important discipline because of the increased interest in the specificity of toxicity of xenobiotics towards key tissues of the body. To fully establish the credibility and relevance of *in vitro* toxicity evaluation of drugs and chemicals, it is essential that *in vitro/in vivo* correlations of toxicity of xenobiotics be determined by toxicologists and cell culture scientists. Thus, close-working relationships must be developed between these scientists so that definitive well-planned studies can be conducted to validate *in vitro* toxicity findings with *in vivo* toxicologic data.

References

Acosta, D., Anuforo, D.C. and Smith, R.V. (1978). *In Vitro Cell. Dev. Biol.* **14**, 428–436.

Acosta, D., Anuforo, D.C. and Smith, R.V. (1980). *Toxicol. Appl. Pharmacol.* **53**, 306–314.

Acosta, D., Sorensen, E.M., Anuforo, D.C., Mitchell, D.B., Ramos, K., Santone, K.S. and Smith, M.A. (1985). *In Vitro Cell. Dev. Biol.* **21**, 495–504.

Acosta, D., Mitchell, D.B., Sorensen, E.M. and Burckner, J.V. (1987). *In* "The Isolated Hepatocyte" (E.J. Rauckman and G.M. Padilla, eds), pp. 189–214. Academic Press, New York.

Ambudkar, I.S., Smith, M.W., Phelps, P.C., Regec, A.L. and Trump, B.F. (1988). *Toxicol. Ind. Hlth.* **4**, 107–123.

Anders, M.W. (1980). *Kidney Int.* **18**, 636–647.

Anuforo, D.C., Acosta, D. and Smith, R.V. (1978). *In Vitro Cell. Dev. Biol.* **14**, 981–988.

Darnell, J., Lodish, H. and Baltimore, D. (1986). *In* "Molecular Cell Biology", pp. 845–848. Scientific American Books, New York.

Davila, J.C., Lenherr, A. and Acosta, D. (1989). *Toxicology* **57**, 267–286.

Davila, J.C., Reddy, C.G., Davis, P.J. and Acosta, D. (1990). *In Vitro Cell. Dev. Biol.* **26**, 515–524.

Federoff, S. (1966). *In* "Cell Tisue and Organ Cultures in Neurobiology" (S. Federoff and L. Hertz, eds), pp. 265–274. Academic Press, New York.

Grisham, J.W. (1979). *Int. Rev. Exp. Pathol.* **20**, 124–210.

Hirsch, G.H. (1976). *Environ. Hlth. Persp.* **15**, 89–99.

Jones, D.P., Sundby, G.B., Ormstad, K. and Orrenius, S. (1979). *Biochem. Pharmacol.* **28**, 929–935.

Kisby, G.E. and Acosta, D. (1985). *Pharmacologist* **27**, 288.

Kisby, G.E. and Acosta, D. (1987). *In Vitro Toxicol.* **1**, 85–102.

Nelson, K.F., Acosta, D. and Bruckner, J.V. (1982). *Biochem. Pharmacol.* **31**, 2211–2214.

Sakhrani, L.M. and Fine, L.G. (1983). *Mineral Electrol. Metab.* **9**, 276–281.

Smith, M.A. and Acosta, D. (1986). *Food Chem. Toxicol.* **24**, 551–556.

Smith, M.A., Acosta, D. and Bruckner, J.V. (1987). *Toxicol. In Vitro* **1**, 23–29.

Stammati, A.P., Silano, V. and Zucco, F. (1981). *Toxicology* **20**, 91–153.

Swann, J.D. and Acosta, D. (1990). *Biochem. Pharmacol.* **40**, 1523–1526.

Swann, J.D., Ulrich, R. and Acosta, D. (1990). *Toxicol. Appl. Pharmacol.* **106**, 38–47.

Trifillis, A.L. and Kahng, M.W. (1988). *Transplan. Proc.* **20**, 717–721.

Discussion

M. Adophe

I agree with Dr Acosta about the use of specific cells for organ toxicity. Does Dr Acosta think it is necessary to perform a primary culture using a complex system of epithelial cornea to test ocular irritancy of drugs? If the results are compared with other results in the literature obtained on a cell line, especially, for example, the SERC cell line from rabbit cornea, they are exactly the same.

D. Acosta

I appreciate those comments. It is particularly important to see the peer review publications of these validation studies in scientific journals, and I am hopeful that we will see them. I understand that many validation studies are being conducted in Europe and the USA. If simpler *in vitro* models can be developed, that would be very good. In my own area of interest I also want to do mechanistic type studies, and there I think perhaps there are problems.

J. Frazier

It is very important to make a signficant distinction between what I would call universal toxins, meaning chemicals that kill every cell by a fundamental mechanism, versus toxins that produce their target organ effects via something unique about that particular tissue. If fibroblasts are used to evaluate ocular irritation, if the toxicity is due to some fundamental effects, say, on mitochondria, the fibroblasts will pick up those toxins that will produce ocular irritation. However, if the ocular irritation is caused by the release of, say, chemotactic factor, the fibroblasts might not pick up that kind of response of that specific cell.

There are arguments on both sides. It is important therefore to keep a clear distinction between universal toxins – something like cyanide, which will kill every cell and do so by basically the same mechanism – and compounds that will elicit a particular target organ response due to some mechanism characteristic of that tissue.

D. Acosta

I wish to add a few more comments to what Dr Frazier said about target organ toxicity. To gain a better understanding of the mechanism of toxicity of a compound to the heart, such as doxorubicin or isoproterenol, our laboratory advocates a primary cell culture system of heart cells to explore the cellular and subcellular actions of the drugs. We do not believe a cell line is an appropriate model for investigating the mechanism of organ toxicity of xenobiotics. The same principle applies to other organs such as the liver, kidneys, brain, etc.

F. Marano

What does Dr Acosta think about the use of transfected cell lines from primary cultures to produce cell lines to investigate the target organ toxicity?

D. Acosta

I think that would be valuable if these cell lines can be characterized in terms of some of their specific functions and characteristic retention. There is more work being done, I think by a group in the Netherlands or Belgium, to establish the validity of some of these cell lines in terms of maintenance of function. I would welcome the utilization of cell lines because to work with primary cell culture systems means using animals. If we are to have strictly an alternative model it would be best to have a cell system with which we do not have to use animals. If we can have cell lines, so much the better; I would welcome that type of progress.

B. Nephrotoxicity

5

In Vitro Techniques for Nephrotoxicity Screening, Studying Mechanisms of Renal Injury and Novel Discoveries about Toxic Nephropathies

P.H. BACH* and M.F. WILKS[†]

*Polytechnic of East London, School of Science, Romford Road, London E15 4LZ, UK
[†]ICI Central Toxicology Laboratory, Alderley Park, Macclesfield, Cheshire SK10 4TJ, UK

Introduction

It is estimated that end-stage renal disease (ESRD) costs Europe approximately 3555 million ECU per year, 20% of which is directly attributable to the use of medicines and exposure to chemicals (CEC-IPCS, 1989). About 50% of cases of ESRD have no defined aetiology (Wing *et al.*, 1989), but chemicals are likely to play a role in the course of degenerative change. The structures of chemicals that produce nephropathies are extensive and diverse (see Hook, 1981; Porter, 1982; Bach *et al.*, 1982, 1985, 1991; Bach and Lock, 1985, 1987, 1989; WHO,

IN VITRO METHODS IN TOXICOLOGY
ISBN 0-12-388175-7

1991), and include natural and synthetic environmental pollutants (such as mycotoxins, heavy metals), work place substances (certain organic chemicals, solvents, heavy metals) and both self-administered and prescribed therapeutic agents (analgesics, antibiotics, anti-cancer drugs).

Some of the prescribed therapeutic agents that cause nephrotoxicity have life-saving potential (cyclosporin A, aminoglycoside antibiotics and several anti-cancer drugs) and the benefit/risk ratio is high enough to warrant their continued use. In addition, there are a wide variety of therapeutic agents (anaesthetics, cisplatin, radiocontrast media) which, if used correctly on non-high-risk patients, produce a maximal beneficial effect with a limited potential for nephrotoxicity. There are, however, some products (such as the analgesics) which can produce ESRD when used inappropriately (Gregg et al., 1989).

This situation highlights the importance of continuing research in the following areas:

    a) better screening for less nephrotoxic drugs
    b) improved understanding of the underlying mechanisms of renal injury
    c) more reliable methods to diagnose such changes
    d) a rational basis by which to limit or treat chemical-related renal injury.

The observation that many renal toxins are nephrogenic suggests that provided the ultimate or proximate toxin is available for investigation, the use of the appropriate target population of kidney cells can provide the necessary tool for both screening and mechanistic investigations. In the past, *in vitro* methods have been used for screening a series of analogues for their potential nephrotoxicity, or as a pivotal technique for studying the mechanisms of target cell injury. There is, however, a need for continual counterpoint between screening and mechanistic studies, and reversion to the *in vivo* situation in order to provide the most important trident by which to approach all aspects of a better understanding of the effects of potentially toxic chemicals on the kidney. As will be outlined below, we believe that it is important to undertake both types of *in vitro* investigations in parallel, and also to revert to the *in vivo* situation, to best use the potential of *in vitro* toxicology investigations. The goal of total replacement cannot be achieved until such time as a diversity of problems has been addressed by this reiterative approach.

Chemicals affect the kidney for a number of reasons, most important of which are the small renal mass in relation to its blood supply and the complex biochemical functions undertaken by the organ, including concentrating processes. The mechanistic basis of renal injury has been explained for several types of chemicals, and can be generalized in terms of the molecular processes outlined in Table 5.1, although these are likely to represent oversimplifications.

Table 5.1

Possible types of molecular mechanism that can give rise to target selective renal injury

---

General mechanism

(1) Agents interact with cell membranes
Bind receptors
Affect transport systems
Disrupt membrane structure and function
(2) Agents interact with a localized intermediary metabolism
(3) Agents interact with specialized metabolic function

Glomeruli

(1) Cation neutralizes anion permselectivity
(2) Immuno deposits in glomerular basement membrane
(3) Metabolic activation
Prostaglandin hydroperoxidase or other peroxidase

Proximal tubule

(1) Organic acid and base transport systems
Direct injury due to high concentration in cell
Competitive inhibitors block the elimination of endogenous toxic metabolites
(2) Interference with mechanisms for acidification
Induce an acidification defect
(3) Absorption by pinocytosis
Concentrated in lysosomes
Digestion by hydrolytic enzymes
Inhibit the hydrolytic process
Drug accumulation
Lysosomal storage
(4) Metabolic activation
β-Lyase-mediated
Cytochrome P-450-mediated
D-amino acid oxidase

Medullary interstitial cells
(1) Metabolic activation
Prostaglandin hydroperoxidase or other peroxidase
Lipid peroxidation polyunsaturated fatty acids

In vitro techniques have been essential to help elucidate our current understanding of the likely mechanisms of nephrotoxicity, but, before the concept of alternatives to animal testing can be validated for screening purposes, there is a need to define the success of extrapolating *in vivo* nephrotoxicity data from animals to man. Only the pig and man have similar renal structural and functional characteristics (Table 5.2). There are substantial differences between all other common laboratory species and man. Thus at first sight it appears inappropriate to extrapolate animal nephrotoxicity data directly to man because of marked species, strain, dietary and sex differences in toxicity (Calabrese, 1985) and the unique absorption distribution, metabolism and excretion profiles of nephrotoxins in each species. Age can also have a profound effect on nephrotoxicity (Calabrese, 1986) as the immature kidney may be resistant to some chemicals (Tune, 1975; Marre *et al.*, 1980), but be more sensitive to others (Hook *et al.*, 1983).

Despite all of these differences, there are, in general, a number of chemical-related nephropathies where the clinical changes are closely paralleled in animals and man (Bach and Hardy, 1985) and presumably have the same mechanistic basis. Other lesions, such as those caused by cyclosporin, and several immunologically mediated changes cannot be

Table 5.2

Comparison between the renal structure and function in man and commonly investigated species

Structure or function	Man	Rat	Dog	Pig[a]
Cortical structure				
Nephrons per g body weight	16	128	45	26
Glomerular radius (μm)	100	61	90	83
Proximal tubular length (mm)	16	12	20	30
Tubular radius (μm)	36	29	33	35
Cortical function				
Glomerular filtration rate (ml/min per m^2)	75	35	104	72
Inulin clearance (ml/min per kg body weight)	2.0	6.0	4.3	2.1
p-Aminohippurate transport maxima (mg/min per kg body weight)	1.3	3.0	1.0	—
Medullary structure				
Number of papillae	15–20	1	1	6–10
Percentage long loops	14	28	100	3
Relative medullary thickness	3.0	5.8	4.3	1.6
Medullary function				
Maximum urine osmolality (mOsmol/kg)	1400	2610	2610	1080

[a] Data from Mudge (1985), Stolte and Alt (1980, 1982) and Gyrd-Hansen (1968).
— No data published on this parameter.

induced in rats easily, without recourse to the use of special species or experimental manipulations (Druet, 1989; Druet *et al.*, 1982, 1987).

Nephrogenic or Extrarenal Nephrotoxicity

A number of kidney functions have extrarenal control, including the concentrating ability. Thus it is possible that a variety of toxins could exert their effects on extrarenal organs, which would be manifested in renal changes. In fact, there appear to be very few examples of extrarenal control of nephrotoxicity *per se*, although the Gunn rat with its hepatic bilirubinaemia also shows renal injury as a result of the local build-up of bilirubin (Axelsen, 1973). Nephrotoxicity may be the consequence of a directly acting chemical or metabolite (Rush *et al.*, 1984) that is formed renally or extrarenally. In general, however, chemicals that are nephrotoxic exert their effects directly. Nevertheless, extrarenal factors (e.g. age, concomitant disease or dehydration) may have a deciding influence on extent, severity and reversibility of the renal damage.

Experience now allows us to argue that the basis of nephrogenic toxicity lies in the properties of the chemical, or its metabolite, its distribution within the kidney and the biochemical/physiological characteristics of the cell that it affects. Thus the concept of target-cell toxicity has been developed, where a chemical produces an adverse effect in one renal cell type but not in adjacent cells.

Concept of Target-Cell Toxicity

The kidney consists of over 20 different cell types, each with specific properties and all working in concert to maintain normal homeostatic function. The selective targeting of chemicals for discrete regions and cell types of the kidney (Table 5.3) is due to the fact that the target cells may have unique biochemical characteristics predisposing them to chemically induced injury. This concept of target cell toxicity, equally applicable to other organs, ensures that the application of *in vitro* methods can provide a most important insight into the underlying processes, and can (once validated) provide the basis for screening for efficacy and toxicity.

The intact and functioning kidney is highly compartmentalized due to localized transport systems, transcellular pH gradients, xenobiotic activating and metabolizing systems and cell organelles. Thus some chemicals are selectively concentrated in (and others actively or selectively excluded

Table 5.3
Examples of target-selective nephrotoxins and likely mechanisms

Target and nephrotoxin	Mechanism
Glomeruli	
Permselectivity barrier	
Polybrene	Charge neutralization
Epithelial cell	
Adriamycin	Membrane binding, redox cycling
Puromycin	
aminonucleoside	Redox cycling
Proximal tubule	
Aminoglycosides	Membrane binding, lysosomal accumulation, disruption of secondary messengers, lipid peroxidation
D-Amino acids	D-Amino acid oxidase-mediated reactive oxygen?
p-Aminophenol	Cytochrome P-450-mediated activation
Cadmium	Binding to a low molecular weight binding protein, lysosomal accumulation
Cephaloridine	Transport-mediated accumulation, oxidative stress
Cisplatin	Oxidative stress?
Chloroform	Cytochrome P-450-mediated activation
Chromium	Oxidative stress?
Haloalkenes*	Transport-mediated accumulation, β-lyase-mediated activation, lipid peroxidation
Mercuric chloride	Sulphydryl binding
Trimethylpentene	Binding to a low molecular weight binding protein
Medullary interstitial cells	
N-Phenylanthranylate	Hydroperoxidase-mediated activation, lipid peroxidation

* Hexachlorobutadiene (HCBD), its glutathione, cysteine and N-acetylcysteine conjugates

from) discrete areas of the kidney (Mudge, 1985). Even when the urinary and the arterial and venous blood concentrations of chemicals are known, there is no certainty of the concentration of a specific metabolite in the target cell, especially if a molecule undergoes metabolism in an adjacent region. This makes it difficult to establish what substance (or its metabolite) reaches a target cell of the kidney. This uncertainty also questions the validity of using the cytotoxicity of a given concentration of a chemical as a useful indicator of toxicological effect *in vivo*. This can be partly addressed by comparing the effects of such a chemical in target and non-target renal cell types (see below).

It is only beginning to be appreciated that there is a cascade of secondary degenerative events involving progressively more of the renal cell types (Bach, 1989a) that invariably follows the primary lesion to the target cells. There have been relatively few attempts to understand the processes underlying the progression to ESRD. While the proximal tubule has a marked repair capacity (Laurent *et al.*, 1988), this is not the case with glomerular or medullary interstitial cells. The secondary degenerative changes develop because of the target-selective nature of certain chemicals towards discrete renal cell types, the malfunction (or loss) of which has a knock-on effect on other cell types with which they normally have a close functional or structural association. This chain reaction may cause renal failure or contribute to a decreased renal functional reserve, which may predispose to the disastrous consequences that arise from subsequent renal insults or disease.

The Development of Toxic Nephropathies

ESRD represents an advanced degenerative state characterized by progression from a normal kidney to one where the function is severely compromised. Despite the progression of such degenerative changes, the kidney has a pronounced capacity to maintain homoeostasis up to the point where renal failure is imminent. Thus, the renal functional reserve normally buffers up to 75% of degenerative changes. Consequently, there are very few clinical indicators of degenerating renal function *per se*, and most non-invasive biochemical pathology techniques that are currently available to diagnose renal injury and disease in man only demonstrate advanced renal injury, many of which are irreversible. They do not identify early or subtle changes. It is for this reason that much of the investigation into the mechanistic basis of chemically related nephropathy has had to be undertaken in experimental animals or *in vitro*.

While exposure to therapeutic agents is usually well defined, the intake of natural toxins or environmental pollutants is difficult to quantify and control in man. Taken together, man is therefore exposed to a great variety of potential nephrotoxicants, the accumulated effects of which may contribute to an age-related compromise of renal function. It is now widely appreciated that the risk of developing a clinically significant nephrotoxicity depends on a number of factors, all of which have to be taken into account for the final risk assessment. These include pre-existing nephrotoxicity, compromised renal functional reserve, loss of renal parenchyma, high protein diet, nephrotoxic chemical and drug exposure, predisposing factors, multiple myeloma, age and other conditions causing proteinuria, hypertension, diabetes, cardiovascular disease, etc. (Bennett,

1983; Porter, 1989; Porter and Bennett, 1989). The impact of these conditions on the development of toxic nephropathies has so far not been systematically investigated. In addition, electrolyte, volume changes, the renin–angiotensin system and a host of other factors affect renal failure (Bennett *et al.*, 1983). An understanding of the risk factors could facilitate their investigation *in vitro*, but considerable *in vivo* investigations are still needed to build appropriate hypotheses.

Nephrotoxicity *In Vitro* – Our Understanding

On the premise that no single *in vivo* or *in vitro* method can elucidate the mechanistic basis of toxicity, there will be an inherent uncertainty as to what should be studied in *in vitro* systems, especially in the kidney. It is therefore advisable not to separate whole animal studies from *in vitro* alternatives or mechanistic investigations from screening procedures. The complexity of the questions that need to be answered (mechanism, cytotoxicity, validity, relevance to man) requires a holistic integrated approach, probably undertaken in several different species, and related to epidemiological and clinical data where these are available. *In vitro* methods have provided information on the mechanism of primary insult and the effect on cell viability appropriate for screening methods. This approach can also be used to develop an understanding of the basis of secondary renal changes that contribute to the cascade of chronic renal degeneration if tissue is harvested over a period of time.

Currently, the rational approaches to studying nephrotoxicity *in vitro* include:

> 1) the use of those compounds with well-documented and understood *in vivo* nephrotoxicity such as the chemicals that specifically target one anatomically discrete cell type *in vivo* (Table 5.3);
> 2) the use of a series of nephrotoxic analogues where a structure–activity relationship can be built;
> 3) the systematic investigation of one or more of these compounds by different *in vitro* methods varying the criteria of cell injury (Table 5.4);
> 4) the study of several cell types each with a defined set of biophysiological characteristics that are thought to contribute to a chemical's cytotoxicity.

In Vitro Technique for Assessing the Kidney and its Cells

In vitro techniques include those where the anatomical integrity of the kidney is maintained (perfusion, micropuncture and slices), and the use of isolated fragments (glomeruli and tubular fragments) or cells. The

Table 5.4
Methods for assessing cytotoxicity in renal cells

Method	Biochemical or morphological parameter	Comment
Light microscopy	Cell growth Cell shape	Non-sensitive and non-specific
Electron microscopy	Organelle and membrane integrity	Gives an insight into target organelle injury, can be used to assess injury dynamics, helps devise other tests
Enzyme leakage Dye uptake/exclusion	Membrane integrity	Reasonably sensitive, but non-specific, good for initial viability assessment
Protein synthesis DNA/RNA synthesis	Labelled amino acid ⎱ Labelled thymidine/ ⎰ uridine	Sensitive, but relatively non-specific, easy to perform
Synthesis-specific macromolecules	Labelled precursor immunoassay	Sensitive and specific, but needs to be appropriate
Oxidative metabolism	Labelled glucose Labelled fatty acids	Less sensitive than protein metabolism synthesis, but more specific
Transport studies	Organic anion uptake	Sensitive for xenobiotica which are actively transported or affect transport processes
Enzyme measurements	Release or inhibition of target enzymes	Can be very sensitive and specific, difficult for areas other than proximal tubule
Lipid peroxidation	Malondialdehyde production Conjugated dienes	Sensitive but prone to artefacts
Synthesis-specific-micromolecules, e.g. glutathione, cytochrome P-450, ATP	Immuno or other sensitive or specific assay	Sensitive and specific, subject to assay, but needs to be appropriate
Ion deregulation	Fluorescent probes	Highly sensitive and specific, potentially high cost of equipment

strengths and weaknesses of each have been reviewed (Bach et al., 1985, 1986; Bach and Kwizera, 1988). Perfusion, micropuncture, microinjection and microperfusion are technically difficult, require sophisticated equipment and are difficult to interpret even in inexperienced hands. They have, however, been applied to important toxicological questions relating to membrane permeability changes, transport processes and the significance of luminal versus peritubular uptake of toxins (Bank et al., 1967; Biber et al., 1968; Tune et al., 1969; Gottschalk and Lassiter, 1973; Roch-Ramel and Peters, 1979; Ullrich and Greger, 1985; Diezi and Roch-Ramel, 1987).

Renal cortical slices have been used extensively to show deleterious effects of chemicals on the kidney, by measuring the accumulation of organic ions p-aminohippurate and tetraethylammonium. While organic ion transport is a sensitive indicator of the toxicity of a variety of compounds such as antibiotics, mercuric ions, chromate ion and hexachlorobutadiene conjugates (Hirsch, 1976; Berndt, 1976, 1981, 1987; Kluwe and Hook, 1978; Kaloyanides and Pastoriza-Munoz, 1980; Bach and Lock, 1982; Kuo and Hook, 1982, 1983; Kuo et al., 1982; Kacew, 1987), the acute toxic effects of other nephrotoxins may not be detected if membrane function and cell metabolism are not early targets.

A number of freshly isolated glomeruli and tubular systems exhibit high initial viability (Cunnaro and Weiner, 1978; Jones et al., 1979; Belleman, 1980; Vinay et al., 1981; Cojocel et al., 1983; Gstraunthaler et al., 1985) and have been used to study metabolism of xenobiotics (Jones et al., 1979) and intermediary metabolism in different species including man (Stumpf and Kraus, 1978; Baverel et al., 1978, 1979, 1980a, b; Schlondorff et al., 1980; Sraer et al., 1980, 1983; Stollenwerk Petrulis et al., 1981; Michoudet and Baverel, 1987; Ormstad, 1987). These systems have also found applications for assessing toxicology (Savin et al., 1985). It is also possible to prepare fragments from a selected region of the nephron, such as the thick ascending limb (Baverel et al., 1980a; Chamberlin et al., 1984; Anand-Srivastava et al., 1986) and collecting tubules (Anand-Srivastava et al., 1986). Fresh tubule or cell suspensions thus offer an important way of studying the mechanisms of nephrotoxicity and screening novel compounds, but have a limited in vitro lifespan (Ormstad, 1982) and the cells lack polarity as a result of which some key transport processes may be lost (Koseki et al., 1988). A spectrum of proximal tubule toxins (ochratoxin A, citrinin, frusemide, cephalosporins, cisplatin, mercuric chloride and potassium chromate) release enzyme markers (Endou et al., 1985) and affect intermediary metabolism (Nakada et al., 1986a,b; Jung et al., 1989; Jung and Endou, 1989) in a time- and dose-dependent manner.

Primary cell cultures allow long exposure to xenobiotics and the choice of appropriate metabolites, as well as ease of manipulating and monitoring of a variety of functional or morphological responses in a dose- and time-related manner (Fry *et al.*, 1978; Belleman, 1980; Fry and Perry, 1981; Bach *et al.*, 1986). The cells may, however, rapidly dedifferentiate (Curthoys and Belleman, 1979) and lose those biochemical characteristics that form part of the molecular basis for target cell toxicity. The modulation of culture media can alter cell biochemistry and morphology and provide an ideal standardized system especially if fully defined (Sato and Reid, 1978). Growth on permeable supports, such as collagen filters (see Jakoby and Pastan, 1979), ensures that cell polarity is expressed. Homogeneous glomerular mesangial and epithelial cells may be cocultured or each derived separately (Kreisberg *et al.*, 1977, 1978; Foidart *et al.*, 1979, 1980, 1981; Striker *et al.*, 1980; Morita *et al.*, 1980; Kreisberg and Karnovsky, 1983). Similarly, defined tubular cell populations can be grown by several methods (see Meezan and Brendel, 1973; Curthoys and Belleman, 1979; Jakoby and Pastan, 1979; Scholer and Edelman, 1979; Belleman, 1980; Striker *et al.*, 1980; Ormstad *et al.*, 1981; Vinay *et al.*, 1981; Pretlow and Pretlow, 1982, 1983, 1984; Boogaard *et al.*, 1989a,b).

Studies on human renal cells have characterized normal and diseased tissue (Roth *et al.*, 1979; Pellett *et al.*, 1984) particularly in glomeruli (Ardaillou *et al.*, 1983; Holdsworth *et al.*, 1978; Scheinman and Fish, 1978; Sraer *et al.*, 1983; Striker *et al.*, 1980). Normal cultured human renal proximal tubular cells have also been exposed to nephrotoxins (Chatterjee *et al.*, 1985; Trifillis *et al.*, 1986).

Established renal lines have properties reminiscent of specific parts of the nephron such as LLC-PK$_1$ and OK (of proximal tubule type) and MDCK (of distal tubule type) (see Saier, 1981; Taub and Saier, 1981), but the exact site of origin is not known and the cells do not totally represent the normal physiological state. LLC-PK$_1$ cells are sensitive to a variety of haloalkene conjugates (Boogaard *et al.*, 1989c, 1990) due to the presence of the brush border enzyme γ-glutamyl transpeptidase (Perantoni and Berman, 1979), which catalyses the breakdown of the conjugate to the proximate toxin, and an organic anion transport system (Handler, 1983), which facilitates the entry of the chemicals into cells.

Organelles, membranes or cytoplasm from defined cells can be used to study a chemical's distribution, interaction between a cellular compartment and a chemical and/or the kinetics of binding or release of substances. This includes specific enzyme inhibition, metabolic activation, covalent binding or the modulation of lipid peroxidation, etc. using purified or commercially available biochemicals; Bach and Bridges (1984, 1985a) provide suitable references for methodology. Isolated brush border membrane vesicles have been used to study aminoglycoside binding and this has been correlated with their *in vivo* nephrotoxicity (Williams *et al.*, 1986).

Toxicity Screening

In vitro methods offer a rapid and economical method of screening specific cell types for specific effects (Williams *et al.*, 1983; Purchase and Conning, 198»). Thus, direct effects of chemicals in well-defined areas can be evaluated and manipulated under precisely controlled experimental conditions, direct and indirect effects can be distinguished, interactions between chemicals can be studied and chemical interactions with cellular organelles and constituents can be monitored.

Mechanisms of Injury

Depending on the questions to be answered, the choice of cell type and *in vitro* system is relatively straightforward (Williams *et al.*, 1983), but the method of assessing cytotoxicity is more complex. Several methods are outlined in Table 5.4, but the implicit weakness of each is that a number of chemicals that target the same region of the kidney could do so via a variety of different mechanisms. There are at least three types of reactive intermediate affecting the proximal tubule. The haloalkanes are thought to damage proximal tubular epithelial cells via reactive intermediates generated from their cysteine metabolites, *p*-aminophenol via the cytochrome *P*-450 system, D-amino acids probably via the amino acid oxidase system and a reactive oxygen species and cephalosporins by oxidative stress (Tune and Fravert, 1980; Tune, 1986). In contrast, aminoglycosides and trimethylpentene damage the proximal tubule by lysosomal accumulation but each on a different carrier molecule (membranes and low molecular weight protein respectively). The exact mechanism of cell death is not clear in any of these examples. Even two closely related compounds could damage the same region of the kidney by different mechanisms and it is not uncommon for structural analogues to target different cell types. Such uncertainties compromise the simplistic concept of finding a "good or valid" test and using it to screen blindly for the toxicity of a series of analogues or for compounds that damage a discrete cell type. It is thus apparent that cytotoxicity should not be assessed by only one method and that both general (enzyme leakage and protein synthesis) and specific (metabolism of specific molecules, organelle function) assays should be used.

Type of Cytotoxicity Tests

Cytotoxicity screening is often performed using simple end points such as membrane integrity (enzyme leakage, dye uptake or release) and the incorporation of radiolabelled precursors into macromolecules (protein, DNA or RNA synthesis). While these methods are often sensitive and allow the rapid screening of large numbers of chemicals at different concentrations, their limitations must be taken into account when interpreting the data thus obtained. The most obvious case is that of compounds that inhibit the activity of enzyme markers or interfere with specrophotometric assays, but there are more subtle pitfalls.

For example, when studying protein synthesis it is important to realize that each amino acid is incorporated into different materials at unique rates which are determined by a variety of factors. Thus, while proline is regarded as an excellent marker for glomerular basement membrane, aromatic amino acids are, in fact, taken up at a much higher rate. Similarly, glycine is very poorly incorporated into both glomerular and tubular protein. In addition, while we have found protein synthesis to be the most sensitive method of assessing cytotoxicity, it is not necessarily specific for the identification of *in vivo* toxins. The cytotoxicity of aminoglycosides towards isolated proximal tubular fragments can be assessed using proline incorporation into *de novo* synthesized protein. However, the ranking of their potential to inhibit protein synthesis (with streptomycin the most potent inhibitor and kanamycin the least effective) is inversely related (Fig. 5.1) to the clinical *in vivo* nephrotoxicity of aminoglycosides (Kwizera *et al.*, 1990). Similar results were obtained when a series of heavy metals was screened for their tubulotoxic potential, where protein synthesis was a more sensitive but less specific parameter of toxicity than the oxidation of fatty acids (Wilks *et al.*, 1990, 1991). These data underline the importance of the choice of suitable parameters for *in vitro* toxicity screening.

It is also possible to undertake very specialized investigations, ranging from chromatographic and mass fragmentation patterns of small molecules handled specifically to immunobased measurements of macromolecules, gene probe studies, etc. to cover the full strengths of molecular and cellular biology. The more specific the assay of cytotoxicity, the more relevant it has to be to a fundamental mechanistic understanding of cell

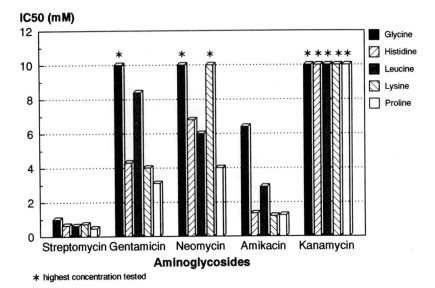

Fig. 5.1 Incubation of freshly isolated rat proximal tubular fragments in Tyrode's solution over 4 h at 37°C in the presence of five aminoglycosides at concentrations ranging from 0.2 to 10 mM. IC_{50} is the estimated concentration of the aminoglycoside that inhibits the incorporation of the five tritiated amino acids by 50% compared with control incubations.

injury and screening for a range of chemicals that affect only this or closely related processes.

Fluorescent Probes

The use of fluorescent probes (see Bach, 1989b) is attractive as they are versatile, more sensitive than conventional biochemical complement methods for assessing cytotoxicity and they demonstrate morphological changes. Plate 5.1 shows viable and damaged cells in freshly isolated glomeruli exposed to 5 μM mercuric chloride for 15 min, compared with control. Glomeruli are removed from media, exposed briefly to a solution of fluorescein diacetate (FDA) and ethidium bromide (EB), final concentration of 100 μg/ml and 6.25 ng/ml respectively. The FDA is hydrolysed to fluorescein in viable cells and the EB enters only those cells where the membranes are damaged, interchelates with nucleic acid and fluoresces red. Perturbations in specific organelles, membranes or the cytoplasm (see Table 5.5) can be linked to subcellular morphological changes. Plate 5.2 illustrates organelle compartmentalization visualizing nuclei or cytoplasm within isolated cells. These undergo changes when

Table 5.5

Selective fluorescent probes that allow subcellular biochemistry and morphology to be interlinked

System being assessed	Fluorescent probes
Enzyme probes	
Esterases	Fluorescein diacetate
Mixed functional oxidase	Ethoxyresorufin
Peroxidase activities	2',7'-Dichlorodihydrofluorescein
Transport probes	
Cationic transport system	4-Acetamido-4'-isothiocyanato-stilbene-2,2'-disulphonic acid
Organelle probes	
Mitochondria	Dimethylaminostyrylmethylpyridinium iodine
Lysosomes	FluoroBora-I[a]
Golgi apparatus	FluoroBora-II[a]
Nucleus	FluoroBora-T[a]
Cytoplasmic probes	
Hydrophobic and hydrophilic regions	FluoroBora P[a]
Ca^{2+} influx	Quin 2
Lipid probes	
Cellular and organelle membranes	5-(N-Hexadecanoyl)aminoeosin
Neutral lipid droplets	Nile Red
Immunological probes	
Cytoskeletal elements	Polyclonal and monoclonal antibodies tagged with a fluorophore
Selective binding proteins	
Microtubular system	Phalloidin tagged with a fluorophore
Carbohydrate constituents	Lectins tagged with a fluorophore

[a] Trademark of Polysciences, Northampton, U.K.

the cells are exposed to chemicals that alter the integrity or function of the specific organelles. Increasingly there is a need to understand cell–cell interaction (Burger *et al.*, 1990), where it is necessary to have morphologically and biochemically different cells in coculture. The application of conventional cytotoxicity tests may make it difficult to distinguish which cell type is undergoing changes. Fluorescent probes offer the potential to compare and contrast adjacent, but different, cell types, which is especially important when target cell toxicity is being studied in a mixed cell population. The immense importance of this rapidly growing topic is, however, beyond the scope of this presentation.

Mechanistic Aspects of Nephrotoxicity

In vitro methods offer a very powerful tool by which the mechanistic basis of chemicals damaging specific renal cell types or chemicals causing a cytotoxic effect to a specific cell type with well-defined characteristics can be assessed. It is possible to use both renal and non-renal cell types based on the interest in interaction between a cell with well-defined characteristics, or a specific set of characteristics, that enhance or ameliorate toxicity.

Glomerular Injury

The glomerulus is the first part of the nephron to come into contact with the majority of xenobiotics, and especially those that are filtered. It is therefore surprising that there is relatively little information on the contribution of chemical injury to the development of glomerular lesions. A model compound which selectively injures glomerular epithelial cells is the anti-cancer drug adriamycin. In rodents, adriamycin causes a nephrotic syndrome within days of administration of a single dose (Bertani *et al.*, 1982). Fluorescent illumination of cultured glomeruli (with outgrowths of both mesangial and epithelial cells) suggests the preferential uptake of adriamycin into epithelial cell nuclei, but not mesangial cell nuclei. Time-lapse recording suggests that nuclear degeneration precedes cell death in these cells (Bach, unpublished data).

Micropuncture studies have shown that the proteinuria originates predominantly from juxtamedullary glomeruli, indicating that cortical glomeruli are less sensitive to the effect of the compound (Soose *et al.*, 1988). These data have recently been supported by a series of *in vitro* experiments in which cortical and juxtamedullary glomeruli from adriamycin-treated animals were separated and incubated with radio-labelled precursors to study protein synthesis and glucose oxidation (Kastner *et al.*, 1991a,b). The results show that glomerular damage by adriamycin is associated with a stimulating effect on glomerular metabolism, which is significantly more pronounced in juxtamedullary than in cortical glomeruli. The mechanistic basis of this heterogeneity of glomerular injury is not fully understood but may be related to differences in oxygen pressure in the outer and inner cortex. The inner cortical Po_2 is considerably higher than that of the subcapsular region (Schurek, 1988), which would enhance oxidative stress on membrane components mediated by adriamycin semiquinone radicals in juxtamedullary glomerular epithelial cells due to the more abundant oxygen supply. Lipid peroxidation is one step in the cascade of adriamycin nephrotoxicity, leading to metabolic alterations in the epithelial cells, which in turn could lead to structural alterations in the glomerular filtration barrier (Fig. 5.2). The effect of adriamycin could also relate to its preferential accumulation in the juxtamedullary nephrons, data that can only be obtained from *in vivo* investigations.

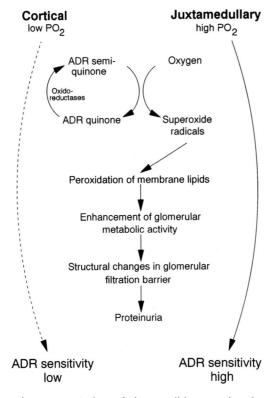

Fig. 5.2 Schematic representation of the possible cascade of events leading to proteinuria in the rat following administration of adriamycin (ADR). The higher oxygen pressure facilitates the formation of oxygen radicals in juxtamedullary glomeruli, whereas superficial glomeruli are better protected by a relative lack of oxygen. This is supported by both *in vitro* (metabolism) and *in vivo* (micropuncture) data.

Aminoglycosides and the Proximal Tubule

Using a combination of *in vivo* and *in vitro* techniques, it has been possible to show that the cationic aminoglycosides bind to the anionic membrane receptor phospholipid (such as phosphatidylinositol; see Sastrasinh *et al.*, 1982). The antibiotic–membrane complex is taken up by adsorptive endocytosis (Silverblatt and Kuehn, 1979) and sequestrated in lysosomes (Morin *et al.*, 1980; Josepovitz *et al.*, 1985) where the aminoglycosides accumulate to high concentrations and cause a number of biochemical effects (Kaloyanides, 1984a). Here the aminoglycosides inhibit the enzymes that normally degrade membrane phospholipid (Laurent *et al.*, 1982; Carlier *et al.*, 1983; Ramsammy *et al.*, 1989a) and cause an increase in renal cortical phosphatidylinositol (Schwertz *et al.*, 1984; Kaloyanides, 1984b) as manifested ultrastructurally by the accumulation of lysosomal myeloid bodies (Josepovitz *et al.*, 1985). The exact cause of cell necrosis is still not clear, but lysosomal phospholipidosis is a critical first step (Tulkens, 1989) dependent on a threshold concentration of aminoglycoside, which if it is not reached does not cause biochemical or morphological evidence of cellular necrosis (Giuliano *et al.*, 1984). In addition, aminoglycosides may also inhibit agonist activation of the phsophatidylinositol cascade (Ramsammy *et al.*, 1988), depress Na^+/K^+-ATPase, adenylate cyclase, alkaline phosphatase and calcium binding (Morin *et al.*, 1980; Williams *et al.*, 1981), impair mitochondrial respiration (Weinberg and Humes, 1980) and decrease the incorporation of leucine into microsomal protein (Bennett *et al.*, 1988). All of these effects could contribute to irreversible cell injury and this emphasizes the multiple sites of interaction between a chemical and a cell.

Using cytotoxicity data alone to screen a series of aminoglycosides can provide conflicting data. The use of the inhibition of protein synthesis by aminoglycosides *in vitro* does not reflect their potential to cause nephrotoxicity *in vivo* (Kwizera *et al.*, 1990), which argues against a major role of this metabolic pathway in the molecular mechanism of the lesion. Similarly, examination of the oxidation of fatty acids also failed to show a good correlation between *in vitro* effects and *in vivo* toxicity (Kwizera *et al.*, 1990). Since renal cortical accumulation of aminoglycosides is believed to be of major importance in the development of renal failure (Luft and Kleit, 1974; Fillastre, 1978), the absence of close clinical toxicity – *in vitro* cytotoxicity correlation and the lack of predictiveness of a single general method of assessing cytotoxicity without relating it to an *in vivo* situatitn and to the intact kidney – is not entirely surprising.

Thus the reiteration between *in vivo* and *in vitro* techniques to investigate aminoglycosides has built up a sufficiently firm foundation of a mechanistic understanding to facilitate the rational choice of methods with which to study these molecules *in vitro*, using appropriate techniques to assess the likely toxicity and to start probing the mechanistic basis of nephroprotectants. Polyaspartic acid protects animals from aminoglycoside nephrotoxicity without inhibiting the proximal tubular cell uptake of the antibiotic (Williams *et al.*, 1986; Gilbert *et al.*, 1989; Ramsammy *et al.*, 1989b). *In vitro* studies show the binding interaction between the polyanionic peptide and aminoglycosides and suggest that this prevents electrostatic interactions between the antibiotic and cellular targets (such as anionic phospholipids) that are central to the development of nephrotoxicity.

Renal Papillary Necrosis

There is now strong morphological evidence (Bach *et al.*, 1983; Bach and Gregg, 1988; Gregg *et al.*, 1989, 1990a,b) to suggest that the renal medullary interstitial cells are the target of most papillotoxic chemicals in animals and probably in man. There are a number of important characteristics that distinguish these cells uniquely from all other renal cells. This includes the high osmolality in which they exist *in vivo*, and the fact that they have an exceptionally high prostaglandin synthetase capacity and a large number of polyunsaturated lipid droplets (Bojesen, 1974). The mechanism of analgesic-induced renal medullary necrosis is thought to be linked to the peroxidative activation of agents to form reactive intermediates (Zenser *et al.*, 1978a,b, 1979a,b,c, 1983; Mohandas *et al.*, 1981a,b; Bach & Bridges, 1984, 1985b). In the presence of high levels of polyunsaturated fatty acids, the reactive analgesic intermediate could cause lipid peroxidation and lead to cell death (Bach and Bridges, 1984).

Rat renal medullary interstitial cells can be isolated and cultured in a hypertonic medium, and have been shown to be sensitive to a number of papillotoxic chemicals (Benns *et al.*, 1985). Plate 5.3 shows the detachment of cultured medullary interstitial cells exposed to 100 mM paracetamol (acetaminophen) at selected time points up to 60 min. These micrographs show the sensitivity to paracetamol, and the heterogeneity of cell response. Fluorescent probes (Plate 5.4) reveal high levels of peroxidase activity and/or peroxides in medullary interstitial cells (Homan-Muller *et al.*, 1975), and Nile Red (Greenspan *et al.*, 1985) confirms the presence of lipid droplets (Plate 5.4a) seen ultrastructurally (Bohman, 1980). The combined use of both probes also demonstrates that cultured rat medullary interstitial cells show heterogeneity in the distribution of lipid droplets and peroxidase activity, with one or other, and both are present simultaneously in some cells. Following exposure to 100 mM paracetamol for 10 min, the probes were used to characterize attached rat medullary interstitial cells (Plate 5.4c). These cells were rich in peroxidase activity, suggesting that the presence of lipid droplets predisposed to cytotoxicity. Recent time-lapse studies on medullary interstitial cells suggest that those cells with lipid droplets are the most sensitive to 2-bromoethanamine (Bach, unpublished data). Medullary interstitial cells are, however, most difficult to culture and do not undergo active division, possibly owing to their highly specialized nature. A number of continuous renal and extrarenal cell lines have been evaluated for their usefulness as surrogates. Medullary interstitial cells are thought to be fibroblastic in origin (Bohman, 1980), hence the comparison with 3T3 cells, whereas HaK (Hull *et al.*, 1976) and MDCK (Herzlinger *et al.*, 1982) represent proximal and distal renal epithelial cells respectively. Both medullary interstitial cells and 3T3 fibroblasts were sensitive to 2-bromoethanamine (Bach *et al.*, 1986), at concentrations as low as 0.2 mM in 4–6 h, whereas MDCK and HaK cells were unaffected by 2 mM for 24 h. The absence of lipid droplets and peroxidase activity from HaK and MDCK cells may explain the lack of 2-bromoethanamine cytotoxicity, confirming the association between peroxidase activity and lipid material as one determinant of cytotoxicity.

Taken together these data add some credence to the proposed mechanism of analgesic-induced renal medullary necrosis being linked to peroxidative activation to form reactive intermediates (Bach and Bridges, 1984, 1985b) and the presence of high levels of polyunsaturated fatty acids in these cells.

From *In Vitro* to *In Vivo* Investigations

Inevitably, *in vitro* investigations must produce a variety of artefacts. These arise because the complex renal system has been disrupted and cell–cell interaction, extrarenal processes (such as the hepatic metabolism of haloalkanes to their cystine derivatives, as shown by Nash *et al.*, 1984), haemodynamic factors and the compartmentalization of the multicellular organ have been lost or changed. It is therefore likely that at least some *in vitro* data will, of necessity, be anomalous, but it is equally possible that subtle cellular abnormalities will be found that reflect *in vivo* processes and are relevant to nephrotoxicity. We have been able to demonstrate two such factors in studies with mycotoxins and heavy metals using freshly isolated glomerular fragments.

Balkan Endemic Nephropathy and Glomerular Injury

Balkan endemic nephropathy is a slow, progressive renal degeneration leading to ESRD and is common in localized areas of Yugoslavia, Romania and Bulgaria. The condition has been well recognized for nearly 40 years, but little progress has been made in understanding the cause, course, prevention, treatment, etc. (WHO, 1979). Pathology of renal material shows proximal tubular lesions, parenchymal damage and fibrosis, and marked glomerular basement membrane thickening and hyalinization (Hall and Dammin, 1978; Hall, 1982). The aetiology of Balkan endemic nephropathy has been controversial, but the role of mycotoxins (particularly ochratoxin A) has emerged as the most likely factor, especially since this mycotoxin causes a renal injury in animals (Krogh *et al.*, 1974, 1977, 1979; Elling *et al.*, 1975; Berndt and Hayes, 1977, 1979; Krogh, 1978; Pavlovic *et al.*, 1979; NTP, 1989) that has similarities to the one seen in patients in the Balkan areas. In the case of the mycotoxin ochratoxin A, the renal target cell is generally considered to be the proximal tubule, but there is evidence to suggest early glomerular involvement. Routine histology has shown, besides the tubular lesion, morphological changes in glomeruli of animals treated with repeated doses of ochratoxin A, such as oedema and prominent periodic acid–Schiff-positive staining, suggesting thickening of the basement membrane. In *in vitro* studies, the mycotoxin decreased *de novo* protein synthesis by isolated rat glomeruli and tubules (Delacruz, 1988). Although ochratoxin A showed a generalized depression of the incorporation of the six amino acids tested, there were differences in their sensitivity to the effect of ochratoxin A. All three aromatic amino acids, phenylalanine, tyrosine and tryptophan, were more sensitive to the effects of ochratoxin A than was proline. Small doses of ochratoxin A stimulated oxidative metabolism of glucose and linolenic acid. Thus, protein synthesis from aromatic amino acids such as phenylalanine and tyrosine appeared to be a sensitive parameter of ochratoxin A toxicity. The sensitivity of the aromatic amino acids to the effect of ochratoxin A (compared with the sensitivity of proline) suggested that glomerular macromolecules other than glomerular basement membrane collagen may be affected. These could include other functional and structural proteins. In addition, the inhibition of the incorporation of aromatic amino acids into glomerular macromolecules by ochratoxin A suggested that the synthesis of specific proteins may be central to the mechanism of target-selective toxicity of ochratoxin A towards the kidney.

Heavy Metals and Acute Renal Failure

Acute toxic renal injury is associated with a number of heavy metal salts, such as mercuric chloride (Zalme *et al.*, 1976), uranyl nitrate (Blantz, 1975) and potassium dichromate (Henry *et al.*, 1968). It is generally believed that the cells of the proximal tubule are the primary target for the majority of these metals, since the earliest morphologically detectable damage occurs most often at this part of the nephron. However, one of the earliest features of acute renal damage is impaired glomerular filtration, frequently seen before any evidence of morphological damage (McDowell *et al.*, 1976).

To compare the toxic effects of heavy metals on the proximal tubule with those that may occur in glomeruli, we have screened a number of heavy metals in an *in vitro* system using inhibition of amino acid incorporation and linolenic acid oxidation in isolated glomeruli and proximal tubular fragments (Wilks *et al.*, 1990, 1991). A most significant finding was a high sensitivity of glomeruli to mercuric chloride (Hg), which exceeded the effect seen in tubular fragments by more than one order of magnitude. Addition of reduced glutathione (GSH) to the incubation medium completely attenuated the toxicity of Hg in both glomeruli and tubular fragments, indicating a non-specific binding of Hg to the SH groups. Preincubation with GSH partially protected tubular fragments, but not glomeruli, against Hg toxicity, possibly because of tubular uptake of GSH (Fig. 5.3).

These *in vitro* data suggested a possible direct glomerulotoxicity of Hg and initiated an *in vivo* study to visualize Hg histochemically in the kidney during the development of acute renal failure (ARF) using the silver enhancement technique (Wilks *et al.*, 1989). We were able to demonstrate Hg deposits in midcortical and juxtamedullary glomeruli during the first 3 h after Hg treatment (Plate 5.5). After this period, Hg was no longer detectable in glomeruli but continued to accumulate in the S2 and S3 segments of the proximal tubule. Subsequent *in vitro* studies, involving the separation of cortical and juxtamedullary glomeruli after *in vivo* treatment with Hg, confirmed an effect of the metal on the juxtamedullary glomerular population, since their metabolism was significantly impaired while cortical glomerular metabolism was unaffected.

These results had their functional expression in the *in vivo* situation as a high molecular weight proteinuria, predominantly albuminuria within 24 h after administration of Hg to female rats (Wilks, unpublished data). Thus, the data show a previously unrecognized early interaction of Hg with glomerular structures and also demonstrate the importance of nephron heterogeneity in the development of Hg-induced acute renal

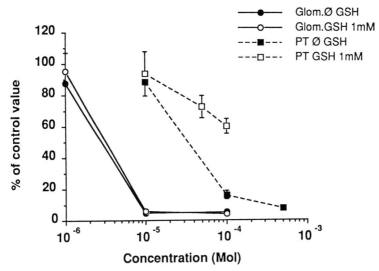

Fig. 5.3 Isolated rat glomeruli (Glom.) and proximal tubular fragments (PT) incubated in Earle's solution with or without ($\emptyset$) 1 mM glutathione (GSH) for 1 h at 37°C. After a change of the incubation medium, incubation was for a further 3 h in the presence of mercuric chloride (1 μM–0.5 mM). In glomeruli, the inhibition of proline incorporation into protein seen with mercury is not ameliorated by preincubation with GSH, whereas proximal tubular fragments are partially protected against mercury effects by GSH preincubation.

failure. A synopsis of both *in vivo* and *in vitro* experiments shows the mercury effects on vasculature, glomerulus and proximal tubule leading to the development of acute renal failure (Fig. 5.4). The relative contribution of damage to each structure will depend on the time and severity of the insult, single or multiple exposure, species, strain and sex differences, age, compromised functional reserve, hydration state, concomitant renal or extrarenal disease, initiation of therapy, etc.

These two examples of unexpected effects of chemicals on isolated glomeruli show the complementary use of data primarily obtained from *in vitro* investigations, which were at first as anomalous, but can in fact be related to *in vivo* findings. Thus the starting point of *in vitro* methods can provide a major input into establishing other aspects of the pathophysiology and molecular mechanisms of nephrotoxicity.

Conclusions

There should be no clearcut boundaries between screening and mechanistic studies and both aspects must often be considered simultaneously

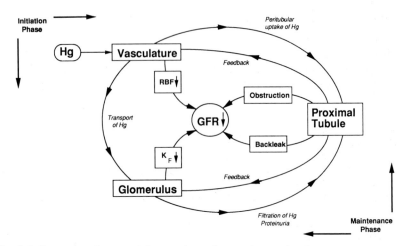

Fig. 5.4 Synopsis of potential vascular, glomerular and tubular effects in the mercuric chloride (Hg) model of acute renal failure. Development of filtration failure is characterized by vascular and glomerular damage in the initial phase leading to a reduction of renal blood flow (RBF) and the ultrafiltration coefficient (K_F). After the initial phase, tubular effects become more prominent and obstruction and backleak are probably the main pathomechanisms in the maintenance phase. However, the situation is aggravated by protein leakage across the glomerular filtration barrier which increases the tubular burden of mercury. Feedback mechanisms may be of crucial importance in this phase. GFR, glomerular filtration rate.

when choosing the appropriate test system to understand and control nephrotoxicity. This does not obviate the necessity for constant comparison with the *in vivo* situation, as the examples mentioned above show. *In vitro* tests are by their very nature likely to over- and mis-interpretation when this link is neglected. The ultimate criterion for using *in vitro* methods must be the applicability to the human situation and the contribution that *in vitro* tests are able to make to the prevention, diagnosis and treatment of nephrotoxicity in the clinical situation.

Acknowledgements

The research reported in this review was supported by The Commission of the European Communities, The Biotechnology Action Programme and the Bridge Programme of the Commission of the European Communities, The Humane Research Trust, The Dr Hadwen Trust for Humane Research and Johns Hopkins Center for Alternatives to Animals in Testing, and in part by The Wellcome Trust, The Smith-Kline Foundation and FRAME. We are indebted to Lisa Breitner, Monique Rivet and Mimps E. van Ek for typing the manuscript and to our colleagues for providing unpublished data or material in press. M.F.W. gratefully acknowledges a fellowship from Deutsche Forschungsgemeinschaft (DFG).

References

Anand-Srivastava, P.M., Vinay, P., Genest, J. and Cantin, M. (1986). *Am. J. Physiol.* **251**, F417–F423.

Ardaillou, N., Nivez, M.-P., Striker, G. and Ardaillou, R. (1983). *Prostaglandins* **26**, 773–784.

Axelson, R.A. (1973). *Pathology*, **5**, 43–50.

Bach, P.H. (1989a). *Toxicol. Lett.* **46**, 237–250.

Bach, P.H. (1989b). *In "In Vitro" Techniques in Research: Recent Advances"* (J.W. Payne, ed.), pp. 91–108. Open University Press, Milton Keynes.

Bach, P.H. and Bridges, J.W. (1984). *Prostaglandins Leukotri. Med.* **15**, 251–274.

Bach, P.H. and Bridges, J.W. (1985a). *Arch. Toxicol. Suppl.* **8**, 173–188.

Bach, P.H. and Bridges, J.W. (1985b). *CRC Crit. Rev. Toxicol.* **15**, 217–439.

Bach, P.H. and Gregg, N. (1988). *Int. Rev. Exp. Pathol.* **30**, 1–54.

Bach, P.H. and Hardy, T.L. (1985). *Kidney Int.* **28**, 605–613.

Bach, P.H. and Kwizera, E.N. (1988). *Xenobiotica* **16**, 685–698.

Bach, P.H. and Lock, E.A. (1982). *In* "Nephrotoxicity: Assessment and Pathogenesis" (P.M. Bach, F.W. Bonner, J.W. Bridges and E.A. Lock, eds), pp. 128–143. Wiley, Chichester.

Bach, P.H. and Lock, E.A. (1985). "Renal Heterogeneity and Target Cell Toxicity". Wiley, Chichester.

Bach, P.H. and Lock, E.A. (1987). "Nephrotoxicity in the Experimental and the Clinical Situation". Nijhoff, Dordrecht.

Bach, P.H. and Lock, E.A. (1989). "Nephrotoxicity: Extrapolation from *in vitro* and *in vivo*, and Animals to Man". Plenum Press, New York and London.

Bach, P.H., Bonner, F.W., Bridges, J.W. and Lock, E.A. (1982). *In* "Nephrotoxicity: Assessment and Pathogenesis". Wiley, Chicester.

Bach, P.H., Grasso, P., Molland, E.A. and Bridges, J.W. (1983). *Toxicol. Appl. Pharmacol.* **69**, 333–344.

Bach, P.H., Ketley, C.P., Benns, S.E., Ahmed, I. and Dixit, M. (1985). *In* "Renal Heterogeneity and Target Cell Toxicity" (P.H. Bach and E.A. Lock, eds), pp. 505–518. Wiley, Chichester.

Bach, P.H., Ketley, C.P., Dixit, M. and Ahmed, I. (1986). *Food Chem. Toxicol.* **24**, 775–779.

Bach, P.H., Gregg, N.J., Wilks, M.F. and Delacruz, L. (1991). "Nephrotoxicity: Mechanisms, Early Diagnosis and Therapeutic Management". Marcel Dekker, New York.

Bank, N., Mutz, E.F. and Aynedijian, H.S. (1967). *J. Clin. Invest.* **46**, 695–704.

Baverel, G., Bonnard, M., D'Armagnac De Castanet, E. and Pellet, M. (1978). *Kidney Int.* **14**, 567–575.

Baverel, G., Bonnard, M. and Pellet, M. (1979). *FEBS Lett.* **101**, 282–286.

Baverel, G., Forissier, M. and Pellet, M. (1980a). *Int. J. Biochem.* **12**, 163–168.
Baverel, G., Genoux, C., Forissier, M. and Pellet, M. (1980b). *Biochem. J.* **188**, 873–880.
Belleman, P. (1980). *Arch. Toxicol.* **44**, 63–84.
Bennett, W.M. (1983). *Nephron* **35**, 73–77.
Bennett, W.M., Houghton, D.C., McCarron, D.A., Elliott, W.C., Porter, G.A. and Gilbert, D.N. (1983). *In* "Acute Renal Failure: Correlations between Morphology and Function" (K. Solez and A. Whelton, eds), pp. 331–358. Dekker, New York.
Bennett, W.M., Mela-Riker, L., Houghton, D.C., Gilbert, D.N. and Buss, W.C. (1988). *Am. J. Physiol.* **24**, F265–F269.
Benns, S.E., Dixit, M., Ahmed, I., Ketley, C.P. and Bach, P.H. (1985). *In* "Alternative Methods in Toxicology" Vol. 3 (A. Goldberg, ed.), pp. 435–447. M.A. Liebert, Baltimore.
Berndt, W.O. (1976). *Environ. Hlth. Perspect.* **15**, 73–88.
Berndt, W.O. (1981). *In* "Toxicology of the kidney – Target Organ Toxicology Series" (J.B. Hook, ed.), pp. 1–29. Raven Press, New York.
Berndt, W.O. (1987). *In* "Nephrotoxicity in the Experimental and the Clinical Situation" (P.H. Bach and E.A. Lock, eds), pp. 301–316. Nijhoff, Dordrecht.
Berndt, W.O. and Hayes, A.W. (1977). *J. Environ. Pathol. Toxicol.* **1**, 93–103.
Berndt, W.O. and Hayes, A.W. (1979). *Toxicology* **12**, 5–17.
Bertani, T., Poggi, A., Pozzoni, R., Delaini, F., Sacchi, G., Thoua, Y., Mecca, G., Remuzzi, G. and Donati, M.B. (1982). *Lab. Invest.* **46**, 16–23.
Biber, T.U.L., Mylle, M., Baines, A.D. and Gottschalk, C.W. (1968). *Am. J. Med.* **44**, 664–705.
Blantz, R.C. (1975). *J. Clin. Invest.* **55**, 621–635.
Bohman, S.-O. (1980). *In* "The Renal Papilla and Hypertension" (A.K. Mandal and S.-O. Bohman, eds), pp. 7–33. Plenum Publishing Corp., New York and London.
Bojesen, I. (1974). *Lipids* **9**, 835–843.
Boogaard, P.J., Mulder, G.J. and Nagelkerke, J.F. (1989a). *Toxicol. Appl. Pharmacol.* **101**, 135–143.
Boogaard, P.J., Mulder, G.J. and Nagelkerke, J.F. (1989b). *Toxicol. Appl. Pharmacol.* **101**, 144–157.
Boogaard, P.J., Commandeur, J.N.M., Mulder, G.J., Vermeulen, N.P.E. and Nagelkerke, J.F. (1989c). *Biochem. Pharmacol.* **38**, 3731–3741.
Boogard, P.J., Zoeteweij, J.P., Berkel, T.J.C. van, Noordende, J.M. van't, Mulder, G.J. and Nagelkerke, J.F. (1990). *Biochem. Pharmacol.* **39**, 1335–1345.
Burger, M.M., Sordat, B. and Zinkernagel, R.M. (1990). "Cell to Cell Interaction". Karker Press, Basel.
Calabrese, E.J. (1985). "Toxic Susceptibility: Male/Female Differences". Wiley Interscience, New York.
Calabrese, E.J. (1986). "Age and Susceptibility to Toxic Substances". Wiley Interscience, New York.
Carlier, M.-B., Laurent, G., Claes, P.J., Vanderhaeghe, H.J. and Tulkens, P.M. (1983). *Antimicrob. Agents Chemother.* **23**, 440–449.
CEC-IPCS (1989). *Toxicol. Lett.* **46**, 1–306.
Chamberlin, M.E., Lefurgey, A. and Mandel, L.J. (1984). *Am. J. Physiol.* **247**, F955–F964.
Chatterjee, S., Trifillis, A.L. and Regec, A.L. (1985). *In* "Renal Heterogeneity

and Target Cell Toxicity" (P.H. Bach and E.A. Lock, eds), pp. 549–552. Wiley, Chichester.

Cojocel, C., Maita, K., Pasino, D.A., Kuo, C. and Hook, J.B. (1983). *Life Sci.* **33**, 855–861.

Cunarro, J.A. and Weiner, M.W. (1978). *J. Pharmacol. Exp. Ther.* **206**, 198–206.

Curthoys, N.P. and Belleman, P. (1979). *Exp. Cell Res.* **121**, 31–45.

Delacruz, L. (1988). "The effect of natural toxicants and other chemicals on the kidney". PhD thesis, Surrey.

Diezi, J. and Roch-Ramel, F. (1987). *In* "Nephrotoxicity in the Experimental and the Clinical Situation" (P.H. Bach and E.A. Lock, eds), pp. 317–358. Nijhoff, Dordrecht.

Druet, P. (1989). *Toxicol. Lett.* **46**, 55–64.

Druet, P., Bernard, A., Hirsch, F., Weening, J.J., Genoux, P., Mahieu, P. and Birkeland, S. (1982). *Arch. Toxicol.* **50**, 187–194.

Druet, P., Jacquot, C., Baran, D., Kleinknecht, D., Fillastre, J.P. and Mery, J.Ph. (1987). *In* "Nephrotoxicity in the Experimental and the Clinical Situation" (P.H. Bach and E.A. Lock, eds), pp. 727–770. Nijhoff, Dordrecht.

Elling, F., Hald, B., Jacobsen, Chr. and Krogh, P. (1975). *Acta Pathol. Microbiol. Scand. Sect. A* **83**, 739–741.

Endou, H., Nonoguchi, Y., Takehara, H., Yamada, H. and Nakada, J. (1985). *Contr. Nephrol.* **47**, 98–104.

Fillastre, J.P. (1978). *In* "Nephrotoxicity. Interaction of Drugs with Membrane Systems; Mitochondria – Lysosomes" (J.P. Fillastre, ed.), pp. 11–23. Mason Publishing, USA.

Foidart, J.B., Deckanne, C.A., Mahieu, P., Creutz, C.E. and De Mey, J. (1979). *Invest. Cell Pathol.* **2**, 15–26.

Foidart, J.B., Dubois, C.H. and Foidart, J.-M. (1980). *Int. J. Biochem.* **12**, 197–202.

Foidart, J.B., Dechenne, C.A. and Mahieu, P. (1981). *Diagnost. Histopathol.* **4**, 71–77.

Fry, J.R. and Perry, N.K. (1981). *Biochem. Pharmacol.* **30**, 1197–1201.

Fry, J.R., Wiebkin, P., Kao, J., Jones, C.A., Gwynn, J. and Bridges, J.W. (1978). *Xenobiotica* **8**, 113–120.

Gilbert, D.N., Wood, C.A., Kohlhepp, S.J., Kohnen, P.W., Houghton, D.B., Finkbeiner, H.C., Lindsley, J. and Bennett, W.M. (1989). *J. Infect. Dis.* **159**, 945–953.

Giuliano, R.A., Paulus, G.J., Verpooten, R.A., Pattyn, V., Pollet, D.E., Tulkens, P.M. and DeBroe, M.E. (1984). *Kidney Int.* **26**, 838–847.

Gottschalk, C.W. and Lassiter, W.E. (1973). *In* "Handbook of Physiology, Sect. 8, Renal Physiology" (J. Orloff and W.R. Berliner, eds), chapter 6. American Physiological Society. Washington D.C.

Gregg, N., Elseviers, M.M., DeBroe, M.E. and Bach, P.H. (1989). *Toxicol. Lett.* **46**, 141–151.

Gregg, N.J., Courtauld, E.A. and Bach, P.H. (1990a). *Toxicol. Pathol.* **18**, 39–46.

Gregg, N.J., Courtauld, E.A. and Bach, P.H. (1990b). *Toxicol. Pathol.* **18**, 47–55.

Greenspan, P., Mayer, E.P. and Fowler, S.D. (1985). *J. Cell. Biol.* **100**, 965–973.

Gstraunthaler, G., Pfaller, W. and Kotanko, P. (1985). *Renal Physiol.* **8**, 38–44.

Gyrd-Hansen, N. (1968). *Acta Vet. Scand.* **9**, 183–198.

Hall III, P.W. (1982). *In* "Nephrotoxic Mechanisms and Environmental Toxins" (G. Porter, ed.), pp. 227–240. Plenum, New York.

Hall III, P.W. and Dammin, G.J. (1978). *Nephron* **22**, 281–300.

Handler, J.S. (1983). *J. Exp. Biol.* **106**, 55–69.

Henry, L.N., Lane, C.E. and Kashgarian, M. (1968). *Lab. Invest.* **19**, 309–314.

Herzlinger, D.A., Easton, T.G. and Ojakian, G.K. (1982). *J. Cell Biol.* **93**, 269–277.

Hirsch, G.H. (1976). *Environ. Hlth. Perspect.* **15**, 89–99.

Holdsworth, S.R., Glasgow, E.F., Atkins, R.C. and Thomson, N.M. (1978). *Nephron* **22**, 454–459.

Homan-Muller, J.W.T., Weening, R.S. and Roos, D. (1975). *J. Lab. Clin. Med.* **85**, 198–207.

Hook, J.B. (1981). "Toxicology of the kidney – Target Organ Toxicology Series". Raven Press, New York.

Hook, J.B., Ishmael, J. and Lock, E.A. (1983). *Toxicol. Appl. Pharmacol.* **67**, 121–131.

Hull, R.N., Cherry, W.R. and Weaver, G.W. (1976). *In Vitro* **12**, 670–677.

Jakoby, W.B. and Pastan, I.H. (1979). "Cell Culture, Methods in Enzymology". Academic Press, New York.

Jones, D.P., Sundby, G.-B., Ormstad, K. and Orrenius, S. (1979). *Biochem. Pharmacol.* **28**, 929–935.

Josepovitz, C., Farruggella, T., Levine, R., Lane, B. and Kaloyanides, G.J. (1985). *J. Pharmacol. Exp. Ther.* **235**, 810–819.

Jung, K.Y. and Endou, H. (1989). *Toxicol. Appl. Pharmacol.* **100**, 383–390.

Jung, K.Y., Uchida, S. and Endou, H. (1989). *Toxicol. Appl. Pharmacol.* **100**, 369–382.

Kacew, S. (1987). *In* "Nephrotoxicity in the Experimental and the Clinical Situation" (P.H. Bach and E.A. Lock, eds), pp. 533–562. Nijhoff, Dordrecht.

Kaloyanides, G.J. (1984a). *Contr. Nephrol.* **42**, 148–167.

Kaloyanides, G.J. (1984b). *Fundament. Appl. Toxicol.* **4**, 930–943.

Kaloyanides, G.G. and Pastoriza-Munoz, E. (1980). *Kidney Int.* **18**, 571–582.

Kastner, S., Wilks, M.F., Gwinner, W., Soose, M., Bach, P.H. and Stolte, H. (1991a). *Renal Physiol. Biochem.* **14**, 48–54.

Kastner, S., Wilks, M.F., Soose, M., Bach, P.H. and Stolte, H. (1991b). *In* "Nephrotoxicity: Mechanisms, Early Diagnosis and Therapeutic Management" (P.H. Bach, N.J. Gregg, M.F. Wilks and L. Delacruz, eds), pp. 467–474. Marcel Dekker, New York.

Kluwe, W.M. and Hook, J.B. (1978). *Toxicol. Appl. Pharmacol.* **45**, 531–539.

Koseki, C., Yamaguchi, Y., Furusawa, ●● and Endou, H. (1988). *Kidney Int.* **33**, 543–554.

Kreisberg, J.I. and Karnovsky, M.J. (1983). *Kidney Int.* **23**, 439–447.

Kreisberg, J.I., Pitts, A.M. and Pretlow, T.G. (1977). *Am. J. Pathol.* **86**, 591–600.

Kreisberg, J.I., Hoover, R.L. and Karnovsky, M.J. (1978). *Kidney Int.* **14**, 21–30.

Krogh, P. (1978). *Acta Pathol. Microbiol. Scand., A. Suppl.* **269**, 1–28.

Krogh, P., Azelsen, N.H., Elling, F., Gyrd-Hansen, N., Hald, B., Hyldgaard-Jensen, J., Larsen, A.E., Madsen, A., Mortensen, H.P., Moller, T., Petersen, O.K., Ravnskov, U., Rostgaard, M. and Aalund, O. (1974). *Acta Pathol. Microbiol. Scand. Suppl.* **246**, 1–21.

Krogh, P., Hald, B., Plestina, R. and Ceovic, S. (1977). *Acta. Pathol. Microbiol. Scand. Sect. B* **85**, 238–240.

Krogh, P., Elling, F., Friis, Chr., Hald, B., Larsen, A.E., Lillehoj, E.B., Madsen, A., Mortensen, P., Rasmussen, F. and Ravnskov, U. (1979). *Vet. Pathol.* **16**, 466–475.

Kuo, C. and Hook, J.B. (1982). *Toxicol. Appl. Pharmacol.* **63**, 292–302.

Kuo, C.-H. and Hook, J.B. (1983). *Life Sci.* **33**, 517–523.

Kuo, C.-H., Braselton, W.E. and Hook, J.B. (1982). *Toxicol. Appl. Pharmacol.* **64**, 244–254.

Kwizera, E.N., Wilks, M.F. and Bach, P.H. (1990). *In Vitro Toxicol.* **3**, 243–253.

Laurent, G., Carlier, M.-B., Rollman, B., VanHoof, F. and Tulkens, P.M. (1982). *Biochem. Pharmacol.* **31**, 3861–3870.

Laurent, G., Toubeau, G., Heuson-Steinnon, J.A., Tulkens, P. and Maldauge, P. (1988). *CRC Crit. Rev. Toxicol.* **19**, 147–183.

Luft, F.C. and Kleit, S.A. (1974). *J. Infect. Dis.* **130**, 656–659.

McDowell, E.M., Nagle, R.B., Zalme, R.C., McNeil, J.S., Flamenbaum, W. and Trump, B.F. (1976). *Virchows Arch B Cell Pathol.* **22**, 173–196.

Marre, R., Tarara, N. and Louton, T. (1980). *Eur. J. Pediat.* **133**, 25–29.

Meezan, E. and Brendel, K. (1973). *J. Pharmacol. Exp. Ther.* **187**, 352–364.

Michondet, C. and Baverel, G. (1987). *FEBBS Lett.* **216**, 113–117.

Mohandas, J., Duggin, G.G., Horvath, J.S. and Tiller, D.J. (1981a). *Res. Commun. Chem. Pathol. Pharmacol.* **34**, 69–80.

Mohandas, J., Duggin, G.G., Horvath, J.S. and Tiller, D.J. (1981b). *Toxicol. Appl. Pharmacol.* **61**, 252–259.

Morin, J.P., Viotte, G., Vanderwalle, A., Van Hoof, F., Tulkens, P. and Fillastre, J.P. (1980). *Kidney Int.* **18**, 583–590.

Morita, T., Oite, T., Kihara, I., Yamamoto, T., Hara, M., Naka, A. and Ohno, S. (1980). *Acta Pathol. Jpn.* **30**, 917–926.

Mudge, G.H. (1985). *In* "Renal Heterogeneity and Target Cell Toxicity" (P.H. Bach and E.A. Lock, eds), pp. 1–12. Wiley, Chichester.

Nakada, J., Yamada, H. and Endou, H. (1986a). *Renal Physiol.* **9**, 213–222.

Nakada, J., Machida, T. and Endou, H. (1986b). *In* "Nephrotoxicity of Antibiotics and Immunosuppressants" (T. Tanabe, J.B. Hook and H. Endou, eds), pp. 179–182. Elsevier, Amsterdam.

Nash, J.A., King, L.J., Lock, E.A. and Green, T. (1984). *Toxicol. Appl. Pharmacol.* **73**, 124–137.

NTP (1989). "NTP Technical Report on the Toxicology and Carcinogenesis Studies of Ochratoxin A (CAS NO. 303-47-9) in F344/N Rats (Gavage Studies) (G. Boorman, ed.), NHI Publication No. 89–2813. U.S. Department of Health and Human Services, National Institutes of Health, Research Triangle Park, NC.

Ormstad, K. (1982). *In* "Nephrotoxicity: Assessment and Pathogenesis" (P.H. Bach, F.W. Bonner, J.W. Bridges and E.A. Lock, eds), pp. 161–168. Wiley, Chichester.

Ormstad, K. (1987). *In* "Nephrotoxicity in the Experimental and the Clinical Situation" (P.H. Bach and E.A. Lock, eds), pp. 405–428. Nijhoff, Dordrecht.

Ormstad, K., Jones, D.P. and Orrenius, S. (1981). *Methods Enzymol.* **77**, 137–146.

Pavlovic, M., Plestina, R. and Krogh, P. (1979). *Acta Pathol. Microbiol. Scand. Sect. B* **87**, 243–246.

Pellett, O.L., Smith, M.L., Thoene, J.G., Schneider, J.A. and Jonas, A.J. (1984). *In Vitro* **20**, 53–58.

Perantoni, A. and Berman, J.J. (1979). *In Vitro* **15**, 446–454.
Porter, G.A. (1982). "Nephrotoxic Mechanisms of Drugs and Environmental Toxins". Plenum, New York.
Porter, G.A. (1989). *Toxicol. Lett.* **46**, 269–279.
Porter, G.A. and Bennet, W.M. (1989). *In* "Nephrotoxicity: Extrapolation from *In Vitro* to *In Vivo*, and Animals to Man" (P.J. Bach and E.A. Lock, eds), pp. 147–170. Plenum Press, New York and London.
Pretlow, T.G. II and Pretlow, T.P. (1982). "Cell Separation: Methods and Selected Applications", Vol. 1. Academic Press, New York.
Pretlow, T.G. II and Pretlow, T.P. (1983). "Cell Separation: Methods and Selected Applications", Vol. 2. Academic Press. New York.
Pretlow, T.G. II and Pretlow, T.P. (1984). "Cell Separation: Methods and Selected Applications", Vol. 3. Academic Press. New York.
Purchase, I.F.H. and Conning, D. (1986). *Fd. Chem. Toxicol.* **24**, 447–818.
Ramsammy, L.S., Josepovitz, C. and Kaloyanides, G.J. (1988). *J. Pharmacol. Exp. Ther.* **247**, 989–996.
Ramsammy, L.S., Josepovitz, C., Lane, B. and Kaloyanides, G.J. (1989a). *Am. J. Physiol.* **256**, C204–C213.
Ramsammy, L.S., Josepovitz, C., Lane, B.P. and Kaloyanides, G.J. (1989b). *J. Pharmacol. Exp. Ther.* **250**, 149–153.
Roch-Ramel, F. and Peters, G. (1979). *Annu. Rev. Pharmacol. Toxicol.* **19**, 323–345.
Roth, K.S., Holtzapple, P., Genel, M. and Segal, S. (1979). *Metabolism* **18**, 677–681.
Rush, G.F., Smith, J.H., Newton, J.F. and Hook, J.B. (1984). *CRC Crit. Rev. Toxicol.* **13**, 99–160.
Saier, M.H. (1981). *Am. J. Physiol.* **240**, C106–C109.
Sastrasinh, M., Knauss, T.C., Weinberg, J.M. and Humes, H.D. (1982). *J. Pharmacol. Exp. Ther.* **222**, 350–358.
Sato, G. and Reid, L. (1978). *Int. Rev. Biochem.* **20**, 219–251.
Savin, V., Karniski, L., Cuppage, F., Hodges, G. and Chanko, A. (1985). *Lab. Invest.* **52**, 93–102.
Scheinman, J.I. and Fish, A. (1978). *Am. J. Pathol.* **92**, 125–139.
Scholer, D.W. and Edelman, I.S. (1979). *Am. J. Physiol.* **237**, F350–F359.
Schlondorff, D., Roczniak, S., Satriano, J.A. and Folkert, V.W. (1980). *Am. J. Physiol.* **239**, F486–F495.
Schurek, H.J. (1988). *Klin. Wochenschr.* **66**, 828–835.
Schwertz, D.W., Kreisberg, J.I. and Venkatachalem, M.A. (1984). *J. Pharmacol. Exp. Ther.* **231**, 48–55.
Silverblatt, F.J. and Kuehn, C. (1979). *Kidney Int.* **15**, 335–345.
Soose, M., Haberstroh, U., Rovira-Holbach, G., Brunkhorst, R. and Stolte, H. (1988). *Clin. Physiol. Biochem.* **6**, 310–315.
Sraer, J., Foidart, J., Chansel, D., Mahieu, P. and Ardaillou, R. (1980). *Int. J. Biochem.* **12**, 203–207.
Sraer, J., Rigaud, M., Bens, M., Rabinovitch, H. and Ardaillou, R. (1983). *J. Biol. Chem.* **258**, 4325–4330.
Stollenwerk Petrulis, A., Aikawa, M. and Dunn, M.J. (1981). *Kidney Int.* **20**, 469–474.
Stolte, H. and Alt, J. (1980). *Contrib. Nephrol.* **19**, 1–249.
Stolte, H. and Alt, J. (1982). *In* "Nephrotoxicity: Assessment and Pathogenesis" (P.H. Bach, F.W. Bonner, J.W. Bridges and E.A. Lock, eds), pp. 102–112. Wiley, Chichester.

Striker, G.E., Killen, P.D. and Farin, F.M. (1980). *Transplant Proc.* **12**, 88–99.
Stumpf, B. and Kraus, H. (1978). *Pediat. Res.* **12**, 1039–1044.
Taub, M. and Saier, M.H. (1981). *J. Cell. Physiol.* **106**, 191–199.
Trifillis, A.L., Regec, A., Hall-Craggs, M. and Trump, B.F. (1986). *Toxicol. Pathol.* **14**, 210–212.
Tulkens, P.M. (1989). *Toxicol. Lett.* **46**, 107–123.
Tune, B.M. (1975). *J. Infect. Dis.* **132**, 189–194.
Tune, B.M. (1986). *Comments Toxicol.* **1**, 145–170.
Tune, B.M. and Fravert, D. (1980). *Kidney Int.* **18**, 591–600.
Tune, B.M., Burg, M.D. and Patlak, C.S. (1969). *Am. J. Physiol.* **217**, 1057–1063.
Ullrich, K.J. and Greger, R. (1985). *In* "The Kidney, Physiology and Pathology" (D.G. Seldin and G. Giebisch, eds), Chapter 20. Raven Press, New York.
Vinay, P., Gougoux, A. and Lemieux, G. (1981). *Am. J. Physiol.* **241**, F403–F411.
Weinberg, J.M. and Humes, H.D. (1980). *Arch. Biochem. Biophys.* **205**, 222–231.
WHO (1979). "World Health Organisation – Environmental Health Criteria Document 11, Mycotoxins". WHO, Geneva.
WHO (1991). "World Health Organisation – IPCS Environmental Health Criteria Document 119, Principles and Methods for the Assessment of Nephrotoxicity Associated with Exposure to Chemicals". WHO, Geneva.
Wilks, M.F., Gregg, N.J. and Bach, P.H. (1989). *Nephrol. Dial. Transpl.* **4**, 448.
Wilks, M.F., Kwizera, E.N. and Bach, P.H. (1990). *Renal Physiol. Biochem.* **13**, 275–284.
Wilks, M.F., Kwizera, E.N. and Bach, P.H. (1991). *In* "Nephrotoxicity: Mechanisms, Early Diagnosis and Therapeutic Management" (P.H. Bach, N.J. Gregg, M.F. Wilks and L. Delacruz, eds), pp. 347–352. Marcel Dekker, New York.
Williams, P.D., Holohan, P.D. and Ross, C.R. (1981). *Toxicol. Appl. Pharmacol.* **61**, 243–251.
Williams, G.M., Dunkel, V.C. and Ray, V.A. (1983). *Ann. N.Y. Acad. Sci.* **407**, 1–482.
Williams, P.D., Hottendorf, G.H. and Bennett, D.B. (1986). *J. Pharmacol. Exp. Ther.* **237**, 919–925.
Wing, A.J., Brunner, F.P., Geerlings, W., Broyer, M., Brynger, H., Fassbinder, W., Rissoni, G., Selwood, N.H. and Tufeson, G. (1989). *Toxicol. Lett.* **46**, 281–292.
Zalme, R.C., McDowell, E.M., Nagle, R.B., McNeil, J.S., Flamenbaum, W. and Trump, B.F. (1976). *Virchows Arch. B., Cell. Pathol.* **22**, 197–216.
Zenser, T.V., Mattammal, M.B. and Davis, B.B. (1978a). *J. Pharmacol. Exp. Ther.* **207**, 719–725.
Zenser, T.V., Mattammal, M.B., Herman, C.A., Joshi, S. and Davis, B.B. (1978b). *Biochim. Biophys. Acta* **542**, 486–495.
Zenser, T.V., Mattammal, M.B. and Davis, B.B. (1979a). *J. Pharmacol. Exp. Ther.* **208**, 418–421.
Zenser, T.V., Mattammal, M.B. and Davis, B.B. (1979b). *J. Pharmacol. Exp. Ther.* **211**, 460–464.
Zenser, T.V., Mattammal, M.B., Brown, W.W. and Davis, B.B. (1979c). *Kidney Int.* **16**, 688–694.
Zenser, T.V., Mattammal, M.B., Rapp, N.S. and Davis, B.B. (1983). *J. Lab. Clin. Med.* **101**, 58–65.

Discussion

P. Tulkens

Dr Bach showed a cascade with respect to analgesic nephropathy. One of the important features of analgesic nephropathy is that it takes many years before eventually leading to the clinical situation that we know. Has Dr Bach any idea how that can be taken into account in models or is this completely impossible?

P. Bach

The interstitial cells are so highly differentiated that we think they do not repair. If a proximal tubule is damaged, some repair will take place, but once the interstitial cells have been knocked out we can find no evidence of any repopulation of that space with equivalent cells. If people are abusing analgesics and knocking out interstitial cells over years, this would be a cumulative effect. The kidney also has a very substantial buffering capacity. It can be severely compromised with 75% of the nephrons damaged before manifesting what will be clinically recognized as the beginning of end-stage renal disease. It is one of those subtle things which develop over a long time and then start to manifest some symptoms.

The point about the cascade is that if the initiating factors and some of the factors that contribute to the cascade are understood, I believe that *in vitro* toxicity studies can have a positive input into chronic toxicity studies – that should be one of our goals.

H. Stolte

Dr Bach said that his *in vitro* systems are also helpful for studying repair mechanisms. This is probably useful because it would be followed by a better understanding of the changes that occur.

P. Bach

That is what I said: we can take those cells from treated animals and start learning more about repair as well as about degenerative changes.

J. Boyer

With regard to the studies with mercury, mercury is a very potent general cell toxin. It illustrates some of the problems in the general field of toxicology in that its toxicity will depend upon both the dose to a given tissue and the presence or absence – or at least the intensity – of the available sulphydryl groups within that tissue.

P. Bach

The glomeruli do not have a lot of glutathione, which may be one of the reasons why the mercury targets for that.

It is also interesting and I think relevant, but possibly confusing, that mercury amalgam fillings are quite safe. If plasma mercury is measured, there is no detectable mercury. Unfortunately, however, some work performed recently on primates with mercury fillings has showed that, on silver intensification it is possible to pick up the passage of mercury down the roots and into the kidney of those animals. It appears that mercury at that level may be good for us but, on the other hand, it also raises the question of the 50% unknown aetiology in end-stage renal disease. Many of us have mercury fillings, and obviously this is just one of the other environmental loads on the kidney. All the mercury was in the proximal tubule in the multi-box electron microscopy studies that are currently being done.

H. Stolte

The time course is important. If we go back to the experimental studies, the tubular effect comes first and the glomerular effect secondarily. From this study the hypothesis could be put forward that the glomerulus is involved primarily, independent of the number of sulphydryl groups present.

P. Bach

There is also the question of levels of exposure and when it occurs – as there is with everything in toxicology and *in vitro*.

Renal Proximal Tubular Cell Culture: Characterization and Use in Nephrotoxicology

H. TOUTAIN, F. COURJAULT and A. CORDIER

Unité de Néphrotoxicologie, Institut de Recherche sur la Sécurité du Médicament, Rhône-Poulenc Rorer SA, 20, Quai de la Révolution, 94140 Alfortville, France

Introduction

A variety of xenobiotic compounds can induce toxic nephropathies and the susceptibility of the kidney to xenobiotics is clearly related to the high renal blood flow, which is equivalent to 25% of the entire cardiac output, and to the glomerular filtration and subsequent intratubular concentration processes of potentially toxic substances. The main site of injury within the kidney is the proximal tubular cell. These cells are located in a portion of the nephron which is involved in the reabsorption and secretion processes and is consequently frequently exposed to high concentrations of xenobiotics or their metabolites. In recent decades, various experimental models have been developed to investigate the mechanisms responsible for drug-induced proximal tubulopathies. These range from intact animals to *in vitro* models, such as the isolated perfused kidney, isolated proximal tubules or isolated proximal tubular cells as

IN VITRO METHODS IN TOXICOLOGY
ISBN 0-12-388175-7

well as cultures of proximal cells, either as primaries or continuous cell lines.

The isolated perfused kidney (IPK) is the only *in vitro* model in which the xenobiotics can be metabolized and, consequently, the only model in which the effects of potentially toxic metabolites on renal function can be assessed in the presence of an intact vasculature and normal anatomical relationships between the nephrons. However, this model suffers from three major limitations: (i) the characteristic metabolic properties of the IPK are preserved only for about 4 h; (ii) this model can be used to assess the function of the whole organ, but cannot identify the drug impact on a specific cell population, which makes it inappropriate for investigating the toxicology of the proximal tubule cell; (iii) the method cannot be used to follow the time-course or dose relationship of the impact of chemicals on a given IPK function, since functional deterioration occurs from the outset of the experiment. The contribution of IPK to renal toxicology has been comprehensively reviewed (Bekersky, 1985; Maack, 1986).

Renal slices have frequently been used over the past 40 years to evaluate the nephrotoxic effects of a variety of xenobiotics. The preparation and use of renal slices in nephrotoxicology has been reviewed (Bach and Lock, 1982; Smith, 1988; Ruegg *et al.*, 1989). Cortical slices offer a method of evaluating proximal nephrotoxicity which despite other drawbacks is both fast and simple to perform. They can be used to evaluate *in vivo* toxic effects by taking slices from animals sacrificed after exposure to drugs or to evaluate *in vitro* effects by using slices from untreated animals exposed to xenobiotics *in vitro*. They can be obtained from a number of mammalian species, including mice, rabbits, rats, dogs, monkeys and humans and therefore make it possible to compare drug-induced proximal dysfunctions in different species. Several authors have identified parameters which can be used to detect the *in vitro* nephrotoxic potential of drugs such as the aminoglycosides, the cephalosporins, cisplatin (Phelps *et al.*, 1987), carbon tetrachloride, mercuric chloride and potassium dichromate (Bach and Lock, 1982; Ruegg *et al.*, 1989). These parameters include the *in vitro* accumulation of *p*-aminohippuric acid, tetraethylammonium and *N*-methylnicotinamide, as well as intracellular K^+ levels, lactate dehydrogenase activity and gluconeogenesis. However, the renal slice method does have several drawbacks and limitations. Firstly, renal cortex slices consist of a heterogeneous population of tubules, which makes it difficult to identify specifically proximal tubular toxicological effects. The tubule lumina collapse soon after slice preparation, limiting the access of incubation medium, oxygen and the test xenobiotics to the apical membrane (Bach and Lock, 1982). In an attempt to overcome this, some investigators have devised more elaborate methods of slice preparation (Brendel *et al.*, 1987; Ruegg *et al.*, 1987), in which ultrathin slices are incubated in optimum oxygenation conditions. Under these incubation conditions, slice viability can be maintained for at least 20 h.

Suspensions of proximal tubules (PT) are currently obtained from several species, including man, by a process involving enzymatic digestion of cortical tissue, followed by purification steps (Vinay *et al.*, 1981), or by mechanical disruption of cortical tissue (Carlson *et al.*, 1978; Toutain *et al.*, 1989b). In spite of the very limited lifespan of these tubules and the fact that solutes have access mainly to the basolateral membrane, it has been shown that the model can be extrapolated to the *in vivo* situation for a variety of xenobiotics, including aminoglycosides, cephalosporins, adriamycin, GSH and cysteine *S*-conjugates (Rylander *et al.*, 1985; Sina *et al.*, 1989).

Isolated proximal tubule cells can be obtained using a variety of methods, including enzymatic digestion combined with isopycnic centrifugation (Boogaard *et al.*, 1989a,b), mechanical disruption (Toutain *et al.*, 1989b, 1991a) and free-flow electrophoresis (Toutain *et al.*, 1989a; Toutain and Morin, 1991). These isolated cells are uniformly exposed to the incubation medium but suffer from a number of inherent limitations, including the absence of polarity and of cell-to-cell interactions. The use of isolated proximal tubular cells is often limited to studies investigating cell-specific biochemical properties or susceptibility to toxicants (Lash, 1989).

The models listed above have all been used extensively in renal toxicology, but they all yield data obtained after short-term incubation with high concentrations of test compounds. The limited relevance of such data to *in vivo* toxicity, which in some cases can be detected only after exposure for several days, constitutes a major drawback. The use of proximal cell cultures provides a method of conducting studies involving prolonged exposure to lower concentrations. This paper will focus on proximal cell cultures derived from mammalian kidneys. We will describe their main characteristics and their use as a complement to animal tests in evaluating nephrotoxicity. We will make no attempt to provide an exhaustive review of the literature, but will concentrate on pivotal studies which highlight the strengths and weaknesses of the methods available.

Renal Proximal Tubule Cell Cultures

Over the past two decades, several renal cell culture models have been developed both from primary cultures and immortal cell lines

(Gstraunthaler, 1988; Kreisberg and Wilson, 1988; Striker *et al.*, 1988). These cultures express differentiated properties of proximal tubular cells (PTC) and provide both cellular specificity and a prolonged lifespan, since they can be maintained satisfactorily under controlled conditions for periods of up to a few weeks. They can be used to investigate the direct effects of prolonged drug exposure on PTC without any interference from extrarenal factors (such as hormonal control, changes in renal haemodynamic or in the glomerular filtration rate). This feature also constitutes the main limitation to extrapolating data obtained from *in vitro* models of this type to the *in vivo* situation. Some of the characteristics of established cell lines of proximal epithelial origin and of PTC primary cultures obtained from various mammalian species are described below.

Characteristics of Established Cell Lines

Several cell lines resembling the renal proximal epithelium have been established. Four of the most commonly used established cell lines are listed in Table 6.1. These cell lines are all grown in serum-supplemented media consisting of either Dulbecco's Minimum Essential Medium (DMEM), Eagle's MEM or a 1:1 mixture of DMEM/Ham's F12 containing 10% fetal calf serum. Their main characteristics, notably hormone responsiveness, specific transport properties and expression of metabolic functions or marker enzyme activities are summarized in Tables 6.1, 6.2 and 6.3 respectively. Cell lines have yielded a lot of information about normal and drug-impaired proximal tubule cell function (Wilson, 1986; Gstraunthaler, 1988). The use of these cell lines has the obvious advantage of cutting out the lengthy preparatory phase required for primary cell cultures, but suffers from many drawbacks, including cellular heterogeneity, an incomplete expression of the PTC phenotype and genetic drift, which leads to changes in characteristics as a result of storage conditions and successive passages (Husted *et al.*, 1986).

The LLC-PK₁ cell line

The LLC-PK$_1$ cell line is of renal tubule epithelial origin and has been derived from the Hampshire pig (Hull *et al.*, 1976); it has been used extensively to study renal PTC function (Gstraunthaler, 1988; Striker *et al.*, 1988). It has been shown that when these cells are grown as a monolayer, they form a polarized epithelium with tight junctions in which domes are formed spontaneously. Microvilli can be seen projecting into the culture medium from the apical surface. LLC-PK$_1$ cells closely resemble proximal tubule cells, and exhibit high activities of apical

Table 6.1
Hormone responsiveness in established cell lines of proximal origin

Cell line	Active Agents[a]	References
LLC-PK₁ (pig) (Hull et al., 1976)	ANF	(Inui et al., 1985b)
	Calcitonin	(Ausiello et al., 1980)
	EGF	(Goodyer and Kachra, 1985)
	Hydrocortisone	(Chuman et al., 1982)
	Insulin	(Roy et al., 1980)
	Oxytocin	(Stassen et al., 1988; Garg et al., 1990)
	Thyroid hormone	(Chuman et al., 1982)
	Vasopressin (V1, V2)	(Ausiello et al., 1987)
	Vitamin D	(Costa and Feldman, 1987)
OK (opossum) (Koyama et al., 1978)	ANF	(Nakai et al., 1988)
	Calcitonin	(Malmström and Murer, 1986)
	Dexamethasone	(Rizzoli and Bonjour, 1987)
	Dopamine	(Cheng et al., 1990)
	Adrenaline	(Cheng et al., 1988; Murphy and Bylund, 1988)
	IGF-I	(Caverzasio and Bonjour, 1989)
	Insulin	(Abraham et al., 1990)
	PGE₂	(Malmström and Murer, 1986)
	PTH	(Teitelbaum and Strewler, 1984)
	Serotonin	(Murphy and Bylund, 1989)
	Thyroid hormone	(Yonemura et al., 1990)
	Vitamin D	(Wald et al., 1989)
JTC12 (monkey) (Takaoka and Katsuta, 1962)	Insulin	(Takuwa and Ogata, 1985a)
	PTH	(Ishizuka et al., 1978)
	PGE₁	—
	Noradrenaline	—
	Vitamin D	(Matsumoto et al., 1985)
RC-SV1 (rabbit) (Vandewalle et al., 1989)	PTH	(Vandewalle et al., 1989)

[a] ANF, atrial natriuretic factor; EGF, epidermal growth factor; IGF-I, insulin-like growth factor I; PGE₂, prostaglandin E₂; PTH, parathyroid hormone.

membrane enzymes such as γ-glutamyl transpeptidase, alkaline phosphatase and leucine aminopeptidase (Gstraunthaler et al., 1985b; Toutain et al., 1990). They also demonstrate high Na^+/K^+ ATPase activity, which is located in the basolateral plasma membrane, as well as a sodium-dependent transport of hexoses, amino acids and phosphate (Mullin et

Table 6.2
Transport properties in established cell lines of proximal origin

Cell line	Characteristics[a]	References
LLC-PK$_1$	Na$^+$/glucose transport	(Mullin et al., 1980; Rabito, 1981)
	Na$^+$/amino acid transport	(Rabito and Karish, 1983a,b)
	Na$^+$ ind. amino acid transport	(Sepulveda and Pearson, 1985)
	Na$^+$/phosphate transport	(Rabito, 1983)
	Na$^+$/H$^+$ exchanger	(Cantiello et al., 1986)
	Cl$^-$/HCO$_3^-$ exchanger	(Chaillet et al., 1986)
	Na$^+$/K$^+$/2Cl$^-$ symport	(Brown and Murer, 1985)
	Na$^+$/Ca^{2+} exchanger	(Parys et al., 1986)
	H$^+$/TEA exchanger	(Inui et al., 1985a; Fauth et al., 1988)
	S-Cysteine conjugates transport	(Schaeffer and Stevens, 1986)
	Lack of PAH transport	(Rabito, 1986)
OK	Na$^+$/glucose transport	(Malmström et al., 1987)
	Na$^+$/amino acid transport	(Schwegler et al., 1989)
	Na$^+$/phosphate transport	(Malmström and Murer, 1986)
	Na$^+$/H$^+$ exchanger	(Helmle-Kolb et al., 1990)
JTC12	Na$^+$/glucose transport	(Takuwa and Ogata, 1985a)
	Na$^+$/amino acid transport	(Takuwa and Ogata, 1985a)
	Na$^+$/phosphate transport	(Takuwa and Ogata, 1985b)
	Cl$^-$/HCO$_3^-$ exchanger	(Fineman et al., 1990)
	Ca^{2+}-activated K$^+$ channel	(Chang et al., 1988)
RC-SV1	Na$^+$/glucose transport	(Vandewalle et al., 1989)
	Na$^+$/H$^+$ exchanger	

[a] TEA, tetraethylammonium; ind., independent; PAH, p-aminohippurate.

al., 1980; Rabito and Karish, 1983a,b; Rabito, 1983). In addition, these cells have been shown to possess an amiloride-sensitive Na$^+$/H$^+$ exchanger, a Na$^+$/K$^+$/2Cl$^-$ cotransport system which is inhibited by bumetamide, and a proton/organic cation exchanger which is inhibited by quinine (Brown and Murer, 1985; Cantiello et al., 1986; Fauth et al., 1988).

The cells do, however, differ from the proximal tubule epithelium in several respects. The hormone response pattern exhibited by the LLC-PK$_1$ cells more closely resembles that of a more distal portion of the nephron, since both calcitonin and vasopressin stimulate cyclic AMP (cAMP) production and adenylate cyclase activity, whereas PTH has a minimal impact (Aussiello et al., 1980; Malmström and Murer, 1986). The absence of certain PCT characteristics, such as a probenicid-sensitive organic anion carrier (Rabito, 1986) and the gluconeogenesis pathway

Table 6.3

Metabolic functions and marker enzymes in established cell lines of proximal origin

Cell line	Characteristics[a]	References
LLC-PK$_1$	Membrane enzyme activities γ-GT, Alk phos, LAP, AAP, NaK-ATPase, trehalase, maltase	(Gstraunthaler et al., 1985b) (Toutain et al., 1990) (Yoneyama and Lever, 1984)
	Lysosomal and peroxysomal activities Ac phos, NAG, cathepsin B, catalase, D-amino-acid oxidase	(Gstraunthaler et al., 1985b) (Toutain et al., 1990)
	Mitochondrial activities Cytox, GDH, MDH, IDH, SDH,	(Gstraunthaler et al., 1985b)
	Transaminase activities Alanine and aspartate aminotransferase	(Gstraunthaler et al., 1985b)
	Biotransformation enzymes GSSG red, GSH perox, GSH aryltrans,UDPGT; DMH demethylase, glutathion-S- transferase	(Siegers et al., 1987) (Stevens et al., 1986)
	Cysteine conjugate β-lyase, lack of Cyclooxygenase	(Lifschitz et al., 1982)
	Glucose metabolism activities HK, LDH, PFK, G6PDH, aldolase, PK	(Gstraunthaler et al., 1985b)
	Gluconeogenesis activities PEPCK, G6Pase, lack of F16BP	(Gstraunthaler and Handler, 1987)
	Ammoniogenesis	(Cole et al., 1986)
	Glucuronide conjugate metabolism	(Stevens et al., 1986)
	Lack of gluconeogenesis	(Gstraunthaler et al., 1985a)
	Plasminogen activator production	(Sudol and Reich, 1984)
	Vitamin D and retinol metabolism	(Napoli and Martin, 1984; Napoli, 1986)
OK	Membrane enzyme activities γ-GT, LAP, lack of alk phos	(Malmström et al., 1987)
	Other marker enzymes NAG, NADH oxidoreductase	(Malmström et al., 1987)
JTC12	Membrane enzyme activities γ-GT, LAP, alk phos, trehalase	(Takuwa and Ogata, 1985a)
RC-SV1	Membrane enzyme activities γ-GT, LAP, NaK-ATPase, DPP IV, endopeptidase	(Vandewalle et al., 1989)

Table 6.3
Continued

---

[a] γ-GT, γ-glutamyl transpeptidase; LAP, leucine aminopeptidase; AAP, alanine aminopeptidase, Alk. phos., alkaline phosphatase; DDP IV, dipeptidylpeptidase; Ac phos, acid phosphatase; NAG, N-acetyl-β-D-glucosaminidase, cytox, cytochrome-C oxidoreductase; GDH, glutamate dehydrogenase; MDH, malate dehydrogenase; IDH, isocitrate dehydrogenase; SDH, succinate dehydrogenase; GSSG red, glutathione reductase; GSH perox, glutathione peroxidase; GSH aryltrans, glutathione aryl transferase; UDPGT, UDP-glucuronyl transferase; DMH demethylase, dimethylhydrazine demethylase; HK, hexokinase; LDH, lactate dehydrogenase; PFK, phosphofructokinase; G6PDH, glucose-6-phosphate dehydrogenase; PK, pyruvate kinase; PEPCK, phosphoenolpyruvate carboxykinase; G6Pase, glucose-6-phosphatase, F16BP, fructose-1,6-biphosphatase.

due to the lack of fructose-1,6-bisphosphatase activity (Gstraunthaler *et al.*, 1985a), raises doubts about the validity of this model for investigating drug-induced PTC toxicity. Indeed, the LLC-PK$_1$ line is obviously inappropriate for studying some nephrotoxic chemicals, such as the cephalosporins (Sina *et al.*, 1989) and N-acetyl-L-cysteine conjugates (Schaeffer and Stevens, 1986), which enter the PTC via the organic anion carrier.

The heterogeneity of the LLC-PK$_1$ line has made it possible to select sublines by simple modifications of the culture medium (glucose concentration, osmolarity). Clones have been isolated from these sublines which exhibit a phenotype distinct from that of the parental cell population (Gstraunthaler and Handler, 1987; Gstraunthaler, 1988). The differences recorded include: an absence of the calcitonin and vasopressin response, resistance to ouabain, an absence of dome formation, an absence of Na^+/H^+ antiport, an ability to grow in serum/insulin-free defined medium or gluconeogenesis activity, due to the induction of fructose-1,6-bisphosphatase by hexose-free medium (Roy, 1985; Agarwal *et al.*, 1986; Jans *et al.*, 1986; Gstraunthaler and Handler, 1987; Rabito *et al.*, 1987). These properties can be turned to experimental advantage by using clones with or without a given function to investigate a particular feature in a complex mechanism (Gstraunthaler, 1988).

The OK cell line

The OK cell line, derived from the American opossum (Koyama *et al.*, 1978), has been characterized in less detail than the LLC-PK$_1$ line. The OK cells also produce monolayers of polarized epithelial cells and express a number of PTC properties, such as dome formation, sodium-dependent transport of glucose, amino acids and phosphate, and responsiveness to

PTH and calcitonin (Malmström and Murer, 1986). However, the alkaline phosphatase activity of these cells is deficient (Malmström *et al.*, 1987). The renal OK cell line is the only established cell line with proximal characteristics which is able to regulate Na^+-dependent phosphate cotransport in response both to fast-acting factors, such as PTH, and long-term stimuli, such as chronic inorganic phosphate deprivation or thyroid hormone stimulation (Quamme *et al.*, 1989; Yonemura *et al.*, 1990). In this cell line, PTH-dependent inhibition of both Na^+/H^+ exchange and Na^+/phosphate cotransport, via adenylate cyclase stimulation, seems to be correlated to a slower V_{max} of both transport systems (Malmström and Murer, 1986; Helmle-Kolb *et al.*, 1990).

The JTC-12 cell line

The JTC-12 cell line, derived from the normal kidney of the Cynomolgus monkey, was established by Takaoka and Katsuta (1962). This cell line was characterized more recently by Takuwa and Ogata (1985a) and demonstrates dome formation by confluent monolayers as well as numerous microvilli on the apical membrane of the cells, which are connected by desmosomes. JTC-12 cells also exhibit marker enzyme activities corresponding to the brush border (γ-glutamyl transpeptidase, alkaline phosphatase, leucine aminopeptidase and trehalase). JTC-12 cells have retained the adenylate cyclase hormone response pattern of the PTC *in vivo*, since they are responsive to PTH but not to vasopressin or calcitonin (Ishizuka *et al.*, 1978; Malmström and Murer, 1986). Furthermore, confluent JTC-12 monolayers retain some of the functional properties of renal proximal epithelial cells, such as sodium-dependent transport of amino acids, glucose and inorganic phosphate (Takuwa and Ogata, 1985a,b) and a chloride/bicarbonate exchanger (Fineman *et al.*, 1990).

The RC-SV1 cell line

This cell line was established recently by Vandewalle *et al.* (1989). It is derived from primary cultures of rabbit cortical cells, which are enriched in proximal cells (Poujeol and Vandewalle, 1985) after SV40 transformation. The RC-SV1 line was initially derived from cultures grown in the presence of fetal calf serum and which exhibit a low degree of proximal differentiation. They were subsequently adapted to grow in serum free hormonally defined medium. In these conditions, RC-SV1 cells exhibit many of the specific properties of proximal tubule cells, including a well-developed apical brush border and the expression of apical hydrolases and also displays sodium-dependent glucose transport and an increase in cAMP production in response to PTH stimulation.

Primary Cell Cultures

Primary cultures of PTC have been successfully obtained from a variety of mammalian species using either isolated proximal tubules or cells prepared by microdissection, immunodissection or preparative fraction-ation techniques (see Table 6.4). The homogeneity and origin of the cells in a primary culture must be checked by appropriate identification methods (morphology, metabolic and transport properties, marker enzyme activities, antigenic pattern and hormone response pattern), as they depend both on the isolation and preparation methods used to obtain the PTC and the cell culture conditions, including culture medium and substratum.

Microdissection techniques

Burg et al. (1966) developed the microdissection technique in order to study transport processes by single tubule perfusion. It remains the most effective method of obtaining pure proximal tubule segments. Several groups have contributed to defining the optimum hormonal and nutritional requirements for the growth of specific nephron segments in primary culture (Horster, 1979, 1980). Almost all the epithelial cell types present in the rabbit and human nephron have now been successfully cultured in hormone-supplemented serum-free medium from individually microdis-sected nephron segments (Wilson et al., 1985, 1987). Primary cultures have been initiated from convoluted proximal tubules (PCT) and from straight proximal tubules (PST) after microdissection of rabbit and human kidney slices, thus avoiding the use of proteolytic enzymes. In contrast, it is apparently impossible to carry out microdissection of the rat kidney without proteolytic pretreatment. This is because the rat kidney contains abundant connecting tissue as well as having smaller nephrons (Jung et al., 1989). To the best of our knowledge, there has not yet been any report of the successful initiation of primary cultures from microdissected proximal tubule fragments obtained from rats.

Once the tubule fragments have been obtained, they are cultured for 3–14 days in a culture medium consisting of either RPMI 1640 or a mixture of equal volumes of DMEM/Ham's F12 supplemented with 3–10% fetal calf serum. Cell proliferation of primary cultures obtained from microdissected proximal tubule fragments begins after a latency period of 4–5 days. Wilson et al. (1987) have clearly demonstrated that

Table 6.4
Characteristics of proximal tubular cells in primary culture

Methods	Species	Characteristics[a]	References
Immuno-dissection	Rat	*Transport properties* Na$^+$/glucose transport Na$^+$/H$^+$ exchange *Hormone responsiveness* EGF *Marker enzymes* γ-GT, Alk phos	(Stanton et al., 1986) — (Stanton and Seifter, 1988)
Micro-dissection	Rabbit (PCT, PST)	*Transport properties* Na$^+$/phosphate transport *Hormone responsiveness* PTH *Marker enzymes* Alk phos, γ-GT, LAP, NaKATPase Cytox, DPP IV, Endopeptidase	(Suzuki et al., 1988) — (Wilson et al., 1987) (Tauc et al., 1989)
	Human (PCT, PST)	*Hormone responsiveness* PTH *Marker enzymes* Alk phos, γ-GT, cytox, NaKATPase	(Wilson et al., 1985)
Macro separation procedures	Rat	*Transport properties* Na$^+$/glucose transport Na$^+$/phosphate transport PAH transport *Hormone responsiveness* PTH, Insulin, EGF *Marker enzymes* Alk phos, γ-GT, NaKATPase 26-hydroxyVitD3-1α hydroxylase	(Chen et al., 1989) — (Boogaard et al., 1990) (Hatzinger and Stevens, 1989) (Larsson et al., 1986) (Chen et al., 1989)
	Mouse	*Transport properties* Na$^+$/glucose transport Na$^+$/phosphate transport Na$^+$/amino acid transport *Metabolic properties* Vitamin D metabolism	(Bell et al., 1988) (Bell et al., 1988) (Kohan and Schreiner, 1988) (Bell et al., 1988)

Table 6.4
Continued

Methods	Species	Characteristics[a]	References
		Hormone responsiveness	
		PTH, AVP, α-IL$_1$, PGF$_{2\alpha}$,	(Kohan and Schreiner, 1988)
		PGE$_1$, PGE$_2$, PGA$_1$, EGF	(Taub and Sato, 1980)
		Marker enzymes	
		Alk phos, LAP	(Bell *et al.*, 1988)
	Rabbit	*Transport properties*	
		Na$^+$/glucose transport	(Sakhrani *et al.*, 1984)
		Na$^+$/phosphate transport	(Sakhrani *et al.*, 1985)
		Na$^+$/amino acid transport	(Friedlander and Amiel, 1989)
		Na$^+$/H$^+$ exchange	(Norman *et al.*, 1987)
		PAH transport	(Yang *et al.*, 1988)
		Metabolic properties	
		PGF$_{2\alpha}$, PGE$_2$, 6-ketoPGF$_{1\alpha,}$ and TxB$_2$ production	(Alavi *et al.*, 1987)
		Hormone responsiveness	
		PTH, EGF, ANG II	(Norman *et al.*, 1987)
		Marker enzymes	
		Alk phos, γ-GT, AAP, NaKATPase	(Toutain *et al.*, 1991b)
		LAP, NAG, cathepsin B, catalase, SDH,	—
		HK, PK, G6Pase, PEPCK, FBP	(Tang *et al.*, 1989)
	Dog	*Transport properties*	
		Na$^+$/glucose transport	(Hruska *et al.*, 1986)
		Metabolic properties	
		Gluconeogenesis	(Goligorsky *et al.*, 1987)
		Vitamin D metabolism	(Yau *et al.*, 1985)
		Hormone responsiveness	
		PTH, ANG II, phenylephrine	(Goligorsky *et al.*, 1987)
		Marker enzymes	
		Alk phos, PEPCK	(Yau *et al.*, 1985)
	Human	*Transport properties*	
		Na$^+$/glucose transport	(Kempson *et al.*, 1989)
		Na$^+$/phosphate transport	(Middleton *et al.*, 1989)
		Na$^+$/amino acid transport	(States *et al.*, 1986, 1987)

Table 6.4
Continued

Methods	Species	Characteristics[a]	References
		Hormone responsiveness	
		PTH, isoproterenol, AVP,	(Middleton *et al.*, 1989)
		NorA, CAL, PGE$_2$	
		Marker enzymes	
		Alk phos, γ-GT, PK,	(Trifillis *et al.*, 1985b)
		G6Pase, FBP	
		NAG, Ac phos,	(Regec *et al.*, 1986)
		sphingomyelinase	
		βGluc,Carb anhydr, 5	(Detrisac *et al.*, 1984)
		nucleotidase	
		Galactosyltr, NADPH-	(Ghosh and
		cytCred, SDH	Chatterjee, 1987)

[a] γ-GT, γ-glutamyl transpeptidase; LAP, leucine aminopeptidase; AAP, alanine aminopeptidase; Alk. phos., alkaline phosphatase; DDP IV, dipeptidylpeptidase; Ac phosp, acid phosphatase; NAG, *N*-acetyl-β-D-glucosaminidase; cytox, cytochrome-*C*-oxido-reductase; SDH, succinate dehydrogenase; HK, hexokinase; PK, pyruvate kinase; PEPCK, phosphoenolpyruvate carboxykinase; G6Pase, glucose-6-phosphatase; FBP, fructose-1,6-biphosphatase; galactosyltr, galactosyltransferase; βGluc, βglucuronidase; Carb anhydr, carbonic anhydrase; NADPH-cytC red, NADPH cytochrome *C* reductase; PTH, parathyroid hormone; AVP, vasopressin; CAL, calcitonin; TxB2, thromboxane B2; ANG II, angiotensin II; NorA, noradrenaline; PG, prostaglandin; α-IL$_1$, α-interleukin$_1$; EGF, epidermal growth factor; PAH, *p*-aminohippurate; PCT, proximal convoluted tubule; PST, proximal straight tubule.

the rapidity with which growth is initiated is inversely proportional to the age of the donor. The proliferating PTC are then maintained in a hormonally defined serum-free medium containing transferrin, hydrocortisone or dexamethasone and insulin (Wilson *et al.*, 1987; Suzuki *et al.*, 1988). Under these conditions, primary cultures of human or rabbit PTC demonstrate high levels of membrane enzyme activity (see Table 6.4). When primary cultures of microdissected PCT are examined by transmission electron microscopy, they display more abundant microvilli and mitochondria and thicker epithelium than cultures of PST cells. Sodium-dependent transport of inorganic phosphate has also been shown to be higher in PCT cultures than in PST cultures, due to an increase in V_{max} of the transporter, but similar K_m values (Suzuki *et al.*, 1988). PTH inhibits Na$^+$/P$_i$ transport in PST cells, but not in PCT cells. The microdissection technique makes it possible to obtain primary cultures from defined portions of the rabbit or human proximal tubule, and some of their differentiated functions are preserved in culture. These highly specific models make it possible to investigate *in vitro* the differing biochemical functions and hormone response patterns found within the proximal tubule (Suzuki *et al.*, 1989). Unfortunately this valuable advantage is more than offset by the limited number of cells it provides, and so these cultures are not widely used to investigate drug-induced proximal toxicity.

Immunodissection techniques

The isolation of defined cell populations within the nephron by means of "immunodissection" is based on the supposition that each type of renal cell possesses at least one specific antigenic site. This technique was first developed by Smith and Garcia-Perez (1985), who prepared monoclonal antibodies using an established canine renal epithelial cell line (MDCK) as antigen. These antibodies were used as an immunoaffinity reagent to isolate cortical collecting duct cells from dogs for culture. More recently, this "immunodissection" technique has been successfully used to culture rat proximal cortical cells, using monoclonal antibodies against microvillus membrane proteins of rat renal cortical cells (Stanton *et al.*, 1986; Stanton and Seifter, 1988). Rat PTC were seeded on fibronectin-coated plastic dishes in a 1:1 mixture of DMEM/Ham's F12 supplemented with 5% fetal bovine serum, insulin, tri-iodothyronine, transferrin and prostaglandin E_1. The cells exhibited brush border enzyme activity, sodium-dependent transport of glucose and a sodium/proton exchanger. This method yields a relatively homogeneous population of renal cells and much larger amounts of material (1000-fold increase) than the microdissection technique. Stanton *et al.* (1986, 1988) have published several papers, but we are not aware of any other reports of primary cultures of immunodissected PTC in the literature.

Preparative fractionation methods

The limited amounts of cellular material which can be obtained for culture from microdissected PTC fragments and the difficulties inherent in obtaining large quantities of the monoclonal antibodies for the immunodissection of PTC has led to the development of preparative fractionation procedures for establishing primary cultures of PTC. Preparations of PTC obtained by preparative methods require complete characterization in order to assess the degree of purity of the structures isolated, since these methods essentially involve successive enrichment rather than the elimination of contaminant cell types. PTC primary cultures have been obtained from several species after macroseparation of well-characterized proximal tubular fragments.

Purified proximal tubular fragments can be prepared from the rabbit kidney by a procedure combining magnetic iron oxide perfusion, mechanical dissociation of the renal cortex and successive sieving steps (Hjelle *et al.*, 1981; Toutain *et al.*, 1989a, 1991b). As shown in Fig. 6.1, this procedure leads to the virtually complete elimination of the glomeruli, which are loaded with iron oxide and attracted to a permanent magnet. On the basis of marker enzyme patterns, hormone responsiveness, metabolic properties and ultrastructural examination, it has been shown that the tubular fragment preparation obtained originates mainly from the convoluted portion of the proximal tubule (Toutain *et al.*, 1989b, 1991a). These findings have recently been confirmed by the separation of two populations of proximal cells by free-flow electrophoresis: 75% of the cells were from PCT and 25% from PST (Toutain *et al.*, 1989a; Toutain and Morin, 1991). Primary cultures from rabbit proximal tubular fragments prepared in this fashion have been successfully grown in hormone supplemented serum-free media (Chung *et al.*, 1982; Sakhrani *et al.*, 1984, 1985; Toutain *et al.*, 1990, 1991b; Morin *et al.*, 1991a). It has recently been reported that the addition of a size-calibration step, by means of forced sieving through a 40-μm mesh nylon gauze, provides more homogeneous monolayers of rabbit PTC and increases the yield, since it has been shown that cell growth is initiated around the tips of proximal tubule fragments (Morin *et al.*, 1991a; Toutain *et al.*, 1991b). Purified proximal tubule fragments have been shown to attach more rapidly and more firmly to untreated plastic dishes after brief exposure to collagenase (H.J. Toutain, personal communication). Hatzinger and Stevens (1989) have shown that this method can be used to prepare rat proximal tubule cells if the cortical fragments are exposed to higher concentrations of collagenase for longer periods.

Rabbit primary PTC cultures, prepared in the way described above, have been extensively characterized and shown to express a number of differentiated properties (see Table 6.4), including dome formation, PTH-sensitive adenylate cyclase activity, sodium-dependent transport of glucose, amino acids and phosphate, as well as a sodium/proton exchanger, an organic cation carrier and prostaglandin synthesis (Sakhrani *et al.*, 1984, 1985; Alavi *et al.*, 1987; Norman *et al.*, 1987; Yang *et al.*, 1988). Using brush border membrane vesicles from the proximal tubule of the rabbit kidney, several authors have demonstrated the existence of two distinct sodium-dependent transporters of glucose within the proximal tubule (Turner and Moran, 1982a,b). The PCT segment transport system exhibits low affinity, with 1:1 sodium/glucose stoichiometry (Turner and Moran, 1982a,b; Barfuss and Schafer, 1981). Surprisingly, sodium/glucose co-transport in primary cultures of rabbit PTC have been found to be of the

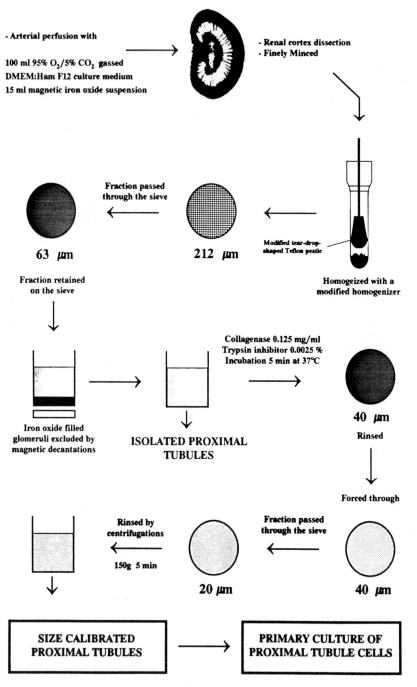

Fig. 6.1

high-affinity type, characteristic of PST, even though the proximal tubule fragments used to establish the culture are mainly of PCT origin (Sakhrani *et al.*, 1984; Alavi *et al.*, 1987). The reason for this discrepancy is not yet understood. Complete time-course analysis of marker enzyme activities has demonstrated that brush-border-associated enzyme activity declines throughout the culture period and particularly alkaline phosphatase activity (Morin *et al.*, 1991a; Toutain *et al.*, 1991b). Different authors attribute the lack of apical hydrolase activities to the confinement of these enzymes within the cytoplasmic vesicle compartment. In contrast, lactate dehydrogenase and hexokinase activities are markedly enhanced, concomitant with increased lactate production (Aleo *et al.*, 1989; Tang *et al.*, 1989; Toutain *et al.*, 1991b). These findings suggest a progressive shift towards the glycolytic pathway. Morin *et al.* (1990, 1991b) have recently demonstrated that this shift does occur and is the result of an adaptation to the high glucose concentration in the culture medium and that it is prevented in fact by total glucose deprivation.

Another effective way of preparing proximal cells or tubules for primary cultures is to subject the renal cortex to proteolytic digestion followed by purification by isopycnic centrifugation. The proteolytic digestion procedure is performed by incubating renal cortical slices with 0.075–0.3% collagenase for about 45 min. The tissue suspension is then strained to remove large debris and glomeruli. After centrifuging, the tubular fragments collected are purified further on a continuous Ficoll gradient (containing a non-ionic polymer of sucrose) or on a Percoll gradient (containing colloidal silica coated with polyvinylpyrrolidone). Discontinuous Ficoll gradients have been successfully used to purify proximal tubular fragments from rat and rabbit kidneys (Rosenberg and Michalopoulos, 1987). The use of a Percoll continuous density gradient to separate proximal tubules was first described by Vinay *et al.* (1981), who applied it to the rat kidney. This technique has since been modified slightly and used to establish primary cultures from rat, rabbit and dog proximal tubules (Chen *et al.*, 1989; Goligorsky *et al.*, 1987; Tang *et al.*, 1989). Primary cultures of PTC from rat kidney have been obtained from suspensions of single PTC purified by isopycnic centrifugation of isolated cortical cells on a discontinuous Nycodenz gradient, containing polyiodinated Percoll of low molecular weight (Boogaard *et al.*, 1989a,b, 1990).

The PTC primary cultures obtained under these conditions retain many of the biochemical properties which are characteristic of proximal tubules (see Table 6.4). For instance, dog PTC cultures express a sodium/glucose cotransport system, gluconeogenesis pathway and vitamin D metabolism (Hruska *et al.*, 1986; Goligorsky *et al.*, 1987; Yau *et al.*, 1985), whereas rat PTC cultures possess sodium-dependent systems for the transport of glucose and phosphate and also exhibit PTH-sensitive cAMP production (Chen *et al.*, 1989; Hatzinger and Stevens, 1989). Brush-border-associated enzymes decrease rapidly with time in primary cultures of rat PTC, which is consistent with results reported for rabbit PTC cultures established by other methods.

Several groups of workers have tried to establish human proximal tubular cells in primary culture using experimental procedures which avoid purification steps. Cortical explants and isolated cortical cells have both been cultured in hormonally defined medium and serum-supplemented medium (Detrisac *et al.*, 1984; Triffilis *et al.*, 1985b). These renal epithelial cell monolayers display dome formation and express other specific PTC properties, such as sodium-dependent transport of glucose, amino acids and phosphate (States *et al.*, 1987; Kempson *et al.*, 1989; Middleton *et al.*, 1989). cAMP production demonstrates PTH, isoproterenol and vasopressin sensitivity (Middleton *et al.*, 1989), which is indicative of heterogeneity within these primary cultures, since *in vivo* PTC cAMP production has been shown to be sensitive to PTH, but not to isoproterenol or vasopressin. These findings contrast with results obtained from human PTC cultures established from microdissected proximal tubule fragments (Wilson *et al.*, 1985). Compared with other species, human renal epithelial cells are easily subcultured and express several PTC functions after multiple passages (Detrisac *et al.*, 1984). However, no successful primary culture system for human PTC obtained from PTC purified by preparative methods has yet been described.

Cell culture conditions

Primary cultures of PTC established by preparative procedures are grown in a 1:1 mixture of DMEM/Ham's F12 supplemented with 2–4 mM glutamine. Hormone-supplemented serum-free medium is used to reduce uncontrolled variables and also to avoid overgrowth by fibroblasts. Primary cultures of PTC have been successfully obtained from various species, including rat, rabbit, mouse and man and cultured in hormone-supplemented serum-free media (see Table 6.5). However, it is possible to culture rat PTC in modified DMEM/Ham's F12 with 10% fetal calf serum (FCS) without any fibroblast contamination (Boogaard *et al.*, 1990) since fibroblast overgrowth is entirely prevented by replacing L-valine by D-valine and L-arginine by L-ornithine in the culture medium (Leffert and Paul, 1973; Gilbert and Migeon, 1975). Goligorsky *et al.* (1987) have demonstrated that primary cultures of dog PTC must be grown on culture medium containing 5% FCS and 5% horse serum during the growth

Table 6.5

Culture conditions of proximal tubule cells in primary culture established by preparative methods

Species	Method/support/additives[a]	References
Mouse	*Collagenase/isolated cortical cells* Untreated plastic dish Transferrin, insulin, PGE1, PS	(Blumenthal *et al.*, 1989)
	Collagenase/isolated proximal tubules Untreated or collagen-coated plastic dish Transferrin, hydrocortisone, insulin, PS	(Bell *et al.*, 1988)
	Collagenase perfusion/Percoll purification Untreated plastic dish Transferrin, hydrocortisone, insulin, Na-Selenite, PS	(Sirivongs *et al.*, 1989)
Rat	*Collagenase perfusion/Percoll purification* Untreated plastic dish Transferrin, hydrocortisone, insulin, EGF, PGE_1 10% FCS, 0.1% BSA, D-valine, L-ornithine	(Chen *et al.*, 1989) (Boogaard *et al.*, 1990)
	Magnetic iron oxide/collagenase treatment Coated plastic dish Cholera toxin, BSA, OA, insulin, EGF, PS	(Hatzinger and Stevens, 1989)
Rabbit	*Collagenase/Percoll purification* Rat tail collagen-coated dish Transferrin, dexamethasone, insulin, T_3, ethanolamine, Na-Selenite, PS	(Bello-Reuss and Weber, 1986)
	Magnetic iron oxide/mechanical dissociation Untreated plastic dish Transferrin, hydrocortisone, insulin, Na-Selenite, PS	(Taub *et al.*, 1989)
Dog	*Collagenase/Percoll purification* Plastic dish or collagen-coated porous filter 5% FCS, 5% horse serum (initiation) Transferrin, hydrocortisone, insulin, PGE_1, T_3 (growth)	(Goligorsky *et al.*, 1987)

Table 6.5
Continued

Species	Method/support/additives[a]	References
Human	*Cortical explant* Collagen-coated dish Transferrin, hydrocortisone, insulin, EGF, T_3, Na-Selenite	(Blackburn *et al.*, 1988)
	Collagenase/isolated cortical cells Untreated plastic dish 10% FCS, PS Transferrin, hydrocortisone, insulin, Selenite, PGE_1, T_3, PS	(Trifillis *et al.*, 1985b) (States *et al.*, 1986, 1987)

[a] PS, Penicillin/streptomycin; EGF, epidermal growth factor; BSA, bovine serum albumin; OA, oleic acid; FCS, fetal calf serum; T_3, tri-iodothyronine; PGE_1, prostaglandin E1.

initiation phase (lasting 1 to 3 days), since some essential growth factors have not yet been identified. Fibroblast-free confluent monolayers of dog PTC can be obtained by using hormone-supplemented serum-free medium during the exponential phase (see Table 6.5). Complete elimination of FCS from the culture medium prevents the phenotypic variations of PTC, which vary with the batch of serum used to promote growth. Elimination of serum also makes it possible to study the long-term effects of specific hormones on cultured PTC.

Table 6.5 reveals that a variety of methods have been used in the attempt to culture PTC. These vary in function of species and isolation method. Transferrin and hydrocortisone (dexamethasone) appear to be required for all species, but other factors required in rat and man include epidermal growth factor and prostaglandins (see Table 6.5). Several studies have clearly demonstrated the key role played by culture medium components on PTC phenotype expression in primary cultures (Chung *et al.*, 1982; Aleo *et al.*, 1989; Morin *et al.*, 1990, 1991b). Most primary culture media include antibiotics (penicillin/streptomycin, 50–200 IU/ml:50–200 μg/ml) at concentrations which may induce toxic effects and delay confluence (Trifillis *et al.*, 1985b; Aleo *et al.*, 1989). Antibiotic-free media must, therefore, be used when PTC primary cultures are used to assess the toxicity of test drugs.

The composition of the substratum can also influence phenotype expression by cultured PTC. Several studies have demonstrated that collagenase-treated proximal tubules or cells are able to grow on an untreated plastic substratum (Yang *et al.*, 1988; Toutain *et al.*, 1991a).

In contrast, rabbit proximal tubules purified by isopycnic centrifugation on Percoll gradients will attach only if the plastic substratum is coated with collagen (Bello-Reuss and Weber, 1986; Friedlander *et al.*, 1990). PTC cultured in this manner are more polarized, have abundant microvilli and show greater responsiveness to PTH compared with rabbit primary cultures of PTC established on an uncoated plastic substratum (Bello-Reuss and Weber, 1986). The recent development of PTC cultures on micropore systems opens the way for specific studies of basolateral transport systems, such as the organic anion *p*-aminohippuric acid carrier. This culture substratum gives nutrients and chemicals ready access to the basolateral membrane of the cells and makes it possible to investigate drug interactions preferentially affecting either the basolateral or apical surface of the cell (Boogaard *et al.*, 1990).

Use of Proximal Tubule Cells to Study *In Vitro* Nephrotoxicity

Primary cultures and continuous cell line cultures of proximal cells are now commonly used to assess the direct toxic effects of xenobiotics on PTC. Compared with other *in vitro* methods, cultured proximal cells are particularly appropriate for the investigation of the impact of xenobiotics, such as the aminoglycosides, which induce toxicity only after prolonged exposure. In the sections that follow, we will cite some examples of the use of cultured PTC to explore xenobiotic-induced nephrotoxicity.

Heavy Metals

Human exposure to heavy-metal-contaminated dusts, fumes or drinking water can result in the progressive accumulation of these metals within the kidney, where they have a biological half-life of between 20 and 30 years. When the heavy metal concentration within the renal cortex reaches a critical concentration, severe tubular damage may occur (Hazen-Martin *et al.*, 1989a). Cultured PTC have been used to determine the nephrotoxic potential of the different heavy metals. Using rat PTC, Cherian (1985) demonstrated that at a concentration of 10 μM, the cellular uptake of Pb^{2+} and of Hg^{2+} is higher than that of Cd^{2+} or Zn^{2+}. There also seems to be a correlation between the uptake of heavy metals and the *in vitro* toxic potential of the substance containing them. The same authors have also reported that the cellular uptake of Cd from Cd-metallothionein, a metal-binding protein, is much lower than that from $CdCl_2$ and that the cytotoxicity of Cd-metallothionein is about seven times greater than that induced by $CdCl_2$ in rat primary PTC cultures. Pretreatment of PTC cultures with 10 μg Cd^{2+} for several days made the cells more resistant to the heavy metals but not to the metallothionein complexes. Cherian (1985) has suggested that Cd-metallothionein injury occurs during its transport across the plasma membrane, whereas the toxic impact of inorganic Cd^{2+} occurs after it has gained access to the cell.

Hazen-Martin et al. (1989b) have shown that irreversible cell injury and death follows the exposure of primary cultures of human PTC to Cd^{2+} at concentrations of between 2 and 10 μg/ml, whereas exposure to lower concentrations (0.5–1 μg/ml) results in the death of only some cells, leaving scope for sublethal injury and possible recovery. Primary cultures of human PTC have been used to study the nephrotoxicity induced by exposure to cadmium for 20 days at low concentrations of between 0.05 and 0.5 μg/ml. At these low concentrations, cell growth and tight junctions are not affected, but changes in transport function were associated with fine structural changes (fewer apical microvilli and more endocytotic vesicles) which are revealed by transmission electron microscopy (Hazen-Martin et al., 1989a,b).

Antibiotics

The aminoglycosides

The aminoglycoside antibiotics (AG) cause a wide range of biochemical, functional and morphological damage to renal proximal tubule cells in many species of laboratory animals and in man (Morin and Fillastre, 1982; Whelton and Neu, 1982; Tulkens, 1989). High concentrations of these drugs accumulate within the PTC lysosomes (Morin et al., 1980). AG also induce phospholipidosis, which is characterized by phospholipid accumulation in the PTC lysosomes. This accumulation results in the formation of myeloid bodies which can be observed by transmission electron microscopy (Tulkens, 1989). These polycationic drugs have been shown to have high binding affinity for anionic phospholipids (phosphatidylinositol-4,5-bisphosphate, PIP_2) found within the apical membrane of PTC. This affinity results from electrostatic interactions and these phospholipids can be considered to be the biological "receptor" for these antibiotics. AG also interact with the plasma membrane, and with intracellular organelles, such as lysosomes and mitochondria, inducing proximal tubule dysfunction which can lead to cell necrosis.

The proximal toxicity of AG has been studied using $LLC-PK_1$ cells and primary cultures of PTC from rat, rabbit and man. Following exposure to AG (at concentrations of 0.1–1 mM), dome formation is inhibited in both LLC-PK$_1$ and PTC cultures and this is correlated to the decrease in Na/K-ATPase activity induced by these compounds (Hori et al., 1984). Changes in PTC biochemistry following AG treatment of animals include a decrease in brush-border-specific enzyme activities (alkaline phosphatase, γ-glutamyl transferase, alanine aminopeptidase) and of specifically lysosomal activities (N-acetyl-β-D-glucosaminidase, sphingomyelinase) (Morin and Fillastre, 1982; Hori et al., 1984; Toutain et al., 1987; Inui et al., 1988). The use of cultured PTC has helped to elucidate the mechanism of AG-induced phospholipidosis. Gentamicin inhibits agonist-stimulated generation of inositol triphosphate (IP$_3$) from PIP$_2$ (Kaloyanides and Ramsammy, 1989) and this inhibition is directly correlated to the inhibition of brush border membrane phosphatidylinositol phospholipase C (Lipsky and Lietman, 1982). This means that AG can inhibit the PI cascade. PIP$_2$ may be involved in transmembrane Ca^{2+} transport, and AG interaction with the apical membrane could affect Ca^{2+} homeostasis (Marche et al., 1987). This hypothesis was confirmed recently by Inui et al. (1988), who demonstrated an increase in the cytosolic concentration of free calcium in LLC-PK$_1$ cells exposed to gentamicin. It would appear that the formation of AG–phospholipid complexes is followed by pycnocytosis and penetration into the lysosomal compartment of the cell, where myeloid bodies are generated. Concentrations of gentamicin which have no effect on protein or DNA synthesis (1 mM) in cultures of rabbit PTC or LLC-PK$_1$ cells have been shown to induce phospholipidosis, characterized by a marked increase in the intracellular levels of phosphatidylinositol (PI and PIP$_2$), phosphatidylcholine (PC) and phosphatidylserine (PS) (Schwertz et al., 1986; Ramsammy et al., 1989). Studies carried out using cultured rabbit PTC suggest that the mechanisms responsible for the increase in intralysosomal levels of phospholipids (PL) in cells exposed to gentamicin may involve an increase in endogenous biosynthesis of PI and PS, associated with a marked decrease in the catabolism of PL (Ramsammy et al., 1989). The mechanism by which the AG inhibit lysosomal phospholipases and catabolism of PL remains to be elucidated. Several authors have postulated a pH-mediated inhibition of intralysosomal phospholipase activities by AG antibiotics, since at least four protons can be bound per molecule, making it possible for the drug to accumulate within these organelles at concentrations of up to 20 mM (Regec et al., 1986; Ghosh and Chatterjee, 1987). Using cultured human proximal tubule cells, Regec et al. (1989) have shown that the decrease in sphingomyelinase activity cannot be explained by an increase in the intralysosomal pH. Indeed, whereas the intralysosomal concentration of AG is dose-dependent, the pH remains constant at all dose levels. Poly-L-aspartic acid (PAA) protects against AG-induced nephrotoxicity (Williams *et al.*, 1986). Kaloyanides and Ramsammy (1989), using the OK cell line, have shown that PAA completely blocks both the accumulation of PL within the lysosomes and the AG-induced inhibition of PL catabolism, whereas it has no effect on intralysosomal accumulation of AG. It appears, therefore, that AG-induced nephrotoxicity is causally linked to modification of PL metabolism by AG, rather than dependent on the intralysosomal concentration of AG.

The exposure of LLC-PK$_1$ cells to AG has been shown to induce a significant decrease in the cellular cAMP content, which is consistent with *in vivo* data reported by Wilson *et al.* (1981), who have demonstrated a decrease in nephrogenic cAMP production due to the inhibition of both basal and forskolin-stimulated adenylate cyclase activity.

Several groups have reported inhibition of the sodium-dependent glucose transporter in both LLC-PK$_1$ cells and cultured rat PTC by gentamicin (10–100 μM) (Inui *et al.*, 1988; Boogaard *et al.*, 1990). Gentamicin does not bind directly to the sodium-dependent glucose transport system, since preincubation of cultured cells with gentamicin does not completely inhibit this transport system, whereas it is totally inactivated by phlorizin (Chung *et al.*, 1982; Inui *et al.*, 1988). Nevertheless, this inhibition, which is not directly related to the toxic mechanism of action of the AG, could provide a useful tool with which to assess the functional impairment of cultured PTC after exposure to low doses of AG. In contrast, LDH release appears to be a relatively insensitive indicator of AG-induced PTC toxicity *in vitro*. Chronic exposure (7–14 days) to gentamicin at 10 mg/ml is required before LDH release is detected, whereas the highest recommended serum concentration in therapeutic use is 12 μg/ml (Regec *et al.*, 1986; Sens *et al.*, 1989). There is a close correlation between the *in vitro* effects of various AG antibiotics on dome formation, cell growth, cellular cAMP content and brush border enzyme activities in cultured PTC and the effects reported *in vivo* (Whelton and Neu, 1982; Hori *et al.*, 1984; Inui *et al.*, 1988; Sens *et al.*, 1989).

The cephalosporins

The first two cephalosporin antibiotics to be discovered (cephalothin and cephaloridine) were found to be nephrotoxic. It has been generally supposed that the numerous cephalosporin antibiotics are all nephrotoxic, but this is in fact far from the case, and most cephalosporins, particularly those of the 2nd and 3rd generations, are not nephrotoxic (Walker and Duggin, 1988). Like all β-lactams, the cephalosporins are weak organic acids. The carboxyl group on the C-4 position is almost entirely ionized at physiological pH values (Fig. 6.2). This anionic state is essential to tubular secretion, which involves the *p*-aminohippurate and other organic anion transporters (Tune, 1986). Cephaloridine is rapidly taken up by the basolateral membrane, but its passage from the cell into the lumen is hampered by the cationic nature of the quarternary nitrogen on the pyridinium side of the ring (Fig. 6.2). The result is that the area under the curve (AUC) of cephaloridine is extremely high compared with other cephalosporins (Tune and Hsu, 1990). The zwitterionic properties of cephaloridine lead to high and sustained intracellular concentrations which almost certainly contribute to the high nephrotoxicity of this drug. However, cephaloridine is not the only nephrotoxic cephalosporin and several other mechanisms have been proposed to account for cephalosporin-induced nephrotoxicity. These include spontaneous acylation of molecular targets by the cephalosporins as a result of the intrinsic reactivity of the β-lactam ring, toxicity affecting mitochondrial respiration and lipid peroxidation of cell membrane.

Cultured PTC have not been extensively used to investigate cephaloridine nephrotoxicity. Using LDH leakage, Smith *et al.* (1987) have shown that the exposure of primary cultures of rat PTC to 20 μM cephaloridine for 4–12 h does not induce severe PTC lethality, but that it does induce impairment of Na/K-ATPase activity, which is indicative of compromised integrity of the plasma membrane and inhibition of mitochondrial succinate dehydrogenase. This study also demonstrated that in response to exposure to cephaloridine, the cellular GSH content, an important factor in cellular protection, was significantly reduced. Boogaard *et al.* (1990) have shown in a recent study that exposure to 10 μM cephaloridine for 12 h reduced α-methylglucoside uptake in rat PTC primary cultures by 30%. These data demonstrate that *in vitro* exposure to the cephalosporins can impair specific functions in cultured cells at concentrations relevant to the *in vivo* situation. These data suggest that primary cultures of PTC provide a reliable way of investigating direct renal cell responses to cephalosporin-induced toxicity. Thus, Williams *et al.* (1990) have reported very close *in*

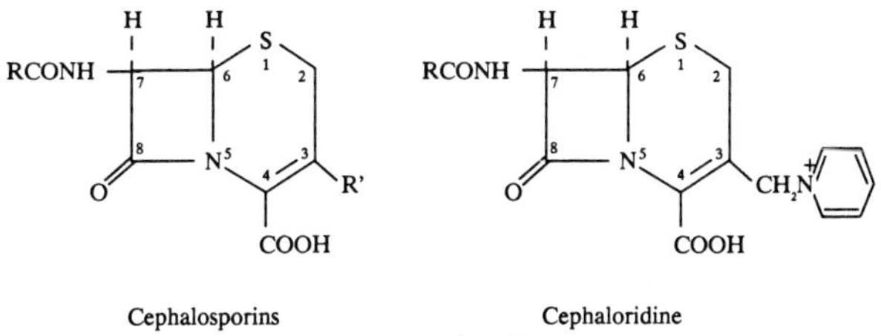

Cephalosporins   Cephaloridine

Fig. 6.2

vivo/in vitro correlation for several cephalosporins between the *in vivo* assessment of the nephrotoxic potential, based on clinical chemistry and histopathology, and the concentration producing 50% lethality in the LLC-PK$_1$ cell line *in vitro*.

Cyclosporin

Cyclosporin A (CSA) is a neutral highly lipophilic cyclic undecapeptide of fungal origin with a novel immunosuppressive action. CSA is now used extensively in solid organ and bone-marrow transplantation. The nephrotoxicity of CSA is associated with dose-dependent renal haemodynamic changes affecting the renal vascular resistance, renal blood flow and glomerular filtration rate and with impaired tubular function (Whiting, 1990).

CSA nephrotoxicity has been investigated *in vitro* using both the LLC-PK$_1$ cell line and primary cultures of human PTC. Exposure of PTC cultures to 0.4–10 μg CSA/ml for 6–7 days increased the number of cytoplasmic vacuoles in a manner which was related to both the concentration and duration of exposure (Becker *et al.*, 1987; Walker *et al.*, 1989). Transmission electron microscopy revealed large amorphous non-membrane-bound cytoplasmic inclusions and increased numbers of lipid droplets (Trifillis *et al.*, 1985a). CSA induced morphological changes in PTC cultures which were similar to the focal tubular cell vacuolization and tubular atrophy observed in renal biopsies from patients on CSA and in kidneys from rats exposed to nephrotoxic doses of CSA (Mihatsch *et al.*, 1989). These morphological changes occurred *in vitro* at concentrations that are relevant to the therapeutic use of the drug, since whole blood levels in rats fed with 25 and 50 mg/kg per day were 4.55 μg/ml and 5.17 μg/ml respectively (Walker *et al.*, 1989).

In the LLC-PK$_1$ cell line, the intracellular concentration of CSA following incubation with 10 μg CSA/ml (5.1–6.7 μg/mg protein) for 2 h was comparable with the renal tissue levels of CSA found in rats fed with 25 and 50 mg/kg per day (7.4 and 8.8 μg/mg protein respectively) (Walker *et al.*, 1989). CSA uptake by the LLC-PK$_1$ cells was rapid, and intracellular levels over a 24 h period varied little from the values reported after 2 h. In view of the highly lipophilic properties of CSA, these findings are consistent with rapid partitioning of the drug by saturable mechanism into the lipid component of the cell membranes.

High concentrations of CSA (10 and 20 μg/ml) inhibit cell growth of the LLC-PK$_1$ cell line, and this is correlated with impairment of DNA and protein synthesis (Becker *et al.*, 1987; Walker *et al.*, 1989). These effects are produced by the same range of concentrations of CSA and the immunologically inert cyclosporin-H (CSH), which differs from CSA by the substitution of the L-isomer of methylvaline for the D-isomer at the 11 position. CSH reportedly induces little or no nephrotoxicity in experimental animals. This suggests that the molecular structure of the cyclosporins may play a key role in determining their cellular toxicity, essentially through modifications of their liposolubility and the extent to which they are bound to cell membranes. The nephrotoxicity demonstrated by CSA is thus probably the outcome of a series of subtoxic changes affecting proximal cell function and other renal functions.

Cisplatin

Cisplatin (*cis*-diamminedichloroplatinum (II)) (cDDP) is a drug widely used in the treatment of human neoplasms. The chemotherapeutic value of this drug is severely hampered by its nephrotoxicity. The exact mechanism of platinum-induced nephrotoxicity has not yet been elucidated, but several studies have shown that cDDP-induced nephrotoxicity is associated with the inactivation of cellular enzymes, impairment of mitochondrial function, interaction with renal membrane transport processes and the formation of lipid peroxides (Tay *et al.*, 1988; Hannemann and Baumann, 1990).

Exposure of rabbit renal cortical cells in primary culture to 12 μM cDDP for 10 h has been shown to inhibit the synthesis of protein, DNA and RNA (Tay *et al.*, 1988; Williams, 1989), which correlates closely with *in vivo* observations. In contrast, LLC-PK$_1$ cells are not very sensitive to cDDP, because toxic effects were detected only after exposure to concentrations in excess of 100 μM for 72 h. Several authors have ascribed this sensitivity difference between LLC-PK$_1$ cells and primary cultures of PTC to the absence of energy-consuming cDDP accumulation in LLC-PK$_1$ cells (Safirstein *et al.*, 1987). However, the synthesis of protein and RNA was inhibited by exposure to cDDP, whereas DNA synthesis remained unchanged. Tay *et al.* (1988) have reported inhibition of both alkaline phosphatase and Na/K ATPase activity in primary cultures of rabbit proximal tubule cells after exposure to 33–100 μM cDDP for 24 h, whereas succinate dehydrogenase activity was unaffected. Inhibition of alkaline phosphatase and Na/K ATPase activities does not occur during an early phase of cDDP-induced nephrotoxicity, since there is no reduction of the activity of either enzyme after incubation for 6 h. The inhibition observed may then be an effect of cDDP-induced nephrotoxicity, rather than the cause of this injury. Boogaard *et al.* (1990) have shown that α-methylglucoside uptake by primary cultures of PTC provides a very sensitive index of cDDP nephrotoxicity, since a 28% inhibition is found after exposure to 0.1 μM cDDP for 40 h.

The high incident of cDDP-induced nephrotoxicity has provided the impetus for the development of biochemical and pharmacological strategies intended to reduce the toxic potential. Sodium thiosulphate and sodium diethyldithiocarbamate (DDTC) are both highly effective in reducing the *in vivo* nephrotoxicity (Borch and Markman, 1989; Borch and Montine, 1990). The *in vitro* toxic effects of cDDP on the LLC-PK$_1$ cell line can also be reduced by these two compounds (Montine and Borch, 1988). Simultaneous exposure of LLC-PK$_1$ cells to cDDP (300 μM) and either sodium thiosulphate or DDTC (3 mM) gave 72-h viability values of 72% and 93%, compared with the 33% viability found after exposure to 300 μM cDDP alone (Borch and Montine, 1990).

It is the stereospecificity of cDDP which determines its toxic potential, so that although cDDP and *trans*-diamminedichloroplatinum (II) (tDDP) result in similar concentrations of platinum, the *trans*-isomer does not produce renal toxicity (Fillastre and Raguenez-Viotte, 1989). The toxicity of tDDP has been demonstrated to be about one-fifth as great as cDDP. Non-nephrotoxic analogues, carboplatin and iproplatin, have no toxic effects on LLC-PK$_1$ cells at concentrations as high as 2 mM (Borch and Montine, 1990; Hannemann and Baumann, 1990).

Conclusion

The development of proximal tubular cell culture systems with which to study the cellular uptake, metabolism and toxicity of chemical-induced nephrotoxicity has markedly intensified during the past decade. Several cultured PTC models have been established from primary cultures derived from various species using a variety of cell culture techniques and conditions, as well as from established cell lines which retain some of the differentiated properties of the original cells. The advantages of using cultured PTC in studies of xenobiotic-induced PTC injury are many and obvious. Cultured PTC systems make it possible to perform studies involving long or short periods of exposure to a wide range of xenobiotic concentrations under strictly controlled conditions without inducing the metabolic, functional or compensatory responses which would occur in the more complex *in vivo* situation. However, they are subject to specific limitations. The expressed phenotype of PTC varies considerably with cell culture conditions (methods of PTC isolation, culture media, presence or absence of serum and growth factors, culture substrata and the nature of the extracellular matrix). Consequently, experimental models of this type can be used to investigate drug-induced nephrotoxicity only after exhaustive characterization of their properties, so that valid conclusions can be drawn from *in vitro* mechanism studies.

Cultured PTC and in particular primary culture systems which exhibit some of the biochemical, functional and morphological characteristics of PTC *in vivo* have demonstrated their usefulness for investigating the mechanisms by which nephrotoxicity is induced by drugs such as the aminoglycosides, cephaloridine and cisplatin. Results from *in vitro* studies at therapeutic concentrations correlate closely with those observed *in vivo*. There have been some reports of the use of cultured PTC in the nephrotoxicity screening of new drugs, but no validation strategy has yet been defined. It will be necessary to define and standardize several parameters for assessment but not necessarily a high level of interpretability regarding mechanism.

It is anticipated that studies of cultured PTC systems will be carried out during the next decade to validate their use in assessing chemical nephrotoxicity. This should establish their credibility as *in vitro* models for use in screening and in mechanism studies as an adjunct to *in vivo* experiments.

Acknowledgements

We thank Roselyne Reibaud for her invaluable assistance with the documentary aspects of this paper.

References

Abraham, M.I., McAteer, J.A. and Kempson, S.A. (1990). *Kidney Int.* **37**, 452.
Agarwal, N., Haggerty, J.G., Adelberg, E.A. and Slayman, C.A. (1986). *Am. J. Physiol.* **251**, C825–C830.
Alavi, N., Lianos, E.A. and Bentzel, C.J. (1987). *J. Lab. Clin. Med.* **110**, 338–345.
Aleo, M.D., Taub, M.L., Nickerson, P.A. and Kostyniak, P.J. (1989). *In Vitro Cell. Dev. Biol.* **25**, 776–783.
Ausiello, D.A., Hall, D.H. and Dayer, J.M. (1980). *Biochem. J.* **186**, 773–780.
Ausiello, D.A., Skorecki, K.L., Verkman, A.S. and Bonventre, J.V. (1987). *Kidney Int.* **31**, 521–529.
Bach, P. and Lock, E.A. (1982). *In* "Nephrotoxicity, Assessment and Pathogenesis" (P.H. Bach, F.W. Bonner, J.W. Bridges and E.A. Lock, eds), pp. 128–134. John Wiley, Chichester.
Barfuss, D.W. and Schafer, J.A. (1981). *Am. J. Physiol.* **241**, F322–F332.
Becker, G.M., Gandolfi, A.J. and Nagle, R.B. (1987). *Res. Commun. Chem. Pathol. Pharmacol.* **56**, 277–280.

Bekersky, I. (1985). *Rev. Biochem. Toxicol.* **7**, 139–157.

Bell, C.L., Tenenhouse, H.S. and Scriver, C.R. (1988). *In Vitro Cell. Dev. Biol.* **24**, 683–695.

Bello-Reuss, E. and Weber, M.R. (1986). *Am. J. Physiol.* **251**, F490–F498.

Blackburn, J.G., Hazen-Martin, D.J., Detrisac, C.J. and Sens, D. (1988). *Kidney Int.* **33**, 508–516.

Blumenthal, S.S., Lewand, D.L., Buday, M.A., Mandel, N.S. and Kleinman, J.G. (1989). *Am. J. Physiol.* **257**, C419–C426.

Boogaard, P.J., Mulder, G.J. and Nagelkerke, J.F. (1989a). *Toxicol. Appl. Pharmacol.* **101**, 135–143.

Boogaard, P.J., Mulder, G.J. and Nagelkerke, J.F. (1989b). *Toxicol. Appl. Pharmacol.* **101**, 144–157.

Boogaard, P.J., Zoeteweij, J.P., VanBerkel, T.J.C., VanTNoordende, J.M., Mulder, G.J. and Nagelkerke, J.F. (1990). *Biochem. Pharmacol.* **39**, 1335–1345.

Borch, R.F. and Markman, M. (1989). *Pharmacol. Ther.* **41**, 371–380.

Borch, R.F. and Montine, T.J. (1990). *Toxicol. Lett.* **53**, 93–96.

Brendel, K., Gandolfi, A.J., Krumdieck, C.L. and Smith, P.F. (1987). *Trends Pharmacol. Sci.* **8**, 11–15.

Brown, C.D.A. and Murer, H. (1985). *J. Membr. Biol.* **87**, 131–139.

Burg, M.B., Grantham, J.J., Abramow, M. and Orloff, J. (1966). *Am. J. Physiol.* **210**, 1293–1298.

Cantiello, H.F., Scott, J. and Robito, C. (1986). *J. Biol. Chem.* **261**, 3252–3258.

Carlson, E.C., Brendel, K., Hjelle, J.T. and Meezan, E. (1978). *J. Ultrastruct. Res.* **62**, 26–53.

Caverzasio, J. and Bonjour, J.P. (1989). *Am. J. Physiol.* **257**, F712–F717.

Chaillet, J.R., Amsler, K. and Boron, W.F. (1986). *Proc. Natl. Acad. Sci. U.S.A.* **83**, 522–526.

Chang, H., Yamashita, N., Matsunaga, H. and Kurokawa, K. (1988). *J. Membr. Biol.* **103**, 263–272.

Chen, T.C., Curthoys, N.P., Lagenaur, C.F. and Puschett, J.B. (1989). *In Vitro Cell. Dev. Biol.* **25**, 714–722.

Cheng, L., Liang, C.T., Precht, P. and Sacktor, B. (1988). *Biochem. Biophys. Res. Commun.* **155**, 74–82.

Cheng, L., Precht, P., Frank, D. and Liang, C.T. (1990). *Am. J. Physiol.* **258**, F877–F882.

Cherian, M.G. (1985). *In Vitro Cell. Dev. Biol.* **21**, 505–508.

Chuman, L., Fine, L.G., Cohen, A.H. and Saier, M.H. (1982). *J. Cell Biol.* **94**, 506–510.

Chung, S.D., Alavi, N., Livingston, D., Hiller, S. and Taub, M. (1982). *J. Cell Biol.* **95**, 118–126.

Cole, L.A., Scheid, J.M. and Tannen, R.L. (1986). *Am. J. Physiol.* **251**, C293–C298.

Costa, E.M. and Feldman, D. (1987). *J. Bone Min. Res.* **2**, 151–159.

Detrisac, C.J., Sens, M.A., Garvin, A.J., Spicer, S.S. and Sens, D.A. (1984). *Kidney Int.* **25**, 383–390.

Fauth, C., Rossier, B. and Roch-Ramel, F. (1988). *Am. J. Physiol.* **254**, F351–F357.

Fillastre, J.P. and Raguenez-Viotte (1989). *Toxicol. Lett.* **46**, 163–175.

Fineman, I., Hart, D. and Nord, E.P. (1990). *Am. J. Physiol.* **258**, F883–F892.

Friedlander, G. and Amiel, C. (1989). *J. Biol. Chem.* **264**, 3935–3941.

Friedlander, G., Le Grimellec, C. and Amiel, C. (1990). *Biochim. Biophys. Acta* **1022**, 1–7.

Garg, L.C., Wozniak, M. and Phillips, I. (1990). *J. Pharmacol. Exp. Ther.* **252**, 552–557.

Ghosh, P. and Chatterjee, S. (1987). *J. Biol. Chem.* **262**, 12550–12556.

Gilbert, S.F. and Migeon, B.R. (1975). *Cell* **5**, 11–17.

Goligorsky, M.S., Osborne, D., Howard, T., Hruska, K.A. and Karl, I.E. (1987). *Am. J. Physiol.* **253**, F802–F809.

Goodyer, P.R. and Kachra, Z. (1985). *Clin. Res.* **33**, 485A.

Gstraunthaler, G. (1988). *Renal Physiol. Biochem.* **11**, 1–42.

Gstraunthaler, G. and Handler, J. (1987). *Am. J. Physiol.* **252**, C181–C185.

Gstraunthaler, G., Pfaller, W. and Kotanko, P. (1985a). *Am. J. Physiol.* **248**, C181–C183.

Gstraunthaler, G., Pfaller, W. and Kotanko, P. (1985b). *Am. J. Physiol.* **248**, F536–F544.

Hannemann, J. and Baumann, K. (1990). *Arch. Toxicol.* **64**, 393–400.

Hatzinger, P.B. and Stevens, J.L. (1989). *In Vitro Cell. Dev. Biol.* **25**, 205–212.

Hazen-Martin, D.J., Sens, D.A., Blackburn, J.G. and Sens, M.A. (1989a). *In Vitro Cell. Dev. Biol.* **25**, 784–790.

Hazen-Martin, D.J., Sens, D.A., Blackburn, J.G., Flath, M.C. and Sens, M.A. (1989b). *In Vitro Cell. Dev. Biol.* **25**, 791–799.

Helmle-Kolb, C., Montrose, M.H., Strange, G. and Muere, H. (1990). *Pflügers Arch.* **415**, 461–470.

Hjelle, J.T., Morin, J.P. and Trouet, A. (1981). *Kidney Int.* **20**, 71–77.

Hori, R., Yamamoto, K., Saito, H., Kohno, M. and Inui, K.I. (1984). *J. Pharmacol. Exp. Ther.* **230**, 742–748.

Horster, M. (1979). *Pflügers Arch.* **382**, 209–215.

Horster, M. (1980). *Int. J. Biochem.* **12**, 29–35.

Hruska, K.A., Goligorsky, M., Scoble, J., Tsutsumi, M., Westbrook, S. and Moskowitz, D. (1986). *Am. J. Physiol.* **251**, F188–F198.

Hull, R.N., Cherry, W.R. and Weaver, G.W. (1976). *In Vitro* **12**, 670–677.

Husted, R.F., Welsh, M.J. and Stokes, J.B. (1986). *Am. J. Physiol.* **250**, C214–C221.

Inui, K., Saito, H. and Hori, R. (1985a). *Biochem. J.* **227**, 199–203.

Inui, K., Saito, H., Matsukawa, Y., Nakao, K., Morii, N., Imura, H., Shimokura, M., Kiso, Y. and Hori, R. (1985b). *Biochem. Biophys. Res. Commun.* **132**, 253–260.

Inui, K., Saito, H., Iwata, T. and Hori, R. (1988). *Am. J. Physiol.* **254**, C251–C257.

Ishizuka, I., Tadano, K., Nagata, N., Niimura, Y. and Nagai, Y. (1978). *Biochim. Biophys. Acta* **541**, 467–482.

Jans, D.A., Resink, T.J., Wilson, L.E., Reich, E. and Hemmings, B.A. (1986). *Eur. J. Biochem.* **160**, 407–412.

Jung, K.Y., Uchida, S. and Endou, H. (1989). *Toxicol. Appl. Pharmacol.* **100**, 369–382.

Kaloyanides, G.J. and Ramsammy, L.S. (1989). *In* "Nephrotoxicity, *In-Vitro* to *In-Vivo*, Animals to Man" (P.H. Bach and E.A. Lock, eds), pp. 193–200. Plenum Press, New York.

Kempson, S.A., McAteer, J.A., Al-Mahrouq, H.A., Dousa, T.P., Dougherty, G.S. and Evan, A.P. (1989). *J. Lab. Clin. Med.* **113**, 285–296.

Kohan, D.E. and Schreiner, G.F. (1988). *Am. J. Physiol.* **254**, F879–F886.
Koyama, H., Goodpasture, C., Miller, M.M., Teplitz, R.L. and Riggs, A.D. (1978). *In Vitro* **14**, 239–246.
Kreisberg, J.I. and Wilson, P.D. (1988). *J. Electron Microsc. Tech.* **9**, 235–263.
Larsson, S., Aperia, A. and Lechene, C. (1986). *Am. J. Physiol.* **251**, C455–C464.
Lash, L.H. (1989). *In* "*In-Vitro* Toxicology Models Systems and Methods" (C.A. McQueen, ed.), pp. 231–262. Telford Press, Caldwell.
Leffert, H. and Paul, D. (1973). *J. Cell. Physiol.* **81**, 113–124.
Lifschitz, M.D. (1982). *J. Biol. Chem.* **257**, 12611–12615.
Lipsky, J.J. and Lietman, P.S. (1982). *J. Pharmacol. Exp. Ther.* **220**, 287–292.
Maack, T. (1986). *Kidney Int.* **30**, 142–151.
Malmström, K. and Murer, H. (1986). *Am. J. Physiol.* **251**, C23–C31.
Malmström, K., Strange, G. and Murer, H. (1987). *Biochim. Biophys. Acta* **902**, 269–277.
Marche, P., Olier, B., Girard, A., Fillastre, J.P. and Morin, J.P. (1987). *Kidney Int.* **31**, 59–64.
Matsumoto, T., Kawanobe, Y. and Ogata, E. (1985). *Biochim. Biophys. Acta* **845**, 358–365.
Middleton, J.P., Dunham, C.B., Onorato, J.J., Sens, D.A. and Dennis, V.W. (1989). *Am. J. Physiol.* **257**, F631–F638.
Mihatsch, M.J., Thiel, G. and Ryffel, B. (1989). *Toxicol. Lett.* **46**, 125–139.
Montine, T.J. and Borch, R.F. (1988). *Cancer Res.* **48**, 6017–6024.
Morin, J.P. and Fillastre, J.P. (1982). *In* "The Aminoglycosides: Microbiology, Clinical Use and Toxicology" (A. Whelton and H.C. Neu, eds), pp. 303–324. Marcel Dekker, New York.
Morin, J.P., Viotte, G., Vandewalle, A., Van Hoof, F., Tulkens, P. and Fillastre, J.P. (1980). *Kidney Int.* **18**, 583–590.
Morin, J.P., Toutain, H., Molon-Noblot, S. and Fillastre, J.P. (1992). *Eur. J. Cell Biol.* in press.
Morin, J.P., Toutain, H., Vauclin-Jacques, N. and Fillastre, J.P. (1991a). *In* "Nephrotoxicity: Early Diagnosis and Therapeutic Management" (P.H. Bach, N.J. Gregg, M.F. Wilks and L. Delacruz, eds), pp. 433–438. Marcel Dekker, New York.
Morin, J.P., Toutain, H., Vauclin-Jacques, N. and Fillastre, J.P. (1991b). *In* "Nephrotoxicity: Early Diagnosis and Therapeutic Management" (P.H. Bach, N.J. Gregg, M.F. Wilks and L. Delacruz, eds), pp. 421–426. Marcel Dekker, New York.
Mullin, J.M., Weibel, J., Diamond, L. and Kleinzeller, A. (1980). *J. Cell. Physiol.* **104**, 375–389.
Murphy, T.J. and Bylund, D.B. (1988). *J. Pharmacol. Exp. Ther.* **244**, 571–578.
Murphy, T.J. and Bylund, D.B. (1989). *J. Pharmacol. Exp. Ther.* **249**, 535–543.
Nakai, M., Fukase, M., Kinoshita, Y. and Fujita, T. (1988). *Biochem. Biophys. Res. Commun.* **152**, 1416–1420.
Napoli, J.L. (1986). *J. Biol. Chem.* **261**, 13592–13597.
Napoli, J.L. and Martin, C.A. (1984). *Biochem. J.* **219**, 713–717.
Norman, J., Badie-Dezfooly, B., Nord, E.P., Kurtz, I., Schlosser, J., Chaudhari, A. and Fine, L. (1987). *Am. J. Physiol.* **253**, F299–F309.
Parys, J.B., DeSmedt, H. and Borghgraef, R. (1986). *Biochim. Biophys. Acta* **888**, 70–81.
Phelps, J.S., Gandolfi, A.J., Brendel, K. and Dorr, R.T. (1987). *Toxicol. Appl. Pharmacol.* **90**, 501–512.

Poujeol, P. and Vandewalle, A. (1985). *Am. J. Physiol.* **249**, F74–F83.
Quamme, G., Biber, J. and Murer, H. (1989). *Am. J. Physiol.* **257**, F967–F973.
Rabito, C.A. (1981). *Biochim. Biophys. Acta* **649**, 286–296.
Rabito, C.A. (1983). *Am. J. Physiol.* **245**, F22–F31.
Rabito, C.A. (1986). *Am. J. Physiol.* **250**, F734–F743.
Rabito, C.A. and Karish, M.V. (1983a). *J. Biol. Chem.* **257**, 6802–6808.
Rabito, C.A. and Karish, M.V. (1983b). *J. Biol. Chem.* **258**, 2543–2547.
Rabito, C.A., Jarell, J.A. and Abraham, E.H. (1987). *J. Biol. Chem.* **262**, 1352–1357.
Ramsammy, L.S., Josepovitz, C., Lane, B. and Kaloyanides, G.J. (1989). *Am. J. Physiol.* **256**, C204–C213.
Regec, A.L., Trifillis, A.L. and Trump, B.F. (1986). *Toxicol. Pathol.* **14**, 238–241.
Regec, A.L., Trump, B.F. and Trifillis, A. (1989). *Biochem. Pharmacol.* **38**, 2527–2534.
Rizzoli, R. and Boujour, J.P. (1987). *J. Cell. Physiol.* **132**, 517–523.
Rosenberg, M.R. and Michalopoulos, G. (1987). *J. Cell. Physiol.* **131**, 107–113.
Roy, C. (1985). *Am. J. Physiol.* **248**, C425–C435.
Roy, C., Preston, A.S. and Handler, J. (1980). *Proc. Natl. Acad. Sci. U.S.A.* **77**, 5979–5983.
Ruegg, C.E., Gandolfi, A.J., Nagle, R.B. and Brendel, K. (1987). *Toxicol. Appl. Pharmacol.* **90**, 261–273.
Ruegg, C.E., Wolfgang, G.H.I., Gandolfi, J.A. and Brendel, K. (1989). *In "In Vitro* Toxicology Models Systems and Methods" (C.A. McQueen, ed.), pp. 197–230. Telford Press, Caldwell.
Rylander, L.A., Gandolfi, A.J. and Brendel, K. (1985). *In* "Renal Heterogeneity and Target Cell Toxicity" (P.H. Bach and E.A. Lock, eds), pp. 531–534. John Wiley, Chichester.
Safirstein, R., Winston, J., Moel, D., Dikman, S. and Guttenplan, J. (1987). *Int. J. Androl.* **10**, 325–346.
Sakhrani, L.M., Badie-Dezfooly, B., Trizna, W., Mikhail, N., Lowe, A.G., Taub, M. and Fine, L. (1984). *Am. J. Physiol.* **246**, F757–F764.
Sakhrani, L.M., Tessitore, N. and Massry, S.G. (1985). *Am. J. Physiol.* **249**, F346–F355.
Schaeffer, V.H. and Stevens, J.L. (1986). *Mol. Pharmacol.* **31**, 506–512.
Schwegler, J.S., Heuner, A. and Silbernagl, S. (1989). *Pflügers Arch.* **414**, 543–550.
Schwertz, D.W., Kreisberg, J.I. and Vankatachalam, M.A. (1986). *J. Pharmacol. Exp. Ther.* **236**, 254–262.
Sens, M.A., Hazen-Martin, D.J., Blackburn, J.G., Hennigar, G.R. and Sens, D.A. (1989). *Ann. Clin. Lab. Sci.* **19**, 266–279.
Sepulveda, F.V. and Pearson, J.D. (1985). *In* "Tissue Culture of Epithelial Cells" (M. Taub, ed.), pp. 87–104. Plenum Press, New York.
Siegers, C.P., Denker, S. and Steffen, B. (1987). *Mol. Toxicol.* **1**, 335–339.
Sina, J.F., Noble, C., Bean, C.L. and Bradley, M.O. (1989). *In "In Vitro* Toxicology Models Systems and Methods" (C.A. McQueen, ed.), pp. 263–290, Telford Press, Caldwell.
Sirivongs, D., Nakagawa, Y., Vishny, W.K., Favus, M.J. and Coe, F.L. (1989). *Am.J. Physiol.* **257**, F390–F398.
Smith, J.H. (1988). *Fundam. Appl. Toxicol.* **11**, 132–142.
Smith, M.A., Acosta, D. and Bruckner, J.V. (1987). *Toxicol. in Vitro* **1**, 23–29.
Smith, W.L. and Garcia-Perez, A. (1985). *Am. J. Physiol.* **248**, F1–F7.

Stanton, R.C. and Seifter, J.L. (1988). *Am. J. Physiol.* **253**, C267–C271.
Stanton, R.C., Mendrick, D.L., Rennke, H.G. and Seifter, J.L. (1986). *Am. J. Physiol.* **251**, C780–C786.
Stassen, F.L., Heckman, G., Schmidt, D., Papadopoulos, M.T., Nambi, P., Sarau, H., Aiyar, N., Gellai, M. and Kinter, L. (1988). *Mol. Pharmacol.* **33**, 218–224.
States, B., Foreman, J., Lee, J., Harris, D. and Segal, S. (1986). *Biochem. Med. Metab. Biol.* **36**, 151–161.
States, B., Foreman, J., Lee, J., Harris, D. and Segal, S. (1987). *Metabolism* **36**, 356–362.
Stevens, J., Hayden, P. and Taylor, G. (1986). *J. Biol. Chem.* **261**, 3325–3332.
Striker, L.J., Tannen, R.L., Lange, M.A. and Striker, G.E. (1988). *In* "International Review of Experimental Pathology" (G.W. Richter and K. Solez, eds), vol. 30, pp. 55–105. Academic Press, New York.
Sudol, M. and Reich, E. (1984). *Biochem. J.* **219**, 917–978.
Suzuki, M., Capparelli, A., Jo, O.D., Kawagushi, Y., Ogura, Y., Miyahara, T. and Yanagawa, N. (1988). *Kidney Int.* **34**, 268–272.
Suzuki, M., Kawaguchi, Y., Kurihara, S. and Miyahara, T. (1980). *Am. J. Physiol.* **257**, F724–F731.
Takaoka, T. and Katsuta, H. (1962). *Jpn. J. Exp. Med.* **32**, 351–368.
Takuwa, Y. and Ogata, E. (1985a). *In Vitro Cell. Dev. Biol.* **21**, 445–449.
Takuwa, Y. and Ogata, E. (1985b). *Biochem. J.* **230**, 715–721.
Tang, M.J., Suresh, K.R. and Tannen, R.L. (1989). *Am. J. Physiol.* **256**, C532–C539.
Taub, M. and Sato, G. (1980). *J. Cell. Physiol.* **105**, 369–378.
Tauc, M., Merot, J., Bidet, M., Koechlin, N., Gastineau, M., Othmani, L. and Poujeol, P. (1989). *Histochemistry* **91**, 17–30.
Tay, L.K., Bregman, C.L., Masters, B.A. and Williams, P.D. (1988). *Cancer Res.* **48**, 2538–2543.
Teitelbaum, A.P. and Strewler, G.J. (1984). *Endocrinology*, **114**, 980–985.
Toutain, H. and Morin, J.P. (1991). *In* "Nephrotoxicity: Early Diagnosis and Therapeutic Management" (P.H. Bach, N.J. Gregg, M.F. Wilks and L. Delacruz, eds), pp. 451–457. Marcel Dekker, New York.
Toutain, H., Olier, B., Fillastre, J.P. and Morin, J.P. (1987). *Nephrol. Dial. Transplant.* **2**, 520–525.
Toutain, H., Fillastre, J.P. and Morin, J.P. (1989a). *Eur. J. Cell. Biol.* **49**, 274–280.
Toutain, H., Vauclin-Jacques, N., Fillastre, J.P. and Morin, J.P. (1989b). *Cell Biol. Int. Rep.* **13**, 701–710.
Toutain, H., Courjault, F., Vauclin-Jacques, N. and Morin, J.P. (1990). *Renal Failure* **12**, 177–182.
Toutain, H., Vauclin-Jacques, N., Fillastre, J.P. and Morin, J.P. (1991a). *In* "Nephrotoxicity: Early Diagnosis and Therapeutic Management" (P.H. Bach, N.J. Gregg, M.F. Wilks and L. Delacruz, eds), pp. 427–432. Marcel Dekker, New York.
Toutain, H., Vauclin-Jacques, N., Fillastre, J.P. and Morin, J.P. (1991b). *Exp. Cell Res.* **194**, 9–18.
Trifillis, A.L., Regec, A.L., Hall-Craggs, M. and Trump, B.F. (1985a). *In* "Renal Heterogeneity and Target Cell Toxicity" (P.H. Bach and E.A. Lock, eds), pp. 545–548. John Wiley, Chichester.

Trifillis, A.L., Regec, A.L. and Trump, B.F. (1985b). *J.Urol.* **133**, 324 329.

Tulkens, P.M. (1989). *Toxicol. Lett.* **46**, 107–123.

Tune, B.M. (1986). *Comments Toxicol.* **1**, 145–170.

Tune, B.M. and Hsu, C.Y. (1990). *Toxicol. Lett.* **53**, 81–86.

Turner, R.J. and Moran, A. (1982a). *Am. J. Physiol.* **242**, F406–F414.

Turner, R.J. and Moran, A. (1982b). *J. Membr. Biol.* **70**, 37–45.

Vandewalle, A., Lelongt, B., Geniteau-Legendre, M., Baudouin, B., Antoine, M., Estrade, S., Chatelet, F., Verroust, P., Cassingena, R. and Ronco, P. (1989). *J. Cell. Physiol.* **141**, 203–221.

Vinay, P., Gougoux, A. and Lemieux, G. (1981). *Am. J. Physiol.* **241**, F403–F411.

Wald, H., Rubinger, D., Sherzer, P., Friedlaender, M.M., Moran, A. and Popovtzer, M.M. (1989). *Kidney Int.* **35**, 397.

Walker, R.J. and Duggin, G.G. (1988). *Annu. Rev. Pharmacol. Toxicol.* **28**, 331–345.

Walker, R.J., Lazzaro, V.A., Duggin, G.G., Horvath, J.S. and Tiller, D.J. (1989). *Transplantation* **48**, 321–327.

Whelton, A. and Neu, H.C. (1982). *In* "The Aminoglycosides: Microbiology, Clinical Use and Toxicology". M. Dekker Inc., New York.

Whiting, P.H. (1990). *Toxicol. Lett.* **53**, 69–73.

Williams, P.D. (1989). *In Vitro Cell. Dev. Biol.* **25**, 800–805.

Williams, P.D., Hottendorf, G.H. and Bennett, D.B. (1986). *J. Pharmacol. Exp. Ther.* **237**, 919–925.

Williams, P.D., Buening, M.K., Gries, C.L., Hanasono, G.K., Laska, D.A., Tamura, R.N. and Heim, R.A. (1990). *Toxicol. in Vitro* **4**, 207–210.

Wilson, P.D. (1986). *Miner. Electrolyte Metab.* **12**, 71–84.

Wilson, P.D., Holohan, P.D. and Ross, C.R. (1981). *Toxicol. Appl. Pharmacol.* **61**, 243–251.

Wilson, P.D., Dillingham, M.A., Breckon, R. and Anderson, R.J. (1985). *Am. J. Physiol.* **248**, F436–F443.

Wilson, P.D., Anderson, R.J., Breckon, R.D., Nathrath, W. and Schrier, R.W. (1987). *J. Cell. Physiol.* **130**, 245–254.

Yang, I.S., Goldinger, J.M., Hong, S.K. and Taub, M. (1988). *J. Cell. Physiol.* **135**, 481–487.

Yau, C., Rao, L. and Silverman, L. (1985). *Can. J. Physiol. Pharmacol.* **63**, 417–426.

Yonemura, K., Cheng, L., Sacktor, B. and Kinsella, J.L. (1990). *Am. J. Physiol.* **258**, F333–F338.

Yoneyama, Y. and Lever, J.E. (1984). *J. Cell. Physiol.* **121**, 64–73.

Discussion

J.P. Morin

Dr Toutain made four very important points:

1) Not only for renal cell culture but also for other cultures we should avoid having antibiotics and other drugs in the media before testing a new drug for its toxicity because of drug interactions which may be important.

2) He has demonstrated the necessity for extensive characterization of the models.

3) Small changes in culture media may be very important and have important impact on the reactions that may be observed in the models.

4) Human renal cultures may lead to some further very interesting studies.

J.E. Trosko

I would like to complement Dr Toutain on the work that he has started.

My colleague and I have developed a primary human epithelial culture system for kidney cells. When we were trying to isolate some particular kidney cells we noticed, as Dr Morin has pointed out, that the culture conditions greatly affect not only the cell types recovered but also the physiology and differentiation of those cells in culture.

We spent about 2 years developing a serum-free antibiotic-free technique, and also a method of isolating the primary stem cells from the kidney, such that when the culture conditions were changed, for example, serum, transforming growth factor (TFG_β) or interesting toxic chemicals added, or calcium levels raised, the differentiation of those cells could be either enhanced or blocked. In effect, the life of the culture could be prolonged, giving the impression that the stem cells have been induced to become transformed or immortal, when in fact all that has been done is to prevent their differentiation. On the other hand, some conditions in the culture would seem to enhance senescence or induce cytotoxicity on gross analysis. On looking closely, however, those chemicals and conditions were inducing differentiation of the stem cells, and therefore enhancing the senescence of the culture.

This attempt of Dr Toutain and others, including ourselves, raises a very important issue with regard to *in vitro* testing. We know that no one cell type can predict the whole organism *in vitro* and also that different cell types within a given tissue cannot predict what will happen within that tissue: it is indeed the interaction of these various cell types that will contribute to our understanding of the ultimate toxic effect.

When we start to do human cultures we have to deal with stem cells. Stem cells are very important for the life of an organism, for the function of any organ. If we have toxic chemicals that not only induce mutations in particular cells which are important, or toxic chemicals that are cytotoxic and kill specific cell types within an organ, we have to start thinking about chemicals that modulate differentiation of the stem cell pool, thereby accelerating the ageing of that particular organ.

P. Tulkens

I would like to take a slightly provocative attitude to Dr Toutain's very interesting work on proximal tubular cells. We know of course that a number of chemicals will interact with the proximal tubular cells. However, the kidney does not only have proximal tubular cells, and Dr Toutain's model therefore ignores many of the interactions that may take place. How far can his model go in ignoring these kinds of relationships, of which I will cite three?

1) *Aminoglycosides* are known to cause necrosis, immediately associated with which is a proliferation of the interstitium. It has been learnt recently that epidermal growth factor distribution is modified on treatment with aminoglycosides by immunoreactivity mostly in the distal tubules back to the proximal tubules. This is one point that the model may not explore.

2) *Cisplatin* also causes proliferation of the interstitium. This is much longer lasting than with the aminoglycosides and leads us to believe that there is some permanent production of either a growth factor or a mitotic factor (or whatever it may be called). Again, there needs to be the interaction between the proximal tubular cell, which is the target, and the interstitium.

3) *Cyclosporin*, as far as I have been able to ascertain, exerts its toxicity clinically mostly through a vascular problem that is possibly associated with the proximal tubular cells.

H. Toutain
What Dr Tulkens has mentioned is not typical of our model. For example, cyclosporin A probably interacts with another part of the kidney. Using this model we can show that cyclosporin A interacts with a glucose transporter. Of course, though, the complete mechanism of drug-induced toxicity cannot be explored with this type of experimental model.

P. Tulkens
Was it possible to identify whether there was a differential toxicity among the cyclosporin A derivatives, including the new Japanese compound, because that would be the ultimate goal? Can the model be used to define which of the derivatives would be less toxic, and prove that to be true?

H. Toutain
No, not for the moment. Cyclosporin A and cyclosporin H, for example, are clearly detected in such an *in vitro* model.

J.P. Morin
By modulating the composition of the culture medium we are now able to have higher levels of brush border marker enzymes, so we are now mimicking the phenotype more closely.

E. Walum
Cultivating the brush border cells in glucose-free media will of course stop the redifferentiation, dedifferentiation or induction of the glycolysis, but it also opens up other metabolic pathways. Cells are probably selected

which are able to use the glutamine usually present in most media. From a toxicological point of view, the reason for preserving the oxidative metabolism of glucose is that compounds may act on that pathway and therefore be toxic. If other metabolic pathways are opened up, that will not be detectable. I cannot therefore understand the reasoning behind cultivating the cells in glucose-free media.

H. Toutain
It has been demonstrated in glucose-free media that when the cell is orientated towards glycolysis the proximal tubular cell seems to be protected against the action of certain xenobiotics. It is interesting to mimic more closely the conditions of the *in vivo* situation because *in vivo* the cell is clearly neoglucogenic and not orientated towards glycolysis.

J.P. Morin
Glucose is not the right fuel for proximal tubules. It provides only 10–15% of their energy. Therefore, exposing proximal tubule cells to 3 g glucose/litre does not seem to be more physiological than removing glucose from the medium.

J.R. Claude
Have the glutathione enzymes been tested as markers of nephrotoxicity?

H. Toutain
That has not been done. We have just measured glutathione *S*-transferase activity and showed that it was maintained at high level compared with established cell lines; for example, in PK-1 cells there is very depressed glutathione transferase activity.

C. Hepatotoxicity

7

In Vitro Approaches to Hepatotoxicity Studies

A. GUILLOUZO and C. GUGUEN-GUILLOUZO

*INSERM U49, Unité de Recherches Hépatologiques, Hôpital
Pontchaillou, 35033 Rennes, Cedex – France*

Introduction

One of the major functions of the liver is to convert chemicals to more water-soluble forms that can be secreted readily from the body. However, several hundreds of xenobiotics may be hepatotoxic either directly or after conversion to a stable or a reactive metabolite (Stricker and Spoelstra, 1985; Biour *et al.*, 1990). In most cases, hepatotoxicity is associated with activation of the toxic compound. Metabolism of xenobiotics is performed by hepatocytes which represent about 65% of the total cell population. These cells are richly endowed with drug-metabolizing enzymes, which are conveniently divided into two groups. Phase I reactions are generally oxidative, reductive and hydrolytic processes; they provide the necessary functional group for phase II reactions, which are generally conjugations. The major phase I enzymes are represented by the cytochrome *P*-450 monooxygenase system which is located in the endoplasmic reticulum. Drug-metabolizing enzymes are not uniformly distributed in hepatic lobules, being usually more abundant or nearly exclusively expressed in centrilobular areas. Like other functions, qualitative and quantitative interspecies differences are common in the metabolism of xenobiotics. Both the rates and the routes of drug

IN VITRO METHODS IN TOXICOLOGY
ISBN 0-12-388175-7

metabolism can vary greatly particularly when comparisons involve laboratory animals and man.

Liver lesions induced by xenobiotics are described as necrosis, steatosis, cholestasis, inflammation and fibrosis. The responses of the liver to hepatotoxins can be analysed at molecular, cellular and tissue levels. Various impaired functions have been identified which are markers of the different types of hepatic lesion. However, because liver functions are under the influence of various endogenous and exogenous factors, complex interactions with other organs exist which make it difficult to distinguish the primary effects of a compound from those induced secondarily. Moreover, for agents which are not given to humans with therapeutic intent, and for potentially toxic foreign chemicals, information on human metabolism or mechanisms of toxicity is fragmentary. The *in vivo* study of such compounds in humans is severely limited by ethical considerations. These drawbacks have led many investigators to turn to simpler experimental models for studying liver functions, including drug metabolism and the response of the organ or the cells to toxic agents.

This chapter reviews the general aspects of hepatotoxicity and the different isolated liver preparations that can be used in toxicity testing with special reference to the isolated hepatocyte model.

General Aspects of Hepatotoxicity

Drugs can induce a variety of liver lesions, the most frequent being hepatitis, which are classified as cytolytic, cholestatic and mixed hepatitis (Benhamou, 1988). Hepatitis is defined as necrosis or dysfunction of hepatocytes resulting in liver failure and/or cholestasis. Acute hepatitis is usually benign, except for the cytolytic form which may lead to fulminant liver failure. Drug-induced chronic hepatitis is far less common than acute hepatitis. Three types can also be distinguished: chronic active hepatitis, alcoholic-like hepatitis and cholestatic hepatitis. Other drug-induced lesions include granuloma which can be associated with hepatitis, storage liver diseases due, for instance, to accumulation of triglycerides (steatosis), vitamin A or iron, vascular and sinusoidal lesions such as peliosis or thrombosis of vessels, and tumours (Benhamou, 1988).

Liver lesions can result from many different mechanisms. Many hepatotoxins require metabolic activation to toxic intermediates, others interfere with metabolic pathways or alter the integrity of cell membranes. Single or short-term dosing may induce necrosis, cholestasis, steatosis or inflammation while repeated doses may result in fibrosis and cirrhosis. Both acute and chronic lesions may have a heterogeneous intralobular distribution (Table 7.1). They all lead to impairment of essential liver functions, that can characterize the different types of hepatic lesions; e.g. increase in serum transaminases (necrosis), in alkaline phosphatase (cholestasis), in acute-phase proteins (inflammation), accumulation of fatty acids (steatosis) and increased production and deposition of matrix proteins (fibrosis and cirrhosis).

Most of the toxic agents induce liver damage in a predictable manner and can be considered as true (predictable) hepatotoxins. However, a few compounds produce hepatic injury only in unusually susceptible humans and have been named idiosyncrasy-dependent (unpredictable) toxins. Idiosyncratic toxicity may be related either to an unusual metabolism or to an immunoallergic phenomenon (Guengerich, 1985; Larrey and Pessayre, 1988; Pessayre and Larrey, 1988).

Drug hepatotoxicity is influenced by various physiological, nutritional and therapeutic factors. In Western countries, the percentage of drug-induced acute hepatitis increases with age. In French adults, it accounts for 10% of cases of acute hepatitis and this rises to 50% or more in

Table 7.1
Mechanisms of hepatotoxicity and liver lesions induced by some toxic agents

Mechanisms of hepatotoxicity	Toxic agent	Acute lesions	Chronic lesions
Mechanism activation	Acetaminophen Bromobenzene Halothane	Centrilobular necrosis	
	Carbon tetrachloride Dimethylnitrosamine	Steatosis, centrilobular necrosis	Fibrosis, cirrhosis
	Thioacetamide		
	Allyl alcohol	Periportal necrosis	
Perturbation of a metabolic pathway	Ethanol Ethionine	Steatosis	Fibrosis, cirrhosis
	Galactosamine	Steatosis, diffuse necrosis	Fibrosis, cirrhosis
	Orotic acid	Steatosis	
Alteration of cellular membrane	Heavy metals Phalloidin	Necrosis	

Data from Siegers (1988).

adults over 50 years of age (Benhamou, 1988). This higher percentage in the elderly may be explained by the higher consumption of drugs or possibly by a greater susceptibility of the subjects. Recent studies have shown that there is no increased susceptibility to the development of adverse drug reactions in elderly subjects when frequency of drug prescriptions is taken into account (Woodhouse *et al.*, 1986; James *et al.*, 1988).

In addition to the above factors, it is now recognized that drug toxicity can be genetically modulated. Oxidation by cytochrome *P*-450 enzymes and acetylation are metabolic pathways that are low or deficient in some subjects, making them more susceptible to the toxic effects of various drugs (Larrey and Pessayre, 1988).

In Vitro Liver Models

In vitro liver preparations are recognized as being very useful experimental models in pharmacotoxicological research; these *in vitro* preparations include isolated perfused organs, tissue slices, isolated cells, subcellular fractions and purified drug-metabolizing enzymes. The isolated hepatocyte is rapidly becoming the most popular of the *in vitro* systems for the toxicologist. Like other preparations, it can be obtained from both animal and human livers and permits a direct evaluation of toxicological effects which were previously based solely on animal experimentation.

Isolated Perfused Liver

This model represents the system closest to the *in vivo* situation. It makes it possible to study hepatic function without interference from the rest of the organism. The perfusate is recirculated and thus simulates blood circulation. Various parameters can be easily measured, e.g. pH, flow rate of the perfusate, oxygen consumption, bile excretion and enzyme release (Bartosek *et al.*, 1973). The perfused liver is a suitable tool with which to study the kinetics and metabolism of new drugs as well as drug interactions, provided that the drugs are rapidly cleared and metabolized.

However, this *in vitro* model is difficult to handle and its functional integrity is not maintained beyond a few hours. Some functions are affected early: e.g. a decrease in glucose and lipid synthesis is observed after 2 h. Moreover, analysis of various experimental conditions is not possible from a single organ.

Tissue Slices

The liver slice was one of the first preparations used to study *in vitro* liver metabolism (Campbell and Hales, 1971). In this system, the anatomical basis for the functional heterogeneity is preserved, since tissue organization, i.e. cell–matrix and cell–cell interactions, is not disrupted. This model is suitable for studies on drug transport and effects of hormones. However, bile secretion cannot be analysed separately. For a long period, tissue slices fell into relative disuse, because they suffered from major limitations due mainly to the poor diffusion of oxygen and nutrients from the incubation medium.

The recent development of a new instrument providing precision-cut liver and kidney tissue has led to new interest in the tissue slice system (Smith *et al.*, 1986). Liver slices of nearly identical dimensions (approximately 250 μm thick) can be prepared under conditions that result in minimum tissue trauma (Smith *et al.*, 1986), and a system has been designed that allows better diffusion of oxygen and nutrients (Goethals *et al.*, 1990). Various studies have shown that liver slices kept in dynamic organ culture express various functions for several hours. These functions are usually depressed right after the slicing process but recover in culture. Thus, the recovery of ATP content takes about 8 h (Goethals *et al.*, 1990). Protein secretion has been shown to be retained for 20 h (Goethals *et al.*, 1990). The cytochrome *P*-450 content is maintained for 8 h (Sipes *et al.*, 1987), and Ghantous *et al.* (1990) have reported biotransformation of halothane through both oxidative and reductive pathways by male guinea-pig liver slices over a 6 h period. It would be important to determine whether the different phase I and phase II drug-metabolizing enzymes are equally preserved. Liver slices could be quite appropriate for studies on human liver since they can be prepared from both whole organs and biopsies.

Isolated Liver Cells

Liver cells were first obtained from explant cultures. However, the proliferating cell population was consistently a mixture of various cell types. Fibroblasts probably at least partly derived from Ito cells and undifferentiated epithelial cells were the most abundant when explants of adult liver tissue were put in culture (Guillouzo *et al.*, 1972).

A considerable step forward in obtaining various liver cell populations was made by the introduction of enzymes as dissociating agents. Techniques have been developed for isolation of hepatocytes (Berry and Friend, 1969), Kupffer and endothelial cells (Knook and Sleyster, 1977),

Ito cells (De Leeuw *et al.*, 1984), pit cells (Bouwens *et al.*, 1987), bile ductular epithelial cells and oval cells (Sirica *et al.*, 1990). Only isolation and culture of hepatocytes which are the critical liver cell type for the toxicologist will be considered here.

Isolation and culture of normal hepatocytes

Hepatocyte isolation
In 1969, Berry and Friend established the basic protocol involving a perfusion of the liver *in situ* to isolate a large number of viable hepatocytes. The protocol, first designed for rat liver, is still used with slight modifications (Seglen, 1975) and has been applied to the liver of various species including man (Guguen-Guillouzo and Guillouzo, 1986). To disaggregate the young adult rat liver, the first step circulates 300 ml of calcium-free Hepes buffer (160.8 mM NaCl; 15 mM KCl; 0.7 mM Na_2HPO_4, 12 H_2O; 33 mM Hepes) at a flow rate of 20 ml/min. The second perfusate consists of 250 ml of the same buffer plus 0.025% collagenase and 0.075% $CaCl_2$. After the digestion, the softened liver is gently minced to disperse the cells. Undigested tissue fragments are removed by filtration through gauze and the cell suspension is allowed to sediment for 20 min. After three washes by centrifuging at 50 g, the preparation usually contains 4 to 6 × 10^8 hepatocytes with a viability of 85% or more as determined by the Trypan Blue exclusion test and with less than 5% non-parenchymal cells.

Hepatocyte suspensions can be further separated according to their degree of ploidy by counterflow centrifugation (Bernaert *et al.*, 1979; Le Rumeur *et al.*, 1981) or their intralobular location by density gradient centrifugation (Bengtsson *et al.*, 1981). However, the use of metrizamide gradients to separate centrilobular and periportal hepatocytes does not result in the obtention of highly purified subpopulations. Major progress has recently been made by perfusing with digitonin which results in the selective destruction of the periportal and the perivenous part of the microcirculation and by applying this principle in combination with collagenase dissociation (Quistorff *et al.*, 1985; Lindros and Penttila, 1985).

The two-step collagenase method is also applied to wedge biopsies (Reese and Byard, 1981; Strom *et al.*, 1982; Clément *et al.*, 1984). Cell yields depend on the size of the biopsy. Cell viability is often high (>90%). However, for human hepatocytes, viability rates depend on various factors related to the organ and the conditions of resection and preservation of the sample before dissociation.

Freshly isolated hepatocytes memorize signals to which they were responding just before organ disaggregation. In addition, they offer the advantages of a homogeneous suspension to allow analysis of multiple parameters from a single cell suspension. However, isolated hepatocytes do not survive in suspension for more than a few hours. In addition, their functional capacity is quite dependent upon the composition of the incubation medium. In an amino-acid-free medium, the cells are in a strong negative nitrogen balance, due to the low rate of protein synthesis which is 10 times lower than that of protein degradation (Seglen, 1977). The protein anabolic state is maintained by using a medium containing a balanced mixture of amino acids (Seglen *et al.*, 1980). This mixture defined by these authors contained 5 mM asparagine and glutamine, 2.5 mM leucine, 2 mM phenylalanine and tyrosine, 1 mM histidine plus all the other amino acids found to be optimal for protein synthesis. The critical role of amino acids has been stressed by others. Synthesis of albumin and angiotensin was found to be diminished by 40% in hepatocyte suspensions after a 5 h incubation in a medium lacking amino acids (Weigand *et al.*, 1977). Hormones also affect protein synthesis in hepatocyte suspensions (for a review see Crane and Miller, 1977; Guillouzo, 1986a).

Hepatocyte survival and function under standard culture conditions
To survive beyond a few hours, hepatocytes must attach to a support. When placed in standard culture conditions they survive for 1–2 weeks but they do not divide and do not remain phenotypically stable. Rodent hepatocytes lose some of their most differentiated functions and attenuation of others occur within a few days (Bissell and Guzelian, 1980; Sirica and Pitot, 1980; Guguen-Guillouzo and Guillouzo, 1983; Guguen-Guillouzo, 1986). At the same time the cells begin to express fetal-like functions such as fetal enzymes and α-fetoprotein (Guguen *et al.*, 1975; Sirica *et al.*, 1979). The rates of transcription of liver-specific genes drop to between 1% and 10% of those found in the liver after 24 h of culture (Clayton and Darnell, 1983; Fraslin *et al.*, 1985).

The unstable functions include cytochrome *P*-450 enzymes. Total cytochrome *P*-450 level decreases by 50% or more during the first 24–48 h of culture (Guzelian *et al.*, 1977; Fahl *et al.*, 1979; Bégué *et al.*, 1984) but cytochrome *P*-450 enzymes, which constitute a gene superfamily (Nebert *et al.*, 1989), are differently affected (Steward *et al.*, 1985; Namiki *et al.*, 1989). Induction of specific *P*-450 enzymes by phenobarbital is difficult to achieve (Newman and Guzelian, 1982), while several other enzymes, although decreased, remain able to respond to inducers (Elshourbagy *et al.*, 1981; Lake *et al.*, 1983; Perrot *et al.*, 1991). However, the response can be different from that observed *in vivo* (Forster *et al.*, 1986; Watkins *et al.*, 1986). As for cytochrome *P*-450 enzymes, differential changes are also observed for UDP-glucuronyltransferase forms (Forster *et al.*, 1986) and glutathione *S*-transferase subunits (Vandenberghe *et al.*, 1988a, 1990).

By contrast, human hepatocytes are more stable than their rat counterparts. More than 50% of the initial cytochrome *P*-450 content is still present after 1 week of culture (Guillouzo *et al.*, 1985) and all cytochrome *P*-450 enzymes hitherto analysed, namely IA, IIC, IIE and IIIA, are expressed (Morel *et al.*, 1990) (Fig. 7.1). Specific inductions have been demonstrated with rifampicin, phenobarbital, 3-methylcholanthrene and omeprazole (Diaz *et al.*, 1990; Morel *et al.*, 1990; Daujat *et al.*, 1991).

Modulation of hepatocyte function in primary culture
In the early years it was assumed that phenotypic changes resulting in preferential loss of the most differentiated functions represent adaptive responses of hepatocytes to an inappropriate environment (Guguen-Guillouzo and Guillouzo, 1983). A number of studies have dealt with the identification of factors that affect cellular functions *in vitro*. Three groups of factors can be distinguished: soluble factors, extracellular matrix components and cell–cell interactions.

Soluble factors   A number of factors have been shown to enhance liver-specific functions in hepatocyte cultures. Physiological factors include hormones, growth factors and trace elements. Several hormonally defined serum-free media have been proposed, which favour maintained plasma protein secretion (Reid *et al.*, 1986), drug-metabolizing enzymes and their response to inducers (Waxman *et al.*, 1990).

Various non-physiological factors also enhance hepatocyte survival and function *in vitro*; they include nicotinamide and isonicotinamide (Paine, 1990), metyrapone (Paine, 1990) and dimethyl sulphoxide (Isom *et al.*, 1985; Muakkassah-Kelly *et al.*, 1987). In the presence of 2% dimethyl sulphoxide, hepatocytes survive and retain specific functions, including secretion of high levels of albumin for several weeks (Isom *et al.*, 1985; McGowan, 1988). Transcriptional activity of albumin gene represents around 8% of that in freshly isolated cells (Isom *et al.*, 1987). This solvent could act at least in part by its strong scavenger properties for hydroxyl radicals, which destroy reactive species of oxygen formed under standard culture conditions (Villa and Guaitani, 1988). Various ligands including ethanol, propan-2-ol, imidazole and 4-methylpyrazole prevent rapid

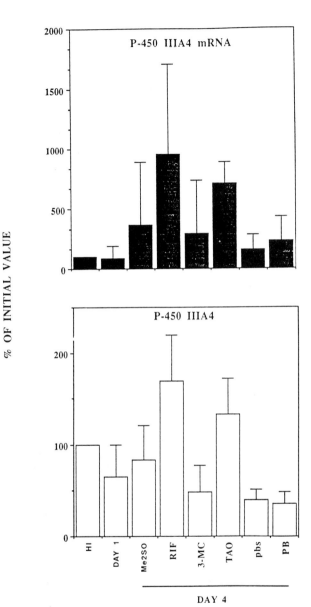

Fig. 7.1 Effects of various inducers on cytochrome *P*-450 IIIA in cultured human hepatocytes. Hepatocytes were treated with 50 μM rifampicin (RIF), 50 μM troleandomycin (TAO), 5 μM 3-methylcholanthrene (3-MC) or 3.2 mM phenobarbital (PB). The inducers were added three times at 24 h intervals with medium renewal. Controls included cultures exposed to 0.2% dimethyl sulphoxide (Me₂SO) used as a solvent (for RIF, TAO and 3-MC) or PBS (pbs) used to dissolve PB. HI, freshly isolated hepatocytes. Day 1, 24 h untreated cultures. The levels of mRNAs and proteins were measured by Northern and Western blotting respectively. The values are means ± S.E.M. of three to five different experiments (from Morel *et al.*, 1990).

decrease of cytochrome *P*-450 IIE1, the ethanol-inducible cytochrome *P*-450 enzyme, for a few days (Eliasson *et al.*, 1988; Wu *et al.*, 1990).

The composition of the medium is also critical for the maintenance of glutathione *S*-transferase (GST). The presence of serum and addition of nicotinamide or dimethyl sulphoxide modify both total GST activity and the relative content of GST subunits (Vandenberghe *et al.*, 1988a,b, 1990).

Extracellular matrix components   The efficiency of attachment of hepatocytes and longevity of cultures are increased when the cells are cultured in plastic dishes coated with various matrix proteins. However, in general these organic substrates either used individually or as a mixture do not markedly delay the occurrence of phenotypic changes (Rojkind *et al.*, 1980; Guguen-Guillouzo *et al.*, 1982; Marceau *et al.*, 1982; Sudhakaran *et al.*, 1986). The substrates that promote cell spreading enhance alterations of liver gene expression, and several authors have come to the conclusion that the preservation of the globular cell shape is a prerequisite for maintenance of liver-specific functions *in vitro* (Guguen-Guillouzo *et al.*, 1982; Ben-Ze'ev *et al.*, 1988).

Recently, it was shown that hepatocyte spreading is prevented and that various specific functions are preserved, including phenobarbital induction of cytochromes *P*-450 IIB1 and IIB2, when hepatocytes are plated on a reconstituted basement membrane gel formed from components extracted from the EHS tumour (Bissell *et al.*, 1987; Schuetz *et al.*, 1988). The mechanisms by which this extracellular matrix substratum regulates liver-specific functions are unclear. This gel, termed matrigel, contains more than 80% laminin and it has been reported that purified laminin added to hepatocytes cultured on type I collagen induces an increase in albumin mRNA levels and albumin secretion (Caron, 1990). Whether laminin is the most effective component of matrigel merits further investigations since contamination of this gel by hormones and/or growth factors cannot be ruled out.

Cell–cell interactions   The first attempts to coculture hepatocytes with other cell types such as human fibroblasts (Michalopoulos *et al.*, 1979) and hepatic sinusoidal cells (Wanson *et al.*, 1979) showed only minor and transient improvement of liver functions. Major progress was made by adding untransformed epithelial cells from 10-day-old rat liver (Guguen-Guillouzo *et al.*, 1983). Coculturing hepatocytes from various species, including man, and from either adults or foetuses with another liver cell type results in their prolonged survival with maintenance of high functional capacities (Guguen-Guillouzo *et al.*, 1983, 1984; Clément *et al.*, 1984;

Lescoat *et al.*, 1985). Among the functions preserved are the production of various plasma proteins (Guillouzo *et al.*, 1984; Conner *et al.*, 1990) and drug-metabolizing enzymes (Ratanasavanh *et al.*, 1986; Vandenberghe *et al.*, 1988a, 1990). Cocultured hepatocytes retain the ability to transcribe specific genes at higher values (20–40%) than in cells cultured with dimethyl sulphoxide or with matrix proteins (Fraslin *et al.*, 1985) and are able to communicate together via gap junctions (Mesnil *et al.*, 1987). The early production and deposition of matrix proteins could favour both high transcriptional gene activity and communication via gap junctions. The enhanced survival and function of hepatocytes cocultured with liver epithelial cells have been confirmed by many other laboratories (Morin and Normand, 1986; Gleiberman *et al.*, 1989; Schrode *et al.*, 1990). Other liver cells as well as non-hepatic cells have also been reported to be effective (Goulet *et al.*, 1988; Mendoza-Figueroa *et al.*, 1988; Donato *et al.*, 1990). However, it would be important to determine whether hepatocytes can easily be separated from these different cell types as shown with liver epithelial cells (Fraslin *et al.*, 1985). The level of the functions in coculture is also dependent on the composition of the medium. As a rule some qualitative and quantitative changes occur and reappearance of foetal-like functions is not totally prevented (Vandenberghe *et al.*, 1990).

Factors affecting replication of hepatocyte in vitro
Various factors may stimulate DNA synthesis *in vitro* (McGowan, 1986; Luetteke and Michalopoulos, 1987). Two groups of humoral growth-promoting agents can be distinguished: the primary mitogenic factors and the co-mitogen factors (Michalopoulos, 1990). Thus, epidermal growth factor requires insulin or angiotensin II for maximal stimulation of DNA synthesis. Serum factors, such as hepatopoietin B and the hepatocyte growth factor which has recently been cloned and sequenced (Nakamura *et al.*, 1989), also stimulate hepatocyte proliferation. In addition, other substances and conditions can modulate the response of hepatocytes to growth stimuli *in vitro*. These include components of the basal medium, e.g. pyruvate, lactate and proline, low cell densities and the extracellular matrix used as substratum (Enat *et al.*, 1984; Sawada *et al.*, 1986). Nicotinamide, which is converted in the cell to NAD and NADP, also stimulates DNA synthesis in rat hepatocytes cultured in a medium with added serum, epidermal growth factor and insulin (Inoue *et al.*, 1989). The ability of hepatocytes to synthesize DNA seems to be related to their intralobular location. Glutamine synthetase-positive hepatocytes located around central veins synthesize less DNA *in vitro* than negative cells (Gebhardt, 1988). Under optimal conditions, more than 80% of

parenchymal cells undergo at least one round of replicative DNA synthesis and about 50% go through one cell cycle of division. A few cells even replicate twice when the cells are grown in serum-free medium containing low Ca^{2+} concentration (0.4 mM) and epidermal growth factor (Eckl *et al.*, 1987).

Current perspectives on drug metabolism by hepatocyte cultures
Clearly, various methods of culture represent a significant advance over conventional cultures. The most suitable culture conditions must take into account that expression of a liver-specific phenotype *in vivo* is regulated by specific humoral factors as well as cell–matrix and cell–cell interactions. A number of conditions favour maintenance of albumin production while other functions are often much less well preserved. In addition, whatever the method of culture, the levels of liver-specific functions depend on cell density and the degree of ploidy. Various functions are increased at low cell densities (Guguen-Guillouzo, 1986) and tetraploid hepatocytes have been shown to synthesize more proteins than their diploid counterparts (Le Rumeur *et al.*, 1983).

Despite these limitations, the potential of hepatocyte cultures as model systems for the study of drug metabolism and toxicity is well demonstrated. In short-term culture, hepatocytes retain their ability to generate metabolites identical with those found *in vivo* from various compounds and therefore to show interspecies variability and potential drug interactions (Bégué *et al.*, 1983; Chenery *et al.*, 1987; Le Bigot *et al.*, 1987; Guillouzo *et al.*, 1988; Le Bot *et al.*, 1988; Rahmani *et al.*, 1988; Seddon *et al.*, 1989). A good *in vivo/in vitro* qualitative correlation is usually found. However, striking quantitative differences are sometimes observed (Berthou *et al.*, 1988; Grislain *et al.*, 1988). Such differences may disappear when the amount of metabolites is expressed per cell, as shown by Berthou *et al.* (1988) for caffeine. This active alkaloid is extensively metabolized *in vivo* and in perfused isolated liver but only at a very limited rate in microsomes and cultured hepatocytes. However, quite similar values are obtained when metabolism is expressed as nmol of metabolite formed/24 h per 10^6 hepatocytes (Table 7.2). Short-term hepatocyte cultures are also very powerful for kinetics studies and for determining metabolism of drug enantiomers (Le Corre *et al.*, 1988). The formation of the main drug metabolites is retained for several days when more sophisticated culture conditions are used, indicating that these are more suitable for drug induction/inhibition studies. Thus Villa *et al.* (1984) found that rat hepatocytes have to be placed in coculture to respond to erythromycin estolate and to form stable complexes between cytochrome *P*-450 and

Table 7.2
Metabolic rates of caffeine calculated from *in vivo* and three *in vitro* models

	Adult human liver microsomes	Adult human cultured hepatocytes	Rat perfused liver	Adult human *In vivo*
Total amount of drug (μmol)	0.5	0.4	1	2800[a]
Percentage of drug metabolized (time)	0.5 (15 min)	7.7 (24 h)	95 (3 h)	50 (6 h)
Total hepatocytes	10^{7b}	2.5×10^6	10^{9c}	150×10^{9d}
Metabolic rate (nmol/24 h per 10^6 cells)	24	12.3	7.6	17

[a] Total amount of drug: plasma concentration × distribution volume, i.e. 80 μM × 0.5 l/kg × 70 kg.
[b] 1 mg of microsomal protein, i.e. 0.1 g of liver.
[c] Whole rat liver: 10 mg.
[d] Whole adult human liver: 1500 g.
Data from Berthou *et al.* (1988).

this macrolide. Other studies have shown that metabolites generated by phase I and phase II reactions are still obtained after 1–3 weeks in hepatocyte cocultures (Bégué *et al.*, 1983; Guillouzo *et al.*, 1988).

Hepatocyte cell lines

Hepatocyte cell lines can be obtained from hepatomas or after transfection of normal hepatocytes with viral or cellular DNA. Hepatoma cell lines are difficult to establish from primary carcinomas and only a few lines of rat or human origin have retained various liver-specific functions including phase I and phase II drug reactions. The most powerful hepatoma cell lines are FaO cells derived from the Reuber rat hepatoma (Deschatrette and Weiss, 1974) and the human HepG$_2$ hepatoma cell line (Knowles *et al.*, 1980). However, none of the established hepatoma cell lines has maintained all the liver-specific markers. Moreover, the levels of the expressed functions depend on the composition of the medium and may vary with time in culture.

Another way to get permanent hepatocyte cell lines is to immortalize normal hepatocytes. Transformed cell lines have been obtained after transfection with SV40 or adenovirus (Isom and Georgoff, 1984). Again, only some liver-specific functions are expressed and they are not stable *in vitro*. No immortalized human hepatocyte cell line has yet been obtained by transfection.

Recently, it has been shown that cultivation of foetal hepatocytes derived from livers of transgenic mice harbouring SV40 early region sequences resulted in the establishment of a non-transformed stable cell line expressing specific hepatic functions (Paul et al., 1988). This approach represents a promising alternative to in vitro transfection when transgenic animals can be obtained.

Subcellular Fractions

Tissue homogenates, microsomes and purified organelles can be prepared from whole livers or liver pieces. These models are useful to study mechanisms of hepatotoxicity. The liver 9000 g supernatant fraction fortified with cofactors is appropriate for expression of the cytochrome P-450-dependent microsomal monooxygenase system and has long been recognized as a good metabolizing system for activation of xenobiotics in in vitro mutagenicity testing procedures (Maron and Ames, 1983). Microsomes are widely used to identify drug-metabolic pathways, covalent binding and lipid peroxidation induced by hepatotoxins. Subcellular liver fractions are also functional for only a few hours but can be prepared from animals pretreated with inducers.

Individually Purified Enzymes

The different phase I and phase II reactions usually involve enzyme families. The different enzymes may have similar sequences and different substrates. Moreover, several enzymes may metabolize the same substrate.

The first attempts to study individual enzymes were made by their immobilization on a support after purification. However, this procedure results in some enzymic denaturation and usually low activity for a short period.

An alternative is to obtain expression of drug-metabolizing enzymes in heterologous cells devoid of interfering enzyme activities. Several studies have been performed on cytochrome P-450 enzymes. Their expresssion has been developed in both mammalian cells and yeasts (Battula et al., 1987; Pompon, 1988). Optimal cytochrome P-450 activity in yeast requires integration of the cytochrome P-450 reductase gene (Pompon, 1990). In the near future it should be possible to create an artificial inducible multienzyme system that mimicks human liver metabolism in yeast and non-hepatic mammalian cells.

Use of *In Vitro* Liver Models in Toxicity Testing

Although all the different *in vitro* models have been used for toxicity studies, isolated hepatocyes, either in suspension or in culture, have so far been the most popular system. Various indicators are currently used for cytotoxicity screening and mechanistic studies.

Cytotoxicity Measures

Since several pathways are possible for chemical-induced cytotoxicity, a wide array of morphological, biochemical and metabolic end points are, consequently, available and potentially applicable to obtain information at the cellular, subcellular and molecular levels (Tyson and Green, 1987). Their specificity, sensitivity, reliability and correspondence to *in vivo* toxicity are, however, related to the experimental conditions.

Cytotoxicity end points

The indicators commonly used in *in vitro* cytotoxicity testing can be classified as non-specific and liver-specific criteria (Tyson and Green, 1987; Guillouzo, 1992).

Non-specific markers may monitor membrane integrity, subcellular perturbations and metabolic functions. Indicators for membrane integrity include cell count and Trypan Blue exclusion, which correspond to irreversible changes, and membrane permeability to ions or small molecules, which can correspond to reversible changes. Cytosolic enzymes are frequently used for monitoring the loss of plasma membrane integrity. The percentage of lactate dehydrogenase release gives a better correlation than that of transaminases or membrane-bound enzymes with morphological changes and cell viability estimated by Trypan Blue exclusion. This parameter is much less reliable for human hepatocyte cultures, and determination of intracellular lactate dehydrogenase is preferred (Le Bot *et al.*, 1988; Mallédant *et al.*, 1990). Subcellular alterations can be demonstrated by electron microscopic examination, but this method is time-consuming. Its choice is justified to confirm or to get more precise information on biochemical changes. Subcellular alterations such as peroxisome proliferation, smooth endoplasmic reticulum proliferation, glycogen depletion, mitochondrion swelling or secondary lysosome accumulation are very informative. The functional markers of organelle disturbance include MTT reduction by mitochondrial dehydrogenases, Neutral Red uptake by lysosomes and whole protein synthesis determination. Other metabolic indicators such as glutathione content, lipid peroxidation and covalent binding are not organelle-specific.

Several liver-specific criteria may also be used. Besides electron microscopic changes which are characteristic of the hepatocyte (peroxisome proliferation, smooth endoplasmic reticulum proliferation), liver-specific alterations can be evaluated quantitatively. The most common functions tested include production of plasma proteins, such as albumin and acute-phase proteins, glycogen synthesis, urea synthesis, induction or inhibition of specific cytochrome *P*-450 enzymes and induction of peroxisomal β-oxidation. These criteria are more sensitive than unspecific ones. However, there is no single indicator for metabolic competence.

Experimental conditions for in vitro toxicity testing

It is obvious that no single protocol, e.g. one single condition, can be used to test any compound and that problems of interpretation can be greatly magnified when tests involving different mechanisms of toxicity or end points are compared.

First, hepatocytes have to retain sufficient drug-metabolizing capacity. Depending on the sex, age or species of the donor, their susceptibility to hepatotoxicants will be potentially different.

Second, the conditions of incubation are critical, particularly the composition of the atmosphere and medium, and the duration of exposure to chemicals. Under anoxic conditions the covalent binding of carbon tetrachloride and halothane, which undergo reductive biotransformation *in vivo*, to cultured hepatocytes is enhanced, whereas that of choroform and 1,2 2-trichloroethane, which undergo oxidative biotransformation, is decreased (Direnzo *et al.*, 1984). The concentration of Ca^{2+} may have a critical role in the magnitude of toxicity induced by various compounds in hepatocyte suspensions. Toxicity is potentiated in the absence of extracellular Ca^{2+} (Smith *et al.*, 1981; Fariss *et al.*, 1984); this is possibly linked to an increase in lipid peroxidation and glutathione depletion (Fariss *et al.*, 1984). Erythromycin estolate which is known to bind to proteins is much more toxic to rat hepatocytes when added in a protein-free medium (Villa *et al.*, 1984). In the choice of the xenobiotic exposure duration, the lack of extrahepatic release of toxic compounds and their accumulation in the culture medium must be considered. Thus, Paine and Hockin (1982) studied different toxins on cultured rat hepatocytes maintained in conditions that resulted in either a low or a high cytochrome *P*-450 content. After a 24 h incubation, compounds which are activated or detoxified by cytochrome *P*-450 were equally toxic regardless of the cytochrome *P*-450 content of the cells. Only when exposure to carbon tetrachloride was limited to 1–4 h and followed by a 20 h incubation in a toxin-free medium was this compound more toxic to rat hepatocytes containing high levels of cytochrome P-450. Coculturing hepatocytes with fibroblasts can overcome the problem of accumulation of toxic metabolites (Fry and Bridges, 1977; Acosta and Mitchell, 1981). The toxicity of cyclophosphamide to fibroblasts, as judged by the 50% inhibition growth, was obtained at concentrations of 16 μg/ml and > 500 μg/ml in the presence and absence of adult hepatocytes respectively (Fry and Bridges, 1979).

Third, the nature of the test compound must also be taken into account. Volatile and liposoluble compounds require appropriate culture conditions. To rank correctly the relative hepatotoxic potentials of five haloalkanes measured in hepatocyte suspensions and *in vivo*, the partition coefficients had to be factored into data to reconcile the differences between solvent volatility and retention into the two systems (Tyson *et al.*, 1983).

Four, there is now the consensus that it is inappropriate to employ a single biochemical parameter as a sensitive indicator of toxic injury. An example, inhibition of protein synthesis by oxytetracycline was not demonstrated in rat hepatocyte suspensions (Vonen and Morland, 1984). A battery of two or more end points, each reflecting one or two features of *in vivo* changes, is more valuable in detecting the early changes in response to chemically induced injury.

In Vitro Toxicity Studies

Detection and comparative evaluation of toxic compounds and hepatoprotectants

Freshly isolated suspensions and primary cultures of hepatocytes are widely used for screening of cytotoxic and genotoxic compounds; they also serve as experimental systems for the evaluation of potential hepatoprotectants (Fry and Bridges, 1979; Klaassen and Stacey, 1982; Guillouzo, 1986b, 1992; Guillouzo *et al.*, 1989, 1990). During the early stages of development of a new chemical, *in vitro* tests provide information used in selection of appropriate candidates from the many that may be available. Such use of *in vitro* tests requires previous adequate validation and the interpretation of results of screening compounds must consider knowledge of the sensitivity and specificity of the test and the structures of the compounds tested (Purchase, 1990).

Screening of cytotoxic compounds

Most of the tests can be carried out in 96-well plates, making it possible to screen various compounds at several concentrations using different end points from a single cell preparation. Dose–response curves are calculated from the results obtained, then the results are summarized as IC_{50} values, i.e. the concentrations of test compounds that modify the values of test wells by 50%.

In general, the *in vivo/in vitro* correspondence in discriminating between hepatotoxicants and non-hepatotoxicants is good. Tyson *et al.* (1980) investigated 23 chemicals and found good correspondence for all but two, thioacetamide and allyl alcohol, using enzyme release to evaluate toxicity. Story *et al.* (1983) came to the same conclusion by studying 34 compounds. A recent multicentre evaluation of 30 compounds using common experimental conditions also led to the conclusion that a few compounds were less toxic *in vitro* than *in vivo* (Fautrel *et al.*, 1991). These compounds, which included cycloheximide, bromobenzene and vincristine, have to be investigated in appropriate conditions, thereby further emphasizing that there is no single protocol to analyse all the compounds.

The suitability of *in vitro* hepatocyte preparations as a screen procedure early in drug development is certainly more convincing when structurally related compounds are ranked. Good examples from our laboratory include neuroleptic agents (Ratanasavanh *et al.*, 1988b) (Fig. 7.2) and macrolides (Villa *et al.*, 1984). Drugs associated with human hepatotoxicity are generally more cytotoxic to rat or human hepatocytes *in vitro* (Ratanasavanh *et al.*, 1988b; Mallédant *et al.*, 1990).

The short-term assay does not reflect the common *in vivo* situation in which drugs induce liver damage after repeated administration lasting weeks or months. Hepatocytes in coculture which retain their drug-metabolic capacity for several days can be used to mimic such a situation. The test compounds are added daily for 1–3 weeks at concentrations equal to or lower than the maximum non-toxic dose defined after a 24 h incubation of these compounds in conventional hepatocyte cultures (Ratanasavanh *et al.*, 1988a; Guillouzo *et al.*, 1990).

The detection of idiosyncratic toxins requires special experimental conditions. Since drug metabolism capacities can be manipulated by exposure to inducers or inhibitors *in vitro* hepatic preparations may be used to determine whether qualitative and/or quantitative alterations in the drug metabolism profile can affect the degree of drug cytotoxicity. Such studies could lead to the detection of chemical-induced cytotoxicity related to an unusual metabolism or to drug interactions.

Up to now there is no *in vitro* liver model to predict drug toxicity related to immune mechanisms.

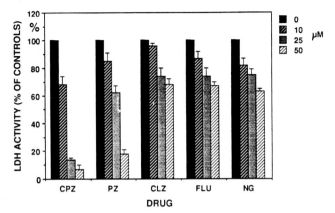

Fig. 7.2 Effects of various neuroleptic agents on intracellular lactate hydrogenase (LDH) content of human hepatocyte cultures. The cells were allowed to acclimate for 20 h before a 24 h exposure to three concentrations of drugs (CPZ, chlorpromazine; PZ, promazine; CLZ, clozapine; FLU, fluperlapine; NG, a new drug in development). As *in vivo*, chlorpromazine is more cytotoxic than the other neuroleptic agents. The values are expressed as percentage of controls; they are means of three experiments in triplicate (from Ratanasavanh *et al.* (1988*b*) with permission).

Studies of genotoxic compounds

In vitro liver models have also long been used to assess the genotoxic potential of chemical and physical agents on the basis of their ability to covalently bind to and damage DNA, induce DNA repair responses, mutate specific genetic loci, induce phenotypically altered cells or induce chromosome or chromatid-level aberrations (Michalopoulos *et al.*, 1986; Strom *et al.*, 1987).

Isolated hepatocytes are well suited for quantification of DNA repair elicited by exposure to genotoxic agents. Since the unscheduled DNA synthesis (UDS) assay requires small numbers of cells, it represents a suitable method for testing genotoxic compounds on human hepatocytes (Butterworth *et al.*, 1989). Surprisingly, the UDS response is usually quite similar in human and rat hepatocytes while marked differences are found when human hepatocytes are compared with hepatocytes of various other animal species (Steinmetz *et al.*, 1985).

Since clonal growth of hepatocytes remains unsuccessful, direct mutagenicity assays with hepatocytes are not possible. To obviate this difficulty, hepatocytes can be cocultured with actively proliferating cells such as human fibroblasts (Strom *et al.*, 1983) or V-79 chinese hamster fibroblasts (Moore and Gould, 1984).

Evaluation of hepatoprotective agents
Various antioxidants and scavengers of free radicals have been tested on *in vitro* liver preparations and found to act as *in vivo*. During the last years, new naturally occurring substances of plant origin and synthetic compounds have also been evaluated (see Guillouzo *et al.* (1989) for review). Their effects may depend on the species studied and the duration of treatment. (+)-Cyanidanol-3 was effective on rat hepatocytes intoxicated by aflatoxin B_1 when added at least 5 min before the mycotoxin but was without effect on human hepatocytes (Bégué *et al.*, 1988). The synthetic compound malotilate, which was reported to protect rats intoxicated with carbon tetrachloride, was without effect on both rat and human hepatocytes even after repeated treatment *in vitro* (Clément *et al.*, 1988) or on active chronic hepatitis in alcoholic patients (personal communication).

Mechanistic studies

Hepatotoxins frequently require metabolic activation to induce cellular damage. The production of reactive metabolites is dependent on a balance of activation and inactivation pathways and consequently the major limitations of *in vitro* liver preparations for mechanistic studies of hepatotoxins are related to the differential stability of drug-metabolizing enzymes and other liver-specific functions *in vitro*. However, many examples have been reported showing similar toxin-induced biochemical changes *in vivo* and *in vitro*; they include toxicity induced by carbon tetrachloride (Long and Moore, 1988), galactosamine (Tran-Thi *et al.*, 1985) and paracetamol (Harman and Fischer, 1983). Species differences in susceptibility to paracetamol have been reproduced *in vitro* (Moldeus, 1978).

The reactive metabolites are often strong electrophiles leading to irreversible alkylation of cellular macromolecules. However, measurement of total covalent binding does not discriminate between potentially critical individual target proteins. Although target proteins which interact with reactive metabolites are highly selective, they have so far received little attention. A recent study, using antibodies directed against paracetamol-bound antibodies, has shown that two proteins of 44 kDa and 58 kDa respectively were covalently associated with paracetamol metabolites (Bartolome *et al.*, 1988).

Isolated hepatocytes could also be used to identify the nature of the antigen recognized by circulating autoantibodies in drug-induced immunoallergic hepatitis. When rabbit hepatocytes pretreated with methyldopa (Neuberger *et al.*, 1985) or halothane (Vergani *et al.*, 1980) were incubated with sera of patients with the corresponding drug-induced hepatitis, a cytotoxic effect was frequently observed, suggesting that the two drugs could generate neoantigenic determinants on hepatocyte plasma membranes which are very similar to those occurring in patients. This conclusion is supported by the study of Loeper *et al.* (1989) who demonstrated the presence of covalently bound metabolites on rat hepatocyte plasma membrane proteins after administration of isaxonine, a drug inducing immunoallergic hepatitis. Recently, Siproudhis *et al.* (1991) incubated normal human hepatocytes with clometacin in the presence of autologous lymphoid cells and then with sera from patients with clometacin-induced hepatitis. Hepatocyte injury was specifically observed with all the sera tested.

Conclusions

Although marked progress has been made in the development of prolonged culture of differentiated hepatocytes by taking into account the critical influence of soluble factors, cell–matrix and cell–cell interactions, it appears that whatever the culture conditions used, hepatocytes undergo some phenotypic changes that do not affect similarly all liver functions. Nevertheless, a number of studies have demonstrated the suitability of hepatocyte cultures for toxicity screening and mechanistic studies of xenobiotics. This model offers the unique possibility for comparing the effects of chemicals on both animal and human cells. However, major problems are encountered when human hepatocytes are used because of their erratic availability. The isolation of viable hepatocytes from long-term hypothermically preserved organs (Guyomard *et al.*, 1990) and the development of cryopreservation protocols (Chesné and Guillouzo, 1988; Chesné *et al.*, 1991) may solve, at least partly, this problem. Obtention of immortalized differentiated hepatocyte cell lines could certainly represent a major progress (Paul *et al.*, 1988).

   Because hepatocytes retain their metabolic competence for several hours and even several days in appropriate culture conditions, they are of great value for screening tests in the selection of compounds early during their development, in defining priorities of selected compounds and in identifying chemicals with particular properties so that *in vivo* experimentation will be optimized (Purchase, 1990). In particular, *in vitro* tests can help in the choice of the species to be studied *in vivo*. Despite the great potential of *in vitro* liver models, it is obvious that they will not totally replace animal studies in the assessment of mammalian hepatotoxicity.

Acknowledgements

We wish to thank Mrs A. Vannier for typing the manuscript. Studies performed by our colleagues and ourselves in the INSERM liver Unit in Rennes were supported by the Institut National de la Santé et de la Recherche Médicale, the Ministère de la Recherche, the Association de la Recherche contre le Cancer, the Ligue contre le Cancer and the Fondation de la Recherche Médicale.

References

Acosta, D. and Mitchell, D.B. (1981). *Biochem. Pharmacol.* **30**, 3225–3230.
Bartolome, J.B., Birge, R.B., Sparks, K., Cohen, S.D. and Khairalla, E.A. (1988). *Biochem. Pharmacol.* **37**, 4763–4774.
Bartosek, I., Guaitani, A. and Miller, L.L. (1973). *In* "Isolated Liver Perfusion and Its Applications". Raven Press, New York.
Battula, N., Sagara, J. and Gelboin, H.V. (1987). *Proc. Natl. Acad. Sci. U.S.A.* **84**, 4073–4077.
Bégué, J.M., Le Bigot, J.F., Guguen-Guillouzo, C., Kiechel, J.R. and Guillouzo, A. (1983). *Biochem. Pharmacol.* **32**, 1643–1646.
Bégué, J.M., Guguen-Guillouzo, C., Pasdeloup, N. and Guillouzo, A. (1984). *Hepatology* **4**, 839–842.
Bégué, J.M., Baffet, G., Campion, J.P. and Guillouzo, A. (1988). *Biol. Cell* **63**, 327–333.
Ben-Ze'ev, A., Robinson, G.S., Bucher, N.L.R. and Farmer, S.R. (1988). *Proc. Natl. Acad. Sci. U.S.A.* **85**, 2161–2165.
Bengtsson, G., Kiessling, K.H., Smith-Kielland, A. and Morland, J. (1981). *Eur. J. Biochem.* **118**, 591–597.
Benhamou, J.P. (1988). *In* "Liver Cells and Drugs" (A. Guillouzo, ed.), p. 3–12. Les Editions INSERM and John Libbey Eurotext, Paris.
Bernaert, D., Wanson, J.C., Mosselmans, R., De Parmentier, F. and Drochmans, P. (1979). *Biol. Cell.* **34**, 159–174.
Berry, M.N. and Friend, D.S. (1969). *J. Cell Biol.* **43**, 506–520.
Berthou, F., Ratanasavanh, D., Alix, D., Carhlant, D., Riché, C. and Guillouzo, A. (1988). *Biochem. Pharmacol.* **37**, 3691–3700.
Biour, M., Poupon, R., Grange, J.D., Chazouilleres, O., Levy, V.G., Bodin, F. and Cheymol, G. (1990). *Gastroenterol. Clin. Biol.* **14**, 263–277.
Bissell, D.M. and Guzelian, P.S. (1980). *Ann. N.Y. Acad. Sci.* **349**, 85–98.
Bissell, D.M., Arenson, D.M., Maher, J.J. and Roll, F.J. (1987). *J. Clin. Invest.* **79**, 801–812.
Bouwens, L., Remels, L., Backeland, M., Van Bossuyt, H. and Wisse, E. (1987). *Eur. J. Immunol.* **17**, 37–42.
Butterworth, B.E., Smith-Oliver, T., Earle, L., Loury, D.J., White, R.D., Doolittle, D.J., Working, P.K., Cattley, R.C., Jirtle, R., Michalopoulos, G. and Strom, S. (1989). *Cancer Res.* **49**, 1075–1084.
Campbell, A.K. and Hales, C.N. (1971). *Exp. Cell Res.* **68**, 33–42.

Caron, J. (1990). *Mol. Cell Biol.* **10**, 1239–1243.
Chenery, R.J., Ayrton, A., Oldham, H.G., Standing, P., Norman, S.J., Seddon, T. and Kirby, R. (1987). *Drug. Metab. Dispos.* **15**, 312–317.
Chesné, C. and Guillouzo, A. (1988). *Cryobiology* **25**, 252–330.
Chesné, C., Guyomard, C., Grislain, L., Clerc, C., Fautrel, A. and Guillouzo, A. (1991). *Toxicol. In Vitro* **5**, 479–482.
Clayton, D.F. and Darnell, J.E. (1983). *Mol. Cell Biol.* **3**, 1552–1561.
Clément, B., Guguen-Guillouzo, C., Campion, J.P., Glaise, D., Bourel, M. and Guillouzo, A. (1984). *Hepatology*, **4**, 373–380.
Clément, B., Dumont, J.M., Ratanasavanh, D., Latinier, M.F., Brissot, P. and Guillouzo, A. (1988). *In* "Liver Cells and Drugs" (A. Guillouzo, ed.), pp. 417–421. Les Editions INSERM and John Libbey Eurotext, Paris.
Conner, J., Vallet-Collom, I., Daveau, M., Delers, F., Lebreton, J.P. and Guilllouzo, A. (1990). *Biochem. J.* **266**, 683–688.
Crane, L.J. and Miller, D.L. (1977). *J. Cell Biol.* **72**, 11–25.
Daujat, M., Fabre, I., Diaz, D., Pichard, L., Fabre, G., Fabre, J.M., Saint-Aubert, B. and Maurel, P. (1992). *Life Sci.*, in press.
De Leeuw, A.M., McCarthy, S.P., Geerts, A. and Knook, D.L. (1984). *Hepatology*, **4**, 392–403.
Deschatrette, J. and Weiss, M.C. (1974). *Biochimie* **56**, 1603–1611.
Diaz, D., Fabre, I., Daujat, M., Saint Laurent, B., Bories, P., Michel, H. and Maurel, P. (1990). *Gastroenterology* **99**, 737–747.
Direnzo, A.B., Gandolfi, A.J., Sipes, I.G., Brendel, K. and Byard, J.L. (1984). *Xenobiotica* **14**, 521–525.
Donato, M.T., Castell, J.V. and Gomez-Lechon, M.J. (1990). *Toxicol. In Vitro* **4**, 461–466.
Eckl, P.M., Whitcomb, W.R., Michalopoulos, G.K. and Jirtle, R.L. (1987). *J. Cell Physiol.* **132**, 363–366.
Eliasson, E., Johansson, I. and Ingelman-Sundberg, M. (1988). *Biochem. Biophys. Res. Commun.* **150**, 436–443.
Elshourbagy, N.A., Barwick, J.L. and Guzelian, P.S. (1981). *J. Biol. Chem.* **256**, 6060–6068.
Enat, R., Jefferson, D.M., Ruiz-Opazo, N., Gatmaitan, Z., Leinwand, L.A. and Reid, L.M. (1984). *Proc. Natl. Acad. Sci. U.S.A.* **81**, 1411–1415.
Fahl, W.E., Michalopoulos, G., Sattler, G.L., Jefcoate, C.R. and Pitot, H.C. (1979). *Arch. Biochem. Biophys.* **192**, 61–72.
Fariss, M.W., Olafsdottir, K. and Reed, D.J. (1984). *Biochem. Biophys. Res. Commun.* **121**, 102–110.
Fautrel, A., Chesné, C., Guillouzo, A., De Sousa, G., Placidi, M., Rahmani, R., Braut, F., Pichon, J., Hoellinger, H., Vintezou, P., Diarte, I., Melcion, C., Cordier, A., Lorenzon, G., Benicourt, M., Vannier, B., Fournex, R., Peloux, A.F., Bichet, N., Gouy, D., Cano, J.P. and Lounes, R. (1991). *Toxicol. In Vitro* **5**, 543–547.
Forster, U., Luippold, G. and Schwarz, L.R. (1986). *Drug Metab. Disp.* **14**, 353–360.
Fraslin, J.M., Kneip, B., Vaulont, S., Glaise, D., Munich, A. and Guguen-Guillouzo, C. (1985). *EMBO J.* **4**, 2487–2491.
Fry, J.R. and Bridges, J.W. (1977). *Biochem. Pharmacol.* **26**, 969–973.
Fry, J.R. and Bridges, J.W. (1979). *Rev. Biochem. Toxicol.* **1**, 201–247.

Gebhardt, R. (1988). *Scand. J. Gastroenterol.* (suppl.) **151**, 8–18.
Ghantous, H.N., Fernando, J., Gandolfi, A.J. and Brendel, K. (1990). *Drug Metab. Disp.* **18**, 514–518.
Gleiberman, A.S., Kudrjavtseva, E.I., Sharovskaya, U.Y. and Abelev, G.I. (1989). *Mol. Biol. Med.* **6**, 95–107.
Goethals, F., Deboyser, D., Lefebvre, V., De Coster, I. and Roberfroid, M. (1990). *Toxicol. In Vitro* **4**, 435–438.
Goulet, F., Normand, C. and Morin, O. (1988). *Hepatology* **8**, 1010–1018.
Grislain, L., Ratanasavanh, D., Moquard, M.T., Raquillet, L., Bégué, J.M., Du Vignaud, P., Génissel, P., Guillouzo, A., and Bromet, N. (1988). *In* "Liver Cells and Drugs" (A. Guillouzo, ed.), pp. 357–363. Les Editions INSERM and John Libbey Eurotext, Paris.
Guengerich, F.P. (1985). *CRC Crit. Rev. Toxicol.* **14**, 259–307.
Guguen, C., Gregori, C. and Schapira, F. (1975). *Biochimie* **57**, 1065–1071.
Guguen-Guillouzo, C. (1986). *In* "Isolated and Cultured Hepatocytes" (A. Guillouzo and C. Guguen-Guillouzo, eds), pp. 259–283. Les Editions INSERM and John Libbey Eurotext, Paris.
Guguen-Guillouzo, C. and Guillouzo, A. (1983). *Mol. Cell Biochem.* **53/54**, 35–56.
Guguen-Guillouzo, C. and Guillouzo, A. (1986). *In* "Isolated and Cultured Hepatocytes" (A. Guillouzo and C. Guguen-Guillouzo, eds), pp. 1–12, Les Editions INSERM and John Libbey Eurotext, Paris.
Guguen-Guillouzo, C., Seignoux, D., Courtois, Y., Brissot, P., Marceau, N., Glaise, D. and Guillouzo, A. (1982). *Biol. Cell* **46**, 11–20.
Guguen-Guillouzo, C., Clément, B., Baffet, G., Beaumont, C., Morel-Chany, E., Glaise, D. and Guillouzo, A. (1983). *Exp. Cell Res.* **143**, 47–54.
Guguen-Guillouzo, C., Clément, B., Lescoat, G., Glaise, D. and Guillouzo, A. (1984). *Dev. Biol.* **105**, 211–220.
Guillouzo, A. (1986a). *In* "Isolated and Cultured Hepatocytes" (A. Guillouzo and C. Guguen-Guillouzo, eds), pp. 155–170. Les Editions INSERM and John Libbey Eurotext, Paris.
Guillouzo, A. (1986b). *In* "Isolated and Cultured Hepatocytes" (A. Guillouzo and C. Guguen-Guillouzo, eds), pp. 313–332. Les Editions INSERM and John Libbey Eurotext, Paris.
Guillouzo, A. (1992). *In* "In Vitro Toxicity Testing. Applications to Safety Evaluation" (J.M. Frazier, ed.), pp. 45–83. Marcel Dekker Inc., New York.
Guillouzo, A., Oudea, P., Le Guilly, Y., Oudea, M.C., Lenoir, P. and Bourel, M. (1972). *Exp. Mol. Pathol.* **16**, 1–15.
Guillouzo, A., Clément, B., Bégué, J.M. and Guguen-Guillouzo, C. (1984). *Biochem. Biophys. Res. Commun.* **120**, 311–317.
Guillouzo, A., Beaune, P., Gascoin, M.N., Bégué, J.M., Campion, J.P., Guengerich, F.P. and Guguen-Guillouzo, C. (1985). *Biochem. Pharmacol.* **34**, 2991–2995.
Guillouzo, A., Bégué, J.M., Maurer, G. and Koch, P. (1988). *Xenobiotica* **18**, 131–139.
Guillouzo, A., Clerc, C., Mallédant, Y., Ratanasavanh, D. and Guguen-Guillouzo, C. (1989). *Gastroenterol. Clin. Biol.* **13**, 725–730.
Guillouzo, A., Morel, F., Ratanasavanh, D., Chesné, C. and Guguen-Guillouzo, C. (1990). *Toxicol. In Vitro* **4**, 415–427.

Guyomard, C., Chesné, C., Meunier, B., Fautrel, A., Clerc, C., Morel, F., Rissel, M., Campion, J.P. and Guillouzo, A. (1990). *Hepatology* **12**, 1329–1336.
Guzelian, P.S., Bissell, D.M. and Meyer, U.A. (1977). *Gastroenterology*, **72**, 1232–1239.
Harman, A.W. and Fischer, L.J. (1983). *Toxicol. Appl. Pharmacol.* **71**, 330–341.
Inoue, C., Yamamoto, H., Nakamura, T., Ichihara, A. and Okamoto, H. (1989). *J. Biol. Chem.* **264**, 4747–4750.
Isom, H.C. and Georgoff, I. (1984). *Proc. Natl. Acad. Sci. U.S.A.* **81**, 6378–6382.
Isom, H.C., Secott, T., Georgoff, I., Woodworth, C. and Mummaw, J. (1985). *Proc. Natl. Acad. Sci. U.S.A.* **82**, 3252–3256.
Isom, H., Georgoff, I., Salditt-Georgieff, M. and Darnell, J.E. (1987). *J. Cell Biol.* **105**, 2877–2885.
James, O.F.W., Rawlins, M.D., Wynne, H. and Woodhouse, K.W. (1988). *In* "Liver Cells and Drugs" (A. Guillouzo, ed.), pp. 13–21. Les Editions INSERM and John Libbey Eurotext, Paris.
Klaassen, C.D. and Stacey, N.H. (1982). *In* "Toxicology of the Liver" (G. Plaa and W.R. Hewitt, eds), pp. 147–179. Raven Press, New York.
Knook, D.L. and Sleyster, C.S. (1976). *Exp. Cell Res.* **99**, 444–449.
Knowles, B.B., Howe, C.C. and Aden, D.P. (1980). *Science* **209**, 497–499.
Lake, B.G., Gray, T.J.B., Stubberfield, C.R., Beamand, J.A. and Gangolli, S.D (1983). *Life Sci.* **33**, 249–254.
Larrey, D. and Pessayre, D. (1988). *In* "Liver Cells and Drugs" (A. Guillouzo, eds.), pp. 143–152. Les Editions INSERM and John Libbey Eurotext, Paris.
Le Bigot, J.F., Bégué, J.M., Kiechel, J.R. and Guillouzo, A. (1987). *Life Sci.* **40**, 883–890.
Le Bot, M.A., Bégué, J.M., Kernaleguen, D., Robert, J., Ratanasavanh, D., Airiau, J., Riché, C. and Guillouzo, A. (1988). *Biochem. Pharmacol.* **37**, 3877–3887.
Le Corre, P., Ratanasavanh, D., Gibassier, D., Barthel, A.M., Sado, P., Le Verge, R. and Guillouzo, A. (1988). *In* "Liver Cells and Drugs" (A. Guillouzo, ed.), pp. 321–324. Les Editions INSERM and John Libbey Eurotext, Paris.
Le Rumeur, E., Beaumont, C., Guillouzo, C., Rissel, M., Bourel, M. and Guillouzo, A. (1981). *Biochem. Biophys. Res. Commun.* **101**, 1038–1046.
Le Rumeur, E., Guguen-Guillouzo, C., Beaumont, C., Saunier, A. and Guillouzo, A. (1983). *Exp. Cell Res.* **147**, 247–254.
Lescoat, G., Thézé, N., Clément, B., Guillouzo, A. and Guguen-Guillouzo, C. (1985). *Cell Diff.* **16**, 259–268.
Lindros, K.O. and Penttilä, K.E. (1985). *Biochem. J.* **228**, 560–575.
Loeper, J., Descatoire, V., Amouyal, G., Letteron, P., Larrey, D. and Pessayre, D. (1989). *Hepatology* **9**, 675–678.
Long, R.M. and Moore, L. (1988). *Toxicol. Appl. Pharmacol.* **92**, 295–306.
Luetteke, N.C. and Michalopoulos, G.K. (1987). *In* "The Isolated Hepatocyte: Use in Toxicology and Xenobiotic Biotransformations" (E.J. Rauckman and G.M. Padilla, eds), pp. 93–118. Academic Press, Orlando.
Mallédant, Y., Siproudhis, L., Tanguy, M., Clerc, C., Chesné, C., Saint-Marc, C. and Guillouzo, A. (1990). *Anesthesiology*, **72**, 526–534.
Marceau, N., Noël, M. and Deschenes, J. (1982). *In Vitro* **18**, 1–11.
Maron, D.M. and Ames, B.N. (1983). *Mut. Res.* **113**, 173–215.
McGowan, J.A. (1986). *In* "Isolated and Cultured Hepatocytes" (A. Guillouzo

and C. Guguen-Guillouzo, eds), pp. 13–38. Les Editions INSERM and John Libbey Eurotext, Paris.

McGowan, J.A. (1988). *J. Cell. Physiol.* **137**, 497–504.

Mendoza-Figueroa, T., Hernandez, A., De Lourdes Lopez, M. and Kuri-Harcuch, W. (1988). *Toxicology* **52**, 273–286.

Mesnil, M., Fraslin, J.M., Piccoli, C., Yamasaki, H. and Guguen-Guillouzo, C. (1987). *Exp. Cell Res.* **173**, 524–533.

Michalopoulos, G.K. (1990). *FASEB J.* **4**, 176–187.

Michalopoulos, G., Russel, F. and Biles, C. (1979). *In Vitro* **15**, 796–806.

Michalopoulos, G.K., Strom, S.C. and Jirtle, R.L. (1986). In "Isolated and Cultured Hepatocytes" (A. Guillouzo and C. Guguen-Guillouzo, eds), pp. 333–352. Les Editions INSERM and John Libbey Eurotext, Paris.

Moldeus, P. (1978). *Biochem. Pharmacol.* **27**, 2859–2863.

Moore, C.J. and Gould, M.N. (1984). *Carcinogenesis* **5**, 1577–1582.

Morel, F., Beaune, P., Ratanasavanh, D., Flinois, J.P., Yang, C.S., Guengerich, F.P. and Guillouzo, A. (1990). *Eur. J. Biochem.* **191**, 437–444.

Morin, O. and Normand, C. (1986). *J. Cell. Physiol.* **129**, 103–110.

Muakkassah-Kelly, S.F., Bieri, F., Waechter, F., Bentley, P. and Staübli, W. (1987). *Exp. Cell Res.* **171**, 37–51.

Nakamura, T., Nishizawa, T., Higiya, M., Seki, T., Shimonishi, M., Sugimura, A., Tashiro, K. and Shimizi, S. (1989). *Nature* **342**, 440–443.

Namiki, M., Degawa, M., Masuki, T. and Hashimoto, Y. (1989). *Jap. J. Cancer Res.* **80**, 126–131.

Nebert, D.W., Nelson, D.R., Adesnik, M., Coon, M.J., Estabrook, R.W., Gonzalez, F.J., Guengerich, F.P., Gunsalus, I.C., Johnson, E.F., Kemper, B., Levin, W., Philipps, I.R., Sato, R. and Waterman, M.R. (1989). *DNA*, **8**, 1–11.

Neuberger, J., Kenna, J.G., Nouri Aria, K. and Williams, R. (1985). *Gut* **26**, 1233–1239.

Newman, S. and Guzelian, P.S. (1982). *Proc. Natl. Acad. Sci. U.S.A.* **79**, 2922–2926.

Paine, A.J. (1990). *Chem. Biol. Interact.* **74**, 1–31.

Paine, A.J. and Hockin, L.J. (1982). *Toxicology* **25**, 41–45.

Paul, D., Höhne, M., Pinkert, C., Piasecki, A., Ummelmann, E. and Brinster, R.L. (1988). *Exp. Cell Res.* **175**, 354–362.

Pessayre, D. and Larrey, D. (1988). In "Liver Cells and Drugs" (A. Guillouzo, ed.), pp. 129–142. Les Editions INSERM and John Libbey Eurotext, Paris.

Perrot, N., Chesné, C., de Waziers, I., Conner, J., Beaune, P. and Guillouzo, A. (1991). *Eur. J. Biochem.* **200**, 255–262.

Pompon, D. (1988). *Eur. J. Biochem.* **177**, 285–293.

Pompon, D. (1990). *Biochimie* **72**, 463–472.

Purchase, I.F.M. (1990). *Toxicol. in Vitro* **4**, 667–674.

Quistorff, B., Grunnet, N. and Cornell, N.W. (1985). *Biochem. J.* **226**, 2189–2197.

Rahmani, R., Richard, B., Fabre, G. and Cano, J.P. (1988). *Xenobiotica* **18**, 71–88.

Ratanasavanh, D., Beaune, P., Baffet, G., Rissel, M., Kremers, P., Guengerich, F.P. and Guillouzo, A. (1986). *J. Histochem. Cytochem.* **34**, 527–533.

Ratanasavanh, D., Baffet, G., Latinier, M.F., Rissel, M. and Guillouzo, A. (1988a). *Xenobiotica* **18**, 773–783.

Ratanasavanh, D., Riché, C. Bégué, J.M. and Guillouzo, A. (1988b). In

"Méthodes *in vitro* en pharmacotoxicologie" (M. Adolphe and A. Guillouzo, eds), vol. 170, pp. 11–16. Les Editions INSERM, Paris.

Reese, J.A. and Byard, J.L. (1981). *In Vitro* **17**, 935–941.

Reid, L.M., Narita, M., Fujita, M., Murray, Z., Liverpool, C. and Rosenberg, L. (1986). *In* "Isolated and Cultured Hepatocytes" (A. Guillouzo and C. Guguen-Guillouzo, eds), pp. 225–258. Les Editions INSERM and John Libbey Eurotext, Paris.

Rojkind, M., Gatmaitan, Z., Mackensen, S., Giambrone, M.A., Ponce, P. and Reid, L.M. (1980). *J. Cell Biol.* **87**, 255–263.

Sawada, N., Tomomura, A., Sattler, C.A., Sattler, G.L., Kleinman, H.K. and Pitot, H.C. (1986). *Exp. Cell Res.* **167**, 458–470.

Schrode, W., Mecke, D. and Gebhardt, R. (1990). *Eur. J. Cell Biol.* **53**, 35–41.

Schuetz, E.G., Li, D., Omiecinski, C.J., Muller-Eberhard, U., Kleinman, H.K., Elswick, B. and Guzelian, P.S. (1988). *J. Cell. Physiol.* **134**, 309–323.

Seddon, T., Michelle, I. and Chenery, R.J. (1989). *Biochem. Pharmacol.* **38**, 1657–1665.

Seglen, P.O. (1975). *Methods Cell Biol.* **13**, 29–83.

Seglen, P.O. (1977). *Biochim. Biophys. Acta* **496**, 182–191.

Seglen, P.O., Solheim, A.E., Grinde, B., Gordon, P.B., Schwarze, P.E., Gjessing, R. and Poli, A. (1980). *Ann. N.Y. Acad. Sci.* **349**, 1–7.

Siegers, C.P. (1988). *In* "Liver Drugs: From Experimental Pharmacology to Therapeutic Application" (B. Testa and D. Perrisoud, eds), pp. 15–29. CRC Press, Boca Raton, FL.

Sipes, I.G., Fisher, R.L., Smith, P.F., Stine, E.R., Gandolfi, A.J. and Brendel, K. (1987). *Arch. Toxicol.* (suppl.) **11**, 20–30.

Siproudhis, L., Beaugrand, M., Malledant, Y., Brissot, P., Guguen-Guillouzo, C. and Guillouzo, A. (1991). *Toxicol. In Vitro*, **5**, 529–534.

Sirica, A.E. and Pitot, H.C. (1980). *Pharmacol. Rev.* **31**, 205–228.

Sirica, A.E., Richards, W., Tsukada, C., Sattler, C. and Pitot, H.C. (1979). *Proc. Natl. Acad. Sci. U.S.A.* **114**, 307–315.

Sirica, A.E., Mathis, G.A., Sano, N. and Elmore, L.W. (1990). *Pathobiology* **58**, 44–64.

Smith, M.T., Thor, H. and Orrenius, S. (1981). *Science* **213**, 1257–1259.

Smith, P.F., Krack, G., McKee, K.L., Johnson, D.G., Gandolfi, A.J., Hruby, V.J., Krumdieck, C.L. and Brendel, K. (1986). *In Vitro Cell. Dev. Biol.* **22**, 706–712.

Steinmetz, K.L., Spak, D.K., Green, C.E. and Mirsalis, J.C. (1985). *Toxicologist* **5**, 20.

Steward, A.R., Dannan, G.A., Guzelian, P.S. and Guengerich, F.P. (1985). *Mol. Pharmacol.* **27**, 125–132.

Story, D.L., Gee, S.J., Tyson, C.A. and Gould, D.H. (1983). *J. Toxicol. Environ. Health* **11**, 483–501.

Stricker, B.H.C.H. and Spoelstra, P. (1985). *In* "Drug-Induced Hepatic Injury". Elsevier, Amsterdam.

Strom, S.C., Jirtle, R.L., Jones, R.S., Novicki, D.L., Rosenberg, M.R., Novotny, A., Irons, G., McLain, J.R. and Michalopoulos, G. (1982). *J. Natl. Cancer Inst.* **68**, 771–778.

Strom, S.C., Novicki, D.L., Novotny, A., Jirtle, R. and Michalopoulos, G. (1983). *Carcinogenesis* **4**, 683–686.

Strom, S.C., Monteith, D.K., Manoharan, K., and Novotny, A. (1987). *In* "The

Isolated Hepatocyte: Use in Toxicology and Xenobiotic Biotransformations"
(E.J. Rauckman and G.M. Padilla, eds), pp. 265–280. Academic Press,
Orlando.
Sudhakaran, P.R., Stamaloglou, C. and Hughes, R.C. (1986). *Exp. Cell Res.*
167, 505–516.
Tran-Thi, T.A., Phillips, J., Falk, H. and Decker, K. (1985). *Exp. Mol. Pathol.*
42, 89–116.
Tyson, C.A. and Green, C.E. (1987). *In* "The Isolated Hepatocyte: Use in
Toxicology and Xenobiotic Biotransformations" (E.J. Rauckman and G.M.
Padilla, eds), pp. 119–158. Academic Press, Orlando.
Tyson, C.A., Mitoma, C. and Kalivoda, J. (1980). *J. Toxicol. Environ. Health*
6, 197–205.
Tyson, C.A., Hawk-Prather, C., Story, D.L. and Gould, D.H. (1983). *Toxicol.
Appl. Pharmacol.* **70**, 289–302.
Vandenberghe, Y., Glaise, D., Meyer, D.J., Guillouzo, A. and Ketterer, B.
(1988a). *Biochem. Pharmacol.* **37**, 2482–2485.
Vandenberghe, Y., Ratanasavanh, D., Glaise, D. and Guillouzo, A. (1988b). *In
Vitro Cell Dev. Biol.* **24**, 281–288.
Vandenberghe, Y., Morel, F., Pemble, S., Taylor, J.B., Rogiers, V., Ratana-
savanh, D., Vercruysse, A., Ketterer, B. and Guillouzo, A. (1990). *Mol.
Pharmacol.* **37**, 372–376.
Vergani, D., Mieli-Vergani, G., Alberti, A., Neuberger, J., Eddleston, A.L.W.F.,
Davis, M. and Williams, R. (1980). *N. Engl. J. Med.* **303**, 66–71.
Villa, P. and Guaitani, A. (1988). *In* "Liver Cells and Drugs" (A. Guillouzo,
ed.), pp. 405–410. Les Editions INSERM and John Libbey Eurotext, Paris.
Villa, P., Bégué, J.M. and Guillouzo, A. (1984). *Biochem. Pharmacol.* **33**,
4098–4101.
Vonen, B. and Morland, J. (1984). *Arch. Toxicol.* **56**, 33–37.
Wanson, J.C., Mosselmans, R., Brouwer, A. and Knook, D.L. (1979). *Biol. Cell*
56, 7–16.
Watkins, P.B., Wrighton, S.A., Schuetz, E.G., Maurel, P. and Guzelian, P.S.
(1986). *J. Biol. Chem.* **261**, 6264–2671.
Waxman, D.J., Morrissey, J.J., Naik, S. and Jaureguy, H.O. (1990). *Biochem.
J.* **271**, 113–119.
Weigand, K., Wernze, H. and Falge, C. (1977). *Biochem. Biophys. Res. Commun.*
75, 102–110.
Woodhouse, K.W., Mortimer, O. and Wiholm, B.E. (1986). *In* "The Effect of
Age in Liver and Ageing" (K. Kitani, ed.), pp. 75–80. Elsevier, Amsterdam.
Wu, D.F., Clejan, L., Potter, B. and Cederbaum, A.I. (1990). *Hepatology* **12**,
1379–1389.

Discussion

P. Laduron
It is somewhat surprising to see that protein synthesis inhibitors like
cycloheximide are not toxic – even less toxic than chlorpromazine. This
means that protein synthesis turnover must be very low – or are there
other reasons for that finding?

A. Guillouzo

This study was performed with coded compounds at certain concentrations and under certain conditions, which is of course a limitation of the study. However, several other studies have shown that in different conditions cycloheximide is cytotoxic. A problem of using a protocol with coded compounds is that we do not know what kind of compound we are testing. It is the same with bromobenzene, for example, with which we found very low cytotoxicity, but in other conditions there is no problem in getting bromobenzene cytotoxicity with isolated hepatocytes. We have to consider that it is a volatile compound. This is why I said that the same protocol cannot be used for all kinds of compounds.

J. Boyer

Dr Guillouzo has presented a lot of very interesting and important data. I am particularly interested in the studies on cell-mediated and antibody-mediated cell cytotoxicity, which looked very exciting. Has he any idea of where the antigen is located in terms of the cell-mediated response? Is there any information on whether the drug is getting into the cell and creating a reactive metabolite that is then being expressed either in the endoplasmic reticulum or on the cell membrane?

A. Guillouzo

That is the next step. It is why I said that these are preliminary results. The first step was to demonstrate that there was a specific cytotoxic effect with all sera tested. We now have to try to understand exactly what is happening. We know that clometacin must be added before adding the serum and that lymphoid cells are needed. I cannot give an answer about a plasma membrane antigen, although we hope it exists.

J. Boyer

Have patients with halothane toxicity been studied?

A. Guillouzo

No, not yet. So far we have studied direct toxicity only. The first step is to define the non-cytotoxic concentration, to be sure that when cytotoxicity is found it is related to the presence of lymphoid cells and not to a direct effect of the drug. The conditions have been set up to study halothane toxicity: specific conditions are required as for bromobenzene.

P. Beaune

If antibodies are directed against cytochrome *P*-450, some cytochrome *P*-450 is expressed on the membrane.

A. Guillouzo

For clometacin only antinuclear or anti-smooth muscle antibodies were found; this differs from Dr Beaune's findings with tienilic acid and some other compounds.

H. Brun

With regard to human hepatocytes, does Dr Guillouzo think that therapeutic drugs, such as corticosteroids which are used to maintain the vital function of the organs, may affect maintenance of hepatocyte function in an *in vitro* model and not enhance the differentiation of the cells?

A. Guillouzo

I think that corticosteroids, for example, are important in the culture medium for maintaining the cells for a long time *in vitro*, so they should have various effects. At the concentration used I do not think that they induce cytochrome *P*-450, but their effect is of course important. Most of the media which are suitable for hepatocyte survival *in vitro* contain various hormones.

N.G. Carmichael

Rather than talking about toxicology problems we often have metabolism problems to bridge from animal to human models. If Dr Guillouzo was able to show differences between his human and animal hepatocyte cultures, how confident would he be, not quantitatively but qualitatively, that it would be representative of the *in vivo* situation?

A. Guillouzo

On the basis of perhaps 40 or 50 compounds, it is possible to say that, in most cases, the main metabolites found *in vivo* are the same as those found *in vitro*. When major differences are found between human and animal hepatocytes, this reflects the *in vivo* situation. We have only one or two examples where some differences were observed.

X. Pouradier Duteil

I am not surprised that when cells are preserved for more than 40 h, defective activity is detected. Every paper on liver transplantation describes the impossibility of preserving hepatic function for more than 10 h in the University of Wisconsin (UW) or in other solutions.

Secondly, Dr Guillouzo said that one advantage of the liver is the great number of cells but, as a result of the huge development of transplantation thanks to cyclosporin, there is great difficulty in obtaining livers. How does he manage to get these cells from human liver?

A. Guillouzo

I agree with the first comment. The same situation arises with an isolated cell suspension. Some functions decrease if we wait for 1 or 2 h before starting experiments.

Of course, getting human hepatocytes is a major problem. We hope that transplantation will not increase in the future as fast as it is increasing now. Also, if we can get hepatocytes from livers preserved for 1 or 2 days in the UW solution (and I hope I have demonstrated that this is possible) there will be more opportunities to use human liver samples.

8

Primary Culture of Hepatocytes in the Investigation of Drug-Induced Steatosis

M.A. IVANOV, E. HEUILLET, P. VINTEZOU, C. MELCION and A. CORDIER

Rhône-Poulenc Rorer, Institut de Recherche sur la Sécurité du Médicament, 20, quai de la Révolution, 94140 Alfortville, France

Introduction

Cultured hepatocytes have been extensively used to investigate the hepatic toxicity of new pharmaceutical compounds. There are three main forms of drug-induced hepatotoxicity: necrosis, cholestasis and steatosis (Zimmerman, 1978). The most common of the three is probably steatosis. An *in vitro* model of drug-induced steatosis could, therefore, be very useful in the prediction of the hepatotoxicity of candidate drugs.

Definition of Steatosis

Steatosis or fatty liver is characterized by the accumulation of lipids (particularly triglycerides) in the hepatocytes. Two types of fatty liver are

IN VITRO METHODS IN TOXICOLOGY
ISBN 0-12-388175-7

distinguished on the basis of the size of the lipid droplets which accumulate in the hepatocytes: macrovesicular steatosis and microvesicular steatosis.

Macrovesicular Steatosis

In macrovesicular steatosis, a few relatively large lipid droplets are formed within the hepatocyte, displacing the nucleus towards the edge of the cell. Fatty liver of this type has been described after the administration of ethanol, methotrexate (Scheuer, 1980), corticosteroids (Steinberg *et al.*, 1952; Hill, 1961; Jones *et al.*, 1965; Alpers and Isselbacher, 1975), L-asparaginase (Biggs *et al.*, 1971; Pratt and Johnson, 1971), mithramycin and colchicine (Dustin, 1941).

Macrovesicular fatty liver is not usually associated with impairment of hepatic function; however, it may be associated with necrosis (Zimmerman, 1987). Following exposure to carbon tetrachloride, chloroform or tannic acid, necrosis is the predominant lesion, whereas following exposure to compounds such as α-amanitin or yellow phosphorus, the main abnormality is fatty liver.

In alcohol-induced hepatitis, fatty liver is associated with necrosis and inflammation. This condition can lead to severe liver failure and cirrhosis (Zimmerman, 1987).

Microvesicular Steatosis

Microvesicular steatosis is considered to be more severe (Flejou *et al.*, 1987). It is characterized by the accumulation of large numbers of small lipid droplets within the hepatocyte, leaving the nucleus occupying its normal central position. The cytoplasm of the cells is foamy and the nucleus is frequently hyperchromatic. Microvesicular fatty liver has been described after administration of valproic acid (Ware and Millward-Sadler, 1980; Zimmerman and Ishak, 1982; Kesterson *et al.*, 1984), pirprofen (Danan *et al.*, 1985), amineptine (Martin *et al.*, 1981; Ramain *et al.*, 1981; Le Dinh *et al.*, 1988), tetracycline (Combes *et al.*, 1972; Symansky and Fox, 1972; Zimmerman, 1978), hypoglycin A (Tanaka and Kean, 1976; Sherratt, 1986), pentenoic acid (Glasgow and Chase, 1975) and methyl salicylate (Meyerhoff, 1930; Eimas and Bridgeport, 1938; Starko *et al.*, 1980; Waldman *et al.*, 1982). Microvesicular steatosis is also seen in Reye's syndrome (Reye *et al.*, 1963) and may occur during pregnancy (Marshall and Kaplan, 1985).

Microvesicular fatty liver is sometimes associated with mild cholestasis, but degeneration or necrosis is very rare. Necrosis has, however, been described after exposure to valproic acid (Zafrani and Berthelot, 1982; Zimmerman and Ishak, 1982) and pirprofen (Danan *et al.*, 1985).

The macro- and micro-vesicular forms of fatty liver can occur simultaneously, but the mechanisms involved remain to be elucidated.

Mechanisms Involved in the Development of Fatty Liver

The high incidence of fatty liver is probably attributable to the central role of the liver in the metabolism of lipids and lipoproteins (Zakim and Boyer, 1990). The liver synthesizes fatty acids from excess sugar and esterifies them to form triglycerides (TG), which are subsequently secreted as very low density lipoprotein (VLDL). The VLDLs are then transported out of the hepatocyte to storage sites in the adipose tissue. During fasting, fatty acids are released from storage in the adipose tissues and can be metabolized by the liver. The accumulation of lipids in the liver is considered to result from an imbalance between the rate of TG synthesis and the rate at which it is utilized by the hepatocytes (secretion and oxidation) (Lombardi, 1966).

Theoretically, then, fatty liver can result from many causes: an increase in the availability of fatty acids from the diet or from adipose tissue, an increase in fatty acid synthesis within the liver (lipogenesis) or a decrease in fatty acid oxidation (β-oxidation within the mitochondria). However, TG is only secreted in the form of very low density lipoprotein if it is associated with apoproteins, cholesterol and phospholipids (Zakim and Boyer, 1990). Therefore, any defect in VLDL lipid or protein synthesis, in protein glycosylation or in the assembly of proteins and lipids and their transportation to the plasma membrane could lead to fatty liver change.

All the mechanisms involved in ensuring normal triglyceride secretion are potential targets for drug toxicity, and this may account for the large number of drugs that induce fatty liver.

Intrahepatic Causes of Fatty Liver

The inhibition of VLDL secretion appears to be a major cause of fatty liver, possibly because it involves many steps, all of which must function correctly if the process is to proceed smoothly. This steatogenic mechanism was first described in the case of CCl_4 (Recknagel *et al.*, 1960; Recknagel and Lombardi, 1961) and has since been shown to be involved in the hepatotoxicity of many other drugs (ethionine, phosphorus, puromycin, tetracycline, orotic acid) and in choline-deficient animals (Lombardi, 1966; Hoyumpa *et al.*, 1975).

As shown in Fig. 8.1, the accumulation of triglycerides may arise as a result of various mechanisms.

Impaired protein synthesis

Many steatogenic molecules have been shown to induce defective protein synthesis and various different steps in the synthetic process may be affected.

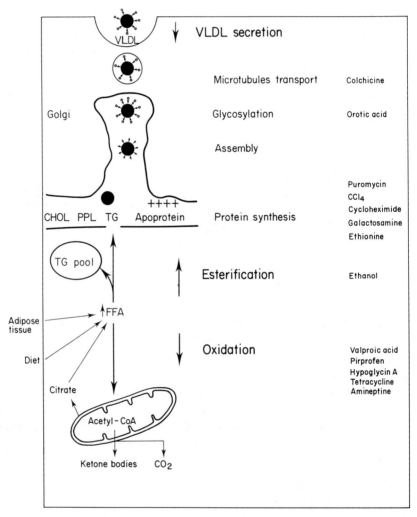

Fig. 8.1 Mechanisms involved in steatosis. FFA, free fatty acids. PPL, phospholipids. CHOL, cholesterol.

Inhibition of mRNA synthesis
Galactosamine has been shown to reduce the synthesis of mRNA and of plasma protein as a result of sequestration of UTP (a precursor of RNA) (Decker and Keppler, 1974).

α-Amanitin blocks the activity of RNA polymerase II (Stirpe and Fiume, 1967; Stirpe and Novello, 1970; Novello *et al.*, 1970; Lindell *et al.*, 1970; Montanaro *et al.*, 1971; Buku *et al.*, 1971).

Inhibition of translation
Many drugs have been shown to inhibit protein synthesis by an inhibitory impact on translation due to a variety of mechanisms. Dimethylnitrosamine induces methylation of ribosomal RNA (Magee and Farber, 1962; Magee and Hultin, 1962). Puromycin blocks the binding of aminoacyl-tRNA to the ribosomal 50S subunit (Yarmolinsky and DeLaHaba, 1959; Nathans and Lipmann, 1961; Nathans, 1964; Reid *et al.*, 1971). Ethionine induces alkylation of both nuclear and cytosolic nucleic acid, but it seems to be more likely that its steatogenic action is related to ATP depletion, since ATP is required for amino acids to be activated and incorporated into proteins (Farber, 1971). Cycloheximide is a potent inhibitor of polypeptide chain elongation and reinitiation (Pestka, 1971). The inhibition of protein synthesis by CCl_4 was first demonstrated by Smuckler *et al.* (1961) and subsequently confirmed by Seakins and Robinson (1963). The mechanism appears to involve inhibition of initiation reactions.

Other mechanisms

The compounds mentioned above all affect protein synthesis, but other mechanisms have also been proposed.

Decreased phospholipid synthesis
Reduced synthesis of the phospholipid lecithin has been demonstrated in fatty liver induced in choline-deficient rats (Lombardi *et al.*, 1964; Lombardi and Ugazio, 1965; Lombardi *et al.*, 1966; Lombardi and Oler, 1967; Lombardi *et al.*, 1969; Oler and Lombardi, 1970).

Inhibition of apolipoprotein glycosylation
It has been suggested that inhibition of apolipoprotein glycosylation could explain the fatty liver induced by a diet containing high levels of orotic acid (see below).

Impaired VLDL transportation
Impairment of VLDL transportation as a result of interaction with microtubules was first demonstrated by Jeanrenaud *et al.* (1977) in the case of colchicine.

Increased fatty acid synthesis
An increase in the synthesis of fatty acid from acetyl-CoA has been proposed as one of the many mechanisms involved in ethanol toxicity (Reboucas and Isselbacher, 1961; Lieber and Schmidt, 1961; Isselbacher and Carter, 1970; Gordon, 1972).

Inhibited fatty acid oxidation
Inhibition of the oxidation of fatty acids (β-oxidation) is commonly observed in microvesicular fatty liver. A mechanism of this type has been demonstrated for valproic acid (Bjorge and Baillie, 1985; Coude *et al.*, 1983; Turnbull *et al.*, 1983; Becker and Harris, 1983), pirprofen (Genève *et al.*, 1987), amineptine (Le Dinh *et al.*, 1988), tetracycline (Freneaux *et al.*, 1988), hypoglycin (Sherratt, 1986) and pentenoic acid (Thayer, 1984). Microvesicular steatosis has also been observed in post-infectious mitochondrial dysfunction (De Vivo, 1987) and in several genetic defects of mitochondrial β-oxidation (Taubman *et al.*, 1987).

Extrahepatic Causes of Fatty Liver

Extrahepatic factors can also be involved in the induction of fatty liver. Hormones such as adrenaline (Elliot and Durham, 1906; MacKay, 1937; Brindle and Ontko, 1986, Herdt *et al.*, 1988), noradrenaline (Aujard, 1953; Luthman and Holtenius, 1972), cortisol (Felt *et al.*, 1962; Moran, 1962; Hill *et al.*, 1965) and adrenocorticotrophin hormone (ACTH) (Paoletti *et al.*, 1961; Ozegovic *et al.*, 1975) and some drugs that activate adenylate cyclase in adipose tissue lead to an increase in the supply of fatty acid to the liver. A similar mechanism of action has been described for caffeine and theophylline (Estler and Ammon, 1966).

The Use of Cultured Hepatocytes in the *In Vitro* Investigation of Lipid Metabolism and Fatty Liver

Investigation of Lipid Metabolism

Cultured hepatocytes have been extensively used to study lipid metabolism and its regulation by hormones. The secretion of VLDL by isolated hepatocytes was first demonstrated by Jeejeeboy *et al.* (1975). The uptake, secretion and degradation of lipoproteins has been investigated in primary cultures of hepatocytes from the rat (Lamb *et al.*, 1977; Davis *et al.*, 1979; Bell-Quint and Forte, 1981; Melin *et al.*, 1984; Vance *et al.*, 1984; Patsch *et al.*, 1986; Rustan *et al.*, 1986; Mangiapane and Brindley, 1986; Sparks and Sparks, 1990), the baboon (Lanford *et al.*, 1989), the rabbit (Kosykh *et al.*, 1989), the chicken (Janero and Lane, 1983; Bamberger and Lane, 1990) and in cultures of human hepatocytes (Kosykh *et al.*, 1985; Edge *et al.*, 1986; Carr, 1987; Bouma *et al.*, 1988). The nascent VLDL secreted is quite similar to serum VLDL, but secretion declines with culture time (Bell-Quint and Forte, 1981; Rustan *et al.*, 1986).

Cultured hepatocytes have also been used to investigate fatty acid metabolism (MacGarry and Foster, 1980; Girard and Malewiak, 1986). The balance between esterification and oxidation seems to depend on the nutritional state of the animal. A high carbohydrate diet leads to the stimulation of lipogenesis, whereas fasting, a high-lipid diet or diabetes leads to stimulation of β-oxidation and inhibition of lipogenesis. The role of hormones in the equilibrium between esterification and oxidation has been extensively studied. Glucocorticosteroids (Agius *et al.*, 1986a,b), thyroid hormones (Saggerson *et al.*, 1982; Stakkestad and Lund, 1984) and the catecholamines (Kosugi *et al.*, 1983; Oberhaensli *et al.*, 1985) have been shown to affect this equilibrium.

Glucagon and cyclic AMP seem to play an important role in regulating fatty acid metabolism by stimulating fatty acid oxidation and ketogenesis (Cole and Margolis, 1974; Witters and Trasko, 1979; Harano *et al.*, 1982; Agius *et al.*, 1986a).

Study of Fatty Liver Induction by Four Steatogenic Compounds; Comparison with *In Vivo* data

Although cultured hepatocytes have been extensively used to investigate lipid metabolism, they have less frequently been used to investigate the mechanisms of drug-induced fatty liver. In this section, we will report data obtained *in vivo* and *in vitro* with four compounds of known steatogenic potential. We will then go on to discuss the contribution of *in vitro* models to the elucidation of the mechanisms involved in fatty liver.

Tetracycline

High-dose levels of tetracylcine have been reported to induce severe microvesicular fatty liver in man (Zimmerman, 1979; Stricker and

Spoelstra, 1985). In experimental animals, tetracyclcine also induces fatty liver (Shauer *et al.*, 1974; Estler and Böcker *et al.*, 1980; Böcker *et al.*, 1981, 1982; Hopf *et al.*, 1985). It is generally thought that defective triglyceride secretion is the mechanism responsible for these changes. This has been demonstrated *in vivo* in animal species (Shauer *et al.*, 1974; Böcker *et al.*, 1985; Hopf *et al.*, 1985) as well as in the isolated, perfused rat liver (Hansen *et al.*, 1968; Breen *et al.*, 1972, 1975) and, more recently, in isolated hepatocytes (Deboyser *et al.*, 1989).

Inhibition of protein synthesis has been reported both *in vivo* and *in vitro* (Yeh and Shils, 1966; Hansen *et al.*, 1968; Infante *et al.*, 1971; Breen *et al.*, 1975; Hopf *et al.*, 1985) and appears to be an important mechanism responsible for fatty liver. Inhibition of the synthesis of apoprotein moiety of lipoprotein could cause a decrease in the secretion of triglycerides. However, in isolated hepatocytes, the inhibition of lipid secretion occurs early and before protein synthesis has been inhibited (Deboyser *et al.*, 1989), suggesting that the inhibition of protein synthesis is not the first effect of the drug. On the other hand, Breen *et al.* (1975) have demonstrated *in vivo* that the decreased lipid secretion accounts for 46% of the accumulation of TG in the liver, suggesting that interference with the fatty acid metabolism could also be a contributing factor.

The latter hypothesis has recently been confirmed. Inhibition of the β-oxidation of fatty acids and of the tricarboxylic acid cycle has been demonstrated *in vivo* in mice and *in vitro* in human and mouse liver mitochondria (Freneaux *et al.*, 1988) and in cultured rat hepatocytes in our laboratory (see below).

Cycloheximide

Cycloheximide is known to induce fatty liver in the rat *in vivo* (Jazcilevich and Villa-Trevino, 1970; Gravela *et al.*, 1971; Bar-On *et al.*, 1972; Garcia-Sainz *et al.*, 1979; Mori, 1983). Inhibition of the biosynthesis of apolipoproteins has been assumed to be the major cause of fatty liver. *In vitro* studies have essentially focused on the inhibition of protein synthesis and triglyceride secretion. This was first demonstrated by Gravela *et al.* (1977) using isolated hepatocytes and was subsequently confirmed by Janero *et al.* (1983), Rustan *et al.* (1986), Nossen *et al.* (1987) and Deboyser *et al.* (1989). These authors have reported that the inhibition of triglyceride secretion appeared between 30 min and 2 h after a marked inhibition of protein synthesis. The effects of protein synthesis are drastic and constitute the first obvious effect of the drug. The period of latency before triglyceride secretion is inhibited is probably explained by the presence of a pool of pre-existing apoprotein B which is sufficient to maintain the normal secretion rate for a period of at least 30 min (Gravela *et al.*, 1977).

The inhibition of protein synthesis in turn has an impact on apolipoprotein B secretion. The disappearance of apolipoprotein B induced by cycloheximide was first demonstrated *in vivo* by Mori (1983), using immunohistochemical methods, and was subsequently confirmed by Keller *et al.* (1986) using cultured rat hepatocytes.

However, Garcia-Sainz *et al.* (1979) have suggested that cycloheximide induces fatty liver via increased fatty acid uptake. These authors have shown that fatty liver is induced by cycloheximide as a result of a decrease in fatty acid uptake without any change in protein synthesis and that it can be prevented by the administration of adenine.

Colchicine

Colchicine inhibits lipoprotein secretion both *in vivo* (Stein and Stein, 1973; Stein *et al.*, 1974) and *in vitro*, in perfused liver (Le Marchand *et al.*, 1973, 1974), in liver slices (Redman *et al.*, 1975), in isolated hepatocytes (Gravela *et al.*, 1977; Deboyser *et al.*, 1989) and in primary cultures of hepatocytes (Davis *et al.*, 1979; Rustan *et al.*, 1986). The mechanism involved must be related to the well-established interference of colchicine with the microtubular system (Wilson, 1975). Colchicine induces the accumulation of lipoprotein in the Golgi complex (Le Marchand *et al.*, 1973). It has been shown in the perfused liver of treated rats that the reduction in hepatocyte microtubules is tightly coupled to the reduction in hepatic VLDL secretion (Reaven and Reaven, 1980). In isolated hepatocytes, the drug has been shown to have no impact on the synthesis of either protein or triglycerides, but to impair the secretion of both protein and lipoprotein (Gravela *et al.*, 1977; Deboyser *et al.*, 1989). This finding would correlate well with inhibition of the microtubular system.

Orotic acid

Orotic acid induces fatty liver in the rat *in vivo* (Standerfer and Handler, 1955). The mechanism involved seems to be the inhibition of VLDL secretion (Windmueller, 1964, 1965; Windmueller and Levi, 1967), probably within the Golgi complex. The inhibition of apolipoprotein glycosylation was first demonstrated *in vivo* by Pottenger *et al.* (1973). Sabesin *et al.* (1977) have demonstrated *in vivo* that fatty liver is associated with an accumulation of VLDL in the Golgi complex, suggesting that the primary secretion defect occurs during the final step of VLDL secretion.

Martin *et al.* (1982) have confirmed the inhibition of glycosylation in liver microsomes isolated from orotic acid-fed rats. However, the importance of glycosylation in the secretion process needs further investigation, since Bell-Quint *et al.* (1981) have shown that tunicamycin, a glycosylation-inhibiting antibiotic, has little or no impact on VLDL secretion in cultured hepatocytes.

These four examples of steatogenic compounds illustrate the fact that steatogenesis can be induced by drugs as a result of impact on a number of different pathways. Possible sites of impact include:

1) Lipid metabolism (inhibition of the β-oxidation of free fatty acids)
2) Protein metabolism (inhibition of the protein synthesis)
3) Carbohydrate metabolism (inhibition of protein glycosylation)
4) VLDL transportation and secretion processes (inhibition of microtubule function).

This means that fatty liver provides a very sensitive tool for the detection of drug-induced toxicity.

Use of Cultured Rat Hepatocytes in the Evaluation of the Steatogenic Potential of Drugs

We have developed a new screening method for evaluating the steatogenic potential of drugs which involves the use of cultured rat hepatocytes. This method was applied to assess the steatogenic potential of a test compound, RP X (Rhône-Poulenc X), which has been developed as an anti-cancer agent and which is known to induce microvesicular fatty liver in animals.

Furthermore, various mechanisms which can induce steatosis were investigated in order to extend our understanding of how steatosis is induced by this compound.

Materials and Methods

Hepatocyte isolation

Liver from Sprague–Dawley rats was perfused with 500 ml of Ca^{2+}-free Hepes buffer (10 mM Hepes, 137 mM NaCl, 2.7 mM KCl, 0.3 mM $Na_2HPO_4.12H_2O$; pH 7.65) at a flow rate of 40 ml/min and then perfused at 20 ml/min with 250 ml of the same buffer containing 0.02% collagenase and 5 mM $CaCl_2$, according to the method described by Guillouzo and Guguen-Guillouzo (1986). The cells were collected and, after being washed several times in the culture medium (see below), they were resuspended in the medium.

Screening for steatogenic potential of drugs

The method used consisted of testing the effects of various drugs with regard to the intracellular accumulation of triglycerides and to cell death, evaluated by means of MTT (3-(4,5-dimethylthiazol-2-yl)-2,5-diphenyltetrazolium bromide) staining. The ratio between the drug concentration inducing a 30% increase in cell death and that producing a 30% increase in intracellular triglyceride levels was used as a predictive index of the steatogenic potential.

Hepatocytes (3×10^6 for triglyceride determinations or 30000 for cell death determination) were cultured on 25 cm^2 flasks or on microtitre plates respectively. In both cases the culture medium used was MEM/199 (2:1,v/v) supplemented with 0.2% bovine serum albumin, 10 μM insulin, 2 mM glutamine, 50 IU penicillin/ml, 50 μg streptomycin/ml and 10% foetal calf serum. A volume of 3 ml was required for the flasks and 100 μl for the wells of the microtitre plates. After 3 h of adherence, the test drugs were added to a medium having the same composition, but without the foetal calf serum. After exposure for 20 h, the triglyceride content and percentage cell death were determined. The triglyceride content was determined using the Boehringer Peridochrom triglycerides, GPO PAP kit (Wahlefeld and Bergmeyer, 1974) and cell death was assessed using MTT staining (Denizot and Lang, 1986). For the MTT staining, 10 μl of MTT 5 mg/ml was added to each well before incubation for 2 h at 37°C. The supernatant was then discarded and the cells were solubilized in 100 μl of dimethyl sulphoxide (DMSO). The optical density was read at 570 nm and the percentage cell death was assessed as follows:

$$\text{cell death} = 100 - \frac{\text{O.D. (treated cells)}}{\text{O.D. (control cells)}} \times 100\%$$

Since the test compound, RP X, interfered with MTT staining, the toxicology end point test used was LDH leakage (Mitchell and Acosta, 1981) using the Enzyline LDH kit (Biomérieux). After exposure for 20 h, the LDH content was determined in the cells and in the supernatant, and the percentage LDH leakage calculated as follows:

$$\text{LDH leakage} = \frac{\text{Extracellular LDH}}{\text{Intracellular LDH} + \text{extracellular LDH}} \times 100\%$$

Determination of VLDL secretion

Hepatocytes (9×10^6) were cultured in 80 cm² flasks containing 10 ml of MEM/199 (2:1,v/v) supplemented with 0.2% bovine serum albumin, 1μM insulin, 2 mM glutamine, 50 IU penicillin/ml and 50 μg streptomycin/ml. After 3 h of adherence, 138 μM of the test compound, RP X, or 100 μM tetracycline or cycloheximide was added to the culture medium. After incubation for 20 h, the medium was centrifuged at 200 *g* for 20 min to eliminate cell fragments. The medium was then concentrated in an Amicon cell. The concentrated medium obtained was then centrifuged again at 100 000 *g* for 16 h at 10°C to separate the VLDLs. The appropriate Boehringer kits were used to test for triglycerides (Peridochrom triglycerides GPO PAP; Wahlefeld and Bergmeyer, 1974), cholesterol (cholesterol C system; Siedel *et al.*, 1983) and phospholipids (Test combination phospholipids; Takayama *et al.*, 1977). The tests for protein were performed as described by Peterson (1979).

Determination of protein synthesis

Protein synthesis was determined using Seglen's method (1976). Hepatocytes (3×10^6) were cultured in 25 cm² flasks containing 3 ml of the same basic medium as above, including the 10% foetal calf serum. After 3 h of adherence, the cells were incubated for 1 h at 37°C in a medium with the same basic composition, containing 0.1 μCi [^{14}C]valine but no foetal calf serum, and containing a range of concentrations of the test compound (RP X) or 100 μM cycloheximide. After incubation, the total proteins were precipitated by adding 0.1 ml of concentrated perchloric acid. The hepatocytes were then scraped off, using a rubber policeman, recovered and the flask was washed with 2 ml of 2% perchloric acid. After centrifuging at 1000 *g*, the pellet was washed twice with 2% perchloric acid and then dissolved in 0.5 ml of 0.1N NaOH. This solution was then transferred to scintillation vials and 8 ml of Ready Solv HP added. The radioactivity was measured using a Rackbeta β-counter (LKB) and the results were expressed as a percentage of the control.

Determination of β-oxidation

The effect of the test compound (RP X) on β-oxidation was compared with that of a well-known inhibitor of β-oxidation, tetracycline (Freneaux *et al.*, 1988). Hepatocytes (3×10^6) were cultured in 25 cm² flasks containing 3 ml MEM/199 (2:1,v/v) supplemented with 0.2% bovine serum albumin, 2 mM glutamine, 50 IU penicillin/ml, 50 μg streptomycin/ml and

10% foetal calf serum. After 3 h of adherence, the cells were incubated with a range of concentrations of the test compound, RP X, or of tetracycline for 20 h in the same medium as before, but containing 1 μM hydrocortisone hemisuccinate and 1 mM-carnitine, but no foetal calf serum, as described by Herbin *et al.* (1987). One hour before the end of the incubation period, the medium was removed by aspiration and the same concentration of drug added together with 500 μM oleate bound to 1% bovine serum albumin. After incubation, 1.5 ml of cultured medium was precipitated by 40% perchloric acid and then centrifuged for 10 min at 2000 **g**. The supernatant was neutralized with 40% KOH and ketone bodies (acetoacetate and 3-hydroxybutyrate) measured at 340 nm as described by Williamson *et al.* (1962), by following the disappearance (acetoacetate) or appearance (3-hydroxybutyrate) of NADH.

3-Hydroxybutyrate, acetoacetate and total ketone bodies were expressed per mg of protein and as a percentage of the control.

Results and Discussion

Screening of the steatogenic potential of drugs

The results obtained with two known steatogenic compounds (tetracycline and cycloheximide) and two compounds which have been shown to have no steatogenic potential (clomipramine and ketoconazole) are shown in Fig. 8.2. All these compounds induced TG accumulation, indicating that this is a sensitive index of drug-induced injury. Triglyceride accumulation was induced by both tetracycline and cycloheximide at much lower concentrations than those that induced cell toxicity. These results demonstrate that these two drugs had an impact on lipid metabolism without impairing cell viability. In contrast, triglyceride accumulation occurred concomitantly with cell death in response to the non-steatogenic compounds clomipramine and ketoconazole, suggesting that in this context, TG accumulation is related to cell necrosis.

The values of the ratio of the concentration which increased cell death (CD) by 30% to that which increased intracellular levels of triglycerides (TG) by 30% are shown in Table 8.1. The ratio calculated for the two steatogenic compounds was high (40 and 50 for tetracycline and cycloheximide respectively), whereas a value of 2 was found for the two non-steatogenic compounds (clomipramine and ketoconazole). This ratio appears, therefore, to provide a good *in vitro* predictive index of the steatogenic potential of drugs.

After exposure to the RP test compound, TG accumulation occurred at a much lower concentration than LDH leakage, yielding a steatogenic

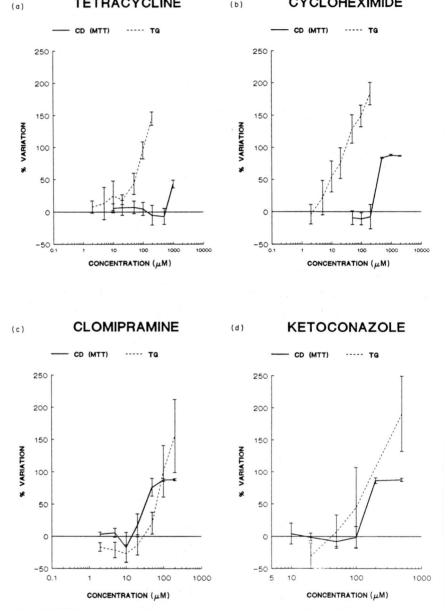

Fig. 8.2 Effect of tetracycline, cycloheximide, clomipramine and ketoconazole on cell death (CD) and on intracellular accumulation of triglycerides (TG) after a 20 h treatment ($n=2$).

Table 8.1
Steatogenic index evaluated by the ratio between the concentrations inducing a 30% increase of cell death and a 30% increase of intracellular triglycerides

		Concentration ratio CD/TG
Tetracycline	(n=2)	40
Cycloheximide	(n=2)	50
RP X	(n=2)	100
Clomipramine	(n=2)	2
Ketoconazole	(n=2)	2

index of around 100, thus providing *in vitro* confirmation of the steatogenic potential of the drug (Fig. 8.3).

This method has been slightly modified and automated, and a large number of steatogenic and non-steatogenic compounds tested in order to confirm the predictive validity of the steatogenicity index (unpublished work).

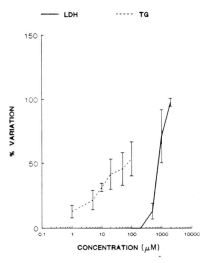

Fig. 8.3 Effect of RP X on LDH leakage and on intracellular accumulation of triglycerides (n=2).

Mechanisms involved in steatosis

*Effects of the RP test compound (RP X), tetracycline and
cycloheximide on VLDL secretion in the culture medium*
As shown in Table 8.2, RP X, like many other steatogenic drugs,
drastically inhibits VLDL secretion to between 10 and 14% of the
corresponding control level. Tetracycline and cycloheximide also inhibited
VLDL secretion, resulting in levels equivalent to 1–4% and 31–38% of
control respectively. These data are consistent with the inhibition of
VLDL secretion observed in the isolated, perfused rat liver reported by
Breen *et al.* (1972) for tetracycline and by Bar-On *et al.* (1972) for
cycloheximide.

*Effects of the RP test compound (RP X) and cycloheximide on
protein synthesis*
As shown in Fig. 8.4, cycloheximide inhibited protein synthesis, as
described in the literature (Gravela *et al.*, 1977). The RP test compound
also induced a dose-related inhibition of protein synthesis. This effect
may be related to the fatty liver induced by the compound, since the
inhibition observed was drastic and occurred early during incubation with
the drug.

*Effects of the RP test compound (RP X) on the β-oxidation of
oleate; comparison with tetracycline*
As shown in Fig. 8.5, tetracycline inhibited the β-oxidation of oleate.
This finding concurred with the inhibition of β-oxidation reported by
Freneaux *et al.* (1988) both *in vivo* in mice and *in vitro* in mouse and

Table 8.2
Effect of RP X ($n=2$), tetracycline ($n=3$) and cycloheximide ($n=3$) on VLDL
secretion and their composition after a 20 h treatment

	VLDL	TG	Composition (%) Cholesterol	PPL	Protein
Control ($n=3$)	100%	100%	100%	100%	100%
RP X ($n=3$) (138 μM)	10–14	8–11	15–32	10–20	66–85
Tetracycline ($n=2$) (100 μM)	1–4	1–3	3–9	2–7	12–30
Cycloheximide ($n=2$) 100 (μM)	31–38	32–34	33–55	21–49	64–66

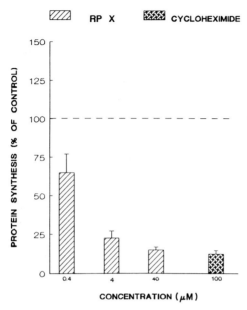

Fig. 8.4 Effect of RP X and cycloheximide on protein synthesis after 1 h of treatment ($n=4$).

human liver mitochondria. In contrast, the RP test compound did not inhibit the β-oxidation of oleate into acetoacetate and hydroxybutyrate, but rather even seemed to stimulate β-oxidation.

The induction of fatty liver by the RP test compound therefore appears to have been secondary to the inhibition of both VLDL secretion and protein synthesis. However, since this compound did not inhibit β-oxidation, it is likely to have only a minor impact on liver function.

Conclusion

Cultured hepatocytes can be used in screening tests to detect the steatogenic potential of candidate drugs and offer an interesting model for use in the study of the mechanisms involved in steatosis.

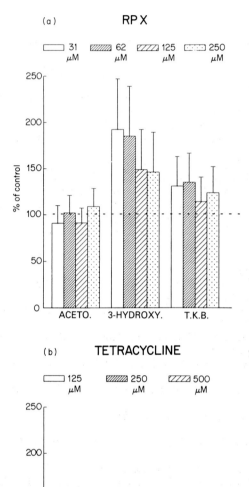

Fig. 8.5 Effect of RP X (*n*=3) (a) and tetracycline (*n*=5) (b) on β-oxidation of oleate after a 20 h treatment. Aceto = acetoacetate; 3-Hydroxy = 3-hydroxy-butyrate; T.K.B. = total ketone bodies.

References

Agius, L., Chowdhury, M.H. and Alberti, K.G.M.M. (1986a). *Biochem. J.* **239**, 593–601.

Agius, L., Chowdhury, M.H., Davis, S.N. and Alberti, K.G.M.M. (1986b). *Diabetes* **35**, 1286–1293.

Alpers, D.H. and Isselbacher, K.J. (1975). *In* "Diseases of the Liver" (L. Schiff ed.), pp. 815–832. Lippincott, Philadelphia.

Aujard, C. (1953). *C.R. Soc. Biol.* **147**, 965–968.

Bamberger, M.J. and Lane, M.D. (1990). *Proc. Natl. Acad. Sci. U.S.A.* **87**, 2390–2394.

Bar-On, H., Stein, O. and Stein, Y. (1972). *Biochim. Biophys. Acta* **270**, 444–452.

Becker, C.-M. and Harris, R.H. (1983). *Arch. Biochem. Biophys.* **233**, 381–392.

Bell-Quint, J. and Forte, T. (1981). *Biochim. Biophys. Acta* **663**, 83–98.

Bell-Quint, J., Forte, T. and Graham, P. (1981). *Biochem. J.* **200**, 409–414.

Biggs, J.C., Chesterman, C.N. and Holliday, J. (1971). *N.Z.J. Med.* **1**, 1–7.

Bjorge, S.M. and Baillie, T.A. (1985). *Biochem. Biophys. Res. Commun.* **132**, 245–252.

Böcker, R., Estler, C.-J., Maywald, M. and Weber, D. (1981). *Arzneim.-Forsch.* **31(II)**, 2118–2120.

Böcker, R., Estler, C.-J., Muller, S., Pfandzelter, C. and Spachmuller, B. (1982). *Arzneim.-Forsch.* **32(I)**, 237–241.

Böcker, R., Strobel, B., Hopf, C. and Estler, C.-J. (1985). *Acta Pharmacol. Toxicol.* **56**, 327–330.

Bouma, M.E., Pessah, M., Renaud, G., Amit, N., Catala, D. and Infante, R. (1988). *In vitro Cell. Dev. Biol.* **24**, 85–90.

Breen, K., Schenker, S. and Heimberg, M. (1972). *Biochim. Biophys. Acta* **270**, 74–80.

Breen, K.J., Schenker, S. and Heimberg, M. (1975). *Gastroenterology* **69**, 714–723.

Brindle, N.P.J. and Ontko, J.A. (1986). *Biochem. Biophys. Res. Commun.* **141**, 191–197.

Buku, A., Campadelli-Fiume, G., Fiume, L. and Wieland, T. (1971). *FEBS Lett.* **14**, 42–44.

Carr, B.R. (1987). *Am. J. Obstet. Gynecol.* **157**, 1338–1344.

Cole, R.A. and Margolis, S. (1974). *Endocrinology* **94**, 1391–1396.

Combes, B., Whalley, P.J. and Adams, R.H. (1972). *In* "Progress in Liver Disease" (H. Popper and F. Schaffner, eds), pp. 589–596. W.B. Saunders Company, Philadelphia.

Coude, F.X., Grimber, G., Pelet, A. and Benoit, Y. (1983). *Biochem. Biophys. Res. Commun.* **115**, 730–736.

Danan, G., Trunet, P., Bernuau, J., Degott, C., Babany, G., Pessayre, D., Rueff, B. and Benhamou, J.P. (1985). *Gastroenterology* **89**, 210–213.

Davis, R.A., Engelhorn, S.C., Pangburn, S.H., Weinstein, D.B. and Steinberg, D. (1979). *J. Biol. Chem.* **254**, 2010–2016.

Deboyser, D., Goethals, F., Krack, G. and Roberfroid, M. (1989). *Toxicol. Appl. Pharmacol.* **97**, 473–479.

Decker, K. and Keppler, D. (1974). *Pharmacol. Rev. Physiol. Biochem.* **71**, 77–106.

Denizot, F. and Lang, R. (1986). *J. Immunol. Method* **89**, 271–277.

De Vivo, D.C. (1987). *Neurology* **28**, 105–108.
Dustin, M.P. (1941). *Bull. Acad. R. Med. Belg.* **6**, 505–529.
Edge, S.B., Hoeg, J.M., Triche, T., Schneider, P.D. and Brewer, H.B. (1986). *J. Biol. Chem.* **261**, 3800–3806.
Eimas, A. and Bridgeport, C. (1938). *J. Pediatr.* **13**, 550–554.
Elliot, T.R. and Durham, H.E. (1906). *J. Physiol.* **34**, 490–498.
Estler, C.J. and Ammon, H.P. (1966). *Experientia* **22**, 589–590.
Estler, C.-J. and Böcker, R. (1980). *Toxicol. Appl. Pharmacol.* **54**, 508–513.
Farber, E. (1971). *Annu. Rev. Pharmacol.* **11**, 71–96.
Felt, V., Röhling, S., Vohnout, S. and Reichl, S. (1962). *J. Endocrinol.* **24**, 309–314.
Flejou, J.F., Degott, C. and Capron, J.P. (1987). *Gastroenterol. Clin. Biol.* **11**, 115–118.
Freneaux, E., Labbe, G., Letteron, P., Le Dinh, T., Degott, C., Genève, J., Larrey, D. and Pessayre, D. (1988). *Hepatology* **8**, 1056–1062.
Garcia-Sainz, J.A., Hernandez-Munoz, R., Santamaria, A. and Chagoya de Sanchez, V. (1979). *Biochem. Pharmacol.* **28**, 1409–1413.
Genève, J., Hayat-Bonan, B., Labbe, G., Degott, C., Letteron, P., Freneaux, E., Le Dinh, T., Larrey, D. and Pessayre, D. (1987). *J. Pharmacol. Exp. Ther.* **242**, 1133–1137.
Girard, J. and Malewiak, M.-I. (1986). *In* "Isolated and Cultured Hepatocytes" (A. Guillouzo and C. Guguen-Guillouzo, eds), pp. 87–112. John Libbey, London.
Glasgow, A.M. and Chase, H.P. (1975). *Pediatr. Res.* **9**, 133–138.
Gordon, E.R. (1972). *Biochem. Pharmacol.* **21**, 2991–3004.
Gravela, E., Pani, P., Ferrari, A. and Mazzarino, C. (1971). *Biochem. Pharmacol.* **20**, 3424–3430.
Gravela, E., Poli, G., Albano, E. and Dianzani, M.U. (1977). *Exp. Mol. Pathol.* **27**, 339–352.
Guillouzo, A. and Guguen-Guillouzo, C. (1986). *In* "Isolated and Cultured Hepatocytes" (A. Guillouzo and C. Guguen-Guillouzo, eds), pp. 313–331. John Libbey, London.
Hansen, C.H., Pearson, L.H., Schenker, S. and Combes, B. (1968). *Proc. Soc. Exp. Biol. Med.* **128**, 143–146.
Harano, Y., Kosugi, K., Kashiwagi, A., Nakano, T., Hidaka, H. and Shigeta, Y. (1982). *J. Biochem. (Tokyo)* **91**, 1739–1748.
Herbin, C., Pegorier, J.P., Duee, P.H., Kohl, R. and Girard, J. (1987). *Eur. J. Biochem.* **165**, 201–207.
Herdt, T.H., Wensing, T., Haagsman, H.P., van Golde, L.M. and Breukink, H.J. (1988). *J. Anim. Sci.* **66**, 1997–2013.
Hill, R.B. Jr. (1961). *N. Eng. J. Med.* **265**, 318–320.
Hill, R.B., Droke, W.A. and Hays, A.P. (1965). *Exp. Mol. Pathol.* **4**, 320–327.
Hopf, G., Böcker, R. and Estler, C.-J. (1985). *Arch. Int. Pharmacodyn.* **278**, 157–168.
Hoyumpa, A.M. Jr., Green, H.L., Dunn, G.D. and Schenker, S. (1975). *Am. J. Dig. Dis.* **20**, 1142–1170.
Infante, R., Koumanov, K. and Caroli, J. (1971). *Gut.* **12**, 765 (abstract).
Isselbacher, K.J. and Carter, Z.A. (1970). *Biochem. Biophys. Res. Commun.* **39**, 530–537.
Janero, D.R. and Lane, M.D. (1983). *J. Biol. Chem.* **258**, 14496–14504.
Jazcilevich, S. and Villa-Trevino, S. (1970). *Lab. Invest.* **23**, 590–594.

Jeanrenaud, B., Le Marchand, Y. and Patzelt, C. (1977). *In* "Membrane Alterations as Basis of Liver Injury" (H. Popper, L. Bianchi and W. Reutter, eds), pp. 247–255. MTP Press, Lancaster.

Jeejeeboy, K.N., Ho, J., Breckenridge, C., Bruce-Robertson, A., Steiner, G. and Jeejeeboy, J. (1975). *Biochem. Biophys. Res. Commun.* **66**, 1147–1153.

Jones, J.P. Jr., Engelman, E.P. and Najarian, J.S. (1965). *N. Engl. J. Med.* **273**, 1453–1458.

Keller, G.-A., Glass, C., Louvard, D., Steinberg, D. and Singer, S.J. (1986). *J. Hist. Cyt.* **34**, 1223–1230.

Kesterson, J.W., Granneman, G.R. and Machinist, J.M. (1984). *Hepatology*, **4**, 1143–1152.

Kosugi, K., Harano, Y., Nakano, T., Suzuki, M., Kashiwagi, A. and Shigeta, Y. (1983). *Metabolism* **32**, 1081–1087.

Kosykh, V.A., Preobrazhensky, S.N., Ivanov, V.O., Tsibulsky, V.P., Repin, V.S. and Smirnov, V.N. (1985). *FEBS Lett.* **183**, 17–20.

Kosykh, V.A., Lankin, V.Z., Podrez, E.A., Novikov, D.K., Volgushev, S.A., Victorov, A.V., Repin, V.S. and Smirnov, V.N. (1989). *Lipids* **24**, 109–115.

Lamb, R.G., Wood, C.K., Landa, B.M., Guzelian, P.S. and Fallon, H.J. (1977). *Biochim. Biophys. Acta* **489**, 318–329.

Lanford, R.E., Carey, K.D., Estlack, L.E., Con Smith, G. and Hay, R.V. (1989). *In vitro Cell. Dev. Biol.* **25**, 174–182.

Le Dinh, T., Freneaux, E., Labbe, G., Letterton, P, Degott, C., Genève, J., Berson, A., Larrey, D. and Pessayre, D. (1988). *J. Pharmacol. Exp. Ther.* **247**, 745–750.

Le Marchand, Y., Singh, A., Assimacopoulos-Jeannet, F., Orci, L., Rouiller, C. and Jeanrenaud, B. (1973). *J. Biol. Chem.* **248**, 6862–6870.

Le Marchand, Y., Patzelt, C., Assimacopoulos-Jeannet, F., Loten, E.G. and Jeanrenaud, B. (1974). *J. Clin. Invest.* **53**, 1512–1517.

Lieber, C.S. and Schmid, R. (1961). *J. Clin. Invest.* **40**, 394–399.

Lindell, T.J., Weinberg, F., Morris, P.W., Roeder, R.G. and Rutter, W.J. (1970). *Science* **170**, 447–449.

Lombardi, B. (1966). *Lab. Invest.* **15**, 1–20.

Lombardi, B. and Oler, A. (1967). *Lab. Invest.* **17**, 308–321.

Lombardi, B. and Ugazio, G. (1965). *J. Lipid Res.* **6**, 498–505.

Lombardi, B., Ugazio, G. and Raick, A. (1964). *Fed. Proc.* **23**, 126.

Lombardi, B., Ugazio, G. and Raick, A.N. (1966). *Am. J. Physiol.* **210**, 31–36.

Lombardi, B., Pani, P., Schlunk, F.F. and Hua, C.S. (1969). *Lipids* **4**, 67–75.

Luthman, J. and Holtenius, P. (1972). *Acta Vet. Scand.* **13**, 31–41.

MacGarry, J.D. and Foster, D.W. (1980). *Annu. Rev. Biochem.* **49**, 395–420.

MacKay, E.M. (1937). *Am. J. Physiol.* **120**, 361–364.

Magee, P.N. and Farber, E. (1962). *Biochem. J.* **83**, 114–124.

Magee, P.N. and Hultin, T. (1962). *Biochem. J.* **83**, 106–114.

Mangiapane, E.H. and Brindley, D.N. (1986). *Biochem. J.* **233**, 151–160.

Marshall, M. and Kaplan, M.D. (1985). *N. Engl. J. Med.* **313**, 367–370.

Martin, D., Bonnet, P.M., Martin, C., Moene, Y. and Ducret, F. (1981). *Gastroenterol. Clin. Biol.* **5**, 1071–1072.

Martin, A., Biol, M.-C., Raisonnier, A., Infante, R., Louisot, P. and Richard, M. (1982). *Biochim. Biophys. Acta* **718**, 85–91.

Melin, B., Keller, G., Glass, C., Weinstein, D.B. and Steinberg, D. (1984). *Biochim. Biophys. Acta* **795**, 574–588.

Meyerhoff, I.S. (1930). *J. Am. Med. Assoc.* **94**, 1751–1753.

186   M.A. Ivanov *et al.*

Mitchell, D.B. and Acosta, D. (1981). *J. Toxicol. Environ. Health* **7**, 83–92.
Montanaro, N., Novello, F. and Stirpe, F. (1971). *Biochem. J.* **125**, 1087–1090.
Moran, T.J. (1962). *Arch. Pathol.* **73**, 300–312.
Mori, M. (1983). *Acta Pathol. Jap.* **33**, 911–922.
Nathans, D. (1964). *Proc. Natl. Acad. Sci. U.S.A.* **51**, 585–592.
Nathans, D. and Lipmann, F. (1961). *Proc. Natl. Acad. Sci. U.S.A.* **47**, 497–504.
Nossen, J.O., Rustan, A.C. and Drevon, C.A. (1987). *Biochem. J.* **247**, 433–439.
Novello, F., Fiume, L. and Stirpe, F. (1970). *Biochem. J.* **116**, 177–180.
Oberhaensli, R.D., Schwendimann, R. and Keller, U. (1985). *Diabetes* **34**, 774–779.
Oler, A. and Lombardi, B. (1970). *J. Biol. Chem.* **245**, 1282–1288.
Ozegovic, B., Rode, B. and Milkivic, S. (1975). *Endokrinologie* **66**, 128–134.
Paoletti, R., Smith, R.L., Maickel, R.P. and Brodie, B.B. (1961). *Biochem. Biophys. Res. Commun.* **5**, 424–429.
Patsch, W., Gotto, A.M. and Patsch, J.R. (1986). *J. Biol. Chem.* **261**, 9603–9606.
Pestka, S. (1971). *Annu. Rev. Biochem.* **40**, 697–710.
Peterson, G.L. (1979). *Anal. Biochem.* **100**, 201—220.
Pottenger, L.A., Frazier, L.E., DuBien, L.H., Getz, G.S. and Wissler, R.W. (1973). *Biochem. Biophys. Res. Commun.* **54**, 770–776.
Pratt, C.B. and Johnson, W.W. (1971). *Cancer* **28**, 361–364.
Ramain, J.P., Labayle, D., Buffet, C., Chaput, J.C. and Etienne, J.D. (1981). *Gastroenterol. Clin. Biol.* **5**, 469–471.
Reaven, E.P. and Reaven, G.M. (1980). *J. Cell Biol.* **84**, 28–39.
Reboucas, G. and Isselbacher, K.J. (1961). *J. Clin. Invest.* **40**, 1335–1362.
Recknagel, R.O. and Lombardi, B. (1961). *J. Biol. Chem.* **236**, 564–569.
Recknagel, R.O., Lombardi, B. and Schotz, M.C. (1960). *Proc. Soc. Exp. Biol. Med.* **104**, 608–610.
Redman, C.M., Banerjee, D., Howell, K. and Palade, G.E. (1975). *J. Cell Biol.* **66**, 42–59.
Reid, I.M., Sarma, D.S.R. and Sidransky, H. (1971). *Lab. Invest.* **25**, 141–148.
Reye, R.D.K., Morgan, G. and Baral, J. (1963). *Lancet* **2**, 749–752.
Rustan, A.C., Nossen, J.O., Blomhoff, J.P. and Drevon, C.A. (1986). *Int. J. Biochem.* **18**, 909–916.
Sabesin, S.M., Frase, S. and Ragland, J.B. (1977). *Lab. Invest.* **37**, 127–135.
Saggerson, E.D., Carpenter, C.A. and Tselentis, B.S. (1982). *Biochem. J.* **208**, 667–672.
Scheuer, P.J. (1980). *In* "Liver Biopsy Interpretation" 3rd edn, pp. 88–101. Williams and Wilkins, Baltimore.
Seakins, A. and Robinson, D.S. (1963). *Biochem. J.* **86**, 401–407.
Seglen, P.O. (1976). *Biochim. Biophys. Acta* **442**, 391–404.
Shauer, B.A., Lukacs, L. and Zimmerman, H.J. (1974). *Proc. Soc. Exp. Biol. Med.* **147**, 868–872.
Sherratt, H.S.A. (1986). *Trends. Pharmacol. Sci.* **7**, 186–191.
Siedel, J., Hagele, E.O., Ziegenhorn, J. and Wahlefeld, A.W. (1983). *Clin. Chem.* **29**, 1075–1080.
Smuckler, E.A., Iseri, O.A. and Benditt, E.P. (1961). *Biochem. Biophys. Res. Commun.* **5**, 270–275.
Sparks, J.D. and Sparks, C.E. (1990). *J. Biol. Chem.* **265**, 8854–8862.
Stakkestad, J.A. and Lund, H. (1984). *Biochim. Biophys. Acta* **793**, 1–9.
Standerfer, S.B. and Handler, P. (1955). *Proc. Exp. Biol. Med.* **90**, 270–271.

Starko, K.M., Ray, C.G., Dominguez, L.B., Stromberg, W.L. and Woodall, D.F. (1980). *Pediatrics* **66**, 859–864.

Stein, O. and Stein, Y. (1973). *Biochim. Biophys. Acta.* **306**, 142–147.

Stein, O., Sanger, L. and Stein, Y. (1974). *J. Cell Biol.* **62**, 90–103.

Steinberg, H., Webb, W.M. and Rafsky, H.A. (1952). *Gastroenterology* **21**, 304–309.

Stirpe, F. and Fiume, L. (1967). *Biochem. J.* **105**, 779–782.

Stirpe, F. and Novello, F. (1970). *FEBS Lett.* **8**, 57–60.

Stricker, B.H. and Spoelstra, P. (1985). *In* "Drug-Induced Hepatic Injury" (M.N.G. Dukes, ed.), p. 157. Elsevier, Amsterdam.

Symansky, M.R. and Fox, H.A. (1972). *J. Pediatr.* **80**, 820–826.

Takayama, M., Itoh, S., Nagasaki, T. and Tanimizu, I. (1977). *Clin. Chim. Acta* **79**, 93–98.

Tanaka, K. and Kean, E.A. (1976). *N. Engl. J. Med.* **295**, 461–467.

Taubman, B., Hale, D.E. and Kelley, R.I. (1987). *Pediatrics* **79**, 382–385.

Thayer, W.S. (1984). *Biochem. Pharmacol.* **33**, 1187–1194.

Turnbull, D.M., Bone, A.J., Bartlett, K., Koundakjian, P.P. and Sherratt, H.S.A. (1983). *Biochem. Pharmacol.* **32**, 1887–1892.

Vance, D.E., Weinstein, D.B. and Steinberg, D. (1984). *Biochim. Biophys. Acta* **792**, 39–47.

Wahlefeld, A.W. and Bergmeyer, H.U. (1974). *Methods Enzym. Anal.* **2**, 1878.

Waldman, R.J., Hall, W.N., McGee, H. and Van Amburg, G. (1982). *J. Am. Med. Assoc.* **247**, 3089–3094.

Ware, S. and Millward-Sadler, G.H. (1980). *Lancet* **2**, 1110–1113.

Williamson, D.H., Mellanby, J. and Krebs, H.A. (1962). *Biochem. J.* **82**, 90–96.

Wilson, L. (1975). *Life Sci.* **17**, 303–310.

Windmueller, H.G. (1964). *J. Biol. Chem.* **239**, 530–537.

Windmueller, H.G. (1965). *J. Nutr.* **85**, 221–229.

Windmueller, H.G. and Levi, R.I. (1967). *J. Biol. Chem.* **242**, 2246–2254.

Witters, L.A. and Trasko, C.S. (1979). *Am. J. Physiol.* **237**, E23–E29.

Yarmolinsky, M.D. and DeLaHaba, G.L. (1959). *Proc. Natl. Acad. Sci. U.S.A.* **45**, 1721–1725.

Yeh, S.D.J. and Shils, M.E. (1966). *Proc. Soc. Exp. Biol. Med.* **121**, 729–734.

Zafrani, E.S. and Berthelot, P. (1982). *Hepatology* **2**, 648–649.

Zakim, D. and Boyer, T.D. (1990). *In* "Hepatology, a Textbook of Liver Disease". pp. 96–123. W. B. Saunders Company, Philadelphia.

Zimmerman, H.J. (1978). *In* "Hepatotoxicity", pp. 91–121. Appleton-Century-Crofts, New York.

Zimmerman, H.J. (1979). *Med. Clin. North. Am.* **63**, 567–582.

Zimmerman, H.J. (1987). *In* "Diseases of the Liver" (L. Schiff and E.R. Schiff, eds), pp. 591–685. J.B. Lippincott Company, Baltimore.

Zimmerman, H.J. and Ishak, K.G. (1982). *Hepatology* **2**, 591–597.

9

Isolated Rat Hepatocyte Couplets: A Model for the Study of Bile Secretion and Cholestasis

J.L. BOYER

Liver Center and Department of Medicine, 333 Cedar St, Yale University School of Medicine, New Haven, CT 06510, USA

Introduction

The isolated rat hepatocyte couplet (IRHC) is a unique cell culture model for the study of bile secretory function and consists of two adjoining hepatocytes that surround a luminal space. The couplets are prepared by collagenase perfusion of rat liver, selecting for hepatocytes that remain attached to one another, as initially described by Oshio and Phillips (1981) and Graf *et al.* (1984). When placed in short-term culture on glass coverslips, certain IRHCs seal off their luminal space with tight junctional elements that have maintained contact between the two adjacent cells. After several hours in culture, the enclosed luminal space expands as a result of incorporation of additional apical membrane and the elaboration of secretion. A unique feature of this model, which represents the primary bile secretory unit, is the maintenance of structural and functional polarity, such that there is continued excretory function, much as exists in the intact organ. In addition, the IRHC has the advantage that the primary

IN VITRO METHODS IN TOXICOLOGY
ISBN 0-12-388175-7

secretory process can be studied in the absence of influences of vascular perfusion or bile duct transport which often confound interpretation of studies of bile secretory function in the perfused liver or bile fistula models. The IRHC is particularly suited for studies using fluorescent microscopic or electrophysiological techniques (Boyer *et al.*, 1990; Graf and Boyer, 1990).

Isolation Techniques

Procedures for preparing hepatocyte couplets have been described elsewhere in detail (Boyer *et al.*, 1990). All procedures begin with collagenase perfusion of the intact liver, and are followed by filtration of cell suspensions through nylon mesh (45–80 μm) in order to remove debris and larger aggregates of undissociated cells. Usually, 10–30% of the filtered cells are in pairs. The cells are allowed to settle on glass coverslips after resuspension in amino acid-containing media together with antibiotics, with or without bicarbonate and appropriate growth factors depending on the application. Foetal calf serum is added (10%) if the cells are to be studied in a flattened state, as is useful for fluorescent microscopic studies, but is to be avoided if electrophysiological experiments are to be performed. A cell concentration of approximately 10^5–10^6 cells/ml is generally used. The hepatocytes are placed on coverslips in 35×10 mm plastic dishes at 37°C. Most preparations deteriorate after 6–8 h but cell viability should exceed 85–90% following cell isolations. Preparations should be discarded if they fail to form expanded canalicular spaces, or demonstrate significant blebbing or cytoplasmic granulation.

Structural Aspects

Fully developed IRHC are highly polarized with respect to the organization of their cytoskeleton and demarcation of apical and basolateral membranes. Fluorescent antibody techniques reveal both actin and tubulin in organized arrays with increased concentrations in the pericanalicular region (Nickola and Frimmer, 1986; Sakisaka *et al.*, 1988). Tight junction-associated proteins (ZO-1) reorganize to the remaining apical (canalicular) domain within several hours after the cultures are initiated as canalicular spaces are expanding. Microtubule-dependent vesicle transcytosis can be demonstrated by horseradish peroxidase staining and remains functionally intact with transcellular transit times of 10–15 min as observed in the intact liver (Sakisaka *et al.*, 1988). Colchicine pretreatment abolishes this phenomenon. Inhibitors of microfilament function (phalloidin and cytochalasins) result in loss of contractility of the canalicular space consistent with a functional role for actin filaments in the bile secretory process (Phillips *et al.*, 1983). Time-lapse cinephotomicrographic studies by Phillips and colleagues have described these phenomena in detail (Watanabe *et al.*, 1985). They suggest that canalicular motility is a highly ordered and purposeful process for facilitating the forward flow of bile.

Functional Studies

Several techniques have been developed for directly measuring the rate of secretion of bile in this isolated bile secretory unit. The first procedure utilizes optical planimetry and video-microscopy techniques (Gautam *et al.*, 1989). When the IRHC is viewed by differential interference contrast microscopy (DIC or Nomarski optics), on the stage of an inverted microscope, multiple cross-sectional images of the expanded canalicular lumen can be obtained in focus at 0.5–2 μm intervals. By recording these images with a high-resolution video camera, the canalicular perimeter can be traced at a later time and the volume determined by knowing the depth of the optical plane. Repeated measurements can be obtained every 3–5 min allowing for determination of choleretic or cholestatic events. However, because the canalicular lumen is an enclosed space, choleretic stimuli usually result in collapse of the space within 10–15 min as volumes expand from 50–100 fl to 300–400 fl. Spontaneous contractions can also occur so that it is important to obtain control measurements prior to initiating the study, to be certain that the IRHC is in an expanding rather than a contracting phase.

An alternative technique for measurement of changes in canalicular volume relies on obtaining continuous video images from a single focal plane (Weinman *et al.*, 1989). This procedure has the advantage of recording rapid changes in canalicular volume but assumes a uniform shape to the canalicular space. A recent modification of this approach adjusts grey scale levels to a threshold that effectively eliminates the surrounding cytoplasm, revealing only the image of the canalicular space (Schild *et al.*, 1991).

Basal rates of secretion vary from couplet to couplet but have been estimated to approximate 40–70% of basal secretory rates in the intact liver when bicarbonate is present in the media and extrapolations are made from two cells to the entire liver (Gautam *et al.*, 1989). These studies suggest that the IRHC functions physiologically with respect to rates of bile formation. In addition to the choleretic effects of bile acids, dibutryl cyclic AMP and forskolin increase bile flow in this model (Nathanson and Gautam, 1988), providing firm evidence for a role of cyclic nucleotides in the elaboration of bile acid-independent bile flow from the hepatocyte. Cholestatic responses can also be assessed in this isolated cell culture system provided that the studies are carefully controlled for spontaneous collapse of the canalicular lumen. Preliminary studies have demonstrated cholestatic effects for stimulators of protein kinase C as well as agents that increase levels of intracellular calcium (Nathanson et al., 1992).

One of the fundamental properties of the excretory system in the hepatocyte is the ability to take up and excrete organic anions. This function is often impaired in hepatocyte monolayer cultures but is retained in the IRHC. This phenomenon is best demonstrated in the IRHC model with fluorescent labelled compounds such as fluorescein or its derivatives (Graf et al., 1984; Weinman et al., 1988). After exposure of the couplets to substances such as fluorescein diacetate, the compound diffuses into the cell where intracellular esterases release the fluorescent organic anion. In couplets with established secretory polarity, the fluorescent anion is rapidly excreted into the bile where it acumulates in higher concentrations as reflected by an increase in fluorescent intensity with the canalicular lumen. The ability to record changes in fluorescent intensity both within the cytoplasm and within the canalicular lumen has provided direct evidence that the intracellular membrane potential serves as a major driving force for the excretion of fluorescent derivatives of bile acids across the canalicular membrane into bile (Weinman et al., 1988). This confirms evidence previously obtained in membrane vesicles (Inoue et al., 1984; Meier et al., 1984).

In other studies, confocal scanning microscopy has been used with the IRHC to demonstrate that animals with genetic deficiencies in organic anion transport (the mutant TR Wistar rat) lack the ability to translocate organic anions across the canalicular membrane but retain the capacity to excrete fluorescent bile acid derivatives (Kitamura et al., 1990).

Fluorescein and its derivatives are also pH indicators and are often utilized to measure intracellular pH. The accumulation of these compounds in bile has enabled estimates of canalicular pH to be obtained (Strazzabosco et al., 1991).

Preliminary studies suggest that fluorescent derivatives of phospholipids may be useful for studying the relationship between biliary excretion of lipids and bile acids. When IRHC are exposed to 6-N-[7-nitro-benz-2-oxa-1,3-diazol-4-yl]aminocaproylsphingosine (C6-NDB-cerimide) or fluorescent derivatives of phosphatidylcholine, these compounds enter the cell and subsequently move to the canalicular domain when taurocholate is added to the medium (Crawford *et al.*, 1991; Bonner and Reuben, 1989).

Electrophysiologic Applications

The development of this cell culture model for the study of bile secretory function has also enabled classic electrophysiological measurements of this secretory process to be made for the first time. Details of these applications are beyond the scope of this review and can be found elsewhere (Graf *et al.*, 1987; Boyer *et al.*, 1988). However, the ability to insert microelectrodes within the canalicular lumen and record the intraluminal electric potential has established a value for the transcanalicular membrane potential of approximately −35 meV. Ion fluxes across the canalicular membrane contribute little to the luminal potential, which appears to be generated by impermeant anions accumulating within the canalicular space and resulting in a Donnan distribution of more permeant ions. The tight junctions offer little discrimination to the conductance of the major ionic species (Na^+, K^+ and Cl^-) and thus have properties of "leaky epithelia". The cell membrane, in contrast, demonstrates considerable resistance, being most permeant to K^+, less to Cl^- and least to Na^+. The sodium pump maintains the ion gradients across the cell membrane and expends energy to establish the major chemical driving forces which include an inwardly directed Na^+ gradient and outwardly directed K^+ gradient. The Na^+ gradient is then used to facilitate the hepatic uptake of organic solutes such as bile acids through a secondary active coupled transport system. The high outward conductance of K^+ generates a negative intracellular potential which in turn serves as an electrical driving force for the hepatic uptake of positively charged solutes and the extrusion of negatively charged substances such as bile acids. Intracellular concentrations of Na^+, K^+, Cl^- and H^+ and the membrane potential can all be determined with ion-sensitive electrodes as well as fluorescent probes not only providing physiological information but allowing sensitive measurements to be made of these basic parameters during injury to the cell. Hepatocytes are electrically coupled to one another by means of gap junctions. The IRHC has been used not only to demonstrate how these junctions are regulated by changes in intracellular pH (acid pH closes the junctions) (Spray *et al.*, 1986), but electrical uncoupling has been demonstrated following exposure of the IRHC to toxins such as carbon tetrachloride (Saez *et al.*, 1987).

Summary

Since the development of the IRHC model as a primary bile secretory unit in cell culture, much has been learned about its electrical properties and cell physiology. These studies demonstrate that these preparations maintain many of the functions of normal hepatocytes, including stable intracellular ion gradients and a normal membrane potential, as well as a structural polarity that allows continued elaboration of secretion while in short-term culture. These background studies suggest that this model should be useful in the future for studying mechanisms of cell injury and for assessing the effects of agents that both stimulate and inhibit bile excretory function.

References

Bonner, G.F. and Reuben, A. (1989). *Hepatol.* **10**, A599.
Boyer, J.L., Gautam, A. and Graf, J. (1988). *Semin. Liver Dis.* **8**, 308–316.
Boyer, J.L., Phillips, J.M. and Graf, J. (1990). *Methods Enzymol.* **192**, 501–515.
Crawford, J.M., Vinter, D.W. and Gollan, J.L. (1991). *Am. J. Physiol.* **260**, G119–G132.
Gautam, A., Ng, O.C., Strazzabosco, M. and Boyer, J.L. (1989). *J. Clin. Invest.* **83**, 565–573.
Graf, J. and Boyer, J. (1990). *J. Hepatol.* **10**, 387–394.
Graf, J., Gautam, A. and Boyer, J.L. (1984). *Proc. Natl. Acad. Sci. U.S.A.* **81**, 6516–6520.
Graf, J., Henderson, R.M., Krumpholz, B. and Boyer, J.L. (1987). *J. Membr. Biol.* **95**, 241–254.
Inoue, M., Kinne, R., Tran, T. and Arias, I.M. (1984). *J. Clin. Invest.* **73**, 659–663.
Kitamura, T., Jensen, P., Hardenbrook, C., Kamimito, Y., Gaitmaitan, Z. and Arias, I.M. (1990). *Proc. Natl. Acad. Sci. USA* **87**, 3557–3561.
Meier, P.J., Meier-Abt, A.S., Barrett, C. and Boyer, J.L. (1984). *J. Biol. Chem.* **259**, 10614–10622.
Nathanson, M.H. and Gautam, A. (1988). *Gastroenterology* **94**, A619.
Nathanson, M.H., Gautam, A. and Boyer, J. (1992). *Am. J. Physiol.* (in press).
Nickola, I. and Frimmer, M. (1986). *Cell Tissue Res.* **243**, 437–440.
Oshio, C. and Phillips, M.J. (1981). *Science* **212**, 1041–1042.
Phillips, M.J., Oshio, C., Miyairi, M. and Smith, C.R. (1983). *Lab. Invest.* **48**, 205–211.
Saez, J.C., Benne, M.V. and Spray, D.C. (1987). *Science* **236**, 967–969.
Sakisaka, S., Ng, O.C. and Boyer, J.L. (1988). *Gastroenterology*, **95**, 793–804.
Schild, L., Giebish, G., Boyer, J.L. and Graf, J. (1991). *Am. J. Physiol.* (Submitted).
Spray, D.C., Ginzberg, R.D., Morales, E.A., Gatmatian, Z. and Arias, I.M. (1986). *J. Cell Biol.* **103**, 135–144.

Strazzabosco, M., Sakisaka, S., Hayakawa, T. and Boyer, J.L. (1991). *Am. J. Physiol.* **260**, G58–G69.

Watanabe, S., Smith, C.R. and Phillips, M.J. (1985). *Lab. Invest.* **53**, 275–279.

Weinman, S.A., Thom, H., Kurz, G. and Boyer, J.L. (1988). *FASEB J.* **2**, A1725.

Weinman, S.A., Graf, J. and Boyer, J.L. (1989). *Am. J. Physiol.* **256**, 826–832.

Discussion

R. Massingham

I was surprised that H7 was able to block the phorbol ester response. What did H7 do by itself and what concentration was necessary to block this effect?

J. Boyer

H7 by itself (10^{-4} M) does not appear to have any significant effect in this system, although in perfused liver preparations it is choleretic and actually stimulates secretion. These studies were preceded by studies in isolated perfused liver which showed that phorbol ester is a cholestatic agent in the perfused liver and can be blocked by H7 couplets. About 10% of the 30% of cells that come through on the final plating out will expand those spaces. We know we are dealing with a good preparation when we begin to see these expanded spaces. We believe that NMR is the best optics to look at them, but phase contrast can be used.

G. Zbinden

Did you look at the effects of hormones in the kind of studies that you presented?

J. Boyer

We have not; for electrophysiological studies the addition of dexamethasone and insulin is required. It somewhat depends upon what we are looking at, but the viability is short term.

J.J. Picard

Are there any major differences in the secretion of molecules or in the metabolism of the couplets as compared to single cells in suspension?

J. Boyer

If single cells are loaded with bile acids or with something we think should be excreted, efflux can be demonstrated. The question always is whether this is efflux across the apical canalicular carrier system or back across the sinusoidal membrane. It has been known for a long time that single cells lose their polarity. The Golgi is no longer between the nucleus and the canalicular membrane but scattered around the cell, they do not carry out transcytosis, and the cytoskeleton is no longer polarized. It remains a question whether isolated cells either in suspension or in culture can be used for excretory studies. They are fine for uptake studies, but the polarity is lost. The unique feature of the secretion-competent couplet is that it retains secretory polarity.

10

Liver Slices for the *In Vitro* Determination of Hepatoxicity

F. GOETHALS, D. DEBOYSER, E. CAILLIAU
and M. ROBERFROID

*Laboratoire de Biochimie Toxicologique et Cancérologique,
Université Catholique de Louvain, UCL 7369, Avenue Mounier
73, 1200 Bruxelles, Belgium*

Introduction

Throughout the late 19th and early 20th century, the application of organ culture methodologies to biomedical research expanded rapidly and included studies spanning a variety of disciplines in cell biology (for review see Fell, 1975). The earliest reports of attempts to culture organs *in vitro* date back to the latter half of the 19th century (Vulpian, 1859; Born, 1897). With regard to culture of mammalian liver, it was not until the early part of the 20th century that attempts were made to maintain it in organ culture. While progress has been made towards this goal, it has been slow and not entirely successful (Trowell, 1959; Sigot-Luizard, 1973; Hart *et al.*, 1983). The major contributions were by Campbell and Hales (1971) and Hart *et al.* (1983). Campbell and co-workers (Campbell and Hales, 1971; Campbell and Siddle, 1973) established an organ culture of mature rat liver which remained hormonally responsive for up to 6

IN VITRO METHODS IN TOXICOLOGY
ISBN 0-12-388175-7

days. On the basis of both morphological and biochemical evidence, they demonstrated the need for proper oxygenation (95% O_2:5% CO_2) of the culture. More recently, Hart *et al.* (1983) have described a system of culture of thin rat liver slices which proved to be successful for the maintenance of the integrity of neonatal but not adult rat liver for up to 72 h. The major limitations of all these systems are the diffusion of O_2 from the gas phase and nutrients from the medium (Reed and Grisham, 1975) into the cultured tissue, a finding which takes on added significance when mouse or rat tissues are used, because these tissues have comparatively higher respiratory rates than the same tissues from larger animals (Krebs, 1950).

These are probably the reasons why organ or slice culture of the adult rat liver have not received as much attention during the last decade or two as cell culture. Indeed, this system has been widely displaced as an experimental tool in biomedical research, including *in vitro* toxicology, by monolayer and suspension cell cultures. However, as compared with cell culture, liver slices in culture offer some advantages which might be highly relevant to *in vitro* toxicology. These are as follows:

1) Preservation of a higher level of tissue organization which may create a better situation for the response of the target tissue to the toxic chemical
2) Preservation of a differentiated state due to the maintenance of "cell–cell" and "cell–matrix" interactions
3) Preservation of the functional heterogeneity
4) Avoidance of exposure of the tissue to proteolytic enzymes necessary for cell isolation which may damage liver cells, in particular those of the centrilobular area (Sweeney, 1983).

A significant breakthrough in the search for a suitable *in vitro* liver slice culture system has been reported recently by the team of Gandolfi and Brendel at the University of Arizona (Smith *et al.*, 1985, 1986 and 1987; Brendel *et al.*, 1987; Sipes *et al.*, 1987). They adapted the Krumdieck tissue slicer (Krumdieck *et al.*, 1980) and developed a dynamic organ culture system.

We have previously demonstrated (Goethals *et al.*, 1990) that, using that mechanical tissue slicer and a suitable incubation system, some functional hepatic parameters such as ATP content, protein synthesis and secretion are maintained for up to 20 h. In this study, we further checked the hepatocellular functional integrity of liver slices by measuring their cytochrome *P*-450 content during the incubation period. Histological evaluation was carried out to assess morphological changes during incubation. The application of this *in vitro* model to the study of cytotoxicity of amitriptyline was investigated. Amitriptyline is a widely used antidepressant which may induce cholestatic or cytolytic hepatitis (Genève *et al.*, 1987).

Methodology

Chemicals

Optimem medium, Ultroser G, penicillin and streptomycin were purchased from Gibco Europe (Gent, Belgium). Methylcellulose membranes were obtained from Millipore (Brussels, Belgium). Amitriptyline was purchased from Sigma Chemical Co. (St Louis, MO, USA). [U-^{14}C]Leucine (specific activity 339 mCi/mmol) was obtained from The Radiochemical Centre, Amersham, Bucks, UK. The liquid-scintillation cocktail was Aquasol from New England Nuclear Corporation.

Preparation of Liver Slices

The major factors that result in uneven oxygen and nutrient diffusion are tissue thickness, lack of uniformity and tissue trauma produced during the preparation of tissue pieces. In order to prevent a spontaneous cellular degeneration in control liver pieces, it was necessary to develop a rapid and precise method for preparing thin liver slices with minimal tissue trauma. The Krumdieck tissue slicer, modified as described by Brendel *et al.* (1987), has been designed to produce rapidly slices of nearly identical thickness and of very similar shape and dimensions under quasi-physiological conditions. Liver slices were prepared from male Wistar rats weighing 280–320 g and fed *ad libitum*. Cylindrical cores were prepared with a sharpened metal tube of 1 cm outer diameter mounted on a motor that turned and advanced the metal tube into the liver lobes, which were suitably positioned on a rubber support. Following the preparation of 10–15 tissue cylinders, up to 120 slices of 250 μm thickness were obtained using the slicer containing cold oxygenated (95% O_2:5% CO_2) Krebs–Henseleit buffer, pH 7.4, supplemented with 25 mM glucose.

Incubation of Liver Slices

In order to improve the diffusion of oxygen and nutrients which is a critical factor in survival of adult liver organ cultures, several authors have underlined the advantages of a constant and gentle stirring of the medium and therefore recommended the use of roller cultures over static cultures (Freshney, 1983). Smith *et al.* (1986) developed a dynamic organ culture system: liver slices are deposited on stainless-steel screens in rotating vials allowing exposure of both sides of the slice alternatively to the gas phase and to the culture medium. We designed an incubation system which also permits both the upper and lower surfaces of the slices to be exposed to oxygen and nutrients during the course of incubation. Slices are deposited on methylcellulose membranes (5 μm pore size) which are submerged in the culture medium. This one is Optimem culture medium, supplemented with 2% Ultroser G, 100 IU penicillin/ml, 0.1 mg streptomycin/ml and glucose to obtain a final concentration of 28 mM. The culture medium is oxygenated by bubbling 95% O_2:5% CO_2 during the whole incubation period.

Analytical Procedures

Lactate dehydrogenase (LDH) leakage

Aliquots of the culture medium were analysed for LDH activity using the method of Wroblesky and Ladue (1955).

Protein synthesis

Protein synthesis was evaluated by measuring the incorporation of [^{14}C]leucine into acid-precipitable protein. The slices were incubated in the presence of [^{14}C]leucine (393 μCi/mmol). They were removed from the incubation system at the appropriate times and immediately homogenized in 1 ml of 2% perchloric acid by sonication (Braunsonic 300S, 60 W, 20s). The homogenate was centrifuged at 11 000 *g* for 5 min (Beckman microfuge). The pellets were washed by suspension and re-centrifugation in 2% perchloric acid and then in water, and finally dissoved in 1 ml of 0.3 N NaOH. After neutralization by HCl, an aliquot was mixed with Aquasol scintillation solution and counted in a Berthold (BF 5000) liquid-scintillator counter. Amount of slice protein was determined in the pellet from centrifugation and data were expressed as c.p.m./mg of protein.

ATP content

ATP levels were evaluated in the supernatant from the centrifugation in the Beckman microfuge and measured spectrophotometrically using the method of Lamprecht and Trautschold (1963). Preincubation values for ATP content were determined on freshly isolated slices (S values). Results were expressed as nmol/mg of slice protein.

Cytochrome P-450 content

Following incubation, slices were homogenized in 0.25 M sucrose buffered with 3 mM imidazole, pH 7.4, with the tight pestle of a Dounce tissue grinder operated up and down five times. The suspension was then centrifuged at 1600 r.p.m. for 10 min (245 *g*); the supernatant was then centrifuged at 15 000 r.p.m. for 16 min (13 000 *g*). The microsomal fraction was obtained by a centrifugation at 39 000 r.p.m. for 30 min (138 000 *g*). Microsomes were resuspended in 0.1 M pH 7.4 phosphate buffer supplemented with 20% glycerol and 1 mM EDTA. The amount of microsomal cytochrome *P*-450 was determined according to Omura and Sato (1964). The value of 91 mM^{-1} cm^{-1} was used as the molar absorption coefficient at 450 nm.

Histology

Slices were fixed in 3.7% formol–0.1% calcium solution, dehydrated and embedded in paraplast+. Microtome sections (7 μm) were stained with haematoxylin and eosin (H&E) and examined by light microscopy.

Statistical Analysis

Data are presented as means ± S.E.M. for values obtained with liver slices from at least three rats. The data were analysed by a two-way analysis of variance (ANOVA); differences between control and treatment means at the same incubation time were determined using Student's *t* test. Differences with $P < 0.05$ were considered statistically significant.

Results

As shown in Fig. 10.1, histological examination of incubated liver slices indicates that the liver architecture is well preserved for up to 20 h. They maintained normal morphology with regard to cytoplasmic staining, nuclear integrity and intercellular contacts. However, after 20 h of incubation, some cytoplasmic vacuolization occurred and peripheral pycnosis or caryolysis appeared which may indicate an alteration caused by the agitation of the culture medium.

The maintenance of cytochrome *P*-450 for *in vitro* toxicity studies is important since many chemicals require metabolic activation to express their potential toxicity. Moreover, it is well known that in rat hepatocyte cultures, a loss of cytochrome *P*-450 occurs very rapidly. The cytochrome

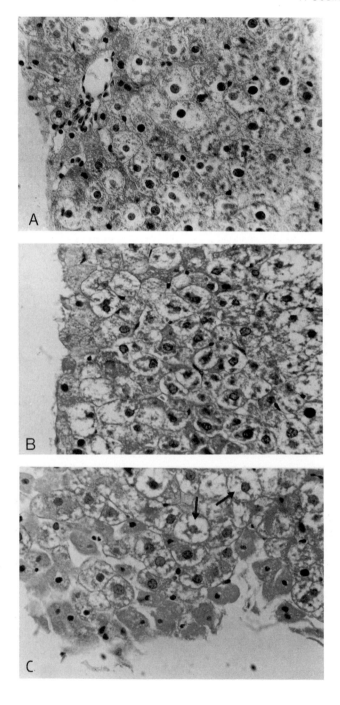

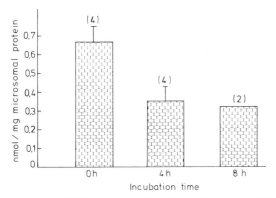

Fig. 10.2 Cytochrome *P*-450 content of rat liver slices over 8 h of incubation.

P-450 content measured in freshly prepared rat liver slices was close to the normal value determined for fresh rat liver (Krack *et al.*, 1980). After 4 h of incubation, the cytochrome *P*-450 content decreased to 52% of that at the initial time point and was maintained at this level for up to 8 h (Fig. 10.2).

The effects of amitriptyline added *in vitro* to rat liver slices were studied. When rat liver slices were exposed to 5×10^{-4} M amitriptyline, a slight, although not significant, increase in LDH leakage from the treated slices was observed as compared with that from control slices. Incubation in the presence of 10^{-4} M amitriptyline did not result in an enhanced release of LDH (Fig. 10.3).

Significant inhibition of protein synthesis immediately occurred when liver slices were incubated in the presence of 5×10^{-4} M amitriptyline. When 10^{-4} M amitriptyline was added to the culture medium, protein synthesis did not significantly differ from that of control slices (Fig. 10.4).

Another sensitive indicator of cellular integrity is the ATP content. While a loss in ATP content was observed between the period of slicing (S value) and the beginning of incubation (zero time value), the ATP level recovered as soon as the liver slices were placed in the incubation system. By 8 h, ATP content rose to a plateau level which was maintained

Fig. 10.1 Haematoxylin and eosin-stained sections of rat liver slices after incubation for 0 h (A), 8 h (B) or 20 h (C). (H&E × 400). In A, hepatocytes are of normal size and have granular, normal-looking cytoplasm. In C, cytoplasmic vacuolization, indicated by arrow, and pycnotic nuclei are observed.

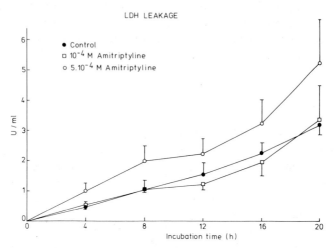

Fig. 10.3 Leakage of lactate dehydrogenase (LDH) into the culture medium following incubation of rat liver slices in the presence of amitriptyline.

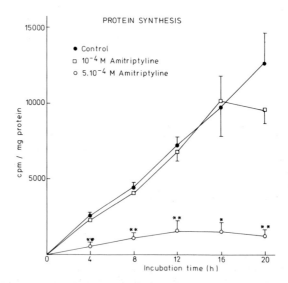

Fig. 10.4 Effect of amitriptyline on protein synthesis in rat liver slices incubated for 20 h. *$P \leq 0.05$ from control. **$P \leq 0.01$ from control.

for 20 h. Incubation in the presence of 10^{-4} M amitriptyline did not modify this parameter. When slices were treated with 5×10^{-4} M amitriptyline, a significant decrease in ATP content was observed from 2 h of incubation until the end of the incubation period (Fig. 10.5).

Discussion

Our results confirm that liver slices represent a biological *in vitro* system in which a relatively high degree of hepatocellular architecture and liver-specific functions is retained. The thinness of the slices as well as the smooth stirring of the culture medium and a sufficient supply of oxygen are necessary for maintaining viable slices for a prolonged period (20 h). These conditions, as already underlined by Smith *et al.* (1985), avoid the appearance of necrosis in the slice centre. The problems arising from limited oxygen and nutrient diffusion associated with earlier culture methods of adult mammalian liver have been overcome.

The measurement of a number of functional parameters demonstrated that the biochemical integrity of the liver slices was retained for several

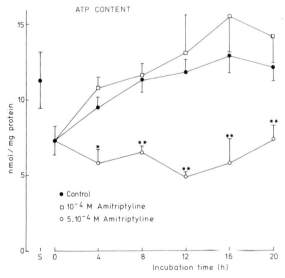

Fig. 10.5 Effect of amitriptyline on ATP content in rat liver slices incubated for 20 h. The S values for ATP content were determined in slices directly after isolation. The zero time values were determined in slices at the beginning of incubation. *$P \leq 0.05$ from control. **$P \leq 0.01$ from control.

hours. After some initial loss of intracellular ATP, the slices recovered and then the ATP concentration remained stable for 20 h. Protein synthesis and secretion, which are complex processes involving uptake of amino acids, incorporation of these amino acids into proteins and the export of newly synthesized proteins from the cells, remained active and constant over 20 h of incubation. However, those culture conditions did not allow the complete maintenance of cytochrome P-450 level, since it decreased down to 50% of the initial value after 4 h of incubation. Nevertheless, it subsequently remained stable until 8 h. According to Sipes *et al.* (1987) the cytochrome P-450 content of cultured rat liver slices is maintained for 8 h of culture at 80% of the initial level. Differences in the culture medium and in the incubation system may explain the difference we observed.

In this study, the liver slice model was used to test for the cytotoxicity of amitriptyline. This drug is mainly metabolized by demethylation into nortriptyline and to a lesser extent by hydroxylation into 10-hydroxyamitriptyline (Mellström *et al.*, 1983, 1986). Prolonged administration of this tricyclic antidepressant is known to increase serum aminotransferase activity in 2–10% of patients (Holmberg and Jansson, 1962) and to induce cholestatic (Morgan, 1969; Larrey *et al.*, 1988) or cytolytic hepatitis (Morgan, 1969; Danan *et al.*, 1984). Whereas at a concentration of 10^{-4} M, amitriptyline did not affect the functional integrity of liver slices, concentrations of 5×10^{-4} M or greater induced signs of cytotoxicity, as shown by depletion of ATP and inhibition of protein synthesis, which were sensitive and early indicators of amitriptyline toxicity in liver slices; LDH leakage increased moderately. Ratasavanah *et al.* (1988) reported that amitriptyline expressed cytotoxicity at progressively lower concentrations, increasing on the duration of treatment. After 24 h exposure of pure rat hepatocyte cultures to amitriptyline, a significant increase in LDH leakage was found at a concentration of 0.8×10^{-4} M. In rat hepatocyte cocultures, LDH leakage was increased with 0.2×10^{-4} M amitriptyline after 8 days.

Our data confirm previous findings (Krack *et al.*, 1983; Goethals *et al.*, 1984) that alteration of a biochemical function of the cells provides a more subtle and sensitive indication of toxic potential than the widely used tests of cytosolic enzyme leakage. Indeed, we assert that if the *in vitro* model is to be used to study a biological reactivity of a chemical, specific for a particular organ, it is necessary to analyse the effects of the chemical on biochemical parameters that express a specific function of the biological system used (Roberfroid and Goethals, 1990).

Acknowledgements

We thank V. Allaeys and R.M. Dujardin for their excellent technical assistance.

References

Born, G. (1897). *Roux Arch. Entwicklung* **4**, 517–623.
Brendel, K., Gandolfi, A.J., Krumdieck, C.L. and Smith, P.F. (1987). *Trends Pharmacol. Sci.* **8**, 11–15.
Campbell, A.K. and Hales, C.N. (1971). *Exp. Cell Res.* **68**, 33–42.
Campbell, A.K. and Siddle, K. (1973). *Diabetologica* **9**, 62.
Danan, G., Bernuau, J., Moullot, X., Dogott, C. and Pessayre, D. (1984). *Digestion* **30**, 179–184.
Fell, H.B. (1975). *In* "Organ Culture in Biomedical Research" (M. Balls and M. Monnickendam, eds), pp. 1–13. Cambridge University Press, Cambridge.
Freshney, R.I. (1983). *In* "Culture of Animal Cells. A Manual of Basic Technique", pp. 225–235. Alan R. Liss Inc., New York.
Genève, J., Larrey, D., Pessayre, D. and Benhamou, J.P. (1987). *Gastroenterol. Clin. Biol.* **11**, 242–249.
Goethals, F., Krack, G., Deboyser, D., Vossen, P. and Roberfroid, M. (1984). *Fundam. Appl. Toxicol.* **4**, 441–450.
Goethals, F., Deboyser, D., Lefebvre, V., De Coster, I. and Roberfroid, M. (1990). *Toxicol. In Vitro* **4**, 435–438.
Hart, A., Mattheyse, F.J. and Balinsky, J.B. (1983). *In Vitro* **19**, 841–852.
Holmberg, M.B. and Jansson, B. (1962). *J. New Drugs* **2**, 361–365.
Krack, G., Gravier, O., Roberfroid, M. and Mercier, M. (1980). *Biochim. Biophys. Acta* **632**, 619–629.
Krack, G., Goethals, F., Deboyser, D. and Roberfroid, M. (1983). *In* "Isolation, Characterization and Use of Hepatocytes" (R.A. Harris and N.W. Cornell, eds), pp. 391–398. Elsevier Science Publishing Co., Inc., Amsterdam.
Krebs, H.A. (1950). *Biochim. Biophys. Acta* **4**, 249–269.
Krumdieck, C.L., Dos Santos, J.E. and Ho, K.J. (1980). *Anal. Biochem.* **104**, 118–123.
Lamprecht, W. and Trautschold, I. (1963). *In* "Methods of Enzymatic Analysis" (H.U. Bergmeyer, ed.), pp. 543–551. Academic Press, New York.
Larrey, D., Amouyal, G., Pessayre, D., Degott, C., Danne, O., Machayekhi, J.P., Feldman, G. and Benhamou, J.P. (1988). *Gastroenterology* **94**, 200–203.
Mellström, B., Bertilson, L., Lou, Y.C., Säwe, J. and Sjöqvist, F. (1983). *Clin. Pharmacol. Ther.* **34**, 516–520.
Mellström, B., Sawe, J., Bertilsson, L. and Smöqvist, F. (1986). *Clin. Pharmacol. Ther.* **39**, 369–371.
Morgan, D.H. (1969). *Br. J. Psychol.* **111**, 1107–1109.
Omura, T. and Sato, R. (1964). *J. Biol. Chem.* **239**, 2370–2378.
Ratasavanah, D., Baffet, G., Latinier, M.F., Rissel, M. and Guillouzo, A. (1988). *Xenobiotica* **18**, 765–771.
Reed, G.B. and Grisham, J.W. (1975). *Lab. Invest.* **33**, 298–304.
Roberfroid, M. and Goethals, F. (1990). *ATLA* **18**, 19–22.

Sigot-Luizard, M.F. (1973). *C.R. Acad. Sci. Paris Ser. D* **276**, 619–620.

Sipes, I.G., Fisher, R.L., Smith, P.F., Stine, E.R., Gandolfi, A.J. and Brendel, K. (1987). *Arch. Toxicol. Suppl.* **11**, 20–33.

Smith, P.F., Gandolfi, A.J., Krumdieck, C.L., Putnam, C.W., Zukowski, C.F., Davis, W.M. and Brendel, K. (1985). *Life Sci.* **36**, 1367–1375.

Smith, P.F., Krack, G., McKee, K.L., Johnson, D.G., Gandolfi, A.J., Hruby, V.J., Krumdieck, C.L. and Brendel, K. (1986). *In vitro Cell. Dev. Biol.* **22**, 706–712.

Smith, P.F., Fisher, R., Shubat, P.J., Gandolfi, A.J., Krumdieck, C.L. and Brendel, K. (1987). *Toxicol. Appl. Pharmacol.* **87**, 509–522.

Sweeney, G.D. (1983). *In* "Drug Metabolism and Distribution" (J.W. Gamble, ed.), pp. 42–48. Elsevier Biomedical Press, New York.

Trowell, O.A. (1959). *Exp. Cell Res.* **16**, 118–147.

Vulpian, M.A. (1859). *C.R. Acad. Sci. Paris* **48**, 807–811.

Wroblesky, F. and Ladue, J. (1955). *Proc. Soc. Exp. Biol. Med.* **90**, 210–231.

Discussion

X. Pouradier Duteil

Dr Goethals' system seems to be very attractive, but could she say slightly more precisely what are the advantages of coculture or slice perfusion with regard to metabolic activity?

F. Goethals

The latter is possibly an easier system to use than coculture. Dr Guillouzo's system is difficult to establish in the laboratory because an epithelial cell line has to be isolated as well as hepatocytes. With tissue slices we have a rather simple system with the advantage that slices can be taken from liver and also from other organs. Also, human liver is increasingly difficult to obtain, but it is easier to get a piece of *normal* human liver. In this way too this model may have some advantages.

There is not enough feedback about the metabolic capacity and maintenance of the biochemical parameters, especially with regard to the biotransformation capacity of the liver slices with time of incubation. I have preliminary data that show the *P*-450 content is maintained to 50%.

M. Adolphe

To me, organ slices present a big disadvantage in that they involve working on cells which are beginning to die. What does Dr Goethals think, for example, about organ culture, which has the same advantage of being able to work on human liver but the cells are able to survive *in vitro*?

F. Goethals
As far as I know, culture of adult liver is almost impossible. It is a highly
differentiated organ and almost impossible to maintain in a differentiated
state. Fetal or perinatal liver may be easier, so, what I have described,
is probably a compromise.

M. Adolphe
Is it perhaps possible to reduce the disadvantages by using a better
medium?

F. Goethals
I agree. Improvement of the medium could perhaps improve the viability
of the cells.

J. Boyer
How many milligrams of tissue does a slice contain, and has the
ultrastructure, the electron-microscopic integrity, been looked at?

F. Goethals
No, that has not been done. One slice is about 1 cm diameter, 200 µm
thickness. There is about 20 mg of tissue, and between 1 and 2 mg of
protein in a slice.

J. Boyer
How long was the light-microscopic integrity maintained with the
haematoxylin/eosin staining?

F. Goethals
It never lasted longer than 20 h.

J. Boyer
At what time during the perfusion does morphological deterioration of
the slice begin to be seen?

F. Goethals
Morphological alterations appear after some biochemical dysfunction has
occurred; for example, the glycogen content dropped after 8 h of
incubation.

D. Neurotoxicity

11

In Vitro Systems for the Determination of Neurotoxicity: Validation Studies with Aluminium and Ethylcholine Mustard Aziridinium (ECMA)

C.K. ATTERWILL and H. JOHNSTON

The CellTox Centre, Division of Biosciences, Hatfield Polytechnic, College Lane, Hatfield, Herts, U.K.

Introduction

In vitro neural systems can be predictive for neurotoxicity (Atterwill and Walum, 1989), with the exception of xenobiotics which act on the central nervous system (CNS) primarily by directly affecting the function or "integrity" of the blood–brain barrier. In general, because of the anatomical and functional complexity of the nervous system, culture systems have been largely used in mechanistic studies, where the neurochemical changes underlying *in vivo* and behavioural phenomena are further investigated *in vitro*. There are currently six acceptable classifications for neurotoxicants (Norton, 1986) consisting of those causing: (i) anoxic damage to CNS grey matter, (ii) myelin damage in

IN VITRO METHODS IN TOXICOLOGY
ISBN 0-12-388175-7

the CNS and peripheral nervous system (PNS), (iii) damage to specialized CNS nuclei or groups of cells in the brain, (iv) peripheral nerve axonopathy, (v) damage to cell bodies (or perikarya) of peripheral neurons, and lastly (vi) functional or structural changes at CNS or PNS synaptic junctions. It is clear then that when interpreting *in vitro* data from mechanistic investigations or developing *in vitro* models as 'prescreens', much attention must be paid to both validation of the proposed system and to the behavioural, pathological and neurochemical correlates of neurotoxicity in the whole animal model.

The wide range of *in vitro* systems at present employed in neurobiological studies is available for use in neurotoxicological investigations, although often, as in neurobiology, the choice of system is usually an arbitrary one. Careful consideration must first be given to the chosen indicators of toxicity which can include cellular viability/death, generic cell functions (such as respiration, ion transport, protein and DNA turnover), differentiated cell functions (e.g. axonal transport, synaptogenesis/myelination, enzyme activities, neurotransmitter function), and lastly, toxicant characteristics (such as neurotransmitter uptake/accumulation/release and metabolism by the neural cells). Both in mechanistic neurotoxicology and when screening for potential neurotoxicants *in vitro* the availability of a more rational 'stepwise' approach is now timely and justifiable.

There are many examples of problems when predicting *in vivo* neurotoxicity from *in vitro* data (see also Goldstein and Shahar, 1987). For example, in the case of carbon disulphide, CNS toxicity may occur after high-dose exposure whereas peripheral neuropathy occurs following long-term low-dose exposure. This highlights the problem of using a single *in vitro* model derived from either the CNS or PNS to predict an *in vivo* neurotoxic effect. As for many other target organ toxicities, metabolic factors are always extremely important. In the case of the well-known dopaminergic neurotoxin, MPTP (1-methyl-4-phenyl-1,2,3,6-tetrahydropyridine) the presence of glial cells is important in a culture system in order to produce the neurotoxic metabolite MPP$^+$ (1-methyl-4-phenylpyridinium ion) (Barnes *et al.*, 1989) from the parent compound and cells from different species also vary in sensitivity. Another factor for consideration is that cells in neural cultures perform little neurophysiological 'work' under standard culture conditions. However, many substances elicit neurotoxicity precisely because some active process is impaired which is expressed only in the working nervous system. Consequently, procedures including excitation of nerve cells should be included in the *in vitro* tests. There are many culture systems now available (Table 11.1) including neural, tumour-derived cell lines, organotypic explant or reaggregation cultures and primary monolayer

Table 11.1
Nervous system culture types

Type	Further detail	Advantages and disadvantages
Dispersed cell cultures (includes 'micromass' type)	*Primary Dispersed* Monolayer – Mixed or enriched in neurons, astrocytes, oligodendrocytes *Secondary Dispersed* Derived from above or cell lines, out-growths from explants	Good reproducibility and large quantities Can perform single cell electrophysiology Differentiation occurs but can dedifferentiate over time. Often not organotypic
Tumorigenic cell lines	Monolayer – neuroblastoma, Schwannoma and glioma	Large quantities of uncontaminated cell types but dedifferentiated
Organotypic explants	'Lying drop' type Different CNS regions	Good cytoarchitectural preservation for morphological studies. Not all CNS areas possible yet. Fairly specialized technique
Whole organ explants	PNS autonomic ganglia	Can culture more 'mature' cells. Limited quantities
Whole embryo culture	Usually rat	Very specialized technique; intact foetal metabolism and near normal brain development. Resource intensive and only narrow development period defined
Rotation-mediated aggregation cultures	Organotypic 'suspension' cultures	Organotypic cell-association and neurochemical characteristics. Highly reproducible; morphological assessment possible; can culture large quantities of tissue. Uses many foetuses

cultures of individual neural cell types: neurons, astrocytes and oligodendrocytes. These are supplemented by various *ex vivo/in vitro* systems, e.g. brain slices and synaptosomes. Much success and insight has been gained in testing and understanding organophosphate-induced delayed neuropathy (OPIDN) through the hen brain assay of neurotoxic esterase

(NTE) enzyme activity *in vitro* following pesticide exposure (Johnson, 1987). From the culture models much success has been achieved using the organotypic explant culture type (Yonezawa *et al.*, 1980), for example when studying excitatory amino acid (β-*N*-oxalylamino-L-alanine from *Lathyrus sativus* or chickling pea (BOAA) or β-*N*-methylamine-L-alanine from *Cycas circinalis* or false sago palms (BMAA)) neurotoxicity. Rotation-mediated aggregating cultures with organotypic characteristics constructed from single cell suspensions of foetal brain have provided much valuable information regarding the neurobiological and neuropharmacological aspects of the developing brain (Atterwill, 1987). The cells within these organotypic cultures change from a population of undifferentiated neuroepithelial cells to an integrated population of differentiated neurons, astrocytes and oligodendroglia organized in a spherical structure of 200–500 μm in diameter (Garber and Moscona, 1972; Atterwill, 1987). Dendritic and axonal growth and synaptogenesis peak at 21–30 days *in vitro*, then myelination occurs and cell division is restricted. The subsequent aspects of neural development in the cultures are as dependent upon thyroid hormone (L-tri-iodothyronine) as they are in the *in vivo* brain (Atterwill *et al.*, 1983).

There is now an increasing number of neurotoxicants with correlations between the functional 'perturbations' produced in developing organotypic brain reaggregate cultures *in vitro* and their known *in vivo* effects. These include methylmercury, cycloheximide and colchicine (Jacobs *et al.*, 1986), 6-hydroxydopamine (6-OHDA), the tricyclic antidepressants (Majocha *et al.*, 1981) and ascorbic acid (Trapp and Richelson, 1980). With respect to cholinergic neurons, the list includes kainic acid (Trapp and Richelson, 1980), the organophosphorus compounds (Wehner *et al.*, 1985) and, in our own laboratory, ethylcholine mustard aziridinium (ECMA) and aluminium (Pillar *et al.*, 1987; Atterwill and Collins, 1988).

A 'tiered' or stepwise *in vitro* CNS neurotoxicity testing procedure was recently proposed by Atterwill (1989a) where the first-stage screen involved neurotoxicant exposure in neural cell lines or in the brain 'micromass' culture model. This would be followed by second-phase testing in a proven organotypic system, such as the whole-brain reaggregate cultures for investigation of the time-course, specificity and mechanisms of neurotoxicity. A third phase would then allow more discrete information on cell type and mechanism to be obtained by using cell-type specific neural cultures and/or alternative cellular systems. Such a scheme is depicted in simple terms in Fig. 11.1. Two known neurotoxins, the cholinotoxin ECMA (Fig. 11.2) and aluminium chloride, have now been tested in our laboratory using the various models described, and the feasibility of such a tiered screen and suggested end points evaluated by

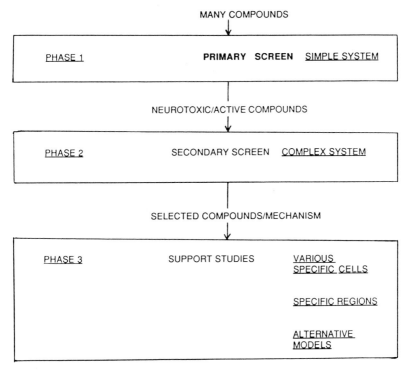

Fig. 11.1 Proposed general "tiered" test model for neurotoxicant detection *in vitro*.

studying the results obtained. The data from the two sets of investigations are summarized in this chapter and a final testing scheme proposed to be used in a (FRAME) (Fund for Replacement of Animals in Medical Experiments) blind validation trial. In the course of these investigations new information on the mechanisms of neurotoxicity of ECMA and aluminium were obtained and these data are also presented here. In particular, the use of peripheral nonneural cells (mast cells) for studying ECMA toxicity has provided a means for studying the action of neurotrophic factors on their receptors.

Methods

The three main methodologies described in this chapter are the whole rat brain reaggregate culture, the rat embryonic midbrain 'micromass' model and the isolated rat peritoneal mast cell preparation.

Whole Brain Reaggregate Cultures

Foetal rat brain reaggregate cultures were prepared from 16–17-day rat foetuses as previously described (Atterwill *et al.*, 1984; Atterwill, 1987) (see Fig. 11.2). The cells were cultured in Dulbecco's Modified Eagle's Medium, supplemented with 10% foetal calf serum and glutamine. ECMA was freshly prepared before use from the precursor *O*-acetylethylcholine mustard by cyclization and hydrolysis (Pillar *et al.*, 1988). Conversion to the aziridinium was found by thiosulphate titration to be consistently 76%. ECMA was added directly to the cultures on the eighth or ninth day *in vitro*, in concentrations similar to those likely in CSF *in vivo* after i.c.v. injection *in vivo* (Leventer *et al.*, 1985).

At various intervals after treatment, aggregates were harvested by sedimentation through buffer and washed. Samples were assayed for choline acetyltransferase (ChAT) activity, muscarinic receptor binding, neurofilament protein, lactate dehydrogenase (LDH) and Na^+/K^+ ATPase activity as previously described (see Atterwill *et al.*, 1985; Woodhams *et al.*, 1986).

Rat Midbrain Micromass Cultures

Rat embryonic midbrain (CNS) cells and limb bud (LB) cells differentiate in culture forming a mixed population of neural cells comprising neurons and glia or chondrocytes (Flint, 1980) respectively. This is the basis of the Micromass Test used successfully as a short-term screen for teratogens and developmental neurotoxicants (Clemedson *et al.*, 1989). For studies on neurotoxicants with other more general toxic effects, this test has made it possible to compare effects on cytotoxicity and differentiation for neural and non-neural cells.

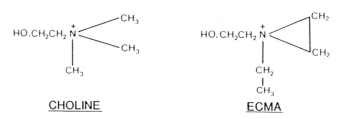

Fig. 11.2 Structural formula of choline and ECMA (ethylcholine mustard aziridinium ion).

Isolation of tissue

Thirteen-day pregnant rats were sacrificed using CO_2 euthanasia and embryo dissection was carried out. The uteri were washed in Earles balanced salt solution (EBSS) and each conceptus released from the uteri. The conceptuses were then transferred to fresh horse serum (HS)/EBSS. The outer membranes still surrounding the embryos were removed. The mesencephalon (midbrain) and forelimb buds were then removed from each embryo and the tissues transferred to separate test tubes using a sterile Pasteur pipette.

Tissue processing

Any excess HS/EBSS was aspirated and the tissue washed three times with a calcium/magnesium-free EBSS (CMF). The tubes were incubated for 20 min at 37°C. CMF was then exchanged for 1%(w/v) trypsin in CMF and the tubes were incubated for a further 20 min at 37°C. The trypsin was then finally washed off using CMF and replaced with 1.3 ml of complete Ham's medium. The tissue was triturated 15 times using a 0.7 mm diameter Pasteur pipette and the cell suspension filtered through a 10 μm nylon mesh. The suspension was divided by transferring 1 ml to a fresh test tube and 20 μl added to 180 μl of CMF and then counted using a Neubauer haemocytometer. The required final cell concentration was, in the case of midbrain, 5×10^6 cells ml and, in the case of limb bud, 2×10^7 cells ml. The final cell suspension was drawn up into a 500 μl combitip and delivered in 10 μl aliquots to 35 mm sterile plastic disposable Petri dishes. Cells were allowed to settle for 2 h at 37°C, forming circular cell islands, and culture dishes (6–8 mm) were then filled to a final volume of 2 ml with culture medium (Ham's F12 with supplements of 10% foetal calf serum, L-glutamine (584.6 mg/l), penicillin (10^6 IU/l) and streptomycin (100 mg/l) and the compounds under test. These cultures were then left until day 2 or 5 *in vitro*.

Determination of cell differentiation—fixing and staining

The medium was removed from both limb bud and midbrain cultures. The limb bud cultures were fixed with 10% formaldehyde containing 0.5% cetylpyridinium chloride for a minimum of 20 min and the midbrain cultures with 10% formaldehyde.

Limb bud

After fixing, the cultures were left for 1 h in 3% acetic acid and then stained for a minimum of 2 h with 1% Alcian Blue in 0.1 M hydrochloric acid. After being washed with tap water, the cultures were air-dried.

Midbrain

Fixative was removed under a running tap. The cells were then stained for 1–3 min with haematoxylin followed by washing with tap water. The cultures were left in water for 2 min, after which time the water was removed and the cultures air-dried. The differentiated foci were counted using an image analyser (AMS 40–10, AMS Cambridge). These data will not be described in detail here.

Determination of cell death (cytotoxicity assay)

Preparation of the cell suspensions and culture medium was as described above. For this assay, cells were plated out in 96-well (10 μl per well) microtitre dishes (Nunclon – Gibco, Paisley, Scotland, UK) which were precoated with 10 μl 0.05% (w/v) collagen in 0.01% (v/v) acetic acid. The collagen layer was air-dried in a laminar flow cabinet before addition of the cells. The first column of wells was left free of cells, to be used later as a blank in the assay. After 2 h settling at 37°C (5% CO_2: 95% air), the volume of culture medium in each well was increased to 200 μl (supplemented with test compound or vehicle). Cultures were left in the incubator for 2 or 5 days (with or without different concentrations of test component) at 37°C under an atmosphere of 5% CO_2: 95% air.

Fixation and staining

The cells were fixed for a minimum of 20 min with 10% formaldehyde solution then washed three times with phosphate-buffered saline (PBS: Dulbecco's phosphate-buffered saline, pH 7.4; Flow Laboratories, Irvine, Scotland, UK). PBS was replaced with 200 μl of Neutral Red stain (0.1% (w/v) Neutral Red in PBS). The blank column was also filled with Neutral Red stain. Cells were stained for 90 min at room temperature, the Neutral Red stain was removed, and the wells were washed with PBS. Stain was then eluted from the cells into 200 μl of acid alcohol (0.5% (v/v) acetic acid in 50% alcohol) per well for a minimum of 2 h. Stain intensity (absorbance) was measured colorimetrically on a Dynatech minireader II (Dynatech, Billingshurst, Kent, UK) at 550 nm. Cell number was directly related to the absorbance of the eluted stain (Flint, 1980; Crapper et al., 1986).

Rat Peritoneal Mast Cells *In Vitro*

These experiments used a mixed population of rat peritoneal cells. In more complex release experiments it is possible to purify the cells by density gradient centrifugation over Percoll.

Rats were killed by CO_2 euthanasia, exsanguinated and then injected intraperitoneally with 10 ml of Hepes-buffered Locke's solution (pH 7.0–7.2) with heparin (5 units/ml). After lavage for 1 min, the abdominal cavity was opened by a midline incision and the fluid collected, using a plastic funnel, in polystyrene tubes chilled on ice.

The cells were recovered by centrifugation (930 r.p.m.) (4°C, 5 min) and washed three times in the ice-cold buffer. Aliquots of equilibrated cells (37°C, 5 min) were incubated (37°C, 15 min) with the releasing agent, nerve growth factor (NGF, from bovine brain; sigma) ± the test compound, in a final colume of 0.5 ml. The secretion reaction was halted by addition of 1.5 ml of ice-cold buffer, immediately before centrifugation (930 r.p.m., 4°C, 5 min). The top 1.0 ml of the supernatant was removed to assay for histamine. Before the histamine assay, residual protein was precipitated using a final concentration of 5% TCA (trichloroacetic acid), tubes were centrifuged (2500 r.p.m., 4°C, 15 min) and supernatants removed.

To determine total amine content, a sample of the tubes from the same population of cells was taken at the incubation stage, cells were disrupted by sonication (50 Hz, 30s). 1.5 ml of ice cold buffer was added and, after centrifugation (2500 r.p.m., 4°C, 10 min), 1 ml was taken for assay. Histamine was measured fluorimetrically using an *O*-phthaldehyde condensate assay (Anton and Sayre, 1969).

Results

Neurotoxicity of ECMA

Brain reaggregate cultures

Previous to the current work with ECMA (Fig 11.2), attempts had been made to damage central cholinergic neurons in brain reaggregates *in vitro* using the excitotoxin, kainic acid. Using cholinergic neuron-enriched telencephalic reaggregates, Honegger and Richelson (1977) demonstrated that 5 μM kainate caused a significant reduction in cholinergic enzyme activities, although its effects were not specific. It was then reported (Sandberg *et al.*, 1985) that a cholinergic neuroblastoma cell line showed marked evidence of generalized cytotoxic effects 18 h after treatment with 100 μM ECMA alongside reductions in ChAT, although this is a higher concentration than generally tested *in vivo* (Leventer *et al.*, 1985; Fisher and Hanin, 1986).

We have now shown that the effects of 12.5–50 μM ECMA in whole brain reaggregate cultures can be divided into two phases, namely a partial loss of ChAT activity (33%) within 2 h of treatment and a longer-term loss (total, 60–80%) evident after 72 h of treatment (Fig. 11.3 for summary of changes). In neither phase did ChAT loss show any marked relation to neurotoxin concentration. Only the initial toxic phase was prevented by prior blockage of choline/ECMA transport using hemicholinium (HC-3; an inhibitor of presynaptic choline transport) suggesting direct inhibition of ChAT by ECMA (Pedder and Prince, 1987): the second phase was not prevented by this blockade and was not, therefore, a consequence of the inhibition of ChAT and would appear to represent actual loss of cholinergic neurons. Since HC-3 prevents ECMA from entering nerve terminals (Pedder and Prince, 1987), it is thought that this second-phase effect must be due to some extracellular action on the cholinergic cells.

An initial direct reduction in muscarinic receptor binding (at 2 h), as measured by [³H]quinuclidinylbenzilate (QNB) binding recovered during this second neurotoxic phase at the lower concentration of 12.5 μM ECMA (72–120 h exposure). Since this second phase probably represents

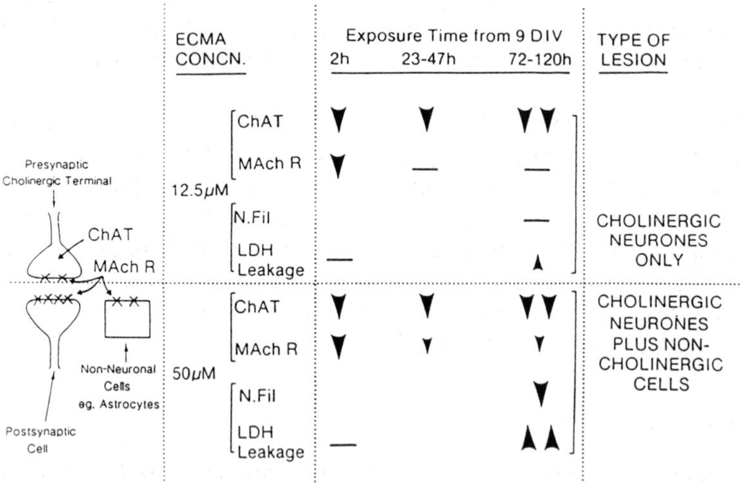

Fig. 11.3 Summary of ECMA-induced neurotoxic changes in whole rat brain reaggregate cultures. MAchR, muscarinic cholinergic receptor; N.Fil, neurofilament protein; DIV, days *in vitro*.

the loss of cholinergic neurons, muscarinic receptor recovery at low concentrations of ECMA would appear to be restricted to cells other than cholinergic neurons (Fig. 11.3). The persistent loss of receptors observed after exposure to the higher concentration of 50 μM ECMA must, therefore, reflect the loss of these non-cholinergic cells as well as of the cholinergic neurons themselves. This confirms that ECMA is more cytotoxic at the higher concentration (Fig. 11.3).

In support of the greater cytotoxicity at higher concentrations of ECMA, neurofilament protein in the reaggregates was found to be reduced after treatment with 25–50 μM but not with 12.5 μM ECMA. LDH leakage was also more pronounced after treatment with 50 μM ECMA (see Fig 11.3) and the Na^+/K^+ ATPase activity of the culture was markedly reduced (approx. 50%). In supporting experiments there was also a marked loss of cells in primary monolayer cultures of non-cholinergic cerebellar granule neurons or astrocytes (for a description of cultures, see Atterwill *et al.*, 1985) after treatment with 50 μM ECMA. There was no such loss after exposure to 12.5 μM ECMA. In agreement with these findings, measurement of 5-hydroxytryptamine function in the reaggregates on the basis of 5HIAA (5-hydroxyindoleacetic acid) levels showed that at 12.5 μM ECMA there is a compensating increase in 5-HT function, suggesting neuronal activation rather than loss (Piller *et al.*, 1989). Furthermore, morphological assessment of ECMA-treated reaggregates showed that astrocytic glial fibrillary acidic protein (GFAP) immunoreactivity (Woodhams *et al.*, 1986) in the outer "glia-limitans" was disrupted and lost in those cultures exposed to the higher concentrations of ECMA. This confirms that astrocyte cytotoxicity occurs at higher concentrations of ECMA.

These findings for ECMA are summarized in Fig. 11.4 in relation to the tiered *in vitro* neurotoxicity testing scheme described in Fig. 11.1. It can be seen that the suggested phases of screening do pick up the neurotoxicity of ECMA, first showing cell death in a neuroblastoma cell line preparation and then concentration-dependent cholinotoxicity using the organotypic reaggregate cultures. Mechanistic information and cell-type specificity information was expanded in phase 3 using other, different *in vitro* cell preparations as described below.

Rat peritoneal mast cells

Regenerative responses to neurotoxin-induced lesions in the nervous system is now a topic of great interest to both neurotoxicologists and neurobiologists. We have previously shown that simultaneous addition of the neurotrophic factor, NGF (50 ng/ml), with cholinotoxic concentrations

EXAMPLE 1   ECMA NEUROTOXICITY

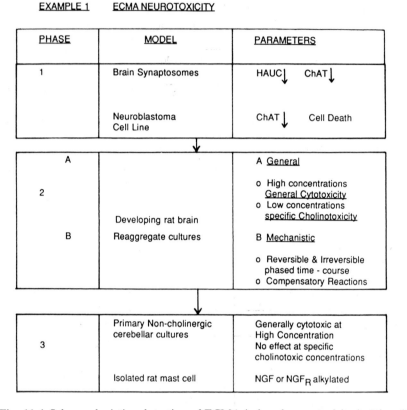

PHASE	MODEL	PARAMETERS
1	Brain Synaptosomes	HAUC↓ ChAT↓
	Neuroblastoma Cell Line	ChAT↓ Cell Death
2	A	A General
		o High concentrations General Cytotoxicity
	Developing rat brain	o Low concentrations specific Cholinotoxicity
	B Reaggregate cultures	B Mechanistic
		o Reversible & Irreversible phased time - course
		o Compensatory Reactions
3	Primary Non-cholinergic cerebellar cultures	Generally cytotoxic at High Concentration No effect at specific cholinotoxic concentrations
	Isolated rat mast cell	NGF or NGF$_R$ alkylated

Fig. 11.4 Scheme depicting detection of ECMA-induced neurotoxicity in "tiered" test model. HAUC, high affinity uptake of choline; NGF$_R$, NGF receptor.

of ECMA (12.5 μM) to rat whole-brain reaggregate cultures failed to effect a reversal of the cholinergic lesioning whereas 'delayed' NGF treatment after ECMA addition to the cultures was able to reverse the cholinotoxin-induced loss of ChAT activity (Atterwill and Meakin, 1990). It was postulated that ECMA may be alkylating NGF and/or its receptor on cholinergic neurons and that this may even bear some relation on its cholinotoxic mechanism of action (Atterwill, 1989a; Atterwill and Meakin, 1990). Thus, a model for testing this hypothesis on live cells bearing NGF receptors was sought. The neuroimmune axis and the interaction of cytokines with trophic factors is currently an active area of research. NGF has been shown to evoke histamine release from isolated peripheral mast cells. Both local and newly formed mast cells may bear NGF receptors (Pearce & Thompson, 1986). Furthermore, NGF-primed spleen cells differentiate into mast cells when introduced into developing rat brain and locate in close proximity to the hippocampus, which is rich in both NGF and cholinergic neurons (Aloe and De Simone, 1989). Although both central cholinergic neurons bear the NGF receptor and mast cells may do so, the mast cells appear to bear predominantly the Type 2 low-affinity type (nanomolar affinity- also on astrocytes) whereas cholinergic neurons have both Type 2 and high-affinity Type 1 (picomolar affinity).

In these preliminary studies, we have confirmed that (a) in the presence of phosphatidylserine NGF evokes a dose-responsive histamine release from the rat peritoneal mast cells *in vitro* with an ED_{50} around 0.1 μg/ml (Fig. 11.5a), (b) the optimum phosphatidylserine concentration for this response is 10 μg/ml (Fig. 11.5b), and (c) ECMA, present before and during the addition of NGF to the mast cells, blocks the NGF-evoked histamine release (Fig. 11.5c) whereas ECMA preincubated with the cells and then washed-off prior to NGF addition has no effect. No effect of ECMA was observed on the spontaneous basal release of histamine from the cells in the absence of NGF, suggesting that there is no direct cellular cytotoxic effect.

Thus, these data have further helped to delineate the likely mechanism of ECMA neurotoxicity seen in the brain culture model. It appears unlikely that ECMA is blocking the NGF response to mast cells by alkylating or inactivating the proposed NGF receptor protein and, therefore, would probably not be expected to produce such a response in central cholinergic neurons. It is able, however, to alkylate the NGF molecule itself (or possibly the histamine exocytotic mechanism) and this would account for the inability of simultaneous NGF ECMA additions to brain reaggregate cultures to reverse the ECMA-induced losses of cholinergic neurons *in vitro* (Atterwill and Meakin, 1990).

Neurotoxicity of Aluminium Chloride

Aluminium ion has been proposed as a contributor to the pathogenesis of several neurological disorders which appear to have an environmental aetiology. Besides its neurotoxic actions, the aluminium ion also has more general toxic effects in both developing and mature tissues (Golub *et al.*, 1987; MacDonald and Martin, 1988). Concern for the potentially toxic effects of chronic exposure has grown due to the increased solubilization from surface waters by acid rain (Driscoll, 1985, Ganrot, 1986; MacDonald and Martin, 1988). Pathologically, high aluminium concentrations have been demonstrated in the nuclear region of neurofibrillary tangle-bearing neurons of the hippocampus in brain tissue from patients with Alzheimer's disease, although it is uncertain whether the aluminium ion has a high

(a)

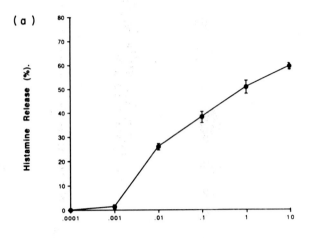

Nerve Growth Factor (µg/ml)

(b)

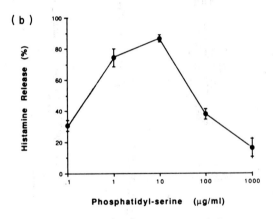

Phosphatidyl-serine (µg/ml)

(c)

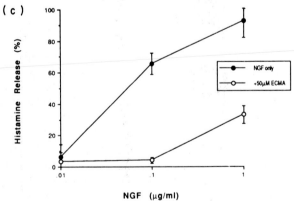

NGF (µg/ml)

affinity for these abnormal neural regions or possesses any aetiological relationship with the disease (Perl and Brody, 1980; Crapper *et al:*, 1986). To date most of the information on the mechanism of neurotoxicity has been gained from *in vivo* models (Troncosco *et al.*, 1986; Johnson and Jope, 1988) or synaptosome and brain slice preparations (Johnson and Jope, 1986).

In the context of the tiered testing scheme (Fig. 11.1), we have utilized the rat embryonic midbrain 'micromass' culture system to define further the neurotoxicity of aluminium, and compared the results with those previously obtained in the organotypic brain reaggregate culture model and with other *in vitro* preparations. Using the micromass model it is possible to detect and quantify time-related effects on neural differentiation as distinct from those producing cytotoxicity. We also investigated as a Phase 1 test whether aluminium had any rapid acute effects on neural function in terms of the bioelectrical properties of *in vitro*-maintained Retzius Cells from the Leech nervous system. This is the largest neuron in the segmental ganglion which can be removed from the animal, maintained *in vitro* for several hours, and has been proposed by Neuropharm Ltd as an early indicator of neurotoxic action (Atterwill *et al.*, 1990). This testing scheme is illustrated in Fig. 11.6. We were able to demonstrate that acute exposure (0–48 h) *in vitro* to high concentrations of aluminium chloride does not appear to perturb neural function in terms of either the electrophysiological properties of lower vertebrate neurons or the cholinergic activity of rat brain reaggregate culture cells (Atterwill *et al.*, 1990). This is despite a reported direct *ex vivo* inhibitory potential on cholinergic transmitter-related enzymes. Longer-term exposure *in vitro* (48 h plus), however, produces neural cytotoxicity in the brain micromass model (Fig.11.7) and inhibits cholinergic function in brain reaggregate cultures at high concentrations (0.5–5 mM). Concentrations of this order can apparently be attained in localized areas in the brains of patients suffering dialysis demention (personal communciation,

---

Fig. 11.5 (a) Effect of different concentrations of NGF incubated for 15 min at 37°C on histamine release from isolated rat peritoneal mast cells *in vitro*. Experiments were conducted in the presence of 10 μg phosphatidylserine/ml, and values are means ± S.E.M. from three experimental runs. (b) Effect of phosphatidylserine concentration on NGF-evoked histamine release from isolated rat peritoneal mast cells *in vitro*. NGF at 0.1 μg/ml was used in these experiments. (c) Effect of 50 μM ECMA on NGF (+phosphatidylserine)-evoked histamine release from isolated rat peritoneal mast cells *in vitro*. ECMA was present both during a 2 h preincubation period and during 15 min NGF exposure. Data represent the means ± s.e.m. for six to eight individual determinations.

EXAMPLE 2   ALUMINIUM NEUROTOXICITY

PHASE	MODEL(S)	PARAMETER(S)	
1	Isolated leech Retzius neurones (Acute Application)	Electrophysiological cell firing pattern and action potential unaltered	
PHASE 2	Developing rat brain reaggregates	Possible Lesion of cholinergic neurones. No general cell death	↑ Reverse ↓
PHASE 3	Midbrain (limb) mixed micromass culture (neurones/ glia)	Brain-specific cytotoxicity at 'clinical' neurotoxic concentrations Immature cells more sensitive	
	Cortical astrocyte monolayer culture	Excitotoxic amino acid (EAA) release increased at sub-cytotoxic concentrations	

Fig. 11.6 Scheme depicting detection of aluminium chloride-induced neurotoxicity in the 'tiered' test model.

J. Albrecht). In terms of the general molecular mechanisms of neurological damage associated with aluminium, a recent study has shown that enhanced lipid peroxidation may be involved (Fraga *et al.*, 1990). More importantly, another study has shown that similar high concentrations of aluminium chloride cause a massive release of excitatory amino acids (EAA) from cultured cortical astrocytes *in vitro* (Albrecht *et al.*, 1990). It is thus highly possible that neuronal cytotoxicity in the mixed culture systems, such as the micromass and reaggregate models, may be due to an excitotoxic mechanism involving amino acid release from astrocytes and sustained activation of EAA receptors on susceptible cholinergic neurons.

Day 2

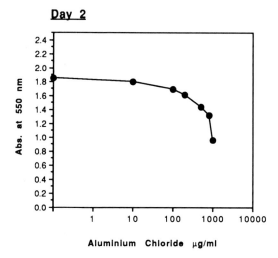

Day 5

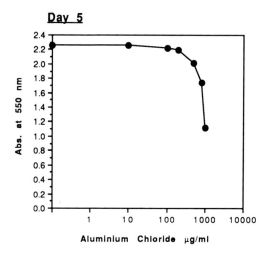

Fig. 11.7 Cytotoxicity profile of rat embryonic mid brain 'micromass' cultures following 2 or 5 days exposure to different concentrations of aluminium chloride. Cultures were prepared as described under Methods in 96-well culture dishes and exposed to 0–1000 μg $AlCl_3$/ml for 2 or 5 days after plating. After this time the cytotoxic potential was determined by the Neutral Red uptake method as described.

Discussion and Conclusions

It becomes apparent from the previous sections that organotypic brain reaggregate cultures have provided an excellent tool with which to study both the mechanism of action of neurotoxicants and the related CNS adaptational changes occurring in response to both neurotrophic factors and neurotoxin-induced lesions. The main advantage of reaggregates is their ease of preparation, reproducibility and representation of the whole brain response rather than just one individual brain area or cell type. By supplementing information gained in this system with observed neurotoxicant actions on primary monolayer cultures of neurons or astrocytes, much information on the mechanism of cholinotoxicity of the two selected examples, ECMA and aluminium chloride, has been obtained.

Brain reaggregates are not the only promising *in vitro* system for a screening procedure. The micromass culture system has also provided interesting data on potential developmental neurotoxins because of its simplicity, and mixed neural cell composition and has presented a useful screening tool to the *in vitro* neurotoxicologist.

A 'tiered' testing scheme can now be proposed utilizing the original proposals by Atterwill (1989b) and the preliminary validation information gained from the described studies with ECMA and aluminium. This full scheme is illustrated in Fig. 11.8 and represents a composite of feasible models and test parameters. This scheme is soon to be tested in a FRAME blind trial.

One of the primary aims of the present work is to utilize relevant general markers for the different neural cell types in the CNS and PNS as indicators of neurotoxicity and/or cytotoxic events. With this objective in mind, the Phase 1 screening models will be assessed for general effects using the Neutral Red and MTT assays (Mosmann, 1983), whereas the Phase 2 organotypic cultures will employ these and more specific neural markers. For the CNS models neuron-specific enolase (NSE), the major enolase isoenzyme found in differentiated neurons, and non-neuronal enolase (NNE) the major form in mature glia and non-differentiated neurons (Marangos *et al.*, 1978, 1986) will be determined as well as neurofilament protein (NFil) and glial fibrillary acidic protein (GFAP) (O'Callaghan and Miller, 1983). When developing a PNS test system, the enzyme, neuropathy target esterase (NTE), will probably be a useful marker (O'Callaghan and Miller, 1983; Johnson, 1987).

The ECMA investigations showed an understanding of the neurotoxicity progressing successfully first through cell lines, then reaggregate cultures and finally through individual cultured cell types. Further mechanistic

GENERAL TIERED SCHEME FOR NEUROTOXICITY TESTING IN VITRO

PHASE	TYPE	MODEL	PARAMETERS
PHASE 1 **(Initial Screen)** ± Metabolic activation	Simple neural systems Cell lines Mixed Monolayer	Neuroblastoma Cell lines (Undifferentiated & Differentiated IMR 32 Neuro 2A Brain Micromass	Cell Death MTT/LDH Neutral Red "
PHASE 2 **Central study** **& Mechanism** ± Depolarisation	Complex Organotypic Culture	Chick/rat Brain Reaggregates	(A) Diameter LDH MTT Protein/DNA NSE/NNE NFIL Na^+K^+-ATPase (B) Neurotransmitter Markers
PHASE 3 **(Support Studies)**	Acute/ex vivo models Specific cell and Regions	eg Isol. leech neurone (Neuropharm Ltd.) Synaptosomes Astrocytes eg Isolated mast cell	Electro- physiology Cells & Regions eg various NGF receptors

Fig. 11.8 Final, proposed "tiered" test model to test for CNS neurotoxicants in a blind "trial" with selected compounds. This trial will be coordinated with FRAME. MTT, 3-(4,5-dimethylthiazol-2-yl)-2,5-diphenyltetrazolium bromide; NSE, neuron-specific enolase; NNE, non-neuronal enolase.

information was gained using the isolated mast cells, which are a good example of a 'designer' Phase 3 model to be included when appropriate. Relating these data to a 'tiered' *in vitro* screening system for potential neurotoxicants, it is also apparent from *in vitro* studies of the neurotoxicity of aluminium (Atterwill *et al.*, 1990) that these further strengthen such proposals. The neurotoxic effects of aluminium were detectable in a 'first-phase' procedure using the micromass culture model (where some indications of cellular specificity and time-course were attained) but not after acute exposure in freshly-isolated *ex vivo* leech neurons. Functional cholinergic neurotoxicity was, furthermore, seen in the organotypic rat brain reaggregate culture model which has been proposed as a second level 'screen'. Further information on neurotoxic mechanisms has been provided by studies using pure glial cultures (Albrecht *et al.*, 1990). It is suggested that the use of preparations such as the *ex vivo* leech cells may better support such investigations at a third-tier than at a first-tier level. The scheme includes the facility for testing both in chick and rat cultures, and including metabolizing and neuronal activation systems.

It must be stressed that these procedures will predominantly give a profile of neurotoxicity in the developing CNS, and extrapolation to the mature CNS must be made with caution. Furthermore, extrapolation from or to the whole animal response *in vivo* must be made with caution. In conclusion, therefore, much work is still required to validate the usefulness of these *in vitro* models and by careful comparison with *in vivo* histopathological, neurophysiological; neurobehavioural and neuropharmacological data using defined series of different neurotoxic xenobiotics in 'blind' trials.

References

Albrecht, J., Simmons, M., Dutton, G.R. and Norenberg, M.D. (1990). *Proc. 8th ESN Meeting*, Leipzig, July 1990: 02.1.

Aloe, L. and De Simone, R. (1989). *Int. J. Dev. Neurosci.* **7**, 565–573.

Anton, A. H. and Sayre, D.F. (1969). *J. Pharmacol. Exp. Ther.* **166**, 285–292.

Atterwill, C.K. (1987). *In* "*In Vitro* Methods in Toxicology" (C.K. Atterwill and C.E. Steele, eds), pp. 133–164. University Press, Cambridge.

Atterwill, C.K. (1989a). *J. Mol. Toxicol.* **1**, 489–502.

Atterwill, C.K. (1989b). *ATLA* **16**, 221–230.

Atterwill, C.K. and Collins, P. (1988). *Br. J. Pharmacol.* **94**, 441.

Atterwill, C.K. and Meakin, J. (1990). *Biochem. Pharmacol.* **39**, 2073–2076.

Atterwill, C.K. and Walum, E. (1989): *Toxicol. In Vitro* **3**, 159–161.

Atterwill, C.K., Kingsbury, A.E. and Balazs, A. (1983). *In* "Drugs and Hormones in Brain Development" (M. Schlumpt and W. Lichtensteiger, eds), pp. 50–61. Karger Press, Basle.

Atterwill, C.K., Kingsbury, A., Nicholls, J. and Prince, A.K. (1984). *Br. J. Pharmacol.* **83**, 89–102.

Atterwill, C.K., Atkinson, D.J., Bermudez, I. and Balazs, R. (1985). *Neuroscience*, **14**, 361–373.

Atterwill, C.K., Davies, W.J. and Kyriakides, M.A. (1990). *ATLA* **18**, 181–190.

Barnes, B.M., Cheng, C.H.K., Costall, B., Jenner, P.G. and Naylor, R.J. (1989). *Br. J. Pharmacol.* **96**, 332.

Clemedson, C., Walum, E. and Flint, O. (1989): *ATLA* **16**, 287–292.

Crapper McLachlan, D.R. and Van Berkum, M.F.A. (1986). *In* "*In Vitro* Methods in Toxicology" (D.F. Swaab, M. Mermisan, W.A. Van Goll and F. Van Haaren, eds), vol. 70, pp. 339–410. Elsevier, Amsterdam.

Driscoll, C.T. (1985). *Environ. Health Perspect.* **63**, 93–104.

Fisher, A. and Hanin, I. (1986). *Annu. Rev. Pharmacol. Toxicol.* **26**, 161–181.

Flint, O. P. (1980): *In* "Teratology of the Limbs" (H.J. Merker, H. Nau and D. Neubert, eds), pp. 325–338. Walker de Gruyter, Berlin and New York.

Fraga, C.G., Oteiza, P.I., Golub, M.S., Gershwin, M.E. and Keen, C.L. (1990). *Toxicol. Lett.* **51**, 213–219.

Ganrot, P.O. (1986): *Environ. Health Perspect.* **65**, 363–441.

Garber, B.B. and Moscona, A.A. (1972). *Dev. Biol.* **27**, 217–234.

Goldstein, A.M. and Shahar, A. (1987). *Alternative Approaches to Animal Testing*. Alan R. Liss Inc., New York.

Golub, M.S., Gershwin, E., Donald, J.M., Negri, S. and Keen, C.L. (1987). *Fund. Appl. Toxicol.* **8**, 346–357.

Honegger, P. and Richelson, E. (1977). *Brain Res.* **133**, 329–339.

Jacobs, A.L., Maniscalco, W.M. and Finkelstein, J.N. (1986). *Toxicol. Appl. Pharmacol.* **86**, 362–371.

Johnson, G.W. and Jope, R.S. (1986). *Toxicology* **40**, 93–102.

Johnson, G.W. and Jope, R.S. (1988). *Brain Res.* **456**, 95–103.

Johnson, M.K. (1987). *TIPS* **8**, 174–179.

Leventer, S. McKeag, D., Clancy, M., Wilfert, E. and Hanin, I. (1985). *Neuropharmacology,* **24**, 453–459.

MacDonald, T.L. and Martin, R.B. (1988). *TIBS* **13**, 15–22.

Majocha, R.E., Pearse, R.N., Baldersarini, R.J., Delong, G.R. and Walton, K.G. (1981). *Brain Res.* **230**, 235–252.

Marangos, P.J., Parma, A.M. and Goodwin, F.K. (1978). *J. Neurochem.* **31**, 727–732.

Marangos, P.J., Schmechel, D.E., Parma, A.M. and Goodwin, F.K. (1986). *Brain Res.* **190**, 185–193.

Mosmann, T. (1983). *J. Immunol. Methods* **65**, 55–63.

Norton S. (1986). *In* "Casarelt and Doull's Toxicology", 3rd ed. (C.D. Klaasen, M.D. Amdur and J. Doull, eds); pp. 359–386. MacMillan, New York.

O'Callaghan, J.P. and Miller, D.B. (1983). *TIPS* **4**, 388–390.

Pearce, F.L. and Thompson, H.L. (1986). *J. Physiol.* **372**, 379–393.

Pedder, E.K. and Prince, A.K. (1987). *In* "Cellular and Molecular Basis of Cholinergic Function" (M.J. Dowdal and J.N. Hawthorne, eds), p. 639. Ellis Horwood, London.

Perl, D.P. and Brody, A.K. (1980). *Science* **208**, 297–299.

Pillar, A.M., Prince, A.K. and Atterwill, C.K. (1987). *Arch. Toxicol. Suppl.* **11**, 243–246.

Pillar, A.M., Atterwill, C.K., Jones, C.A. and Prince, A. (1989). *J. Pharmacol.* **96**, 35.

Sandberg, K., Schnaar, R.L., McKinney, M., Hanin, I., Fisher, A. and Coyle, J.T. (1985). *J. Neurochem.* **44**, 439–445.

Trapp, B.P. and Richelson, E. (1980). *In* "Experimental and Clinical Neurotoxicology" (P.S. Spencer and H.H. Schaumberg, eds,), pp. 803–819. Williams and Wilkins, Baltimore and London.

Troncosco, J.C., Sternberger, N.H., Sternberger, L.A., Hoffman, P.N. and Price, D.L. (1986). *Brain Res.* **364**, 295–310.

Wehner, J.M., Smolen, A., Ness-Smolen, T. and Murphy, C. (1985). *Fund. Appl. Toxicol.* **5**, 1104–1109.

Woodhams, P.L., Atterwill, C.K. and Balazs, R. (1986). *Neuropathol. Appl. Neurobiol.* **12**, 577–592.

Yonezawa, T., Bernstein, M.B. and Peterson, E.R. (1980). *In* "Experimental and Clinical Neurotoxicology" (P. S. Spencer and H.H. Schaumburg, eds.), pp. 788–802. Williams and Wilkins, Baltimore and London.

Discussion

I. Purchase
First, in regard to ECMA neurotoxicity, from the evidence presented here it appeared that there was non-specific toxicity on specific cell types at the same concentration as Professor Atterwill claimed to have found the specific cholinotoxic effects.

C. Atterwill
In terms of concentration-dependent toxicity, at the highest 50 μM concentration, the cholinergic cells as well as non-specific cell types including astrocytes, non-cholinergic neurons and cholinergic cells were killed. At the lower concentrations of 12.5 μM and less, there was specific cholinotoxicity which affected neither the cultured astrocytes nor the other neurons present in the cultures.

I. Purchase
Secondly, if 40 chemicals were to be tested for neurotoxicity in an animal system, quite a number of end points might be measured, including pathological end points, with perhaps multiple potential end points within the brain and behavioural effects – a very rich possibility of outcomes. How will it be decided whether you are successful and that the culture system is effective? What is the final test that will be applied if 40 random compounds are put through three tiers involving 6 or 10 different cell culture systems?

C. Atterwill
As I said at the beginning, the use of such an *in vitro* tiered test system has to be in conjunction with *in vivo* information. The list of compounds used to evaluate the system would have to include a number of positive neurotoxicants for which the exact mechanism and range of *in vivo* effects were known. Against that would be included non-neurotoxic analogues of those compounds and totally non-neurotoxic compounds. Only by doing this could the true performance of such a tiered test system be judged. A totally random chemical list for testing in such a system that might contain a neurotoxicant could not be properly evaluated with the hope of predicting its full neurotoxic *in vivo* profile. However, such a

tiered system might be extremely useful for prescreening *in vitro* for potential neurotoxicants whose full profile could then be evaluated *in vivo*.

I. Purchase
I understand that, but are you going to take, say, level 2 culture (organotypic cultures) as an indication of behavioural effects, and level 1 culture as a primary indicator? How will it actually be decided whether the system is giving results that are of value?

C. Atterwill
The compounds for the validation studies will progress through the three tiers as you describe, and at the end of the day it will be decided whether, using the parameters we have selected, a compound has proven to be neurotoxic. Only then will it be known whether the predictivity of the test is good or bad.

I should add that in the industrial setting (which I believe, is what Dr Purchase is alluding to here) the integration of such data into a regulatory "package" is not quite as simple as I have presented it, but would have to be done in a phased fashion. We would have to decide whether to test a group of related analogues through such an *in vitro* system as a "prescreen" (and which suitable end points to use) or whether to use these tests elsewhere simply as mechanistic adjunct tests to *in vivo* studies. This system used in a blind fashion, such as for irritancy testing, may eventually prove to be predictive as a replacement test for neurotoxicity. We have actually been quite surprised as to how many of the compounds whose effects have been compared in this system come out positive if they are taken through the three phases of a tiered *in vitro* procedure.

M. Balls
We have to start somewhere. If we see somebody beginning a journey, it is not fair to ask why he has not arrived at his destination yet. The question is whether he is on the right road that will lead him there.

I. Purchase
My question was how will he know whether he is at his destination when he gets there?

G. Zbinden
At a recent talk I gave on alternative research, a well-known British neurologist in the audience said that MPTP would certainly not show any neurotoxicity in an *in vitro* neural system. I have performed no work on

this and do not know about it, but I would think it could. Did Professor Atterwill pick up at least some toxic effect with MPTP?

C. Atterwill
All through the tiered system that I have described the toxic effect would be detected to a degree, but a complex system has to be included somewhere in the tiers since with MPTP there is need for a glial metabolizing system to produce the neurotoxic metabolite MPP^+.

G. Zbinden
Did you try any of the cells with neural melanin in them?

C. Atterwill
We have not looked at those. Dr Thomas, who is working on MPTP and MPP^+ in my group, has tested this in a cultured cell line preparation. She has shown that cell lines respond to MPP^+ *in vitro* in a species-dependent fashion. A mixed-cell culture system is needed for MPTP neurotoxicity to be manifested because, of course, it is converted into MPP^+ by the glial cell.

12

Biochemical Approaches to Neurotoxicology *In Vitro*: Attempts to Develop a Test System for Chemically Induced Axonopathy

E. WALUM*, L. ODLAND*, L. ROMERT†,
G. EKBLAD-SEKUND*, M. NILSSON,*
C.J. CALLEMAN,‡ E. BERGMARK‡
AND L.G. COSTA‡

*Unit of Neurochemistry and Neurotoxicology and †Department of Genetic and Cellular Toxicology, Stockholm University S-106 91 Stockholm, Sweden. ‡Department of Environmental Health, SC-34 University of Washington, Seattle, WA 98195, USA

Introduction

The synapse can be said to be the functional unit of the nervous system. All functions responsible for signal transmission, modulation and transduction are found at the synapse. These functions include synthesis and release of transmitters, regulators and modulators, their combination with receptors and their inactivation. Receptor–receptor, receptor–ion channel and receptor–transport mechanism interactions in the pre- and

IN VITRO METHODS IN TOXICOLOGY
ISBN 0-12-388175-7

post-synapse, as well as in surrounding glial elements, contribute to the modulation of signals. Second messengers (cyclic nucleotides, calcium ions and inositol phosphates) transduce the signal into cellular responses. Consequently, detection of alterations in synaptic properties should be ideal for the identification of neurotoxic compounds. However, this might not always be the case. The vast number of possible parameters for a test system based on specific neurochemical assays will make the system too extensive to be operational in the practical test situation. This problem can possibly be dealt with by the application of stepwise or hierarchical procedures (Atterwill, 1989; Pichon, 1990; Walum *et al.*, 1990a). Furthermore, our knowledge of the functional reality of the synapse is limited. The complexity of the brain is accentuated by the fact that each synapse does not function independently, but as part of a neuronal network in which neurons are activated as assemblies (Palm, 1990). An alteration in a certain neurochemical property may thus cause a functional disturbance or may be compensated for. Therefore, neurotoxicological studies on a very sophisticated level become ineffective for risk identification.

Often more general biochemical studies are better suited for the detection of neurotoxic effects and the assessment of health risks. We know that a number of basal functions of the nerve and glial cell must be maintained, otherwise severe signs of neurotoxicity will occur. The neuronal cells may share these functions with most other cells in the body, but owing to the special requirements of the neuron, impairment of these functions first becomes critical in the nervous system. Among these functions are oxidative phosphorylation, protein synthesis, calcium homoeostasis, intracellular transport and turnover of cytoskeletal elements. An example to illustrate this point: we found that, among 20 chemicals, the most neurotoxic ones were the 10 inhibiting respiration in a neuroblastoma cell line (Varnbo *et al.*, 1985). The ability of the nervous system to transform chemicals into more active metabolites or to deactivate them represents a special issue with respect to general biochemical properties.

Distal Axonopathy

Axonopathy, the degeneration of axons, is a most common sign of neurotoxicity. Several chemicals are known to cause different types of axonopathies, e.g. acrylamide, carbon disulphide, *n*-hexane, tri-*o*-cresyl phosphate (distal) and ββ-iminodipropionitrile (proximal). Distal axonopathy, a state where degeneration starts in the most distal part of the axon and proceeds proximally, may be caused by insufficient supply of essential material to the far end of the axon. This could be due to either impaired axonal transport or inhibited metabolism in the nerve cell body. Newly synthesized proteins, e.g. enzymes, plasma membrane proteins or structural elements in vesicles and mitochondria, are actively transported along the axon down a gradient. Abnormalities in the synthesis, transport, turnover or deposition of those molecules could shift the gradient downwards. Consequently, the amount of transported material would reach a critical level at a point proximal to the nerve terminal. This will result in a degeneration distal to the critical point (McLean, 1984).

According to Cavanagh (1988), the most important mechanisms for the development of distal axonopathies are energy deprivation (arsenic, thallium, misonidazole, metronidazole, nitrofurantoin) defects in anti-oxidant availability (isoniacid, acrylamide) and defects in cytoskeletal functions (vincristine, carbon disulphide, 2,5-hexanedione). Since axonopathy is a common toxic response in the nervous system and since it results in a serious impairment of neuronal functions, it is important to develop test procedures that are able to identify chemicals that may induce axonopathy.

Acrylamide

The acrylamide monomer produces central-peripheral distal axonopathy in experimental animals and man. Nerve terminal deformation, distal axonal swelling and retrograde axonal disintegration are some of the morphological characteristics of acrylamide-induced axonopathy. We have found that these signs of the neurotoxic disease can be reproduced in a cultured model of mouse neuroblastoma N1E115 cells (Walum and Peterson, 1984).

Axonal degeneration is considered to be due to an effect on the neuron itself (see above) and not secondary to demyelination, compromise of glial cell functions or impairment of vascular integrity. In several publications (Sterman and Sheppard, 1983; Jones and Cavanagh, 1984; Sterman, 1984), it has been suggested that the first signs of acrylamide intoxication are to be found in the nerve cell body. These authors reported that acrylamide causes an increase in mitochondrial size and number in neurons of exposed animals. We have previously found that acrylamide causes a marked stimulation of the oxygen consumption and in the uptake of 2-deoxy-D-glucose in cultures of mouse neuroblastoma N1E115 cells (Nyberg and Walum, 1984). Furthermore, acrylamide causes a twofold increase in the carbon dioxide production in N1E115 cells when glucose or pyruvate is used as substrate (Walum et al., 1987), whereas lactate production remains unchanged (Nyberg et al., 1991). Obviously, the inhibition of the glycolytic enzyme glyceraldehyd-3-phosphate dehydrogenase reported earlier (Sabri and Spencer, 1980; Nyberg and Walum, 1984) does not prevent a rise in glycolytic activity in the cell body. It can, however, not be excluded that this enzyme, in an inhibited state, could become rate-limiting in distal parts of the axon. It is not known whether the stimulation of energy metabolism is related to the immediate action of acrylamide or represents a later stage of compensation. Jones and Cavanagh (1984) have suggested that an increased energy demand in nerve cells, as a result of acrylamide intoxication, could be secondary to an abnormal influx of calcium ions. This theory is consistent with our findings that increased oxygen consumption after exposure to acrylamide is correlated to an elevation of the basal level of intracellular free Ca^{2+} in N1E115 cells (Walum and Ekblad-Sekund, unpublished observations).

Despite a large number of studies on the toxicity of acrylamide, little is known about its metabolism, and direct structural evidence for putative active metabolites is missing. In vivo, acrylamide appears to be detoxified through conjugation with glutathione (Miller et al., 1982). Acrylamide has also been shown to react with glutathione in vitro (Hashimoto and Aldridge, 1970). Several reports in the literature have also provided circumstantial evidence that acrylamide does undergo oxidative metabolism mediated by the cytochrome P-450 system, and Hashimoto et al. (1988) have suggested glycidamide to be a hypothetical epoxide metabolite of acrylamide. Since then, Calleman et al. (1990) have presented results strongly indicating that acrylamide is indeed metabolized by cytochrome P-450 to form glycidamide.

N1E115 Cells as Models in a Test System for Distal Axonopathy

Acrylamide is a highly reactive compound and can therefore be expected to bind to a number of sites in the nerve cell. For instance by forming derivatives with biologically important functional groups on macromolecules, acrylamide may cause a multitude of biochemical lesions. Thus, it can be assumed that acrylamide-induced axonopathy arises from a complex combination of mechanisms. Nevertheless, acrylamide is water-soluble and freely diffuses through membranes and therefore it should be possible to study its effects on a cellular level in clonal cell lines. This assumption presupposes, however, that it is acrylamide itself, that is responsible for the neurotoxic effects, and not one or several of its metabolites. Furthermore, the biochemical properties with which acrylamide interferes *in vivo* must be expressed in a representative manner in the cultured cells. It appears that the mouse neuroblastoma cell line C1300, clone N1E115, may serve as a model for mechanistic studies concerning the neurotoxic action of acrylamide. These cells have been shown to attain a high degree of neuronal maturation with respect to morphology (Seeds *et al.*, 1970), electrophysiology (Spector, 1981) and biochemistry (Kimi, 1981). These data combine to suggest that N1E115 cells may be a suitable biological model to be used in a test system for prediction of chemically induced axonopathy.

Further Biochemical Studies in N1E115 Cells

It is known that a close relationship exists between glutathione depletion, lipid peroxidation, increased intracellular levels of Ca^{2+} and cellular disintegration in some cell systems (for a review see Walum *et al.*, 1990b). Furthermore, it has been suggested that acrylamide causes an increase in cytosolic Ca^{2+} in nerve cells (Jones and Cavanagh, 1984; Walum *et al.*, 1987): Acrylamide is also known to react with glutathione *in vivo* and *in vitro* (Cavanagh, 1988). We therefore investigated if a connection could be demonstrated between neurite degeneration in N1E115 cells and alterations in the levels of glutathione, lipid peroxides and Ca^{2+}. To be of significance for the mechanism behind distal axonopathy, such a relationship should be present at doses of acrylamide causing no signs of general cytotoxicity. Therefore we reduced the incubation time from 14 days, as used in the experiments described above, to 3 days. At a concentration of 0.25 mM acrylamide, neurite degeneration was visible, at 1.0 mM it was obvious and at 2.5 mM almost all cells were stripped of their processes. These morphological changes were accompanied by a concentration-dependent decrease in the rate of protein synthesis (Fig. 12.1) However, none of the concentrations affected cell survival, as judged by the total protein content in the cultures (Fig. 12.2). From these observations we concluded that this exposure procedure caused selective degeneration of neurites.

In N1E115 cells exposed to 1.0 mM acrylamide for 3 days, no increase in intracellular free Ca^{2+} could be observed (control: 86 ± 10 nM; exposed: 67 ± 13nM) nor was there any change in the respiratory activity (control: 69 ± 7 nl O_2/min per culture; exposed: 83 ± 5 nl O_2/min per culture). When considering the previous results from the 14-day exposure together with these from the 3-day exposure, one may conclude that there does exist a relationship between the increase in free Ca^{2+} and in

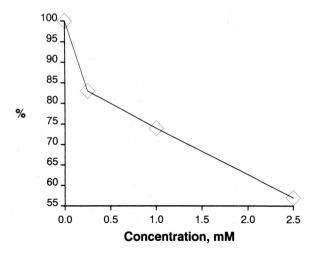

Fig. 12.1 Effects of acrylamide on the rate of protein synthesis in mouse neuroblastoma N1E115 cultures. Cells were plated in plastic tissue culture dishes at a density of 6700 cells/cm^2. Seven days later the growth medium was changed to one containing 0, 0.25, 1.0 or 2.5 mM acrylamide and incubation continued for another 3 days. The cultures were then washed, incubated in a phosphate-buffered balanced salt solution containing 0.5 μCi tritiated leucine/ml for 2 h, washed and extracted 2 × 15 min with 10% trichloroacetic acid (TCA). Rate of protein synthesis was calculated according to: (total protein (mg) × TCA-insoluble radioactivity (c.p.m.))/TCA-extractable radioactivity (c.p.m.). Values are expressed as percentage of control (no acrylamide exposure), and each value represents the mean of three duplicate independent experiments.

respiratory activity (cf. Denton and McCormac, 1990), but that these changes are secondary and not directly related to neurite degeneration.

As can be seen from Fig. 12.3, acrylamide caused a concentration-dependent decrease in the level of glutathione in the N1E115 cells. The glutathione S-transferase activity was found to be somewhat decreased at 1.0 mM acrylamide (control: 32 ± 5 nmol/min per mg of protein; exposed: 23 ± 5 nmol/min per mg of protein), whereas 2.5 mM increased the activity considerably (exposed: 90 ± 21 nmol/min per mg of protein). These findings are in general agreement with previous observations *in vivo* and *in vitro* (Hashimoto and Aldridge, 1970; Edwards, 1975; Srivastava *et al.*, 1984; Hashimoto *et al.*, 1988). The reduction in glutathione levels was not accompanied by any increase in lipid peroxidation (Fig. 12.4). Thus, there seems to be no obvious connection between neurite degeneration and alterations in the levels of glutathione, lipid peroxides or Ca^{2+} in N1E115 cells. However, acrylamide exerts similar effects in N1E115 cells, with respect to glutathione/glutathione S-transferase, as it

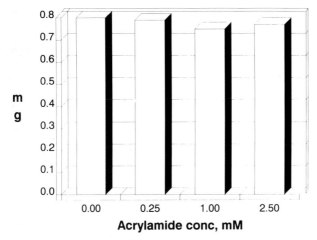

Fig. 12.2 Total protein content in mouse neuroblastoma N1E115 cultures exposed to 0, 0.25, 1.0 and 2.5 mм acrylamide. Cultures were prepared and exposed as described in Fig.12.1. Protein determinations were made using bovine serum albumin as standard. Values are expressed as mg of protein/dish, and each value represents the mean of three duplicate independent experiments.

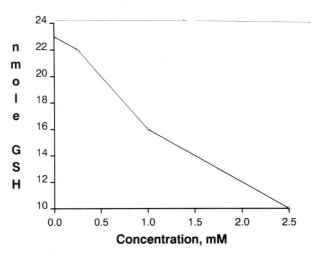

Fig. 12.3 Glutathione levels in mouse neuroblastoma N1E115 cultures exposed to 0, 0.25, 1.0 and 2.5 mм acrylamide. Cultures were prepared and exposed as described in Fig.12.1. Glutathione was determined using high-pressure liquid chromatography and values are expressed as nmol of glutathione/mg of protein. Each value represents the mean of four independent determinations.

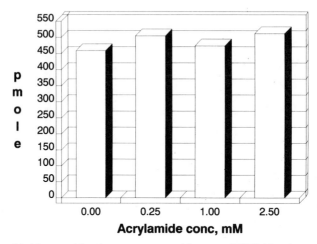

Fig. 12.4 Lipid peroxides in mouse neuroblastoma N1E115 cultures exposed to 0, 0.25, 1.0 and 2.5 mM acrylamide. Cultures were prepared and exposed as described in Fig.12.1. The level of lipid hydroperoxides in the cultures was estimated as the amount of malondialdehyde (MDA). Values are expressed as pmol MDA/mg of protein. Each value represents the mean of five independent experiments.

does in animals. This further strengthens the idea that N1E115 cells could be useful in an *in vitro* test system for axonopathies.

Specificity of Neurite Degeneration in N1E115 Cells

The general cytotoxic effect of acrylamide was compared with that of methylene-bis-acrylamide and glycidamide using a lipid staining method (Walum and Flint, 1990) to detect changes in growth and survival. Methylene-bis-acrylamide is a structural analogue of acrylamide and is often used as a control substance in studies of acrylamide-induced distal axonopathy, since it produces no signs of neurotoxicity in the brain. Little is known about the toxicity of glycidamide and we found it therefore interesting to include it in the comparison. Figure 12.5 shows that the general cytotoxicity of glycidamide was very similar to that of acrylamide. Also in animals, glycidamide and acrylamide produce similar toxic effects (Hashimoto *et al.*, 1988). Methylene-bis-acrylamide was found to have higher cytotoxicity than the other two compounds tested. We have previously shown that methylene-bis-acrylamide is more cytotoxic than acrylamide in primary cultures of rat embryo midbrain (Walum and Flint, 1990). On the basis of the concentration–effect curves in Fig. 12.5, three

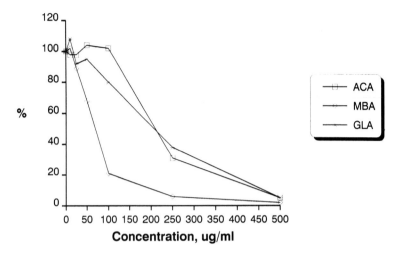

Fig. 12.5 Cytotoxicity of acrylamide (□), methylene-bis-acrylamide (◇) and glycidamide (×) in mouse neuroblastoma NB41A3 cells. Cells were plated in 96-well plates at a density of 10000 cells/cm². Two days later the growth medium was removed and the test substances were added with new medium. After another 48 h the cells were washed, fixed in glutaraldehyde, stained with Neutral Red, eluted with acid alcohol and the absorbance read at 540 nm. Results are expressed as absorbance in percentage of control (no exposure). Each value represents the means of six determinations.

concentrations of the test compounds were chosen. These concentrations all produced minimal effects: 25, 50 and 100 μg/ml for acrylamide and glycidamide and 7.5, 15 and 30 μg/ml for methylene-bis-acrylamide. At these concentrations, the effects of the three compounds on the morphology of highly differentiated N1E115 cells (Fig. 12.6a) were investigated. In agreement with previous observations (Walum and Peterson, 1984), we found that acrylamide drastically reduced the number of neurites without affecting the overall appearance of the cell bodies (Fig. 12.6b). Glycidamide and methylene-bis-acrylamide did not produce this effect (Fig. 12.6c and d). Calleman *et al.* (1990) have reported that glycidamide appears to be less potent in producing neurotoxicity than acrylamide, as judged by the performance of rats on a rotarod apparatus.

Conclusions

From the results presented here we conclude:

1) Mouse neuroblastoma cells N1E115 are suitable biological models for studying acrylamide-induced distal axonopathy.

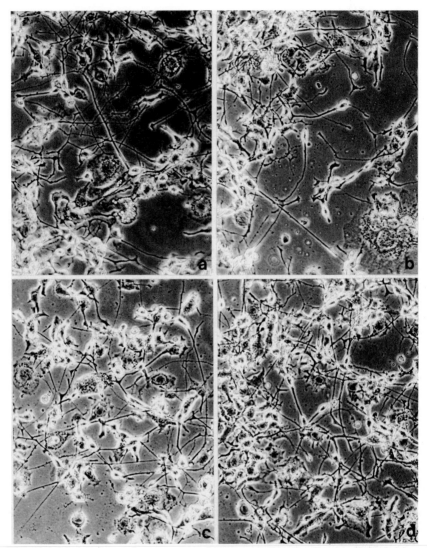

Fig. 12.6 Morphology of mouse neuroblastoma N1E115 cells, unexposed (a) or exposed to 50 μg of acrylamide/ml (b), 15 μg of methylene-bis-acrylamide/ml (c) or 50 μg of glycidamide/ml (d). Cultures were prepared and exposed as described in Fig.12.1. Photographs of living cells have been taken in a Leitz inverted microscope. Enlargement: 174 ×.

2) No obvious or direct relationship exists between the acrylamide induced neurite degeneration in N1E115 cells and alterations in respiration or changes in the levels of intracellular free Ca^{2+} or lipid peroxides. However, a reduced level of glutathione and the induction of glutathione *S*-transferase, might be of toxicological significance.

3) An *in vitro* test system based on N1E115 cells could utilize the difference in concentration–effect curves, for general cytotoxicity and neurite degeneration, i.e. differential nerve cell toxicity, to identify potentially axonopathy-inducing chemicals.

4) Glycidamide does not, according to the idea of differential nerve cell toxicity, produce distal axonopathy at concentrations comparable with those at which acrylamide is active.

Acknowledgements

This study was supported by the Swedish Work Environment Foundation, the National Board for Laboratory Animals, the National Swedish Environmental Protection Board, Draco AB, Sweden, the Swedish Cancer Society, the Swedish Tobacco Company, NIEHS and the Department of Environmental Health, University of Washington. We thank Mrs Inger Varnbo and Ms Homa Hasanvan for their excellent technical assistance.

References

Atterwill, C.K. (1989). *ATLA* **16**, 221–230.
Calleman, C.J., Bergmark, E. and Costa, L.G. (1990). *Chem. Res. Toxicol.* **3**, 406–412.
Cavanagh, J.B. (1988). *In* "Recent Advances in Nervous System Toxicology" (C.L. Galli, L. Manzo and P.S. Spencer, eds), pp. 23–42. Plenum Press, New York.
Denton, R.M. and McCormac, J.G. (1990). *Annu. Rev. Physiol.* **52**, 451–466.
Edwards, P.M. (1975). *Biochem. Pharmacol.* **24**, 1277–1282.
Hashimoto, K. and Aldridge, W.N. (1970). *Biochem. Pharmacol.* **19**, 2591–2604.
Hashimoto, K., Hayashi, M., Tanii, H. and Sakamoto, J. (1988). *J. UOEH* **10**, (suppl.), 209–218.
Jones, H.B. and Cavanagh, J.B. (1984). *Neuropathol. Appl. Neurobiol.* **10**, 101–121.
Kimi, Y. (1981). *In* "Excitable Cells in Tissue Culture" (P.G. Nelson and M. Lieberman, eds), pp. 170–245. Plenum Press, New York.
McLean, G. (1984). *TIPS* **5**, 243–246.
Miller, M.J., Carter, D.E. and Sipes, I.G. (1982). *Toxicol. Appl. Pharmacol.* **63**, 36–44.
Nyberg, E. and Walum, E. (1984). *ATLA* **11**, 194–203.
Nyberg, E., Ekblad-Sekund, G. and Walum, E. (1991). *ATLA* **19**, 199–203.
Palm, G. (1990). *Concepts Neurosci.* **1**, 133–147.

Pichon, Y. (1990). Abstract 50, Sixth International Workshop on *In Vitro* Toxicology, October 1–6, Seillac, France.

Sabri, M.J. and Spencer, P.S. (1980). *In* "Experimental and Clinical Neurotoxicity" (P.S. Spencer and H.H. Schaumburg, eds), pp. 206–219. Williams & Wilkins, Baltimore.

Seeds, N.W., Gilman, A.G., Amano, T. and Nirenberg, M. (1970). *Proc. Natl. Acad. Sci. U.S.A.* **66**, 160–167.

Spector, I. (1981). *In* "Excitable Cells in Tissue Culture" (P.G. Nelson and M. Lieberman, eds), pp. 247–277. Plenum Press, New York.

Srivastava, S.P., Das, M., Mukhtar, H., Malhotra, O.P. and Seth, P.K. (1984). *Bull. Environ. Contam. Toxicol.* **32**, 166–170.

Sterman, A.B. (1984). *Neuropathol. Appl. Neurobiol.* **10**, 221–234.

Sterman, A.B. and Sheppard, R.C. (1983). *Neurobehav. Toxicol. Teratol.* **5**, 151–159.

Varnbo, I., Peterson, A. and Walum, E. (1985). *Xenobiotica* **15**, 129–138.

Walum, E. and Flint, O.P. (1990). *Acta Physiol. Scand.* **140**, suppl. 592, 61–72.

Walum, E. and Peterson, A (1984). *ATLA* **12**, 33–41.

Walum, E., Ekblad-Sekund, G., Nyberg, E. and Gustafsson, L. (1987). In "Model Systems in Neurotoxicology: Alternatives to Animal Testing" (A. Shahar and A.M. Goldberg, eds), pp. 121–136. Alan R. Liss Inc., New York.

Walum, E., Hansson, E. and Harvey, A. (1990a). *ATLA* **18**, 153–179.

Walum, E., Stenberg, K. and Jenssen, D. (1990b). *In* "Understanding Cell Toxicology: Principles and Practice", p. 206. Ellis Horwood, London.

Discussion

H. Baron

First, does Dr Walum feel reasonably comfortable that a mouse neuroblastoma cell line can predict peripheral neuropathy in humans due to drugs?

Secondly, how well equipped does he think his model is to deal with other mechanisms of peripheral neurotoxicity, such as alterations in axonal flow and cytoskeletal proteins, etc.?

E. Walum

I can draw conclusions only about acrylamide because, with the exception of the last little study I reported, we have worked only with acrylamide. Acrylamide produces exactly the same effects in man and in animals, so there we can be confident. I suggested that a model based on our ideas must be validated or evaluated. I have no specific idea about the reliability of such a system in a general sense. However, the performance of these cells as models in general neurobiology and neurochemistry leads to a certain amount of confidence in the possibility of using the cells. They possess most of the neurochemical processes and reactions. If we take a compound like 2,5-hexanedione, for which the mechanism and its cross-linking on neurofilaments are known, these cells have a very normal expression on neurofilaments. I cannot be sure, but I think it will work for other compounds too.

M. Adolphe
Is the cell line cultivated in serum-free medium?

E. Walum
No.

M. Adolphe
Is serum added?

E. Walum
Yes.

M. Adolphe
It has been said that a neuroblastoma cell line is able to differentiate better if the serum is suppressed. In these conditions, this cell line can produce neurotransmitters and so on, and the differentiation is better.

E. Walum
That is absolutely true. In our initial studies with 14-day exposure, the cells were not in serum-free medium but in a reduced concentration, 0.5% instead of 14%, for the reasons outlined by Dr Adolphe. When we became doubtful about our results and started to change the dosing regime, the presence of serum was found not to influence the degeneration – the fixed point of our studies was to maintain what seems to be a model of the degeneration *in vivo*. We tried to maintain that, and if some serum was present it did not interfere with it.

X. Pouradier Duteil
It has been clearly shown that the presence of serum in medium in toxicity studies has a detoxifying effect on many molecules. How is it possible to prevent that effect when culturing cells?

E. Walum
We did not prevent it in this study. To a certain extent the dose is not controlled because the active concentration at the cell is not known. A reactive molecule such as acrylamide will be partially bound to serum proteins. The good thing about a cell culture is that things can be controlled, and to make proper use of a cell culture the serum should be

taken out because that is an uncertainty factor. On the other hand, plenty of serum is present in the body. We can argue to and for about what to do. In the type of cytotoxicity test that I showed we do both: we use a defined medium which is almost protein-free (it is serum-free) and compare the results to ordinary serum. In one respect, this gives valuable information that is needed to extrapolate to the *in vivo* situation. One of the parameters in toxicokinetics, of course, is the binding of a compound to proteins in the serum.

J. Boyer
One of the earliest signs of cell injury is often a change in the permeability of the membrane to ions. Did Dr Walum look to see whether the sodium pump was increased as a possible explanation for the increased oxygen consumption? Could it be due to an increase in sodium permeability?

E. Walum
We measured the intracellular level of calcium. The A2 receptor was activated to open up the current-dependent calcium channels. In the first type of experiments there was a tremendous increase in the calcium influx, but that also disappeared in the second type of experiments that were performed.

P. Laduron
What is the concentration of acrylamide in tissue *in vivo* to produce neurotoxicity? I assume it is not a millimolar concentration.

E. Walum
The first concentration that we used was based on what is found *in vivo*. There is a fairly steady level of about 25 µg/ml (equal to 0.35 mM) of acrylamide in the blood. At that level, there is severe hind limb paralysis in the rat within 14 days.

G. Moonen
In that particular neuroblastoma cell line, is neurogenesis spontaneous or does it have to be induced?

E. Walum
In the last picture I showed it was spontaneous. Serum can be reduced or many different compounds added to stress the cells into switching on certain genes to increase the differentiation. I think that is a slightly dangerous situation when studying neurotoxicology because if, say, dibutyrlcyclic-AMP is added, it will have membrane effects. We were

pleased to find that we do not have to stress the cells, but when they reach, not confluency (because these cells will not be confluent), but a certain density they will spontaneously differentiate beautifully.

13

Neuron and Glia Interrelationships in Developmental Neurotoxicology *In Vitro*

A. VERNADAKIS, S. KENTROTI, C. BRODIE,
N. SAKELLARIDIS, D. MANGOURA
and D. DAVIES

*Departments of Psychiatry and Pharmacology, University of
Colorado School of Medicine, Denver, CO 80262, USA*

Introduction

Numerous studies have confirmed that CNS drugs given to the pregnant organism exert variable degrees of neurotoxicity to the foetus (for review see Vernadakis and Parker, 1980; Rodier, 1990). It has been generally accepted that the effects of drugs on the developing central nervous system are dependent on the stage of brain maturation at the time the drug is administered. Thus, frequently drugs that are relatively safe in the adult organism exhibit severe neurotoxicity in the developing organism. However, despite considerable research using a variety of animal models, the mechanisms of developmental neurotoxicity remain to be understood. The lack of understanding of neural toxicity partially rests on the fact that the brain is very complex, consisting of cells which reach maturation

IN VITRO METHODS IN TOXICOLOGY
ISBN 0-12-388175-7

at different stages during development and that their interactions play a vital role not only for brain growth but for brain homoeostasis throughout the lifespan. The brain consists of neurons, neuroglia and a variety of connective tissue cells, (endothelial cells, fibroblasts, mesenchymal cells) and it is the interactions among these cell types and with their microenvironment which maintain normal brain homoeostasis (Fig. 13.1).

Embryonic morphogenesis depends on the aggregation and organization of individual cells and cell groups into characteristic multicellular patterns which give rise to distinct tissues and organs. Considerable evidence (not to be reviewed here) has established that the complex organization of the nervous system depends on cell–cell recognition or cellular affinities. Failure of the mechanisms of cell recognition prevents cells from becoming organized correctly and may lead to defective morphogenesis in the affected parts of the nervous system. Cell recognition affinities involve not only those between identical cells, but also between different cells that cooperate developmentally, such as the contacts between glia and neurons, between neurons and muscle cells and among different kinds of neurons. Extensive evidence derived from *in vitro* studies has established

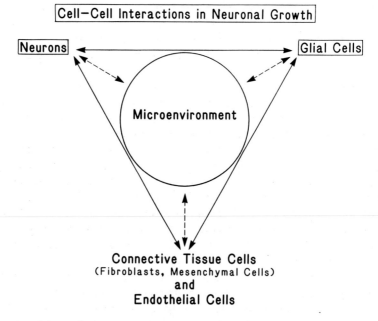

Fig. 13.1 Schematic representation of cell–cell interactions in the central nervous system tissue (from Vernadakis and Sakellaridis, 1985).

the role of neuron–glia interrelationships (for review see Vernadakis, 1988).

Neural culture systems have been useful tools to investigate cell growth and differentiation and also epigenetic factors, including xenobiotics, which influence neuronal plasticity and neuron–glial interactions. In this chapter we will present studies from our laboratory which have focused on understanding the cellular neurotoxicity of two xenobiotics, opioids and ethanol, on neuronal and glial cell growth and differentiation during early neuroembryogenesis.

Neuronal Cultures as a Model System

We have studied extensively neuronal growth patterns in dissociated monolayer cultures derived from 3-day-old whole chick embryo (E3WE) or 6- and 8-day-old chick embryo cerebral hemispheres (E6CH or E8CH) (Vernadakis *et al.*, 1986; Mangoura *et al.*, 1988a,b; Mangoura and Vernadakis, 1988; Mangoura *et al.*, 1990). We use the dissociation method originally described by Booher and Sensenbrenner (1972) which we have modified according to the chick embryonic age from which the tissue derives. For cultures derived from embryonic day 3, embryos are dissociated by sieving through a 48 μm (pore diameter) nylon mesh. The outside of the mesh is stroked with a glass rod, releasing the cells into the culture medium, Dulbecco's Modified Eagle's Medium (DMEM) plus 10% fetal calf serum (FCS). Cells are counted and accordingly plated into Petri dishes of various sizes, depending on whether the cultures are to be used for immunocytochemistry (chamber/slides) or biochemistry (dishes 60 or 100 mm). For cultures derived from embryonic day 6 or 8, whole brain or cerebral hemispheres (we use whole brains instead of cerebral hemispheres when we need to obtain a maximum number of tyrosine hydroxylase neurons) are removed from 6-day-old chick embryos, cleaned of adhering meningeal membranes and mechanically dissociated through a 48 μm nylon mesh in DMEM plus 10% FCS at a plating density of one pair of cerebral hemispheres per 60 mm Petri dish. Culture dishes and chambers are coated with 30 000-70 000 M_r poly-L-lysine (Sigma). All cultures are incubated at 37°C in an atmosphere of 5% CO_2 and 95% air, saturated with water. Cultures are changed at day 4 for the first time and every third day thereafter. For cultures grown in chemically defined medium, we use the medium described by Aizenman *et al.* (1986).

The E3WE culture system consists primarily of neuroblasts and is a very suitable model to study such development-regulating processes as adhesion and neuronal differentiation. In E3WE cultures on poly-L-lysine, the neuronal primary growth patterns are aggregation with neuritic fasciculation. The presence of growth cones with microspikes and very few flat cells is also noted (Vernadakis *et al.*, 1986; Mangoura *et al.*, 1988a,b). In E6CH or E8CH cultures (Fig . 13.2), single, isolated neurons attach quickly on the poly-L-lysine substrata and tend to aggregate or form neuronal networks. Completely formed aggregates with radiating neuritic outgrowth – single processes of fascicles – are first seen at day 3 in culture and although the outgrowth zones overlap, the aggregates are distinctly confined from each other. Fasciculation takes over later. Neurons in E6CH cultures are of various sizes and shapes, round oval or pyramidal and exhibit long thin processes (Mangoura and Vernadakis, 1988; Mangoura *et al.*, 1988a).

We have detected biochemically choline acetyltransferase (ChAT) activity as early as embryonic day 3 *in ovo* (Mangoura *et al.*, 1988b; Kentroti and Vernadakis, 1990a). In E3WE cultures, ChAT activity shows a continuous sharp rise reaching a peak between 5 and 7 days in culture. When cells are dissociated from 6-day-old chick embryo, activity is detectable from day 2 in culture. It increases progressively up to day 6 in culture and rises sharply up to day 15 when ChAT activity is six times greater than at 2 days in culture. In contrast, when cells are dissociated from 8-day-old chick embryo cerebral hemispheres, ChAT activity is present but at low levels up to day 9; then it slowly but progressively increases up to day 15 (Mangoura *et al.*, 1988b). ChAT-like immunoreactivity is expressed by day 6 in E3WE cultures (Fig. 13.3). In E6CH or E8CH cultures (Figs 13.4 and 13.5), neurons are stained first at day 3 in culture, and, besides perikarya and proximal processes, some fine processes are also positively stained.

We have also characterized the expression of GABAergic neurons (GABA is γ-aminobutyric acid) in culture both biochemically and immunocytochemically (Mangoura and Vernadakis, 1988). Neurons exhibiting GABA-like immunoreactivity are present as early as 4–6 days in culture (Figs 13.6, 13.7 and 13.8). The developmental profile of glutamic acid decarboxylase (GAD) activity, a biochemical marker used for GABAergic neurons, has also been examined in cultures derived from 3-day-old whole chick embryos or 6- or 8-day-old chick embryo cerebral hemispheres (Mangoura and Vernadakis, 1988).

In early studies we examined the development of the adrenergic system in the chick embryo and in the chicken up to 3 years. We reported high-affinity uptake of [³H]noradrenaline (10^{-7}M) inhibited by cocaine and reserpine to be present in 15-day-old chick embryo cerebral hemispheres (Kellogg *et al.*, 1971; Vernadakis, 1973, 1974). In a later study, we found [³H]noradrenaline uptake (5×10^{-9}M) in 6-day-old chick embryo brain

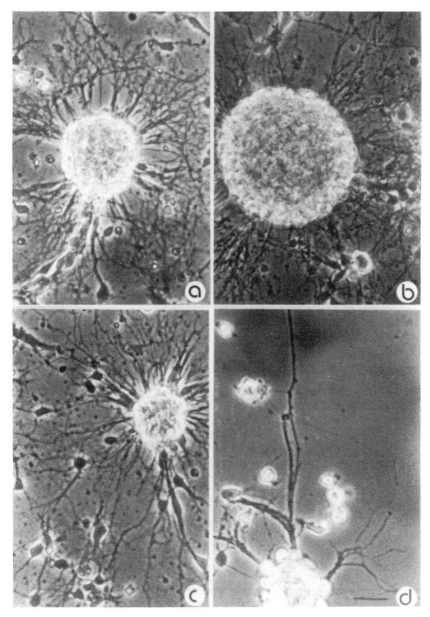

Fig. 13.2 Neuron-enriched cultures derived from 6-day-old chick embryo cerebral hemispheres. Cultures were grown in DMEM plus 10% FCS on poly-L-lysine-coated dishes. (a) 3 days in culture; (b) 7 days in culture; (c) 11 days in culture; (d) 30 days in culture. Neuronal aggregates with rich neurite outgrowth and single cell networks.

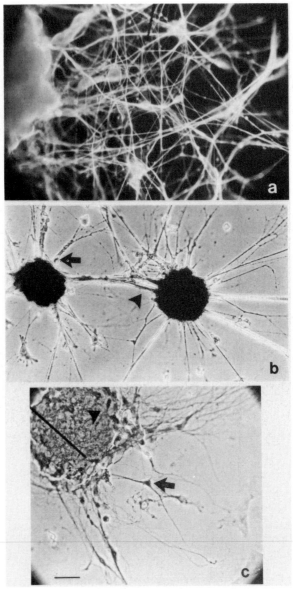

Fig. 13.3 Primary neuronal cultures derived from 3-day-old whole chick embryo and plated on poly-L-lysine. (a) Cultures stained with anti-neurofilament antibody and fluorescein-conjugated IgG at day 10 in culture (C10). (b) Cultures stained for acetylcholinesterase (AChE) at C10: neuronal somata in aggregates are heavily stained as well as somata of isolated neurons extending from aggregates (arrow) and also bundles (arrowhead). (c) PAP method was used to stain neurons for ChAT, at C6. The substrate solution contained $NiCl_2$, thus the colour of the final product is purple. Triangular (arrow) or bipolar neurons and their main processes are stained. Positive perikarya can also be noted in the main bulk of the aggregate (arrowhead). Bar: a = 13.82, b = 33.85, c = 19.74 μm (from Mangoura *et al.*, 1988b).

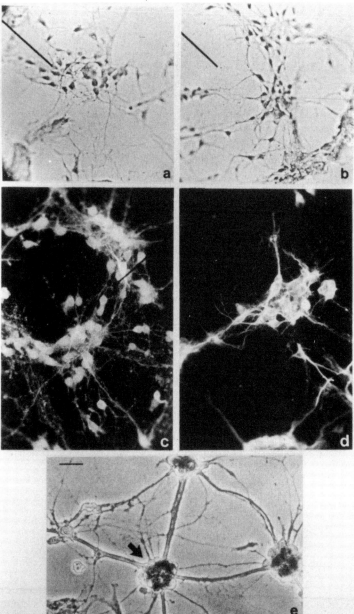

Fig. 13.4 Primary neuronal cultures derived from 6-day-old chick embryo cerebral hemispheres. (a,b) Cultures stained for ChAT with the peroxidase–antiperoxidase (PAP) method at day 3 in culture 9C3. Perikarya and the proximal parts of their processes of small-sized neurons are distinctly stained, although fine processes are also decorated with the antibody. The majority of neurons exhibited positive staining. (c) Cultures stained for neurofilament and fluorescein-conjugated IgG, at C7. (d) Cultures stained for tubulin and rhodamine-conjugated IgG, at C7 also. (e) Cultures stained for AChE, at C14. Note heavily stained, weakly stained and unstained neurons within the aggregates (arrow). Bar: a = 12.9, b = 13.63, c = 14.03, e = 30.04 μm (from Mangoura *et al.*, 1988b).

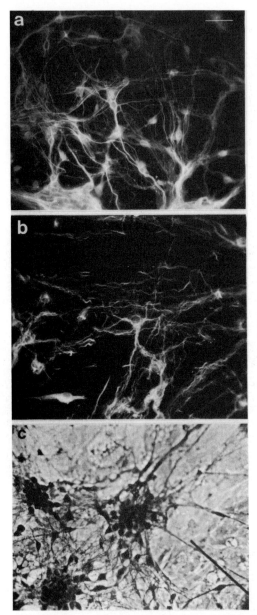

Fig. 13.5 Primary neuronal cultures derived from 8-day-old chick embryo cerebral hemispheres. (a) Neuronal networks positively stained for neurofilament (immunofluorescence) at day 5 in culture (C5). (b) Cultures stained for tubulin and rhodamine conjugated IgG, at C7. The fine structure of neurons of varying shapes and sizes is revealed. (c) Cultures stained for ChAT with the PAP method, at C13. The majority of neurons, forming an aggregate or lying independently, exhibited ChAT-like immunoreactivity. The neuronal somata were stained heavier than the processes, although varying staining density can be noted. Bar: a = 13.83, b = 14.36, c = 13.8 μm (from Mangoura *et al.*, 1988b).

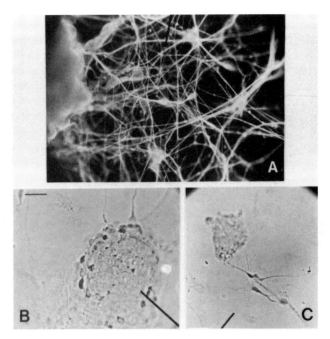

Fig. 13.6 Phase-contrast photomicrographs of primary neuronal cultures derived from 3-day-old whole chick embryo and plated on poly-L-lysine. (A) Indirect immunofluorescence of neurofilament and IgG-fluroescein isothiocyanate (FITC), at 10 days in culture (C10). (B,C) PAP staining for GABA, at C6. The common pattern consisted of bipolar and, rarely, pyramidal neurons in the periphery of the aggregate (B) or extending from it. Both somata and processes were stained (bar: A = 14.61, B = 14.68, C = 17.35 μm) (from Mangoura and Vernadakis, 1988).

and also in cultures derived from 8-day-old chick embryo whole brain (Hoffman and Vernadakis, 1979). We have also reported that tyrosine hydroxylase (TH), the rate-limiting enzyme of catecholamine synthesis, is present in chick embryo brain (Arnold and Verandakis, 1979) and in cultures derived from 8-day-old chick embryo cerebral hemispheres (Arnold and Vernadakis, 1979; Vernadakis and Kentroti, 1989). More recently, using a more sensitive method developed by Masserano *et al.* (1983), we were able to detect TH activity as early as 4 days of embryonic age (Fig. 13.9) (Kentroti and Vernadakis, 1989).

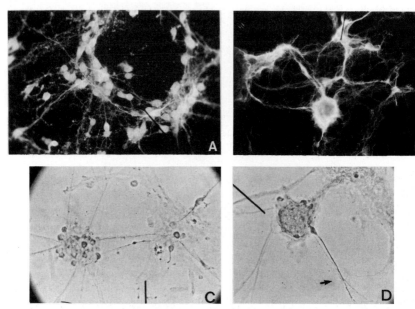

Fig. 13.7 Primary neuronal cultures derived from 6-day-old chick embryo cerebral hemispheres (E6CH), plated on poly-L-lysine and stained for: (A) neurofilament and IgG-FITC, at C7 (same as in Fig. 13.3c); (B) tubulin and IgG–rhodamine at C7; (C) GABA with PAP technique, at C4; the most common features were bipolar neurons with long processes interconnecting aggregates; (D, arrow see text) as (C) at C15; the percentage and morphology of stained neurons was similar between the ages of C4 and C15 (bar: A = 13.1, B = 12.1, C = 10.71, D = 13.13 μm) (from Mangoura and Vernadakis, 1988).

Effects of Xenobiotics on Neuronal Phenotypes

Opiates

It has been established that infants born to mothers addicted to opiates exhibit physiological dependence on narcotics and develop symptoms of withdrawal at birth (for review see Vernadakis and Parker, 1980). We have used the chick embryo as an animal model to investigate some of the neurotoxicity of narcotic drugs during embryogenesis.

Numerous pharmacological studies have demonstrated that the effects of opiates *in vitro* and *in vivo* reflect their interaction with specific neuronal receptors (see references in Gibson and Vernadakis, 1982). Therefore, the ontological development of opiate receptors is relevant to our understanding of the effect of opiates during early development. In our early studies

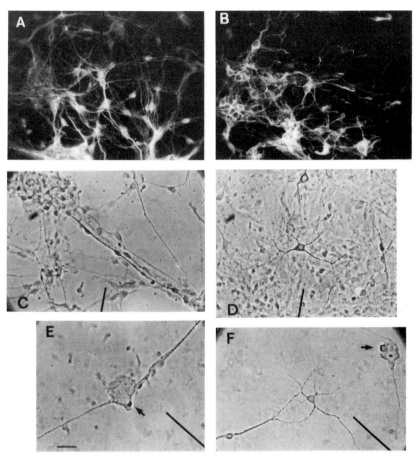

Fig. 13.8 Primary neuronal cultures derived from 8-day-old chick embryo cerebral hemispheres (E8CH), plated on poly-L-lysine (A,B,C,E,F) or collagen (D) and stained for: (A) neurofilament and IgG-FITC, at C5 (same as in Fig. 13.4a); (B) tubulin and IgG–rhodamine; (C) GABA with PAP technique, at C4; most of the neurons expressing GABA-like immunoreactivity were bipolar and extending between aggregates; (D–F) GABA; by C13 large, multipolar neurons were laying on top of flat cells grown on collagen substratum (D) or directly on poly-L-lysine substratum, as in (F); bipolar neurons were also present (D–F) in the periphery of an aggregate (E,F, arrows) or in connection with another neuron (F). Bar: A = 14.13, B = 13.85, C = 13.76, E = 14.3, F = 12.04 μm) (from Mangoura and Vernadakis, 1988).

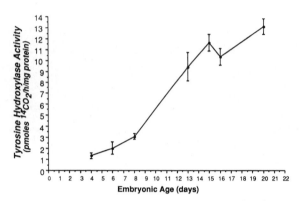

Fig. 13.9 Developmental profile of tyrosine hydroxylase (TH) activity in the chick embryonic brain. TH activity was first detectable at 4 days of embryonic age. Values shown are means ± S.E.M. of five to nine samples (from Kentroti and Vernadakis, 1989).

(Gibson and Vernadakis, 1983) we reported that stereospecific [³H]etorphine binding is detected in the chick embryonic brain as early as day 4 of incubation, a time when there is active neuronal proliferation and differentiation. We were therefore one of the first groups to propose that interaction of the opiate receptors with endogenous opioid substances, also reported to be present early in the chick embryo, may be critical during early neuroembryogenesis. In this chapter we will present a brief account of our view that endogenous opioids may play a role in early neuro-embryogenesis.

Neuroregulatory role of endogenous opioids

Localization of opioids in neuronal populations during neuroembryogenesis (see references in Vernadakis *et al.*, 1990) supports the view that these peptides may be involved in early neuronal differentiation. Using neuron-enriched cultures derived from 6-day-old chick embryonic brain, we have detected enkephalin-like immunoreactivity in several neurons (Vernadakis *et al.*, 1990) (Figs 13.10, 13.11 and 13.12). In addition, in an earlier study we have found [³H]etorphine specific binding sites in similar neuron-enriched cultures (Fig. 13.13) (Gibson and Vernadakis, 1983). Convincing evidence has been reported that opioids and neurotransmitter substances coexist in several neuronal populations: enkephalin in cholinergic neurons (Chang *et al.*, 1987; Altschuler *et al.*, 1984) enkephalin and serotonin-like substance (Kanagawa *et al.*, 1986), opioid peptides and co-transmitters in noradrenergic sympathetic nerves (Wilson *et al.*, 1980). We have, therefore, initiated

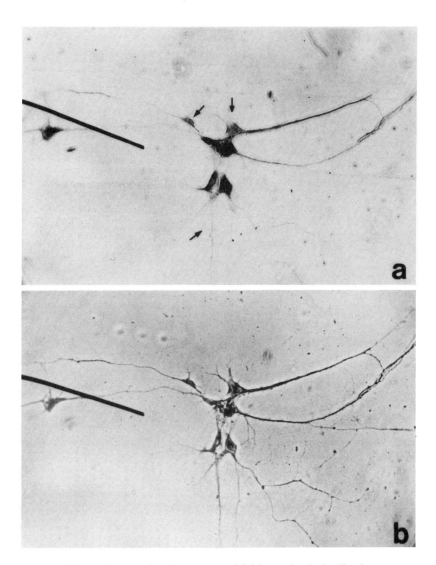

Fig. 13.10 Photomicrographs of neurons exhibiting enkephalin-like immunoreactivity (Enk-LI) (PAP method). Neuronal cultures were derived from 6-day-old chick embryo cerebral hemispheres and grown in chemically defined medium. At day 7 in culture, cells on coverslips were fixed with 4% paraformaldehyde and 1% glutaraldehyde and processed for immunocytochemistry. Primary antibody was Met-enkephalin (rabbit origin, Amersham) at 1/3000 in PBS. (a) Light microscopy, lens 40×. Arrows indicate non-stained neuronal somata and processes. (b) Phase contrast 2, lens 40×; both stained and non-stained neurons (from Vernadakis *et al.*, 1990).

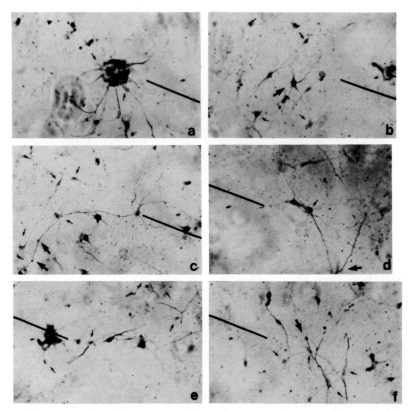

Fig. 13.11 Neuronal cultures as in Fig. 13.10. (a) Neuronal aggregate exhibiting Enk-LI on neuronal somata. Light arrows indicate some of the non-stained neurons (a–f); (b) heavy arrow indicates neuron positive for enkephalin, with Enk-LI being polarized on the right side of the neuron; (c,d,e) heavy arrows indicate Enk-LI on varicosities of processes; (f) heavy arrow indicates growth cone exhibiting Enk-LI (from Vernadakis *et al.*, 1990).

studies to examine the possible interrelationship among enkephalin-like substances and cholinergic and catecholaminergic neurons (Vernadakis and Kentroti, 1990). Neuron-enriched cultures were prepared from 3-day-old whole chick (E3WE) which, as we have reported, consists of proliferating neuroblasts (Vernadakis *et al.*, 1986; Mangoura *et al.*, 1988a). Cultures were grown in serum-free chemically defined medium (CDM) described by Aizenman *et al.* (1986), and bacitracin (50 μg/ml) was added to inhibit cell peptidase activity and preserve levels of test substances in cultures. All test substances were added at day C0 when cultures were changed to CDM,

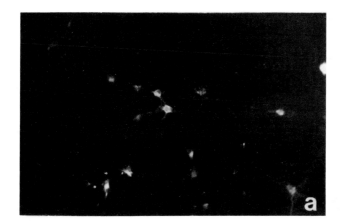

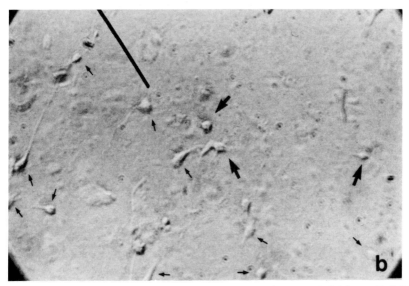

Fig. 13.12 Fig.   13.12 Photomicrographs   of   neurons   exhibiting   Enk-LI
(immunofluorescence). Neuronal cultures as in Fig. 13.10. (a) At day 3 in culture,
cells on coverslips were stained with enkephalin antibody and IgG conjugated
with fluorescein; (b) phase-contrast photomicrograph of exactly the same field as
in (a). Heavy arrows indicate neurons exhibiting Enk-LI shown on (a). Light
arrows indicate non-stained neurons (print of (b) is magnified ×2) (from
Vernadakis *et al.*, 1990).

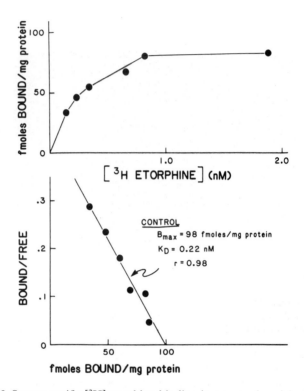

Fig. 13.13 Stereospecific [³H]etorphine binding in neuronal-enriched cell cultures dissociated from 6.5-day-old chick embryo whole brain and plated on polylysine-coated dishes; 9 days in culture. Upper half: Saturation curve. Lower half: Scatchard analysis (from Gibson and Vernadakis, 1983).

3 h after plating. In one experimental series normal rabbit serum 1:1000 dilution was used instead of [Met]enkephalin antiserum (anti-Met) as control. At day 4 (C4), cultures were boosted with the appropriate treatment substance and were harvested at day 6 (C6). Again, we used ChAT activity as a cholinergic marker and TH activity as a catecholaminergic marker. The preliminary findings we report here (Table 13.1) show that [Met]enkephalin (Met), an endogenous opioid, had no effect on ChAT activity but markedly increased TH activity and that this increase was blocked by naloxone, an opiate receptor antagonist. Therefore, this effect of Met is receptor mediated. These findings are preliminary and cannot be fully evaluated or explained. However, the present paradigm is that in E3WE cultures with proliferating neurons, the increase in TH activity, interpreted to reflect increased expression of catecholaminergic neurons, could be due to either (a) an

Table 13.1

Neurotransmitter enzyme activity in neuron-enriched cultures exposed to opioid
agonists and antagonists

Treatment	Enzyme activity	
	Choline acetyl transferase (nmol acetylcholine formed/h per mg of protein)	Tyrosine hydroxylase (pmol CO_2 formed/h per mg of protein)
Control	1.195 ± 0.09	6.24 ± 0.68
Naloxone		
10^{-11}M	1.46 ± 0.07	6.74 ± 0.78
10^{-9}M	1.253 ± 0.06	6.97 ± 0.81
10^{-7}M	0.58 ± 0.03	9.77 ± 1.27
[Leu]Enkephalin		
10^{-7}M	1.40 ± 0.14	9.36 ± 0.74
[Met]Enkephalin		
10^{-7}M	1.18 ± 0.09	10.66 ± 1.49
[Leu]Enk. + naloxone	1.46 ± 0.05	10.48 ± 0.85
[Met]Enk. + naloxone	0.97 ± 0.06	5.98 ± 1.46
[Met]Enkephalin in antiserum (1:1000)	2.60 ± 0.68	12.63 ± 1.60
Normal rabbit serum (1:1000)	1.01 ± 0.07	

Neuron-enriched cultures were prepared from 3-day-old whole embryos and grown in
chemically defined serum-free medium. Cultures were treated with the various substances
at culture day 1 and 4 and harvested at day 6. Values are means ± S.E.M. of two to three
experiments, each experiment consisting of four to six cultures (from Vernadakis and
Kentroti, 1990).

increase in neuronal proliferation and/or survival of catecholaminergic
neurons in culture and/or (b) an effect of this opioid substance on the
expression of TH mRNA and thus to enhanced phenotypic expression.
(These questions can be partially answered by comparing [^{3}H]thymidine
uptake into DNA in cultured neurons in the presence of absence of opioid
treatment.) Of interest is the observation that in the cultures treated with
anti-Met, both ChAT and TH activities were increased (Table 13.1). We
interpret this enhancement of enzyme activity as suggesting that opioids and
neurotransmitters are colocalized. Moreover, cultures grown in the presence
of anti-Met in the medium exhibited markedly different growth patterns
from those in CDM alone: well-organized neuronal aggregates with long
neurites and fasciculations (Fig. 13.14). This is not due to the serum factors
present in anti-Met since when we replaced anti-Met with normal rabbit
serum of the same dilution, the growth pattern was similar to CDM

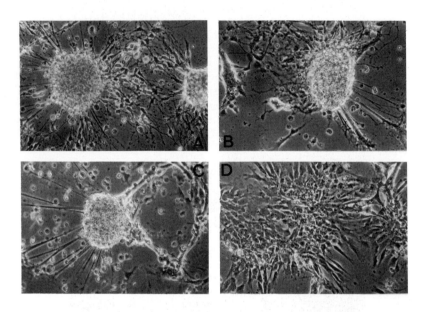

Fig. 13.14 Photomicrographs of neuron-enriched cultures derived from 3-day-old whole chick embryo. Cultures were grown in chemically defined medium (CDM) supplemented with [Met]enkephalin antiserum (anti-Met), at a final dilution of 1:1000, (A,B); or with naloxone, 10^{-7}M final concentration (C); or CDM alone (D). Test substances were administered at culture day 1 and cultures were photographed at culture day 4. ×589. (From Vernadakis and Kentroti, 1990.)

controls. On the basis of these preliminary findings, we have proposed that opioids may have several functions in modulating neuronal growth: colocalized opioids and neurotransmitters may have one function and opioids released into the microenvironment may have another function.

Cholinotoxic effects of narcotics on neuron-enriched cultures

In an earlier study we examined the effects of morphine and methadone on the growth of cholinergic neurons in neuron-enriched cultures derived from 6-day-old chick embryo cerebral hemispheres using ChAT activity as a marker (Sakellaridis *et al.*, 1986). We found that ChAT activity was reduced by both morphine and methadone and that to our surprise, methadone was more potent than morphine (10^{-6}M vs 10^{-5}M respectively). In contrast, morphine exerted more severe morphological changes than methadone. Specifically, we observed an increased number of flat cells, assumed to be immature glial cells, and neuronal aggregates surrounded

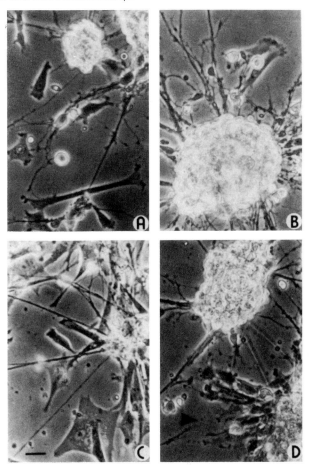

Fig. 13.15 Phase-contrast micrographs of neuron-enriched cultures derived from a 6-day-old chick embryo whole brain and plated on a poly-L-lysine-coated surface (8 days in culture). (A) Treated with 10^{-6}M morphine from day 4 to day 6; (B) treated with 10^{-6}M morphine from C6 to C8; (C) treated with 10^{-5}M morphine from C4 to C6; (D) treated with 10^{-5}M morphine from C6 to C8. Arrowhead indicates the side of an aggregate that consists of glial cells and bears no neurite outgrowth. Bar = 26 µm. (From Sakellaridis *et al.*, 1986.)

by flat cells, and devoid of the thick bundles of neuritic processes that normally characterize neuron-enriched cultures (Fig. 13.15). We suggest that morphine exerts a general neurotoxic effect, whereas methadone may affect some specific cholinergic function. Of importance is the comparison of the effects of these exogenous opiates, morphine and methadone, with those of endogenous opioids, the enkephalins, in neuron-enriched cultures reported above. It appears from our observations that exogenous opiates have cholinotoxic effects, whereas endogenous opioids, such as [Met]enkephalin, stimulate cholinergic neuronal expression as assessed by increased ChAT activity (Table 13.1). Whether exogenous opiates interfere with the actions of endogenous opioids (i.e. down-regulation of receptors) can only at present be speculated.

Ethanol Neurotoxicity

The effects of prenatal exposure to ethanol have been abundantly documented both in humans and animals. CNS dysfunction is the most frequent and adverse outcome of *in utero* alcohol exposure. In addition to mental retardation, hyperactivity, irritability and fine-motor dysfunction, morphological alterations in the brain of children characterized as fetal alcohol syndrome (FAS) have been observed. These alterations include microcephaly, leptomeningeal and neuroglial heterotopias, aberrant neuronal and glial cell maturation, retarded maturation of the cerebral hemispheres and agenesis of the corpus callosum and the anterior commissure (Vernadakis and Parker, 1980).

The neuroteratogenicity of alcohol has also been observed in laboratory animals exposed to alcohol *in utero* and morphological changes include: microcephaly, reduction in the size of the cerebral hemispheres, agenesis of the corpus callosum and olfactory bulbs, dysplasia of the hypophysis (Diaz and Samson, 1980) and cerebellum (Nathaniel *et al.*, 1986; Stolterburg-Didinger and Spohr, 1983), decreased number of hippocampal pyramidal cells (Davies and Smith, 1980) and of dendritic spines in the hippocampus (Abel *et al.*, 1983) and cerebral cortex (Reyes *et al.*, 1983; Stoltenberg-Didinger and Spohr, 1983). *In vitro* studies have also confirmed the effects of ethanol on neuronal maturation (Blakley and Fedoroff, 1985; Dow and Riopelle, 1985) and also glial growth and differentiation (Davies and Vernadakis, 1984, 1986; Kennedy and Mukerji, 1986a,b), as we will discuss below.

Neurotoxicity of ethanol in chick embryos: neuropeptide beneficial influence

In a recent series of studies we have been investigating the neurotoxic effects of ethanol using two experimental paradigms: the chick embryo and neural cultures derived from chick embryonic brain. In this chapter we will present some of our data derived from the *in vitro* culture studies. However, in order for these *in vitro* findings to be more meaningful in relation to *in vivo* ethanol neurotoxicity, we will briefly state some of our *in vivo* results using the chick embryo (Kentroti and Vernadakis, 1990b; Brodie and Vernadakis, 1990; Brodie *et al.*, 1990). We found that ehtanol (5–20 mg/50 μl per day) administered to embryos *in ovo* from day 1 to day 3 of development produced a dose-dependent decrease in ChAT activity, while TH activity exhibited a dose-dependent increase when embryos were sacrificed at embryonic day 8. The optimal neurotoxic dose of ethanol following this paradigm was 15 mg/day and the LD_{50} was 17.5 mg/day for 3 days. Subsequently, embryos were administered ethanol (15 mg) either alone or concomitantly with growth hormone-releasing hormone (GHRH; 100 ng/50 μl per day). Previous studies from this laboratory have demonstrated both potent cholinotrophic and catecholaminotrophic effects for this neuropeptide (Kentroti and Vernadakis, 1989, 1990a). Co-administration of ethanol and GHRH resulted in a significant increase in ChAT activity as compared with both saline- and ethanol-treated controls when examined at day 8 of embryonic growth. No additive effect was observed in TH activity following co-administration of ethanol and GHRH. The findings from this study are interpreted to mean that GHRH represents a potent secondary signal to undifferentiated neuroblasts which may lead to a restoration of the cholinergic neuronal population following neurotoxic insult by ethanol.

The apparent differential sensitivity of cholinergic versus catecholaminergic neuroblasts may reflect the earlier ontogeny of cholinergic neuronal elements. As we and others have previously shown, the cholinergic phenotype arises earlier in embryogenesis than the catecholaminergic phenotype (Kentroti and Vernadakis, 1989, 1990; Mangoura *et al.*, 1988b), leaving cholinergic neuroblasts more susceptible to the neurotoxic effects of ethanol at this stage of development. Alternatively, presumptive cholinergic neuroblasts may be arrested at an intermediate stage of differentiation. The absence of or decrease in cholinotropic signals allows neuroblasts to respond to alternative signals. This shift in response results in an increase in the expression of the catecholaminergic phenotype.

In view of the well-known neurotrophic effects of nerve growth factor (NGF) and epidermal growth factor (EGF) we were also interested in examining the possibility that NGF may prevent the cholinotoxic effects of ethanol (Brodie *et al.*, 1991). We found that concomitant administration of either NGF or EGF with ethanol eliminated the decrease in ChAT activity produced by ethanol. Moreover, NGF or EGF treatment at embryonic days 4–7 to embryos treated with ethanol at embryonic days 1–3 raised ChAT activity to control levels. Thus these growth factors can reverse the ethanol-induced cholinergic insult and restore the cholinergic neuronal population to normal.

Neuronotoxic effects of ethanol in neuron-enriched cultures

As discussed earlier, neuron culture has provided a useful tool to examine both the mechanisms of actions and the neurotoxic effects of xenobiotics at the neuronal level. Neuron-enriched cultures were prepared from 3-day-old whole chick embryos which, as we stated earlier and have also reported (Vernadakis *et al.*, 1986; Mangoura *et al.*, 1988a), consist primarily of proliferating neuroblasts. Cultures were grown in the presence of ethanol (50 mM) in the medium beginning on day 2 until day 10, the end of the experimental period. As in other studies, we used the biochemical activity of choline acetyltransferase and of glutamic acid decarboxylase as markers for cholinergic and GABAergic neurons respectively. We found that ethanol exposure markedly affected these two neuronal populations in culture (Kentroti and Vernadakis, 1991a). However, on the basis of these findings we cannot conclude whether ethanol affected phenotypic expression, i.e. enzyme activity *per se*, and/or neuronal survival in culture. The results discussed in the following section provide some evidence that ethanol exerts marked neuronotoxic effects (Table. 13.2) (Kentroti and Vernadakis, 1991b). Moreover, it appears

Table 13.2

Neuronotoxic effects of ethanol treatment in neuron-enriched cultures derived from 3-day-old chick embryo

Days in culture	Treat-ment	Protein (μg/μl)	ChAT activity (nmol Ach formed/h per culture)	ChAT activity (nmol Ach formed/h per mg of protein)	GAD activity (nmol CO_2/h per mg protein)
3	Control	8.52 ± 0.73	5.42 ± 0.46	0.64 ± 0.03	0.68 ± 0.08
6	Control	8.00 ± 0.18	4.96 ± 0.17	0.83 ± 0.10	0.76 ± 0.01
	50 mM EtOH	6.32 ± 0.94	4.91 ± 0.15	0.62 ± 0.02	0.45 ± 0.05§§
10	Control	5.30 ± 0.54	4.61 ± 0.12	0.90 ± 0.08	1.04 ± 0.17
	50 mM EtOH	5.95 ± 0.22	3.16 ± 0.38**	0.43 ± 0.01§§	0.37 ± 0.04§
13	Control	5.65 ± 0.41	5.79 ± 0.33	1.06 ± 0.12	0.42 ± 0.07
	50 mM EtOH	7.08 ± 0.39*	5.35 ± 0.07	0.76 ± 0.03§§	0.56 ± 0.07

Choline acetyltransferase (ChAT), glutamate decarboxylase (GAD) activity and protein content were determined in neuronal cultures derived from 3-day-old whole chick embryo and grown in DMEM + 10%FCS. On culture day 3, medium was replaced with DMEM + 10%FCS with or without ethanol (50 mM) in which they were grown for the remainder of the culture period. Cells were harvested on culture day 3, 6, 10 and 13.
$*P < 0.05$; $**P < 0.02$; $§P < 0.01$; and $§§P < 0.002$ versus controls within the same group.

from these preliminary findings that GABAergic neurons are more sensitive than cholinergic neurons, showing sensitivity to ethanol by day 6 in culture. This differential sensitivity may be partially explained by the state of differentiation of these neurons at day 3, the time of first ethanol exposure. We have reported in other studies that GABAergic neurons are detected biochemically by 3 days in the chick embryonic brain (Mangoura and Vernadakis, 1988), whereas cholinergic neurons are at a high activity by day 2 in the chick embryonic brain (Vernadakis *et al.*, 1986; Kentroti and Vernadakis, 1990). These findings are supportive evidence that differentiating neuroblasts are most sensitive to the ethanol insult.

Neuronal survival in culture is affected by in ovo treatment with ethanol

In order to determine whether ethanol interferes with neuronal survival, the following paradigm was adopted (Kentroti and Vernadakis, 1991b). Neuronal survival was examined in (E3WE) neuron-enriched cultures prepared from embryos treated with ethanol (10 mg/50µl) *in ovo*, on embryonic days 1 and 2. Control cultures were prepared from embryos receiving the vehicle (saline). Neuronal survival was assessed by incorporation of [^{3}H]thymidine into DNA. Pretreatment with ethanol resulted in a significant decrease in neuronal survival *in vitro*. Only 33% of neurons derived from ethanol-treated embryos survived from C2 to C6 as compared with 100% in cultures derived from saline-treated embryos. Again, we were interested in examining the effects of neuropeptides in rescuing cells following neuronal insult by ethanol. Thus, cultures derived from ethanol-treated embryos were grown in the presence of somatotrophin (somatostatin release inhibitory factor, SRIF) in the medium. SRIF partially reversed the effects of ethanol pretreatment. By 13 days in culture, 46% of labelled cells had survived in cultures from saline-treated embryos as compared with 19% in cultures from ethanol-treated embryos and 24% in cultures derived from ethanol-treated embryos and grown in SRIF (Fig. 13.16). These preliminary data suggest that ethanol may enhance the natural neuronal death which occurs in culture. The fact that SRIF attenuated the effects of ethanol suggests the possibility that SRIF provides neurotrophic signals to reverse the deficits produced by ethanol on neuroblastic elements. The naturally occurring phenomenon of cell death during early neuroembryogenesis has received considerable attention and several functions have been put forward including morphogenesis, the regulation of target innervation, removal of cells that make projection or synaptic errors, removal of transient synaptic targets, and the removal

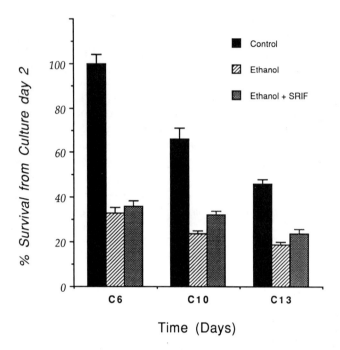

Fig. 13.16 Cell survival in neuron-enriched cultures derived from 3-day-old whole chick embryos treated on embryonic days 1 and 2 with saline (control) or ethanol (10 mg/day). One group of cultures derived from ethanol-treated embryos received 50 nM somatostatin (SRIF) at culture day 3. All cultures were incubated for 24 h with 0.1 μCi of [³H]thymidine at culture day 2 and harvested at culture days 6, 10 and 13 for assay of [³H]thymidine incorporation into DNA. Barograms with bracketed lines are means ± s.e.m. of 46 cultures. (Adapted from Kentroti and Vernadakis, 1991b.)

of cells that provide transient guidance cues for axonal pathway formation (Oppenheim *et al.*, 1990). One theory is that the death of neurons that accompanies many of these developmental events may result from loss of trophic support. A classic candidate for the promotion of neuronal survival is NGF. However, recent research by others and also now by us shows that other neurotrophic molecules, such as neuropeptides, can serve as environmental signals to regulate the developmental fate of cells.

Glial Cell Culture Systems

It is not our intent to discuss the large body of literature characterizing glial cells in culture systems. We will focus only on our own studies, in which we use two glial cell enzymes as markers of astrocytes and oligodendrocytes: glutamine synthetase (GS), used as a marker for astrocytes (Norenberg and Martinez-Hernandez, 1979), and 2',3'-cyclic nucleotide 3'-phosphohydrolase (CNP), used as a marker for oligodendrocytes (Poduslo and Norton, 1972; Poduslo, 1975). We have studied the developmental aspects of these two markers both *in vivo* in the chick embryo and in glial-enriched cultures derived from embryonic chick brain (Sakellaridis *et al.*, 1983). Glial-enriched cultures are prepared from 15-day-old chick embryo cerebral hemispheres by dissociation through a nylon mesh of 75 μm. In these cultures we and others (Booher and Sensenbrenner, 1972) have shown that neuronal cells do not survive after 5 days in culture and that by 15 days the cultures consist predominantly of glial cells and about 10% fibroblasts (after removal of meninges). The developmental GS and CNP profiles in the glial-enriched cultures are shown in Figs 13.17 and 13.18. There is a marked rise in astrocytic proliferation during the first few days in culture followed by a plateau.

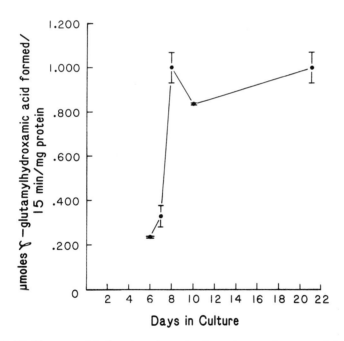

Fig. 13.17 Changes with days in culture in glutamine synthetase activity in glial-enriched cultures dissociated from cerebral hemispheres of 15-day-old chick embryos. Activity is expressed in μmol of γ-glutamylhydroxamic acid formed in 15 min/mg of protein and plotted vs days in culture. Points represent means ± s.e.m. of three to four separate culture dishes. (From Sakellaridis *et al.*, 1983.)

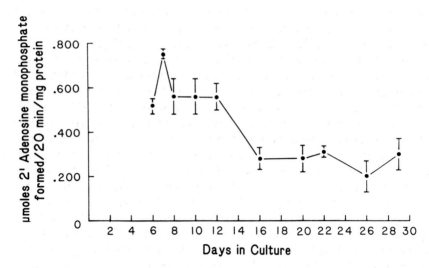

Fig. 13.18 Changes with days in culture in 2′,3′-cyclic nucleotide 3′-phosphohydrolase activity in glial-enriched cultures dissociated from cerebral hemispheres of 15-day-old chick embryos. Activity is expressed in μmol of 2′-adenosine monophosphate formed in 20 min per mg of protein and plotted vs days in culture. Points represent means ± s.e.m. of three to four separate culture dishes. (From Sakellaridis *et al.*, 1983.)

The plateau phase in astrocytes (Fig. 13.17) coincides with a decline in oligodendrocytic expression (Fig. 13.18). We have proposed that the decline in oligodendrocytes may be due to the absence of neuronal input and that the plateau in astrocytic expression may reflect the dependence of astrocytes on interactions with oligodendrocytes, which are declining in culture. Several groups of investigators are focusing their research on understanding those cell–cell interactions (for review, see Vernadakis, 1988).

Gliotoxic Effects of Ethanol

In view of the intimate relationship between neurons and glial cells in maintaining brain homoeostasis, it is important to understand the sensitivity of glial cells to xenobiotics and neurotoxins.

It has been suggested that the neurotoxicity of ethanol may be partially attributed to a perturbation of the glutamate/glutamine system (Clarke *et al.*, 1975). A component of this system is glutamine synthetase, localized in astrocytes. Thus, glial cells have been implicated in the termination of the excitatory activity of glutamic acid by taking up this amino acid and converting it to glutamine (Hertz, 1979). We initiated studies to examine the sensitivity of glial cells to ethanol and their possible role in ethanol-induced neuronal toxicity (Davies and Vernadakis, 1984). Glial-enriched cultures were prepared from 15-day-old chick embryo cerebral hemispheres. As stated earlier, this time period corresponds to rapid glial cell proliferation and differentiation in the chick. On day 6 *in vitro*, a group of cultures was exposed to a range of ethanol doses (0.1–2%, w/v, or 21.7–434 mM) and were compared with untreated controls. After 10 days *in vitro*, control cultures approach confluency and areas of the cultures are densely packed with cells. The cultures are formed of a carpet of epithelioid cells; numerous smaller non-neuronal cells having branched processes appear to be attached to the flat cells, as shown in Fig. 13.19. The flat cells are considered to be astrocytes because of the manner in which the cultures were prepared and the resemblance of these cells to epithelioid cells shown to be GFA-positive. The multibranched cells are considered to be oligodendrocytes in view of their morphology and their position above the flat cells. Phase-microscopic comparisons of cultures on day 10 *in vitro* show that cultures exposed to 0.1% and 0.5% ethanol are morphologically similar to controls (Fig. 13.19b and c). In contrast, cultures treated with 1% or 2% ethanol appear to have sparser cell populations, but no greater incidence of vacuolated or necrotic cells (Fig. 13.19d and e). Especially evident in cultures treated with 2% ethanol are patches of Petri dish floor devoid of cells. The cultures treated with 1% and 2% ethanol contain both flat cells and multibranched cells, similar to controls. Cells resembling reactive astrocytes are depicted in cultures treated with 1% and 2% ethanol, but are not observed with lower concentrations of ethanol or in control cultures. The somata of these astrocytes are hypertrophied, and numerous, thin branching processes radiate from the somata. A characteristic feature is that these cells reside as a single cell within a lacuna bordered by epithelioid cells (Fig. 13.20a, b). The presence of reactive astrocytes in cultures treated with the high doses of ethanol cultures is interpreted to reflect the responsiveness of glial cells to this neurotoxin, a cellular phenomenon observed in several pathological conditions (Duchesne *et al.*, 1981). The reduction in GS activity caused by ethanol (Fig. 13.21) is interpreted to be significant on the basis of the proposal that this enzyme is involved in the detoxification of ammonia in the brain, and glial cells have been implicated in glutamate/glutamine compartmentation (Hertz, 1979). Hertz and colleagues have suggested that glutamate released from neurons is taken up into astrocytes, where it is converted to glutamine by glutamine synthetase. Glutamine released from astrocytes can be taken up into neurons where it is hydrolysed by glutaminase to glutamate. Rosenberg and Aizenman

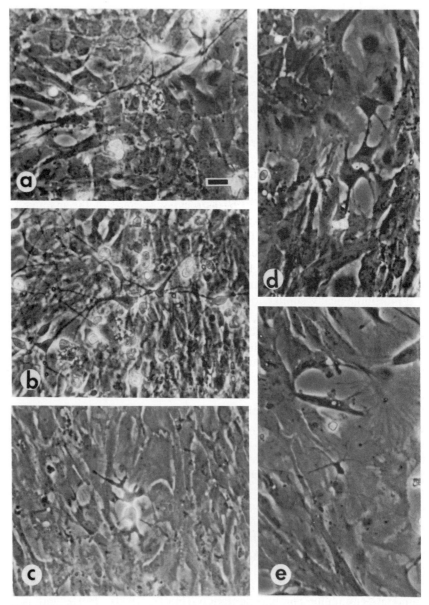

Fig. 13.19 Phase-contact micrographs of glial-enriched cultures derived from 15-day-old chick embryo cerebral hemispheres. Control (a), 0.1% ethanol-treated (b) and 0.5% ethanol-treated (c) cultures consist of densely packed epithelioid cells having smaller somata and numerous branches. Cultures exposed to 1.0% (d) and 2% ethanol (e) contain sparser cell populations. Magnification bar = 25 μm. (From Davies and Vernadakis, 1984.)

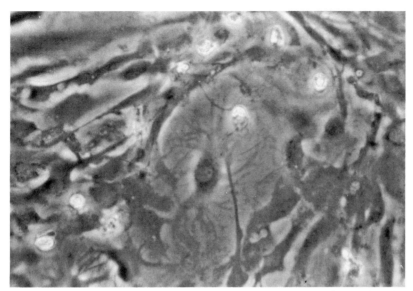

Fig. 13.20 Phase-contrast micrographs of glial-enriched cultures (as in Fig. 13.19) exposed to 2.0% ethanol. Individual cells in a space enclosed by epitheloid cells resemble reactive astrocytes and exhibit enlarged somata extending numerous branching processes. Magnification = 857×. (From Davis and Vernadakis, 1984.)

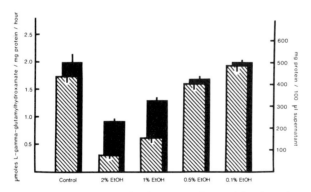

Fig. 13.21 Glutamine synthetase (GS) activity (striped bars) and protein content (solid bars) in control and ethanol-treated cultures. Cultures were treated daily with ethanol, beginning on day 6, and harvested on day 10. GS activities in 1.0% and 2.0% ethanol-treated cultures were significantly lower compared with controls ($P < 0.001$); protein contents of these cultures were also significantly reduced ($P < 0.01$ and $P < 0.001$ respectively). Data represent means ± s.e.m. of five cultures.

(1989) have found a hundredfold increase in vulnerability to glutamate toxicity in astrocyte-poor cultures of rat cerebral cortex. Considering that we have not as yet studied any other enzymes involved in glutamate/glutamine metabolism, we cannot propose a direct effect on GS. Rather, we suggest that astrocytes rich in GS are sensitive to ethanol and thus delayed in their differentiation. Recent studies by Kennedy and Mukerji (1986a,b) have also shown that ethanol markedly reduced GS activity in glial cultures prepared from newborn Swiss-Webster mice cerebral hemispheres. As also discussed earlier, astrocytes play a significant role in neuronal migration and guidance, neurite outgrowth and neuronal phenotypic expression (for review see Vernadakis, 1988). Changes, therefore, in their functional state, growth and differentiation will be manifested as a severe neuronal impact.

General Conclusions

We have presented two pharmacological examples where *in vitro* models can contribute important information concerning the sensitivity and responsiveness of brain cells to xenobiotics. In the case of ethanol neurotoxicity, the *in vitro* findings are very similar to *in vivo* results. Although we do not claim that either the chick embryo or the *in vitro* model simulate the fetal alcohol syndrome, our findings provide evidence that ethanol has both neuronotoxic and gliotoxic effects. Interruption of neuron–glia interrelationships during early neuroembryogenesis will have severe neurological consequences. Finally, for the first time it is reported that growth factors such as neuropeptides may prevent the ethanol insult.

References

Abel, E.L, Jacobson, S. and Sherwin, B.T. (1983). *Neurobehav. Toxicol. Teratol.* **5**, 363–366.

Aizenman, Y., Weichsel, M.E. and de Vellis, J. (1986). *Proc. Natl. Acad. Sci. USA* **83**, 2263–2266.

Altschuler, R.A., Fer, J., Parakkal, M.H., Eckenstein, F. (1984). *J. Histochem. Cytochem.* **8**, 819–843.

Arnold, E.B. and Vernadakis, A. (1979). *Dev. Neurosci.* **2**, 46–50.

Blakley, M.M. and Fedoroff, S. (1985). *Int. J. Dev. Neurosci.* **3**, 69–76.

Booher, G. and Sensenbrenner, M. (1972). *Neurobiology* **2**, 97–105.

Brodie, C. and Vernadakis, A. (1990). *Dev. Brain Res.* **56**, 223–288.

Brodie, C., Kentroti, S. and Vernadakis, A. (1991). *Dev. Brain Res.* in press.

Chang, H.T., Penny, G.R. and Kitai, S.T. (1987). *Brain Res.* **426**, 197–203.

Clarke, D.D., Roman, E.J., Dicker, E. and Tirri, L. (1975). *In* "Metabolic Compartmentation and Neurotransmission" (S. Berl, D.D. Clarke and D. Scheider, eds), pp. 449–460. Plenum Press, New York.

Davies, D.L. and Smith, D.E. (1980). *Neurosci. Lett.* **26**, 49–54.

Davies, D.L. and Vernadakis, A. (1984). *Dev. Brain Res.* **16**, 27–35.

Davies, D. and Vernadakis, A. (1986). *Dev. Brain Res.* **24**, 253–260.

Diaz, J. and Samson, H.H. (1980). *Science* **20**, 751–753.

Dow, K.E. and Riopelle, R.J. (1985). *Science* **228**, 591–593.

Duchesne, P.Y., Gerebtzoff, M.A. and Brotchi, J. (1981). *Anatomy* **19**, 313–316.

Gibson, D.A. and Vernadakis, A. (1982). *Dev. Brain Res.* **4**, 23–29.

Gibson, D.A. and Vernadakis, A. (1983). *Neurochem. Res.* **8**, 1197–1202.

Hertz, L. (1979). *Progr. Neurobiol.* **13**, 277–323.

Hoffman, D. and Vernadakis, A. (1979). *Neurochem. Res.* **4**, 731–746.

Kanagawa, V., Matusyama, T., Wanaka, A., Yonedo, S., Kimura, K., Kamado, T., Steinbasch, H.W.M. and Tohyama, M. (1986). *Brain Res.* **379**, 377–379.

Kellogg, C., Vernadakis, A. and Rutledge, C.O. (1971). *J. Neurochem.* **18**, 1931–1938.

Kennedy, L.A. and Mukerji, S. (1986a). *Neurobehav. Toxicol. Teratol.* **8**, 11–15.

Kennedy, L.A. and Mukerji, S. (1986b) *Neurobehav. Toxicol. Teratol.* **8**, 17–21.

Kentroti, S. and Vernadakis, A. (1989). *Dev. Brain Res.* **49**, 275–280.

Kentroti, S. and Vernadakis, A. (1990a). *Dev. Brain Res.* **512**, 297–303.

Kentroti, S. and Vernadakis, A. (1990b). *Dev. Brain Res.* **56**, 205–210.

Kentroti, S. and Vernadakis, A. (1991a). *J. Neurosci. Res.* **30**, 484–492.

Kentroti, S. and Vernadakis, A. (1991b). *J. Neurosci. Res.* **30**, 641–648.

Mangoura, D. and Vernadakis, A. (1988). *Dev. Brain Res.* **40**, 25–35.

Mangoura, D., Sakellaridis, N. and Vernadakis, A. (1988a). *Int. J. Dev. Neurosci.* **6**, 89–102.

Mangoura, D., Sakellaridis, N. and Vernadakis, A. (1988b). *Dev. Brain Res.* **40**, 37–46.

Mangoura, D., Sakellaridis, N. and Vernadakis, A. (1990). *Dev. Brain Res.* **51**, 95–101.

Masserano, J.M., Takimoto, G.S. and Weiner, N. (1983). *Alcohol Clin. Exp. Res.* **7**, 294–298.

Nathaniel, E.J.H., Nathaniel, D.R., Mahmed, S.A., Nahngbida, L. and Nathaniel, L. (1986). *Exp. Neurol.* **93**, 610–620.

Norenberg, M.D. and Martinez-Hernandez, A. (1979). *Brain Res.* **161**, 303–310.

Oppenheim, R.W., Prevette, D., Tyrell, M. and Homma, S. (1990). *Dev. Biol.* **138**, 104–113.

Podulso, S.E. (1975). *J. Neurochem.* **24**, 647–664.

Poduslo, S.E. and Norton, W.T. (1972). *J. Neurochem.* **19**, 727–736.

Reyes, E., Rirarch, M., Saland, L.C. and Murray, Y.M. (1983). *Neurobehav. Toxicol. Teratol.* **5**, 263–267.

Rodier, P. (1990). *Toxicol. Pathol. ISSN* **18**, 89–95.

Rosenberg, P.A. and Aizenman, E. (1989). *Neurosci. Lett.* **103**, 162–168.

Sakellaridis, N., Bau, D., Mangoura, D. and Vernadakis, A. (1983). *Neurochem. Int.* **5**, 685–689.

Sakellaridis, N., Mangoura, D. and Vernadakis, A. (1986). *Int. J. Dev. Neurosci.* **4**, 293–302.

Stolterburg-Didinger, G. and Spohr, H.L. (1983). *Dev. Brain Res.* **11**, 119–123.

Vernadakis, A. (1973). *Mech. Aging Dev.* **2**, 371–379.
Vernadakis, A. (1974). *In* "Drugs and the Developing Brain" (A. Vernadakis and N. Weiner, eds), pp. 133–148. Plenum Press, New York.
Vernadakis, A. (1988). *Int. Rev. Neurobiol.* **30**, 149–224.
Vernadakis, A. and Kentroti, S. (1990). *J. Neurosci. Res.* **26**, 342–348.
Vernadakis, A. and Parker, K. (1980). In "Pharmacology and Therapeutics" (J.F. Papp, ed.), pp. 593–647. Pergamon Press, Oxford.
Vernadakis, A. and Sakellaridis, N. (1985). *In* "Progress in Neuroendocrinology" (H. Parvez, S. Parvez and D. Gupta eds), vol. 1, pp. 17–44. VNU Science Press, The Netherlands.
Vernadakis, A., Sakellaridis, N. and Mangoura, D. (1986). *J. Neurosci. Res.* **16**, 397–407.
Vernadakis, A., Sakellaridis, N., Geladopoulos, T. and Mangoura, D. (1990). *In* "A Decade of Neuropeptides: Past, Present Future" (G.F. Kook, C. Sandman and F.L. Strand, eds), vol. 579, pp. 109–122. Ann. N.Y. Acad. Sci., New York.
Wilson, S.P., Klein, R.Z., Chang, K.J., Casparis, M.S., Vireros, D.H. and Yang, W.H. (1980). *Nature* **288**, 707–709.

Discussion

C. Atterwill

Has Dr Vernadakis tried to see whether corticosteroids which induce glutamine synthetase also reverse ethanol lesions by bringing the levels of the enzyme back to normal?

A. Vernadakis

No, that has not been done. It is an interesting suggestion which we will investigate. However, it depends upon where the corticosteroids are put in these glial cultures. If they are used at the glioblastic stage, they have their own neurotoxic effect.

H. Baron

How do you explain the observation, at the same time, of the maturation arrest in astrocytes and of the presence of astrocytes reactive to injury, which are very nicely reacting like true astrocytes in producing glial fibrillary acidic protein?

A. Vernadakis

I do not know whether these reactive astrocytes are the same reactive astrocytes as those seen in brain injury, for example, where several studies have been done. This is neuro*toxic* injury. It shows the potential of the astrocytes to rescue the system. I feel strongly that astrocytes are there to protect the neurons from all kinds of problems that are encountered. I consider the reactive astrocyte is a rescuing cell. It is trying to protect the neurons, and therefore it picks up all kinds of toxins or it reacts to them – although in the glioblastic state some of them escape and become reactive, which is puzzling and something we will be investigating to see how often reactive astrocytes are seen.

H. Brun
The action of ethanol and opioid substances on gonadal function is known. What is the action of these drugs on neurons and hypothalamic cells which secrete this hormone?

A. Vernadakis
We have not done hypothalamic cultures. However, Anna Taylor, at UCLA, has done some beautiful work on the effects of opioids on the hypothalamic gonadal system.

I think ethanol is a universal neurotoxin which affects all kinds of systems. I do not know whether anybody has looked at this; probably someone has. I am not familiar with it, and only know about the opioids.

E. Cardiotoxicity

14

Single Heart Cells as Models for Studying Cardiac Toxicology

G. BKAILY

Department of Physiology and Biophysics, Faculty of Medicine, University of Sherbrooke, Sherbrooke, Quebec, Canada J1H 5N4

Introduction

The first report using cultured heart cells was given by Burrows (1912), who concluded that the independent pacemaker activity of single cells was direct confirmation of the myogenic theory of heart muscle. On the basis of studies on cultured heart cells, Lewis (1928) rejected the concept of a branching syncytium in favour of cellular independence. Since then the potential usefulness of freshly isolated or cultured single heart cells as a model for studying cardiac toxicology has been recognized (for review see Sperelakis, 1967, 1978; Schanne and Bkaily, 1981; Bkaily *et al.*, 1984; Jacobson and Piper, 1986; Sperelakis and Bkaily, 1987). The freshly isolated or the freshly cultured single heart cells possess electrical properties and pharmacological receptors virtually identical to those of cells from the original myocardium from which they were derived. However, single cells cultured for more than 3 days may change their electrophysiological properties or revert back to the early embryonic

IN VITRO METHODS IN TOXICOLOGY
ISBN 0-12-388175-7

state. Such reverted ventricular heart cells develop pacemaker potentials which make them a good model for cardiac nodal cells.

The fact that single ventricular cells may be considered as a very small and simple model for the whole heart makes them a highly suitable alternative to animal experimentation for studying direct toxicity of drugs and chemicals in the heart.

The data presented here come mainly from my own laboratory, but the reader is referred to books edited by Lieberman and Sano, and by Atterwill and Steele for results from other laboratories and to review articles by several investigators (Sperelakis, 1978; Schanne and Bkaily, 1981; Farmer *et al.*, 1983; Bkaily *et al.*, 1984; Mitra and Morad, 1985; Jacobson and Piper, 1986). The present chapter is an updated and expanded version of recent articles written by Schanne and Bkaily (1981), Bkaily *et al.* (1984) and Sperelakis and Bkaily (1987).

Advantages of Using Single Heart Cells

Single cells offer several advantages over the intact heart for studies on the myocardial effect of drugs and chemicals. Additional advantages of using single heart cells could be added to those already summarized in Table 14.1. For example, single cells can be obtained from embryonic heart at all stages of development, thus allowing determination of cardiac toxicity of a substance at the foetal heart level. Also, early single foetal heart cells possess pacemaker activity similar to that of nodal cells. Therefore, this preparation is a good model for studying the effect of drugs on pacemaker activity. In addition, single heart cells can be cocultured with nerve cells to study nerve–muscle interaction or cocultured with endothelial cells to study endothelium–heart interaction. Since a high yield of pure single heart cells can be obtained, this preparation constitutes an ideal model for biochemical assays. Finally, the use of single heart cells permits the deployment of state of the art techniques that enable us to determine not only the exact site of action of a substance but may also aid in the design of new drugs that have a high safety ratio. The reader is referred to articles by Sperelakis (1981) and Schanne and Bkaily (1981) which summarize the effects of numerous agents on heart cells. In summary, the use of freshly isolated or freshly cultured single heart cells offers a unique opportunity to use several state of the art techniques to answer many types of questions that cannot be answered using intact cardiac muscle.

Table 14.1

Some advantages of cultured single heart cells for studying cardiac toxicology

1. Low cost and easy to obtain
2. Can be obtained from human biopsy material
3. Large number of pure cardiac cell population for *in vitro* study
4. Denervated and no blood flow
5. Direct effects of substances
6. Direct observation of pacemaker activity
7. Retain functional receptors and electrical properties similar to cells in intact hearts
8. Permit the intracellular injection of substances
9. Excellent for ion flux studies
10. Excellent for molecular biology and biochemical assay
11. Excellent for measuring the whole-cell and single-channel currents
12. Excellent for measuring macroscopic and microscopic variations of $[Ca]_i$, $[Na]_i$, $[pH]_i$ and $[K]_i$ using fluorescence dyes
13. Excellent for spatial intracellular ionic distribution studies using fluorescence imaging technique
14. Allow simultaneous measurement of ionic channels and intracellular ionic concentrations
15. Allow direct observation of cells coupling through a gap junction using fluorescence dye
16. Metabolically active
17. Decrease the number of animals to be used
18. Could be established as a standard cultured cell line
19. Reduce the risk of killing a perfectly valid compound
20. Permit easily the application of a new high technology to biomedical testing
21. Permit comparison of results obtained from animals and man
22. Permit a better testing of genotoxicity of substances
23. Give a good therapeutic ratio that is similar to those obtained *in vivo*
24. Predict the potential toxic effect of drug
25. Permit easily the identification of the target organ of the drug
26. Permit the use of very small amount of a drug
27. Permit the use of high doses and long periods of chronic testing

Some Caveats to Using Single Heart Cells

If single heart cells are to become a valuable tool for studying drug cardiotoxicity, scientists must take into account the caveats that are associated with this preparation. Most of these caveats are not directly related to the isolated single heart cells themselves, but to the measurement techniques and experimental conditions used.

Some of the caveats related to the preparation itself include the following. The use of enzymes during cell separation that may damage the cell membrane and influence the electrical and pharmacological properties of the isolated heart cells. Therefore, the use of single heart cells for cardiotoxicity studies requires the determination of the basic electrical and pharmacological properties of ionic currents and receptor function. Most embryonic single heart cells and the reverted cultured single ventricular heart cells show spontaneous contractions. The fact that the rate of spontaneous activity varies in these cells confuses the interpretation of the effect of substances on pacemaker activity. This problem can be overcome by stimulating the single cells electrically. Also using the whole cell patch clamp technique (Marty and Neher, 1983), one could record the action potential; reaggregated single heart cells also constitute an excellent preparation which can be used to record pacemaking action potentials.

Most of the problems and potential pitfalls associated with single heart cells can be overcome if the following reasonable precautions are taken into account: (1) animals of an appropriate age, (2) mild enzymic dispersion, (3) pure cardiac preparation, (4) correct temperature, (5) freshly isolated or freshly cultured single cells and (6) the right serum and culture medium.

Isolation of Single Heart Cells

Two methods are currently employed either alone or in combination: these are enzymic digestion and mechanical disintegration. The effectiveness of these methods differs: enzymic digestion is widely used but some controversy still exists as to which enzyme causes optimal digestion of extracellular connections while causing minimum damage to the cells.

Embryonic and Newborn Single Heart Cells

Since Burrows (1912) first investigated cultured fragments of embryonic chick heart, many techniques have been developed to isolate single heart cells from different animal species at different ages. Embryonic chick hearts and newborn rat hearts have been widely used because at these stages of development, the single heart cells can be easily dispersed enzymically and cultured. Trypsin, collagenase and hyaluronidase are used at present. The use of trypsin alone at low concentration together with gentle stirring was found less damaging to single embryonic heart cells (DeHaan, 1967; Goshima, 1970; Glick et al., 1974; Gordon and Brice, 1974).

Rapid addition of serum to the medium before centrifugation and after cell isolation inactivates the trypsin (Weiss, 1959; Poste, 1971). For the newborn rat, collagenase-dispersed heart cells seem to be a more valuable model of the intact heart than cells treated with trypsin. However, cell disintegration is usually performed in media containing very low Ca^{2+} concentrations and this can damage the cells. Collagenase is more effective when dispersing cells from adult animals whereas trypsin is more efficient when separating neonatal or mainly embryonic cardiac cells. Moreover, cell damage is almost exclusively assessed by studying ultrastructural changes. These alterations, however, when induced by trypsin treatment seem to be reversible.

It is important that studies on single cells isolated from chick embryos or human foetuses should be conducted after between 1 h and 2 days in culture to avoid collecting of data from cells that have reverted to the early embryonic state.

For cultured chick heart cells, fertilized chicken eggs can be obtained from a local hatchery on a weekly basis and incubated in an egg incubator at 37°C with daily rotation. The eggs are opened when the embryos are between 3 and 20 days old (hatching occurs at 21 days), and the hearts removed. The hearts from approximately 12 embryos are pooled (in chilled Ringer solution) to make one preparation. The hearts are washed free of blood in Ringer solution (5 °C), and the atria dissected and discarded (unless atrial cultures are desired). The ventricles are then minced with small scissors. Cell separation is carried out by stirring (with a magnetic stirring bar) in Ca^{2+}-free, Mg^{2+}-free Ringer solution (37 °C) containing glucose (100 mg%) and 0.05% trypsin.

During the dissociation process, at intervals of 5–15 min, the cloudy cell-containing supernatant is decanted into chilled culture medium (containing normal levels of Ca^{2+} and Mg^{2+}). The combination of low temperature and the presence of serum rapidly inactivates the trypsin, thus minimizing the exposure of the already-freed cells to trypsin. Fresh dissociation solution is added to the undissociated tissue, and the process is repeated from five to seven times. The first one or two harvests are discarded because they contain a high proportion of non-muscle cells, and the subsequent ones are pooled. The cells are washed by mild centrifugation (50–200 g for 5–10 min) into a pellet. Then the supernatant is aspirated or decanted, replaced with fresh culture medium, and the cells are resuspended. Washing is often repeated for a second or third time to remove the dissociating enzymes completely. Embryonic heart cells usually become round immediately after cell separation, but this does not mean that they have been severely damaged, as in the case of the adult heart cells.

The usual composition of the culture medium is 10% or 15% serum (foetal calf or horse), 40% nutrient solution (such as Puck's N-16 or

Medium 199), and 45–50% balanced salt solution (Hank–Ringer). The chemical compositions of the various synthetic media, such as Medium 199, Puck's N-16 NCTC-135, basal medium Eagle (BME), modified Eagle medium (MEM), Dulbecco's modified Eagle medium (DMEM), Hanks Minimum Essential Medium (HMEM), L-15, etc., are usually given in the catalogues of the companies that supply the media. In general, these media contain various amino acids, glucose, vitamins, inorganic salts and a variety of other components. Some media are claimed to promote the growth and well-being of specific types of cells. The type of serum used may be important as well, and it is thought that foetal serum contains a higher concentration of a factor that promotes cell division. Some investigators also add chick embryo extract (CEE), bought commercially or prepared in their own laboratory, to the culture medium to promote cell growth and viability. In order to facilitate the sealing of a patch clamp microelectrode, a low serum concentration (2–5%) is sometimes used to prevent the cells from becoming too thin.

Antibiotics, such as penicillin plus streptomycin (50 units/ml) or gentamicin, may be added to the medium, but if scrupulously sterile procedures are used throughout, antibiotics and fungicides (e.g. fungizone) may be avoided. All the solutions used are sterilized by passing through filters with pore diameters of approximately 0.2 μm. All glassware and dissecting instruments are sterilized by autoclaving; plasticware used for culture vessels is purchased presterilized and wrapped, and all dissections and procedures are carried out under a laminar-flow hood (presterilized with ultraviolet irradiation).

The washed pellet of cells is diluted with sufficient culture medium to give a concentration of approximately 0.5×10^6–1.0×10^6 cells/ml for plating into the culture vessels or for gyrotation. The optimal plating density can be determined by serial dilution and assaying for some selected parameter, e.g. rate of cell proliferation. Some workers pass the cell suspension through a small-pore nylon mesh to disrupt any large multicellular aggregations before plating.

In some case, the dissociation solution is modified to contain elevated levels of K^+ (10–25 mM) and ATP (5 mM), because this modification may facilitate the production of electrically highly differentiated cells (McLean and Sperelakis, 1974). The addition of insulin to the culture medium also appears to promote a state of high electrical differentiation, including high tetrodotoxin (TTX) sensitivity (LeDouarin et al., 1974; Suignard, 1979). A very simple method (Bkaily et al., 1988a,b,c,d) to separate single cells from chick embryo heart preparation consists of using a solution of HMEM (Gibco) containing 0.1% trypsin and 1.8 mM Ca^{2+}.

This solution (without trypsin, with 5% serum) can be used for culturing the cells, and helps protect them against enzyme damage.

To produce monolayer cultures, the cells are plated into the desired type of culture vessels (e.g. modified Carrell flasks with removable lids (Bellco), plastic Petri dishes or plastic Falcon flasks). A glass coverslip can be placed in the culture vessel so that the coverslip with adhering cells can be removed and placed into another chamber for experimentation. A volume of 1–3 ml of cell suspension is added per culture vessel. The cells settle to the bottom of the culture dish over a period of 12–48 h if left undisturbed, and become attached to the substrate. They make contact with one another to form various monolayer patterns, such as loose random networks, strands, rosettes and confluent sheets. Confluent sheets are usually produced when the cells are plated at higher densities. Usually the myocardial cells in suspension contract spontaneously, each with its own independent rhythm. Shortly after the monolayer cells make morphological contact with one another (within 10–50 min), they contract synchronously, indicating that they have formed functional junctions. One or more cells acts as a pacemaker to drive the others. At low plating densities, regions of isolated single cells are often found. Such isolated single cells are suitable for whole-cell voltage clamping. Monolayer cells can be impaled with one or two microelectrodes to examine their electrophysiological properties, or the patch electrode technique can be used (Bkaily et al., 1988a,e; Sperelakis, 1972a; Sperelakis and McLean, 1978a).

Since fibroblasts and endothelioid cells adhere to the substrate much faster than do myocardial cells, if the plated cells are allowed to settle for only 30–90 min and then poured off carefully, many of the fibroblasts will remain stuck to the dish and can thus be discarded. If this procedure of differential adhesion is serially repeated three to six times, a myocardial-enriched fibroblast-depleted culture can thus be produced (Horres et al., 1979). In addition, an inhibitor of fibroblasts can be added to the culture medium. Such "pure" cultures are not necessary for most electrophysiological studies, but could facilitate interpretation of biochemical experiments. But even without such procedures, the percentage of beating myocardial cells in a monolayer culture is often 70–90%; thus the proportion of non-muscle cells may be quite low.

The cultures may be "fed" once or twice a week with fresh culture medium, if desired, but primary cultures of heart cells survive quite well for several weeks without such feeding. In fact, some types of cells prefer "conditioned medium" (medium in which other cells are growing or have grown). For example, it has been reported that the ratio of the number of cells to the volume of the medium has a critical value below which the cells will not proliferate because they are unable to "condition the medium" adequately (Earle *et al.*, 1951). Since the volume of culture medium (e.g. 3 ml) is relatively large compared to the volume of cells (wet weight of approximately 1–3 mg). there is almost no acidosis produced (pH indicator added to the culture medium or medium pH checked with a pH meter) after 1–3 weeks in culture.

The cultures survive very well even if the culture vessels are sealed to the incubator atmosphere (compressed air and 5% CO_2, filtered and washed). Presumably the amount of oxygen available in the culture vessel (e.g. about 8 ml of air in a Carrell flask) is sufficient to last the cells for several weeks. The oxygen tension may be important in determining the rate of cell proliferation (Hollenberg, 1971) and the relative activity of glycolytic versus oxidative metabolism. Cultured chick heart cells, while primarily dependent on glucose for energy metabolism, retain a capacity to utilize fatty acids, whereas cultured mammalian foetal heart cells lack this ability (Rosenthal and Warshaw, 1973). Mammalian foetal heart cells in culture seem to adapt to low environmental oxygen tension by diminished synthesis of contractile proteins and a shift in the lactate dehydrogenase isozyme pattern, without a decrease in cellular energy stores (Karsten *et al.*, 1973). Some laboratories place a group of open culture vessels in a large closed plastic box, which can be "flushed" daily with any desired gas mixture.

Wenzel *et al.* (1970) showed that the spontaneous beating of cultured neonatal rat heart cells (confluent monolayers and multilayers) is maintained for a longer time if the plating concentration is high (e.g. 0.5×10^6 cells/ml) than when it is low (e.g. 1.3×10^3 cells/ml). In addition, the higher the proportion of muscle cells to non-muscle cells in the culture, the longer the period that beating is maintained. The addition of nicotine (0.016–0.6 mM) to the culture medium also prolongs the beating period. Similarly, it was found that high carbon monoxide (75% of atmosphere for periods up to 26 days) not only inhibits the overgrowth of muscle cells by endothelioid cells, but also prevents the usual time-dependent reduction in spontaneous beating rate (Brenner and Wenzel, 1972).

In addition to the monolayer preparations and fibreglass strands described above, the single cells can also be reaggregated into small spheres of about 100–500 μm in diameter by either of two methods. (1) The cells can be plated into glass culture dishes containing cellophane squares on the bottom. Since the cells do not adhere very well to cellophane, they pull free and form small (0.1–0.5 μm) spherical reaggregates spontaneously (Halbert *et al.*, 1971; McLean *et al.*, 1976;

Nathan *et al.*, 1976). (2) Alternatively, the cell can be placed into Ehrlenmeyer flasks and rotated on a gyrotatory shaker for about 48 h (Mettler *et al.*, 1952). The cells make contact with one another in the vortex of the solution and stick together. The longer the gyrotation period, the larger the spherical reaggregates become. Rotation for 24–48 h produces reaggregates varying between 50 and 400 μm in diameter. Larger reaggregates are not desirable because of a tendency for the cells in the core to become hypoxic and necrotic. After the rotation period, the spherical reaggregates can be transferred to a regular culture vessel and cultured for up to 6 weeks. The reaggregates will stick lightly to the substrate (or tightly in some cases with outgrowth). The entire reaggregate contracts synchronously.

The spherical reaggregates are transferred to a heated (37 °C) bath containing fresh culture medium or Ringer solution for microelectrode impalement. There are several advantages of spherical reaggregates over monolayers, the most notable of which is that microelectrode impalement is much easier because of the three-dimensional packing of cells and to isolation from vibrations (shock-mounting). An advantage of spherical reaggregates ("mini-heart") over an intact heart is that the contractions are more feeble, so that it is often possible to remain in the same cell for a prolonged period. In addition, since there are no blood vessels in the reaggregates, the effect of a drug under investigation cannot be dependent on the rate of perfusion.

Reaggregates that are composed of highly electrically differentiated cells usually do not contract spontaneously, but do contract in response to electrical stimulation. Reaggregates that are composed of reverted cells generally contract spontaneously at a rate of approximately 1 s^{-1}. The properties of the cells do not seem to change very much, if at all, during incubation periods of 5–30 days. The number of TTX-sensitive reaggregates can be increased if Ca^{2+} is replaced by Sr^{2+} or Ba^{2+} during the trypsin dispersion (Bkaily *et al.*, unpublished results).

Scanning electron microscopy has been done on heart reaggregates at various stages of formation by Shimada *et al.* (1974) and Shimada and Fischman (1976). These authors showed that a thin fibroblastic coat eventually completely covers the reaggregate. Fibroblasts from within the centre of the reaggregate work their way out to the surface.

Cells Dissociated from Adult Hearts

Isolated adult myocytes can be prepared by enzymic perfusion of adult hearts (Berry *et al.*, 1970; Vahouny *et al.*, 1970, 1979; Pretlow *et al.*, 1972; Nag *et al.*, 1977; Carlson *et al.*, 1978; Altschuld *et al.*, 1980) or by mechanical disaggregation (Bloom et al., 1974). The methods used are similar to those developed to disperse and culture heart cells from embryonic and neonatal animals (for review see Sperelakis, 1982; Kuzuya et al., 1983). For preparing isolated adult cardiomyocytes, the species that have been used include rat, mouse, dog, rabbit, guinea pig, human beings, cattle and cat (Berry et al., 1970; Vahouny et al., 1970, 1979; Pretlow et al., 1972; Nag et al., 1977; Carlson et al., 1978; Altschuld et al., 1980; Bkaily et al., 1984).

Numerous investigators have obtained isolated adult mammalian cardiomyocytes by a variety of techniques. In 1970, Berry et al. obtained morphologically intact myocytes by perfusing hearts with collagenase and hyaluronidase. Vahouny et al. (1970) used trypsin and collagenase in their incubation medium to obtain isolated cardiac cells. Powell and Twist (1976) isolated cardiomyocytes by perfusing hearts with collagenase and albumin. In general, isolated cardiomyocytes are prepared by perfusing or incubating whole adult hearts or fragments with a Ca^{2+}-free solution. This solution washes out residual blood and weakens the intracellular cement. Tissues are then treated with solutions of various Ca^{2+} concentrations that contain multiple enzymes to remove the glycocalyx. Finally, the cells are dispersed by one of a variety of mechanical procedures (for review see Bkaily et al., 1984; Farmer et al., 1983; Mitra and Morad, 1985).

Type I and type II collagenase are used by most investigators preparing isolated cardiomyocytes. This crude collagenase requires Ca^{2+} for activation, and is inhibited by cysteine and EDTA. Therefore, many investigators add some Ca^{2+} to the medium (e.g. 1 μM) to activate the collagenase. However, ventricular myocytes obtained by these methods are often rounded cells that have been damaged. Some cells, although rod-shaped, exhibit the calcium paradox (cells going into contracture, becoming spherical and dying). Other cells beat spontaneously, indicative of damage during dispersion. The rod-shaped cells generally do not survive for more than a few hours. Although these isolated cells usually have a resting potential (RP) of only about −30 to −50 mV, normal resting potentials can be obtained by exposing the cells to high concentrations of calcium (5–10 mM) (Powell et al., 1981) or by incubating them for a period in a high-K^+ medium (Isenberg and Klockner, 1982).

Clark et al. (1978) reported a procedure for dissociating cells from adult rat hearts without causing major cell damage. These investigators used a combination of collagenase (0.5%) and hyaluronidase (0.2%), followed by a solution containing EDTA (0.5 mM) and dimethyl sulphoxide (DMSO; 10%, v/v). They reported that the DMSO protected the cells against degeneration during the isolation, and permitted physiological levels of $[Ca]_o$ to stimulate rhythmic contractions without inducing cell damage. The ultrastructure of the isolated cells was normal. The cells remained intact for up to 1 h if stored at 4 °C; longer storage periods produced some degeneration of the cells. Other investigators also have succeeded in preparing by enzymic digestion isolated cardiac cells that tolerate external $[Ca]_o$ in the millimolar range (Glick et al., 1974; Powell and Twist, 1976; Farmer et al., 1977; Powell et al., 1978; Rajs et al., 1978). However, these isolated cells usually beat spontaneously.

Isenberg and Klockner (1980) demonstrated that the RPs and action potentials (APs) of isolated rat heart myocytes (dissociated by collagenase (1 mg/ml) and hyaluronidase (1 mg/ml) in a Ca^{2+}-free solution) were similar to those of cells in intact rat hearts. The calcium paradox was avoided by incubating the cells in high K^+ (>100 mM) and substrate-enriched solutions before stepwise elevation of $[Ca]_o$ to 3.6 mM. Voltage clamp experiments were also done on these myocytes (using a single microelectrode method), and the inward slow current (I_{si}) was measured.

Lee et al. (1979), using the dispersal method of adult rat hearts described by Powell and Twist and drawing the isolated single cells (cylinders, approximately 15–25 μm diameter by 100 μm length) into a suction pipette (about 20 μm diameter), reported that the cells had high RPs (-70 to -90 mV), pacemaker potentials and fast-rising TTX-sensitive APs. Using internal perfusion of the cells and with blockade of I_k (by Cs^+), I_{Ca} (by Co^{2+} or Ca^{2+}-free), and I_{Cl} (Cl-free solution), they were able to measure the fast inward Na^+ current (I_{Na}) in voltage clamp experiments. Because the surface area of the cell could be measured accurately, the current densities were obtained.

Bkaily et al. (1984) used a modified bristle method (Jacobson, 1977; Jacobson et al., 1983) for mechanical dispersion of adult single heart cells with enzyme-free medium containing Sr^{2+} or Ba^{2+} as a replacement for Ca^{2+}, and obtained healthy rod-shaped Ca^{2+}-tolerant single adult cells. These myocytes did not contract spontaneously, had a normal RP and were TTX-sensitive (Fig. 14.1). The yield was improved by the following modification (Bkaily et al., 1984): a Ca^{2+}-free medium containing 0.1% trypsin and 1.8 mMSr^{2+} was used for perfusion of the whole heart, which was stimulated electrically during the enzymic perfusion. When the contraction of the heart became greatly weakened, the perfusing solution was replaced by trypsin-free medium. After a few minutes, the ventricle was minced and bristle dispersion was begun. This method gave a large number of dispersed cells. Recently, a uniform enzymic method for dissociation of myocytes from adult hearts was described by Mitra and Morad (1985).

Brown et al. (1981b) used one-electrode and two-electrode suction

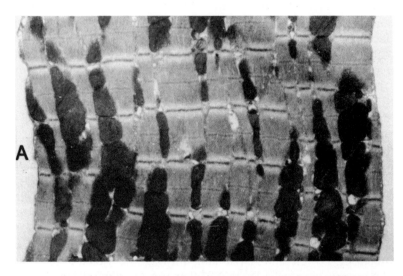

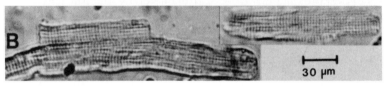

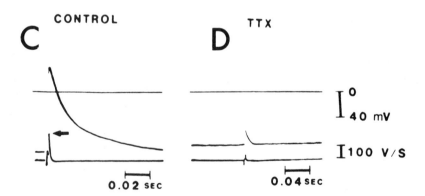

pipettes to record the fast Na^+ current. Patlak and Ortiz (1985) found three types of Na^+ channels: fast, slow and ultraslow. Several types of K^+ channels were reported in single myocytes, such as inward rectifier, outward rectifier, ATP-dependent, Ca^{2+}-dependent, Na^+-dependent, 4-AP sensitive and acetylcholine-activated K^+ currents. Single adult myocytes retain insulin receptors and a strong Na^+/K^+ pump.

Experimental Examples

Developmental Changes in Membrane Electrical Properties

The anterior half of the flat 16–20 h-old chick embryo blastoderm contains bilateral "precardiac" areas (mesoderm) whose cells are destined to form the heart (Rosenquist and DeHaan, 1966). Twin tubular primordia are formed bilaterally from the precardiac mesoderm and fuse to form a single tubular heart (Patten, 1956). The tubular heart begins contracting spontaneously at 30–40 h (9–19 somite stage) (Romanoff, 1960). The blood pressure is very low (1–2 mmHg), and propagation of the peristaltic contraction wave is very slow (approx 1 cm/s in 3-day hearts) (Romanoff, 1960). Chambers first appear in the heart on about day 5, and circulation to the chorioallantoic membrane is established, so that metabolism of the embryo becomes aerobic at that time. The nerves arrive at the heart on about day 5 (Romanoff, 1960), but they do not become functional with respect to neurotransmitter release until considerably later (Enemar et al., 1965; Pappano, 1976): The heart rate of the chick embryo increases from approximately 50 beats/min on day 1.5 to 220 beats/min on day 8.

Electron microscopy of young chick hearts shows that there are only few and short myofibrils (Sperelakis et al., 1976; Sperelakis and McLean,

---

Fig. 14.1 Light photomicrograph and high-power electron micrograph of single myocytes mechanically dispersed in the presence of Sr^{2+} (replacing Ca^{2+}) and in the absence of enzymes. Cells were bathed in 1.8 mM Ca^{2+} Tyrode solution and did not show spontaneous contractile activity. (A) high-power electron micrograph ($\times$ 11 200) of isolated adult cells showing normal arrangement of myofilaments and T tubules located at the Z-line level of adjacent sarcomeres. Note the presence of abundant mitochondria. (B) Light photomicrograph of isolated adult rat myocytes after 8 h in 1.8 mM Ca^{2+} Tyrode. (C) These myocytes do not contract spontaneously but respond to electrical stimulation by firing a fast action potential that is blocked within 60 s by tetrodotoxin (D). (C,D) Upper solid line, zero potential level. Lower trace is dV/dt. Stimulation rates, 0.5 Hz. (Modified from Bkaily et al., 1984.)

1978a, b). The sarcomeres are not complete, and the myofibrils run in all directions, including perpendicular to one another. There is an abundance of ribosomes and rough endoplasmic reticulum, and large pools of glycogen are found in the cells. As development progresses, the number of myofibrils increases and they become aligned. By day 18, the ultrastructure of the myocardial cells is similar to that of cells in adult hearts.

In order to determine the state of membrane differentiation of the cultured cells, comparison should be made with the properties of intact chick hearts at different stages of development *in situ*. The electrical properties of the heart undergo sequential changes during development (Sperelakis, 1967; Ishima, 1968; Shigenobu and Sperelakis, 1971; Schneider and Sperelakis, 1975; Bernard, 1976). The myocardial cells in young (2–3 days *in vivo*) hearts possess slowly rising (10–30 V/s) action potentials (APs) preceded by pacemaker potentials. The upstroke is generated by Na^+ influx through slow Na^+ channels which are insensitive to TTX and Mn^{2+} (Figs. 14.2A and 14.2B). Kinetically fast Na^+ channels that are sensitive to TTX make their initial appearance on about day 4, and increase in density until about day 18. The maximal rate of rise of the AP ($+V_{max}$) increases progressively from day 3 to day 18, when the adult V_{max} of approximately 150 V/s is attained. From day 5 to day 7, fast Na^+ channels coexist with a large complement of slow Na^+ channels. TTX reduces $+V_{max}$ to the value observed in 2-day hearts, i.e. 10–20 V/s, but the APs persist. After day 8, the APs are completely abolished by TTX (Fig. 14.2C), and depolarization to less than -50 mV now abolishes excitability. This indicates that the AP-generating channels consist predominantly of fast Na^+ channels (Fig. 14.2D), most of the slow Na^+ channels having been lost (functionally) so that insufficient numbers remain to support regenerative excitation.

Single heart cells from 3-day-old embryonic chick heart cells exhibit three types of slow Na^+ inward current (Fig. 14.3). The first type, a fast transient (ft) slow Na^+ inward current ($I_{si(ft)}$), is activated from a holding potential (HP) of -80 mV and shows fast activation and inactivation. The maximal mean ft I_{Na} activated from an HP of -80 mV with a voltage step (VS) to -20 mV averaged 93.5 ± 14.5 $\mu A/\mu F$ (Bkaily et al., 1991). This value is lower than that reported for the TTX-sensitive fast I_{Na} in heart muscle (Freeman et al., 1984; Brown and Yatani, 1986). The low current density of the ft I_{Na} may explain in part the low V_{max} of these single cells. The ft I_{Na} is responsible for the rising phase of the slow action potential in 3-day-old embryonic chick hearts (Figs. 14.2A and 14.2B). This type of ft I_{Na} exists during the development of the foetal human heart and disappears completely at a foetal age of 20 weeks. In

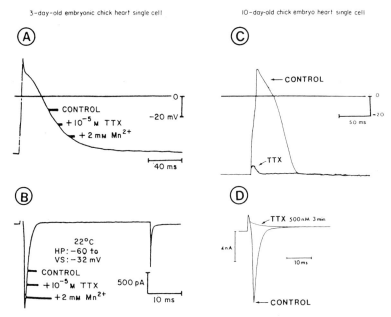

Fig. 14.2 Characteristics of the action potentials (APs) and the inward currents in single embryonic chick hearts at different stages of development. (A–D) Action potentials (A and C) and inward currents (B and D) recorded from single cells by switching between current clamp and voltage clamp modes. (A,B) The APs and the inward slow current of single 3-day-old embryonic chick ventricular cells in culture were insensitive to 10^{-5}M TTX and 2 mM Mn^{2+}. (C,D) Blockade of APs (C) and inward current by 500 nM TTX in single heart cells from 10-day-old embryonic chick. The frequency of stimulation was 0.02 Hz. HP = holding potential and VS = voltage step. Current traces in panels (C) and (D) were taken from two different single cells.

both 3-day-old chick embryonic heart cells and in 10–19-week-old foetal human heart cells, the decay phase of the ft I_{Na} fits well to the sum of two exponentials (Bkaily *et al.*, 1991) as in adult animal cardiac cells (Brown *et al.*, 1981a; Patlak and Ortiz, 1985; Follmer *et al.*, 1987). The kinetics of the ft I_{Na} in young embryonic heart cells is similar to that of the TTX-sensitive I_{Na} (Follmer *et al.*, 1987) or the TTX-insensitive (Anderson, 1987) and TTX-resistant (Bossu and Fletz, 1984; Ikeda and Schofield, 1987) Na^+ currents (Sperelakis, 1980; Sperelakis and Shigenobu, 1972; Sperelakis *et al.*, 1988).

The TTX- and Mn^{2+}-insensitive ft inward Na^+ channel in young embryonic heart seems to share a few characteristics with the Ca^{2+} channel: (1) it is completely insensitive to the fast Na^+ channel blocker,

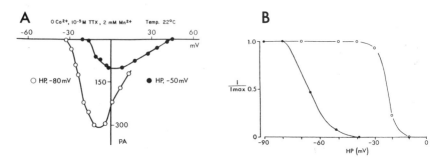

Fig. 14.3 Presence of two types of TTX- and Mn^{2+}-insensitive slow Na^+ currents in single cells from 3-day-old embryonic chick hearts. (A) Separation of the current voltage curves for the fast transient (ft,○) and the slow transient (sts,●) channels in single cells that show overlapping of the slow inward Na^+ currents. (B) Inactivation curves of the ft (●) and the sts (○) slow inward Na^+ currents (I_{Na}). For the ft slow I_{Na}, 50% of these channels are inactivated at a holding potential (HP) of −65 mV. For sts, 50% of these channels are inactivated at a HP of −23 mV. (Modified from Bkaily *et al.*, 1988b.)

TTX; (2) it is highly sensitive to one calcium blocker, apamin (Bkaily *et al.*, 1988e); and (3) it is highly permeable to the divalent cation Ba^{2+}. However, these two types of channels do not seem to share many other properties such as: (1) threshold and reversal potential (Bkaily *et al.*, 1988b,e); (2) insensitivity of the ft I_{Na} to Mn^{2+}, Ni^{2+}, Cd^{2+}, Co^{2+}, La^{3+} and $[Ca]_0$; (3) low sensitivity of the ft inward Na^+ current to verapamil, D-600, (−)D-888 and nifedipine; (4) high permeability of the ft I_{Na} to Na^+ and Li^+; (5) stability of the current in whole-cell voltage clamp conditions; the ft inward Na^+ current is much more stable than I_{Ca} (Bkaily *et al.*, 1988b,e); (6) the time-course of the ft I_{Na} activation is different from that reported for the T-type Ca^{2+} channels in heart muscle (Bean, 1985; Fox *et al.*, 1987a,b). The decrease observed in 10.7% of the single cells tested (Fig. 14.2) cannot be due to the presence of TTX and Mn^{2+}, since similar results were obtained in single cells that were not exposed to these blockers. This decrease in the ft I_{Na} could be due to the rundown of the current in some single cells. Also, our results showed that the lack of effect of TTX, Mn^{2+} and high $[Ca]_0$ on the ft I_{Na} is not due to the low stimulation frequency used in our experiments. This TTX- and Mn^{2+}-insensitive ft inward Na^+ channel resembles the TTX- resistant fast Na^+ chennel (Ikeda and Schofield, 1987) only in that it is permeable to Na^+ and Li^+ and impermeable to Ca^{2+}.

As with the TTX-sensitive fast I_{Na}, the slow Ca^{2+} current coexists with the slow Na^+ current at the embryonic age of 10 days for chicks and in

10-week-old foetal human heart cells. At least two types of Ca^{2+} currents were found in 10-day-old embryonic chick heart cells, 10–20-week-old foetal human heart cells and heart cells of newborn hamster (Fig. 14.4, 14.5 and 14.6). These slow Ca^{2+} currents are similar in voltage ranges and kinetics to the Ca^{2+} channels characterized in adult cardiac cells, neurons and other cell types (Bean, 1985; Fox et al., 1987a,b). In embryonic chick heart (Fig. 14.4) as well as in foetal human heart (Fig. 14.5) and hamster heart cells (Fig. 14.6), the high-threshold inward Ca^{2+} current (L-type current) was induced by holding potentials (HP) of −50 mV. The L-type threshold potential was near −30 mV, it reached maximum amplitude at about +10 mV and decayed very slowly (within 300 ms). The low-threshold (T-type current) I_{Ca} activated from HP of −80mV, decayed more rapidly than the L-type I_{Ca} (within 30 ms), had a threshold potential close to −40 mV and reached maximum amplitude at about −20 mV. Both types of Ca^{2+} current had a reversal potential at about +70 mV. The half-inactivation voltage was at about −65 and −15 mV for the T- and L-types respectively (Fig. 14.4B, 14.5B and 14.6B). The mean T-type Ca^{2+} current amplitude in all the three preparations was greater than the mean L-type Ca^{2+} current.

As with the TTX-sensitive I_{Na} and the slow Ca^{2+} currents, the inwardly rectifying K^+ channel that is important is determining the resting potential

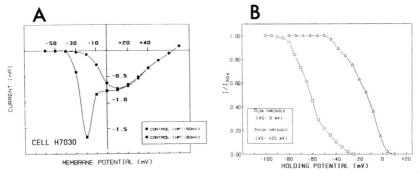

Fig. 14.4 Separation of low-threshold- (T) and high threshold- (L) type inward Ca^{2+} currents. (A) Current-voltage (I/V) relationship of Ca^{2+} currents in 10-day-old chick embryonic heart cells. The single cell was stimulated in steps of 10 mV from a holding potential (HP) of −80 mV (■) and −50 mV (●). Current traces at three different voltage steps (VS) for the I/V curve at an HP of −80 mV are in (A). (B) Steady-state inactivation curves of the T- (□) and L- (△) type of Ca^{2+} currents. The T- and L-types had a $V_{0.5}$ of −63 and −13 mV respectively. Only one type of I_{Ca} was found in each of these cells. The T-type current curve was taken from the cell no. E8205 and the L-type current curve from the cell no. A8505. (Bkaily et al., unpublished results.)

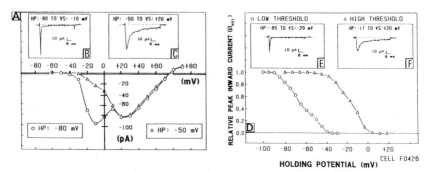

Fig. 14.5 Two types of Ca^{2+} currents in ventricular single cells of 17-week-old human foetuses. (A) Voltage-dependence of the low-threshold I_{Ca} (○) and separation of the high-threshold I Ca (△). (B) Peak current trace of the low-threshold I_{Ca} recorded from holding potential (HP) of -80 mV with a voltage step (VS) to -10 mV. (C) Current trace of the high-threshold I_{Ca} recorded from a HP of -50 mV with a VS to $+20$ mV. (D) Steady-state inactivation relationship of the low- (○) and high-threshold (△) I_{Ca}. (E) Low-threshold current trace recorded from HP of -65 mV with a VS to -20 mV. (E) High-threshold current trace recorded from HP of -17 mV with a VS to $+20$ mV. All records were taken from cell no. F0426. Currents were measured at the peak. (Bkaily *et al.*, unpublished results.)

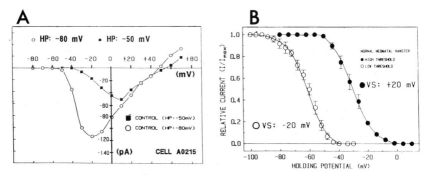

Fig. 14.6 Two types of Ca^{2+} currents in single ventricular heart cells of neonatal hamster. (A) Voltage-dependence of the low-threshold I_{Ca} (○) and separation of the high-threshold I_{Ca} (■). (B) Steady-state inactivation relationship of the low- (○) and high- (●) threshold I_{Ca}. All records were taken from the cell no. A0215. Currents were measured at the peak. (Bkaily *et al.*, unpublished results.)

in chick heart cells was found to be absent from 3-day-old embryonic chick hearts but present in older hearts (Fig. 14.7). This finding is consistent with the low resting potential and high input resistance in the young hearts.

The Na^+/K^+ ATPase specific activity and the intracellular cyclic AMP level also undergo changes during the development of the heart. The Na^+/K^+ ATPase activity is low in 3-day-old chick hearts and increases progressively during development, reaching the final adult value by about day 18 (Sprerelakis, 1972b). Although the Na^+/K^+ pump activity is low in young hearts, it is sufficient to maintain a relatively high $[K]_i$. The cyclic AMP level is very high in young embryonic hearts, and decreases during development to reach the final adult level by about day 16 (McLean *et al.*, 1975; Renaud *et al.*, 1978; Thakkar and Sperelakis, 1987).

The sarcoplasmic reticulum (SR) seems to be present and functional in young embryonic heart cells and in foetal human heart cells. The SR caffeine-sensitive Ca^{2+} channel can be observed in all young embryonic and foetal single heart cells. There was no difference in the response to caffeine-induced release of Ca^{2+} in both young and adult embryonic heart cells (Bkaily, unpublished results).

In 3-day-old embryonic hearts, Ca^{2+} channels are very few in number

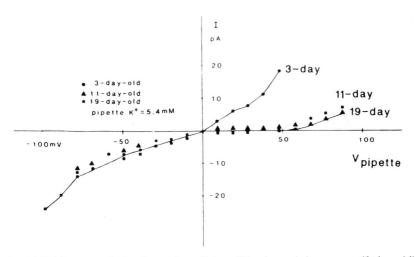

Fig. 14.7 Absence of the inward-rectifying K^+ channel in young (3-day-old) embryonic chick hearts. To characterize the age-related changes in K^+ channel-kinetic properties, cell-attached patch clamp experiments were conducted on embryonic chick myocytes prepared from three different embryonic stages: 3-day-old (●), 11-day-old (▲) and 19-day-old (■). The *I–V* curve of steady-state K^+ currents attained 1 min after changes in pipette potential are shown. Data plotted are the mean values ($n = 4$–6) of the channel current amplitude for each age. As can be seen, the inward-going rectification was substantial at potentials higher than 0 mV for 11-day-old and 19-day-old hearts, but absent from 3-day-old hearts. (H. Sada, G. Bkaily and N. Sperelakis, unpublished observations).

or are not present at all. This raises questions about the underlying mechanism(s) behind the spontaneous contractions and its source of Ca^{2+} of these single cells. It is possible that the low Na^+/K^+ pump activity allows a build up of $[Na]_i$ via the slow Na^+ channels, which in turn may allow Ca^{2+} entry via the Na^+/Ca^{2+} exchanger. Also, we have recently identified, in both young and adult heart cells, a new type of voltage-dependent Ca^{2+} channel which was called a "resting calcium channel" (R-type). This type of channel is highly active during depolarization and stays open while depolarization of the membrane is maintained (Bkaily et al., 1992a). Since 3-day-old embryonic chick heart cells have a low resting potential, the activity of this new Ca^{2+} channel should be correspondingly high and may contibute to entry of Ca^{2+} at rest as well as during the action potentials of these cells. The activity of the channel is very low at hyperpolarized membrane voltages and is insensitive to cyclic nucleotides and ATP but is blocked by the calcium blocker PN 200–110 and activated by insulin (Bkaily et al., 1992a).

Pacemaker Activities of Embryonic Chick Single Heart Cells

Most of the single cells isolated from 3-day-old chick embryonic hearts show pacemaker activity. However, fewer single heart cells from older embryonic chicks show spontaneous activity. Heart cells isolated from newborn animals also show spontaneous activity (Sperelakis, 1978). However, adult heart cells do not contract spontaneously unless they are damaged during the enzymic dispersion or after several days in culture (Jacobson and Piper, 1986). Reaggregates of single heart cells from old chick embryos also contract spontaneously after 4 days in culture. Some of the reaggregated single heart cells show spontaneous action potentials (Fig. 14.8A) that are blocked by the fast Na^+-channel blocker, TTX (Fig. 14.8B). Superfusion with the β-agonist isoproterenol (ISO) induces bursts of slow Ca^{2+} APs (Fig. 14.8C). These slow APs induced by ISO or those occurring naturally in cultured heart-cell reaggregates (see Fig. 14.14A) are blocked by organic and inorganic Ca^{2+} channel blockers (Sperelakis, 1978). As in reaggregated single heart cells, quiescent freshly isolated single heart cells from 10-day-old embryonic chick show spontaneous increases in intracellular free Ca^{2+} during the ISO-induced burst of slow APs. This burst of $[Ca]_i$ is not due to SR Ca^{2+} release (SR depleted by caffeine) but is blocked by the L-type Ca^{2+} channel blocker nifedipine.

Spontaneous activity and intracellular free Ca^{2+} concentration can be monitored and measured using the fura-2 Ca^{2+} imaging technique and Plate 14.1 shows an example. As can be seen, freshly isolated single heart cells from a 3-day-old chick embryo show a spontaneous increase in free

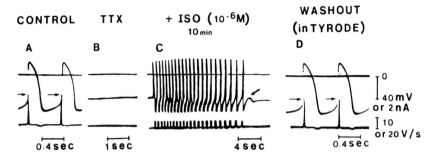

Fig. 14.8 Burst of spontaneous slow action potentials (APs) induced by isoproterenol in highly differentiated cultured chick heart cells (reaggregates). (A) Control fast APs in normal Tyrode solution. (B) Tetrodotoxin (TTX, 3.3 μM) blocks fast APs. (C) Addition of 10^{-6}M isoproterenol (ISO) induces bursts of slow APs each followed by a delayed after-depolarization (DAD). (D) Washout with Tyrode solution (no TTX) restores completely the fast APs. Upper solid line, zero potential level. Lower trace is dV/dt, the maximum excursion of which gives $+V_{max}$. All records are from the same impalement. (Modified from Bkaily *et al.*, 1984.)

[Ca]$_i$ during the spontaneous contraction of the cell (Plate 14.1A–E). The spontaneous contraction and the spontaneous increase in [Ca]$_i$ are blocked by a low concentration of isradipine (PN 200-110; 10^{-8}M; Fig. Plate 14.1F). This compound was found to be a highly potent pacemaker channel blocker.

Therefore, spontaneously active 3-day-old embryonic chick heart cells could be considered as a good model for studying nodal pacemaker heart cells. As mentioned above, these single heart cells of young embryonic chick hearts do not possess active Ca^{2+} channels and the inward current is carried by Na^+ ions. This preparation can also provide a model for studying the effect of drugs and substances on young foetal human hearts.

Calcium-Channel Blockers

The effect of isradipine (PN 200–110) on the L-type I_{Ca} of 10-day-old embryonic chick heart cells is summarized in Fig. 14.9 (filled circles). At low concentration (0.02 μM), it increased the peak amplitude of the L-type I_{Ca} by 5 ± 2.0% ($n = 4$). Increasing the concentration to 0.05 μM decreased the peak I_{Ca} amplitude by 22 ± 4.0% ($n = 4$), and a larger decrease (86 ± 1.0%, $n = 4$) of I_{Ca} peak amplitude was obtained at 0.15μM. A complete block of the L-type I_{Ca} was achieved with 5 μM.

The high-threshold (L-type) Ca^{2+} current was also recorded from single

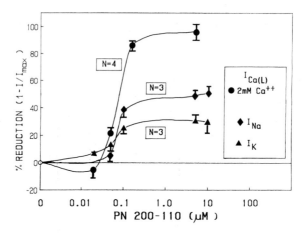

Fig. 14.9 Dose-dependence of PN 200-110 blockade of ionic currents in chick embryo heart cells. PN 200-110 decreased all the ionic currents in a dose-dependent manner. However, while the L-type I_{Ca} (●) was completely blocked at concentration of 5 μM the delayed outward K^+ current (▲) decreased by 22% and the TTX-sensitive fast Na^+ current (◆) decreased by 43%. (Bkaily *et al.*, unpublished results.)

cells of 20-week-old foetal human hearts, and Fig. 14.10 shows a typical example. After 30 s of superfusion with 10^{-6}M PN 200-110 there was a gradual decrease in the L-type I_{Ca} amplitude (Fig. 14.10, open triangles) and the inward tail Ca^{2+} current (not shown). By 5 min, the decreases in the L-type I_{Ca} peak amplitude (Fig. 14.10 left panel and curve with open triangles) and the inward tail Ca^{2+} current were very marked. Exposing PN 200-110 to a flash of light immediately and completely abolished the block of the L-type I_{Ca} peak amplitude (Fig. 14.10 right panel and curve with open squares). Turning off the flash of light (for 4 min) did not restore the blocking activity of PN 200-110 (not shown). However, addition of a low concentration of PN 200-110 (in the presence of the inactivated drug) substantially reduced the peak amplitude of the L-type I_{Ca} within 11 min.

The low-threshold (T-type) I_{Ca} was recorded from a holding potential (HP) of -80 mV with a voltage step (VS) to -20 mV. Superfusion with a low concentration of PN 200-110 (10^{-9}M) increased the peak amplitude of the T-type I_{Ca} within 2 min. Increasing the concentration of the drug to 10^{-8}M decreased the T-type I_{Ca} back to the control level. Superfusion with higher concentrations of PN 200-110 (up to 10^{-6}M) did not affect the peak T-type I_{Ca} amplitude.

The effect of different concentrations of PN 200-110 on the delayed

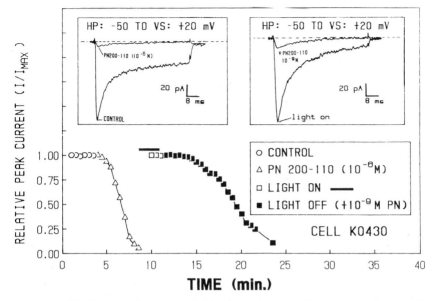

Fig. 14.10 Blockade of the L-type Ca^{2+} current in single foetal human heart cells by PN 200-110. The L-type I_{Ca} was activated from holding potential (HP) of -50 mV with a voltage step (VS) to $+20$ mV. Superfusion with 10^{-6}M PN 200-110 completely blocked the L-type I_{Ca} within 5 min ($\triangle$ and current traces in the left panel). Inactivation of PN 200-110 with a flash of light returned the L-type I_{Ca} amplitude to the control level ($\square$ and right panel current trace). After turning off the light, very low concentrations of PN 200-110 (10^{-9}M) decrease the L-type I_{Ca} by 88% within 11 min ($\blacksquare$ and current trace in right panel). (Bkaily *et al.*, unpublished results.)

outward K^+ current (I_K) and the TTX-sensitive I_{Na} of 10-day-old chick embryonic heart single cells was studied. Fig. 14.9 shows the dose–response curve of PN 200-110 on peak I_{Na} (curve with filled diamonds) and peak I_K (curve with filled triangles) amplitudes. As shown in this figure, at a concentration that decreased L-type I_{Ca} by 22% (0.05 μM), PN 200-110 decreased I_{Na} amplitude only by $6 \pm 1.0\%$. At a concentration that decreased the L-type I_{Ca} by $86 \pm 1.0\%$ (0.15 μM), PN 200-110 decreased I_{Na} amplitude by $38 \pm 3.0\%$ and the next concentration (5 μM) decreased I_{Na} by $43 \pm 2.0\%$ (Fig. 14.9, curve with filled diamonds). At the highest concentration used [complete blockade of cell-type I_{Ca} (10 μM)], PN 200-110 did not further decrease I_{Na} amplitude $48 \pm 4.0\%$.

At a low concentration (0.02 μM), PN 200-110 was found to decrease I_k peak amplitude by $7 \pm 1.0\%$. Increasing the concentration up to 0.05 μM, 0.1 μM and 5 μM and 10 μM respectively decreased I_K amplitude by $13 \pm 4.0\%$, $25 \pm 1.0\%$ and $31 \pm 2.0\%$ respectively (Fig. 14.9, curve with filled triangles). As for I_{Na}, the high concentration of PN 200-110 (10 μM) did not further decrease I_k ($33 \pm 4\%$, $n = 3$).

PN 200-110 was found to block the L-type I_{Ca} in both 10-day-old embryonic chick heart cells and human foetal heart cells in a dose-dependent manner. The effect is completely reversible upon washout or a light flash. The fact that very low concentrations of PN 200-110 (10^{-9}M) blocked the L-type I_{Ca} after light exposure could be due to the incomplete or reversibility of the photobleaching of the 10^{-6}M concentration of this drug. PN 200-110 blocked 50% (ID_{50}) of the L-type I_{Ca} channels at a concentration close to 8×10^{-8}M. When compared with nifedipine (not shown), PN 200-110 is a more potent blocker of ventricular heart L-type I_{Ca} than nifedipine. As with PN 200-110, a very low concentration of nifedipine increased the L-type I_{Ca}. This effect could be due to the Bay K 8644-like effect of these two dihydropyridine drugs. High concentrations of PN 200-110 did not affect the T-type I_{Ca}. Thus, PN 200-110 seems to be a highly specific L-type I_{Ca} blocker. If the T-type Ca^{2+} current is a pacemaker Ca^{2+} current (Bean, 1985, 1989), then this drug would be an ineffective blocker of the pacemaker T-type I_{Ca} in old embryonic ventricular heart cells.

The blockade of the TTX-sensitive I_{Na} and of the L-type I_{Ca} by PN 200-110 was also reported by Brown's group (Yatani et al., 1988a). However, the concentration for the half-maximal block (IC_{50}) (1.25×10^{-5}M) reported here is lower than that reported by Yatani et al. (1988a). PN 200-110 was reported to be ineffective in blocking I_{K1} and I_x in single heart cells (Yatani et al., 1988a), while our results showed that the delayed outward rectifier in 10-day-old embryonic chick heart cells (Bkaily et al., 1988a,b,c,e; Renaud et al., 1988) was sensitive to this drug.

Brown's group suggests that Na^+ channels, like Ca^{2+} channels, have dihydropyridine (DHP) receptors. If this is true, our results may suggest that the delayed outward rectifier K^+ channels may also have DHP receptors. The high sensitivity of the L-type I_{Ca} and the low sensitivity of I_{Na} and I_K to PN 200-110 may also suggest either (1) a non-specific effect of this drug on I_{Na} and I_K or (2) the presence of a low-affinity DHP receptor site on the Na^+ and K^+ channels (Yatani et al., 1988a). As with Bay K 8644, PN 200-110 effects on Ca^{2+}, Na^{2+} and K^+ currents may suggest a complicated binding pattern of this drug for cardiac membranes (Yatani et al., 1988a).

Finally, when the effect of PN 200-110 on the L-type I_{Ca} is compared with that on the T-type I_{Ca}, we can conclude that PN 200-110 is a highly potent and specific L-type I_{Ca}-channel blocker. However, when the effect of this drug on the L-type I_{Ca} is compared with that on I_{Na} and I_K, we can only state that PN 200-110 is a highly potent and relatively specific L-type I_{Ca} blocker.

As previously cited, we very recently found a new voltage-dependent Ca^{2+} channel (R-type) that is responsible for the Ca^{2+} influx during prolonged depolarization of the cell membrane (Bkaily, unpublished results). Using fura-2 Ca^{2+} measurement (Fig. 14.11), depolarizing the cell membrane of freshly isolated single heart cells from 10-day-old chick embryo (or from 20-week-old foetal human heart) induced a rapid increase in $[Ca]_i$. This increase in $[Ca]_i$ is due to the opening of the L-type Ca^{2+} channel. The transient $[Ca]_i$ increase is followed by a sustained component that is insensitive to the L-type Ca^{2+} blocker nifedipine (Figure 14.11A). As in old embryonic chick heart cells (not shown), pre-exposing the single heart cells from 20-week-old human foetuses to nifedipine blocked the transient increase of $[Ca]_i$ induced by high $[K]_o$ (30 nM) without affecting the sustained increase of $[Ca]_i$ (Fig. 14.11B). The sustained increase in Ca^{2+} influx by high $[K]_o$ is blocked by EGTA (Fig. 14.11B) which suggests that the increase in $[Ca]_i$ is due to Ca^{2+} entry through a channel that is blocked by PN 200-110. Using a fura-2 Ca^{2+} imaging technique, the sustained increase in $[Ca]_i$ caused by high $[K]_o$ is blocked by PN 200-110. Plate 14.2 shows an example: the colour ratio (0.29–0.46) level of $[Ca]_i$ is low when the cell membrane is not depolarized by $[K]_o$ (Plate

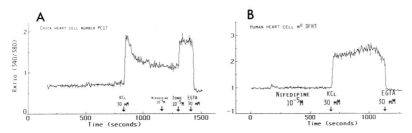

Fig. 14.11 Blockade by nifedipine of the high $[K^+]_o$-induced transient increase in intracellular free Ca^{2+} ($[Ca]_i$) recorded with fura-2. (A) Increasing the concentration of $[K]_o$ from 5.4 mM up to 30 mM caused an immediate transient increase in $[Ca]_i$ followed by a sustained one. Addition of 10^{-5}M L-type Ca^{2+}-channel blocker nifedipine had no effect on the late sustained increase in $[Ca]_i$ induced by high $[K]_o$. Ionomycin (IONO) and EGTA were added subsequently to obtain maximal and minimal fluorescence respectively. (B) Addition of 10^{-5}M nifedipine did not affect the resting $[Ca]_i$; however, this drug prevented the transient increase in $[Ca]_i$ induced by high $[K]_o$ leaving behind the sustained component. Reduction of extracellular Ca^{2+} concentration with EGTA reduced the $[Ca]_i$ below the control level. The experiments were carried out using a PTI microfluorimeter.
(Bkaily *et al.*, unpublished results.)

14.2). Upon membrane depolarization by 30 m$M[K]_o$, there is a fast transient increase in $[Ca]_i$ as expected (not shown) followed by a sustained increase (Plate 14.2B) in the colour ratio from 0.71 to 1.75. Addition of PN 200-110 (10^{-6}M) reduced $[Ca^{2+}]_i$ close to that seen in the control (Plate 14.2C, ratio between 0.46 and 0.71). At rest, $[Ca^{2+}]_i$ seems lower in the middle of the cells than near the internal cell membrane. During the sustained depolarization of the membrane, the intracellular free Ca^{2+} seems to be homogeneously distributed.

Natural Toxin

Several toxins were reported to be highly specific blockers of a single type of ionic channel. A good example of this is tetrodotoxin (TTX), the highly specific fast Na^+-channel blocker (Hille, 1975). Like TTX, scorpion toxins have become important tools for studies on Na^+ channels (Wheeler et al. (1983) and references therein). However, different scorpion venoms have different types of action on this channel (Carbone et al., 1982; Wheeler et al., 1983; Yatani et al., 1988b): Saxotoxin (STX) was also reported to be a specific fast Na^+ channel blocker (Kao and Nishiyama, 1965; Hille, 1975; Strichartz, 1984). Some natural toxins do not inhibit the fast Na^+ channel but rather activate or open this type of channel. These include gonioporatoxin (GPT; Nishio et al., 1988), batrachotoxin (BTX; Garber, 1988) and grayanotoxin (GTX; Seyama et al. (1988) and references therein). Several other types of toxin were found to be specific for different types of K^+ channels. Examples are charybdotoxin (ChTX), apamin, dendrotoxin, noxiustoxin and gaboon viper venom (for review, see Castle et al. (1989) and references therein). Recently our laboratory, as well as other laboratories, reported that some toxins may affect specifically the L-type Ca^{2+} channels (Bkaily et al., 1985) as well as the early embryonic ft slow Na^+ channels (Bkaily et al., 1988b,e; 1991) in heart muscle. Another toxin, the ω-conotoxin (ω-CgTx) was reported to block the L-type and N-type Ca^{2+} channels but with only transient inhibitory effects on T-type Ca^{2+} channels in neurons and not in heart muscle (McCleskey et al., 1987). Maitotoxin (MTX) was found to activate a new class of voltage-independent Ca^{2+} channel or an entirely modified form of voltage-gated Ca^{2+} channel in heart cells (Kobayashi et al., 1987).

Recently, apamin was reported to block specifically the L-type I_{Ca} in old embryonic chick hearts and the early cardiac embryonic ft slow Na^+ channels (Bkaily and Sperelakis, 1985; Bkaily et al., 1988e, 1991) This toxin, at a very low concentration (10^{-10}M), decreased the overshoot and the duration of the action potentials recorded from isolated 19-day-old embryonic chick hearts (Fig. 14.2D) and blocked completely the slow

Ca^{2+} action potential of old single heart cell reaggregates (Figure 14.2A–C). This toxin of the bee venom decreased the slow Ca^{2+} action potentials (Bkaily and Sperelakis, 1985) and the L-type Ca^{2+} current in a dose-dependent manner (Fig. 14.13). Very low concentrations of this toxin (10^{-12}M) decreased the L-type I_{Ca} amplitude by 10%, and 50% blockade of this current was achieved at 10^{-10}M) apamin. At this low

CULTURED CHICK HEART CELL REAGGREGATES

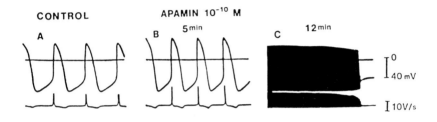

INTACT NON-CULTURED EMBRYONIC CHICK HEART

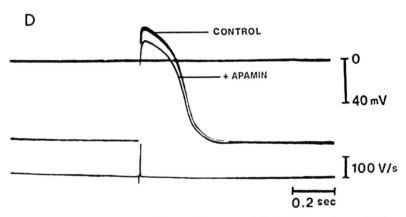

Fig. 14.12 Apamin decreased the action potential (AP) overshoot (OS) and duration in intact heart and blocked the naturally occurring slow Ca^{2+} APs in reaggregated single heart cells of old embryonic chick. (A) Control slow Ca^{2+} APs. (B) Superfusion with Tyrode solution containing 10^{-10}M apamin for 5 min increased the OS and $+V_{max}$. (C) After 12 min, there was a complete block of the slow Ca^{2+} APs. Washout of apamin did not restore the slow APs, and recovery was only possible when quinidine was added to the superfusion medium. (D) Normal fast AP recorded in the absence (upper trace) and presence (lower AP trace) of 10^{-10}M apamin. Upper solid line is the zero potential, lower trace is dV/dt, the maximum excursion of which gives $+V_{max}$. A and B calibration is 0.8 s and in C is 20 s. (Modified from Bkaily *et al.*, 1985.)

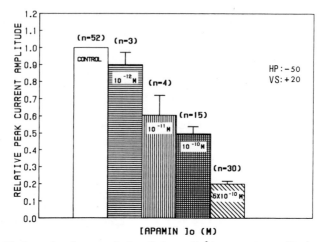

Fig. 14.13 Apamin decreased the L-type Ca^{2+} current amplitude in a dose-dependent manner in 10-day-old chick embryo heart single cells. The ED_{50} for apamin was $10^{-10}M$. Data presented are the means $\pm$ S.E.M. and n is the number of cultured single cells tested (Bkaily *et al.*, unpublished results).

concentration ($10^{-10}M$, apamin also decreased the L-type I_{Ca} by 50% in 20-week-old single human foetal heart cells; Fig. 14.14 shows an example. Apamin decreased the L-type and the tail current within 5 min. This toxin had no effect on the TTX-sensitive I_{Na} (Bkaily *et al.*, 1991) and the T-type I_{Ca} of heart muscle. Apamin was also found to block specifically the early embryonic and foetal ft slow Na^+ channels (Bkaily *et al.*, 1991). This type of channel does not exist in older embryronic or foetal heart but continues to function in Duchenne muscular dystrophy (Bkaily *et al.*, 1990) and single heart cells of hereditary cardiomyopathic hamsters (Bkaily *et al.*, 1991). Also another toxin in bee venom, melittin, at low concentrations ($10^{-8}M$) was found to block the early embryonic ft slow Na^+ channels (Bkaily *et al.*, 1988b). However, this toxin was less potent that apamin in blocking this type of early embryonic slow Na^+ current. Also melittin, but not apamin at high concentration ($10^{-4}M$), blocked completely the slow transient (st) Na^+ current without affecting the sustained type of the slow I_{Na} (Bkaily *et al.*, 1988b).

Local Anaesthetics

Local anaesthetics usually act by blocking Na^+ and K^+ channels in heart muscle (for review, see Hondeghem and Katzung, 1984; Clarkson and

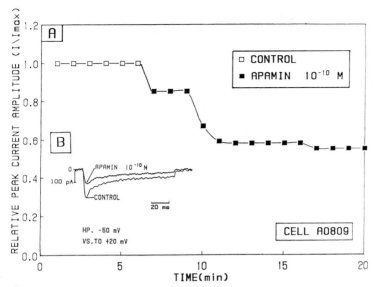

Fig. 14.14 Blockade of the L-type I_{Ca} in single foetal human heart cells by apamin. (A) Time course of the block of the L-type I_{Ca} by 10^{-10}M apamin. (B) Current traces showing the block of the L-type I_{Ca} after 5 min in the presence of apamin. A concentration of apamin that decreased by 50% the amplitude of the L-type I_{Ca} in 10-day-old embryonic chick heart cells, also decreased by 50% this type of current in single foetal human heart cells. (Bkaily *et al.*, unpublished results.)

Hondeghem, 1985). However, some local anaesthetics have also been reported to block the Ca^{2+}-mediated slow action potentials in ventricular muscle (Coyle and Sperelakis, 1987).

Bupivacaine, a popular local anaesthetic, is used widely because of its high anaesthetic potency, relative specificity for sensory fibres and prolonged duration of action. However, bupivacaine is also a highly cardiotoxic agent (Albright, 1979; Davis and deJong, 1982; Marx, 1984). It is known to produce serious cardiac arrhythmias and even death if it accidently gains access to the cardiovascular system (Albright, 1979; Kotelko *et al.*, 1984): One of the most severe forms of arrhythmias initiated by bupivacaine, the sino-atrial block, is known to be reversed by noradrenaline (Wheeler *et al.*, 1988). Bupivacaine is also known for its potent negative inotropic action on heart muscle (Lynch, 1986).

Bupivacaine was found to be a highly potent L-type Ca^{2+}-channel blocker in single cells of 10-day-old chick embryo hearts (Fig. 14.15). Bupivacaine at a concentration of 25 μM completely blocked the L-type I_{Ca} (Figure 14.15, open diamonds). However, this concentration also

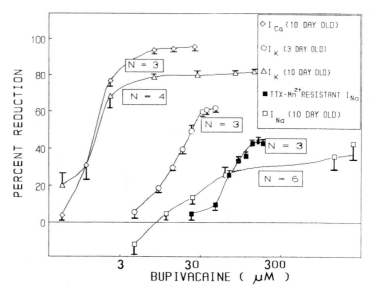

Fig. 14.15 Dose-dependence of the bupivacaine blockade of ionic currents in chick embryo heart cells. Bupivacaine blocks all the ionic currents studied in a dose-dependent manner. However, while I_{Ca} and I_K of 10-day-old chick embryonic heart are almost completely blocked at concentrations less than 3 μM, the I_K in 3-day-chick embryo heart cells, the slow I_{Na} and the fast I_{Na} are only partially blocked at concentrations of bupivacaine ranging from 3 to 300 μM. The order of potency of the block of the latter ionic currents by bupivacaine is: I_K (3-day-old), slow I_{Na} (3-day-old) followed by the fast TTX-sensitive I_{Na} in 10-day-old chick embryo heart (Bkaily *et al.*, unpublished results).

decreased the delayed outward K^+ current by 80% (Fig. 14.15, open triangles). At low concentrations, bupivacaine was more effective in blocking the L-type I_{Ca}. What is surprising, however, is that at concentrations that block I_{Ca}, this local anaesthetic did not affect the TTX-sensitive I_{Na} (Fig. 14.15, open squares). This compound seems to be a less effective blocker of the ft slow I_{Na} in young embryonic hearts (Fig. 14.15, closed squares). The reduction of fast I_{Na} by bupivacaine may account for its local anaesthetic effects. This drug, like lidocaine, decreases I_K and purportedly has an antiarrhythmic action in the heart; this, however, appears to be untrue. Finally, the arrythmogenic effects of bupivacaine could be due to its non-specific effects on ionic currents of the heart muscle when it is used at a concentration that blocks Na^+ channels.

Potassium-Channel Openers

The first report concerning K^+-channel activators as a new class of antihypertensive drugs was made by Bkaily et al. (1988a). This modulation of K^+-channel opening is not a novel physiological mechanism (Hamilton and Weston (1989) and references therein). Recently, several compounds, such as cromakalim (BRL 34915), pinacidil and nicorandil, have been reported to be activators of an ATP-dependent K^+ channel in vascular smooth muscle. Other compounds such as the antifibrillatory drug bethanidine have been reported to open cyclic GMP-sensitive K^+ channels and to relax vascular smooth muscle (Bkaily et al., 1988a; Bkaily 1990). These K^+-channel activators also affected heart muscle function. For example, in heart cells, bethanidine blocks the delayed outward K^+ current, increases the fast I_{Na} and slow I_{Ca} and induces a positive inotropic effect (Bkaily et al., 1988c). This drug also increases the duration of the action potential (Bkaily et al., 1988c). However, all other K^+-channel activators, including cromakalim, decrease the duration of the action potential and produce a negative inotropic effect on heart muscle (Grossett and Hicks, 1986; Cohen and Colbert, 1986; Yanagisawa et al., 1988; Escande (1989) and references therein).

Earlier studies have established that the decrease in the action potential duration of cardiac muscle (Escande et al., 1988) induced by high concentrations of cromakalim ($10^{-6} - 10^{-4}$M) is due to activation of an ATP-dependent K^+ channel. However, the changes reported (negative inotropic) are observed at concentrations of K^+-channel openers higher than those required to produce K^+-channel opening in vascular smooth muscle, and this effect is also temperature-dependent (Cohen and Colbert, 1986; Weston and Abbott, 1987; Hamilton and Weston, 1989). The reason for the low sensitivity of heart muscle to cromakalim was attributed to the poorly developed delayed outward K^+ current in a guinea-pig myocardium (Osterrieder 1988). This is probably true, since in 10-day-old chick ventricular cells, at a concentration similar to that used in vascular smooth muscle (10^{-8}M), cromakalim (as well as pinacidil; unpublished results) increased a delayed outward K^+ current in these single cells.

Pinacidil, as well as cromakalim, has been reported to induce spontaneous activity in ventricular muscle (Steinberg et al., 1988), electrocardiographic T-wave abnormalities (Callaghan et al., 1988), tachycardia and palpitations (Goldberg, 1988). Visual microscope observation as well as fura-2 Ca^{2+} measurement (Fig. 14.16) revealed that quiescent 10-day-old embryonic ventricular as well as single heart cells from 19-week-old human foetus developed spontaneous activity in the

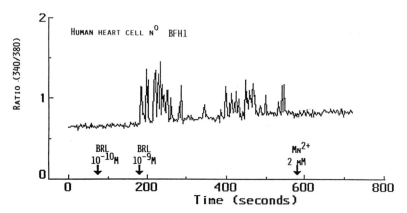

Fig. 14.16 Cromakalim (BRL 34915) induced spontaneous transient increases in calcium in ventricular heart cells from 19-week-old human foetus. Traces shows fluorescence signal ratio from a single cell loaded with fura-2. At the point indicated, addition of 10^{-10}M cromakalim had no effect on the resting level of $[Ca]_i$. Increasing the concentration of cromakalim to 10^{-9}M immediately induced spontaneous contraction associated with spontaneous transient increase in $[Ca]_i$. Addition of the inorganic Ca^{2+}-channel blocker Mn^{2+} (2 mM) completely blocked the cromakalim-induced spontaneous transient increase of $[Ca]_i$. (Bkaily *et al.*, unpublished results.)

presence of 10^{-8}M cromakalim. This pacemaker activity is due to stimulation of a T-type I_{Ca} that plays a pacemaking role in almost all cells (Hagiwara *et al.*, 1988; Bean, 1989). It is very likely that stimulation of the T-type I_{Ca} (Fig. 14.17B), accompanied by an increase in the TTX-sensitive I_{Na} (Fig. 14.17C) caused by cromakalim, could be responsible for the spontaneous activity of heart cells (Fig. 14.16). This may in part explain the cardiac side effects of this drug.

It is difficult to explain the mechanism by which cromakalim activates the T-type I_{Ca}, the TTX-sensitive I_{Na} and the delayed outward I_K. It is certain that the mechanism of action of cromakalim cannot be mediated via cyclic nucleotide stimulation (Yanagisawa *et al.*, 1988), which is mainly known to regulate the L-type I_{Ca} (Bean, 1985, 1989). However, it is possible that cromakalim may act via the mechanism which regulates both the T-type I_{Ca} and the TTX-sensitive I_{Na}.

Angiotensin II, Atrial Natriuretic Factor (ANF) and Insulin

Single heart cells in culture possess functional receptors for a variety of agents such as hormones. For example, angiotensin II (Ang II) is known to be a vasoconstrictive hormone that blocks K^+ currents and increases

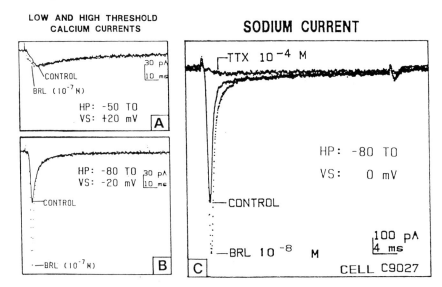

Fig. 14.17 Stimulation of the T-type I_{Ca} and the TTX-sensitive fast I_{Na} by cromakalim (BRL 34915) in 10-day-old chick embryo single heart cells. (A) Addition of 10^{-7}M of BRL 34915 had no effect on the L-type I_{Ca}. (B) Upper trace shows the T-type I_{Ca} recorded in the absence of BRL 34915 and the lower current trace shows the large increase in amplitude of this current caused by 10^{-7}M of BRL 34915. (C) The fast Na^+ current (middle current trace) was recorded in presence of Mn^{2+} (Ca^{2+}-channel blocker) and TEA (K^+-channel blocker). Addition of 10^{-8}M BRL 34915 within a minute markedly increased the peak I_{Na} (lower current trace) and addition of 10^{-4}M TTX (fast Na^+-channel blocker) completely inhibited the fast inward Na^+ current (upper current trace).
(Bkaily *et al.*, unpublished results.)

Ca^{2+} currents in vascular smooth muscle (Bkaily *et al.*, 1988d). This peptide induces a rapid phospholipase C-mediated breakdown of phosphatidylinositol bisphosphate (PIP_2), the formation of inositol trisphosphate (IP_3) and hydrolysis of *sn*-1,2-diacylglycerol (DG) which in turn stimulates C-kinase. IP_3 has been proposed to act as a second messenger for the mobilization of $[Ca]_i$ and the C-kinase activation may stimulate protein phosphorylation. This hormone induces slow Ca^{2+} action potential in cardiac preparations in which the fast I_{Na} is blocked by TTX or by depolarizing the membrane with high $[K]_o$ (Freer *et al.*, 1976). The stimulation of a pacemaking T-type (Fig. 14.18A and 14.18B) Ca^{2+} current could be responsible for the induced slow Ca^{2+} action potential in heart single cells. This increase of the T-type I_{Ca} is blocked by specific angiotensin II receptor-blocking agents (Fig. 14.18B).

Another hormone, ANF, secreted mainly by the atria, is known to be

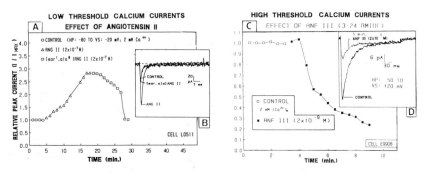

Fig. 14.18 Angiotensin II (Ang II) increased T-type I_{Ca} and atrial natriuretic factor (ANF) blocked L-type I_{Ca} in 10-day-old chick embryo single heart cells. (A, B) The single cell (L0511) showed only a T-type I_{Ca}. (A) Time-course effect of Ang II on the T-type I_{Ca}. Open circles are the control relative peak inward current. Addition of Ang II progressively increased the T-type peak amplitude ($\triangle$). Addition of the Ang II antagonist, [Sar^1, Ala^8]Ang II (2×10^{-7}M) largely reversed the Ang II effect ($\square$). (B) Control current traces (upper trace), after addition (14 min) of Ang II (lower trace) and after addition of the Ang II antagonist (middle trace). (C) Time-course effect of ANF III on the L-type I_{Ca}. Addition of 2×10^{-9}M ANF III progressively decreased the relative peak L-type current amplitude induced from a HP of -50 mV. (D) Current traces showing the effect of ANF III. (Bkaily *et al.*, unpublished results.)

involved in reducing blood volume and blood pressure (Pandey *et al.*, 1987), inhibition of agonist-induced activation of vascular smooth muscle (Cauvin *et al.*, 1987; Delaflotte *et al.*, 1989) and control of electrolyte and fluid homoeostasis (Bolli *et al.*, 1987). Stimulation of ANF secretion activates the membrane-bound form and guanylate cyclase without altering the activity of the soluble form of the enzyme. Most of the proposed effects of ANF are attributed mainly to the stimulation of a cyclic GMP (cGMP)-dependent pathway that may regulate cell functions. ANF (10^{-7}M) was reported to inhibit the isoprenaline-elevated L-type I_{Ca} without affecting the basal L-type I_{Ca} in frog and guinea pig single heart cells (Gisbert and Fischmeister, 1988; Sorbera and Morad, 1989) and both isoprenaline-elevated and basal L-type I_{Ca} in foetal human and 10-day-old embryonic chick heart cells (Fig. 14.18C and 14.18D). The L-type I_{Ca} in foetal human and 10-day-old chick embryonic single heart cells is more sensitive to blockade by ANF (2×10^{-9}M, Fig. 14.18D) than the Ca^{2+} current of frog and guinea pig heart single cells (10^{-7}M; Gisbert and Fischmeister 1988; Sorbera and Morad, 1989). The blockade of the L-type I_{Ca} by ANF is due to the increase in [cGMP]$_i$ caused by this hormone.

ANF was also found to activate a delayed outward K$^+$ current in

10-day-old embryonic chick heart cells in a dose-dependent manner (Fig. 14.19). The increase in K^+ current caused by ANF is not due to the increase in $[cGMP]_i$ caused by this hormone. Neither the T-type I_{Ca} nor the TTX-sensitive I_{Na} in either foetal human or 10-day-old embryonic chick heart single cells is affected by ANF. It is possible that the activation of K^+ current by ANF could be due to direct coupling of ANF receptor to K^+ channels. The L-type Ca^{2+} antagonist and the K^+ agonist effect of ANF in single heart cells may explain the decrease in the duration of the action potential and the negative inotropic effects of this hormone.

Insulin, a very well known hormone, is also reported to affect ion movement across the plasma membrane. This hormone also increases glucose and amino acid transport as well Na^+ efflux and hyperpolarizes the membrane potential (Moore (1983) and references therein). It is worth pointing out that the concentrations of insulin used in the literature were much greater than the normal plasma concentration of about 0.5 nM. The action of insulin upon membrane functions such as glucose transport and Na^+/K^+ pump has been proposed to be mediated by an increase in cytoplasmic Ca^{2+} (Moore (1983) and references therein).

In cultured single atrial cells from diabetic patients, insulin had no effect on the L-type I_{Ca}; however, in 10-day-old embryonic chick single heart cells, as well as in single cells of foetal human heart and atrial cells from diabetic patients, relatively low concentrations of insulin were found

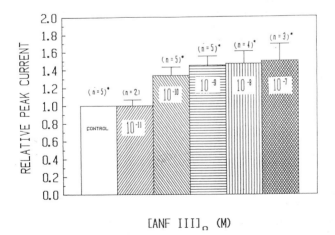

Fig. 14.19 Dose-dependence of ANF III effect on I_K in 10-day-old chick embryo heart single cell. The relative peak I_K amplitude increased by $43 \pm 3.0\%$ in the presence of 10^{-10}M ANF. Further increase was seen with 10^{-9}M ANF III. At concentrations of 10^{-8} and 10^{-7}M, there was no additional increase in I_K amplitude. ($*P<0.005$). (Bkaily *et al.*, unpublished results.)

to increase intracellular free Ca^{2+} by activating R-type Ca^{2+} channels (Fig. 14.20). The insulin-sensitive Ca^{2+} influx was sensitive to the dihydropyridine Ca^{2+}-blocker PN 200-110 (Bkaily et al., 1992a) (Plate 14.3) but insensitive to nifedipine, ATP and cyclic nucleotide. The activation of Ca^{2+} influx in heart cells by insulin may in part explain the positive inotropic action in heart muscle and the hypertensive action of this hormone.

Cardiomyopathy

Single heart cells can also be isolated from biopsy material of diseased hearts or from hearts of animal models such as streptozotocin-induced diabetic rats (Horackova and Murphy, 1988) and hereditary cardio-myopathic hamster (Fig. 14.21C, D, G and H).

Hereditary cardiomyopathy in hamsters provides unique possibilities for studying the pathology and clinical course of primary congestive cardiomyopathies. This autosomal recessive disorder is readily transmiss-ible with 100% incidence in the offspring, although the defective gene has not yet been identified. The cardiomyopathy develops in characteristic well-defined predictable stages (Jasmin and Proschek, 1984). Verapamil (an L-type Ca^{2+} blocker) and isoproterenol (an L-type Ca^{2+} activator),

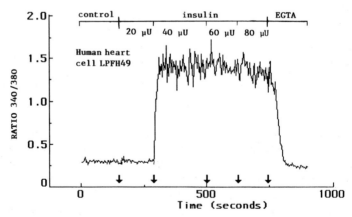

Fig. 14.20 Insulin induced a sustained increase in intracellular free Ca^{2+} by opening R-type Ca^{2+} channels in single heart cells. Using the fura-2 Ca^{2+} measurement technique, addition of 20 μU of insulin had no effect on $[Ca]_i$ in heart cells from a 20-week-old human foetus. Increasing the concentration of insulin up to 40 μU immediately caused a fast sustained increase in $[Ca]_i$. Reduction of extracellular Ca^{2+} with EGTA reversed the effect of the insulin-induced increase in $[Ca]_i$. (Bkaily et al., unpublished results.)

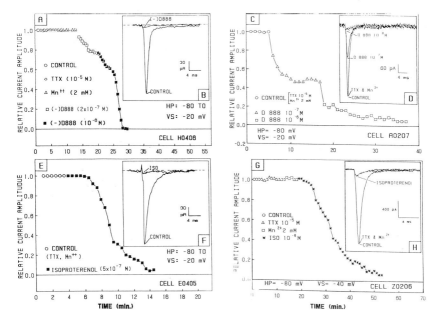

Fig. 14.21 Blockade of the fast transient TTX- and Mn^{2+}-insensitive Na^+ current in single heart cells from a 10-week-old human foetus and newborn cardiomyopathic hamster by $(-)$ D888 and isoproterenol (ISO). (A,C) Time-course of inhibition of the peak TTX- and Mn^{2+}-insensitive Na^+ current by $(-)$ D888 in heart single cells of both human foetus and newborn cardiomyopathic hamster respectively. (B,D) Current traces in the absence and presence of $(-)$ D888. (E,G) Time-course of inhibition of the peak TTX- and Mn^{2+}-insensitive I_{Na} by the L-type Ca^{2+} channel activator, isoproterenol, in single cells of both 10-week-old human foetus and newborn cardiomyopathic hamster respectively. (F,H) Current traces in the absence and presence of isoproterenol. (Bkaily *et al.*, unpublished results.)

which have opposing effects on L-type I_{Ca}, were highly efficient in preventing the development of cardiac necrotic changes in cardiomyopathic hamster (Jasmin *et al.* (1991) and references therein). Necrotic changes in cardiomyopathic hamsters become fully expressed at the critical age of 55 days. However, no biochemical or morphological changes were found in young cardiomyopathic hamsters. At this stage of development, early-embryonic TTX- and Mn^{2+}-insensitive ft slow Na^+ channels were detected in newborn cardiomyopathic hamster (Jasmin *et al.*, 1991). This ft slow I_{Na} has the same kinetics as the one reported in 3-day-old chick embryonic heart cells (Fig. 22A). A similar TTX- and Mn^{2+}-insensitive slow I_{Na} was found in 10–19-week-old human foetal single heart cells. This early foetal slow Na^+ current was similar in its kinetics and

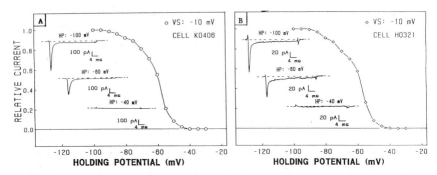

Fig. 14.22 Steady-state inactivation curves of the ft TTX- and Mn^{2+}-insensitive Na^+ current in single cells of 10-week-old human foetus (A) and newborn cardiomyopathic hamster (B). (Bkaily *et al.*, unpublished results.)

pharmacology to the slow Na^+ channels in newborn cardiomyopathic heart cells (Fig. 14.22A and B and Table 14.2). This current in both early fetal human and new born cardiomyopathic hamster heart cells was blocked by the L-type Ca^{2+} current blocker $(-)$D888 and the L-type Ca^{2+} current activator isoproterenol (Fig. 14.21). The blockade of this

Table 14.2

Pharmacology of the TTX- and Mn^{2+}-insensitive Na^+ current in human foetus, 3-day-old chick embryo and cardiomyopathic hamster

Human fetus	3-day-old chick embryo	Conc. (M)	Substances	Conc. (M)	Cardiomyopathic hamster
N.D.	+	10^{-5}	Nifedipine	10^{-5}	+
−	−	10^{-3}	Cadmium	10^{-3}	−
−	−	10^{-4}	Nickel	10^{-4}	−
−	−	10^{-4}	Lanthanum	10^{-4}	N.D.
−	−	10^{-3}	Cobalt	10^{-3}	−
+++	+++	10^{-4}	Azelastine	10^{-4}	+++
+++	+++	10^{-5}	D-88	10^{-7}	+++
N.D.	− +	10^{-5}	Verapamil	10^{-5}	− +
N.D.	− +	10^{-5}	D-600	10^{-5}	− +
+++	+++	10^{-10}	Apamin	10^{-6}	+++
N.D.	+++	10^{-8}	Melittin	10^{-8}	+
++	++	10^{-3}	8Br-cAMP	10^{-3}	N.D.
++	+++	10^{-3}	8Br-cGMP	10^{-3}	N.D.
+++	+++	10^{-8}	Isoproterenol	10^{-8}	+++
+++	+++	10^{-8}	Propranolol	10^{-8}	+++

+, inhibition; −, no effect; N.D., not determined.

early foetal slow Na^+ channel by the L-type Ca^{2+} blockers and Ca^{2+} activator may explain the prevention of cardiac necrotic development in cardiomyopathic hamster by these agents. Thus, single heart cells from diseased hearts are a good model for studying the beneficial effects as well as toxicity of substances.

Discussion and Conclusions

This chapter attempts to give a brief, and perhaps oversimplified, summary of cultured heart cells as model systems for studying the physiology, pharmacology and toxicology of myocardial cells. The general techniques used are briefly described, and references are given so that the reader can study any specific topic in greater detail. The types of single cell preparations commonly used are given, and some of the advantages and disadvantages of working with single heart cells are summarized.

In order to provide the reader with a reference point with which to assess the functional state of myocardial cells in culture, a brief description is given of some of the key properties of the cells that change during normal development of the heart *in situ*. It is demonstrated that the cells in standard monolayer cultures (primary) initially isolated from old embryonic hearts usually possess the characteristics of cells in intact young embryonic hearts, that is, they tend to revert back to the young embryonic state ("partial differentiation"). Reverted cultured heart cells possess few or no functional fast Na^+ channels and have a low P_K, thus resulting in a low RP, automaticity and slow-rising TTX-insensitive and Mn^{2+}-sensitive APs. In contrast, cells in spherical reaggregate cultures often retain (or regain) their initial highly differentiated electrical properties: they have stable RPs and fast-rising TTX-sensitive APs. However, some spherical reaggregates contain cells that possess reverted properties. Many factors, some unknown, appear to influence the degree of differentiation observed in cultured heart cells. These factors may include: the embryonic age of the hearts, possible damage during cell separation, plating density, reaggregation, composition of the culture medium, period in culture and presence of fibroblasts. The cultured cells retain their pharmacological receptors. The ultrastructure of the cultured myocardial cells reverts to the early embryonic state even in those cases in which the cell membrane remains highly differentiated.

It is apparent from the data presented in this chapter that the electrophysiology as well as the pharmacology of single heart cells from different species including man are very similar. These single heart cells can be obtained from necropsy or biopsy material. Thus, these preparations permit toxicological evaluation of compounds in animals and man on an equal basis which cannot be achieved in conventional *in vivo* toxicological testing. The results presented in this chapter demonstrate that it is possible to obtain responses *in vitro* using single heart cells that can explain results obtained *in vivo*. The most important feature of using single heart cells is that this preparation not only gives results close to responses obtained *in vivo* but also explains why, how and where the drug is acting. This preparation is also the only model that can be used to check whether the drug is acting directly on heart muscle or not. An example of this was given in the section dealing with the K^+-channel opener, cromakalim. This new drug was reported *in vivo* to lower blood pressure and produce reflex tachycardia (Buckingham *et al.*, 1986). Using single heart cells, it has been shown that at clinical concentrations it acts directly on heart cells.

In order to determine the cardiotoxicity of a substance, one must study the effect of a compound not only on a single type of receptor or channel but also on other channel types. This will permit us to obtain a relatively good picture of the possible degree and nature of the toxicity of a drug. If human heart cells are not used, species specificity must be ascertained by using single heart cells of a variety of animal species.

In conclusion, single heart cells can be used to study and to answer a wide variety of multidisciplinary questions that are difficult or impossible to answer using intact cardiac muscle or *in vivo*. This macroscopic small heart model permits the use of new techniques for measuring the biological activity of heart muscle and enables a better understanding of cellular mechanisms of toxicity. It therefore provides a perfect screening model for assessing new compounds in both animals and human beings. Nevertheless, this *in vitro* model should be used in conjunction with animal testing.

Acknowledgements

The work on which this chapter is based was supported by grants from the CRMC (MT 16496) and FQMC. The work dealing with PN 200-110 was supported by a grant from Sandoz Canada Inc. I am a Merck-Frosst-FRSQ Professor. These studies were performed in my laboratory by Mr A. Sculptoreanu, Miss D. Jacques, Miss L. Potvin and Miss N. Perron. I thank Dr C. Fong for reading the manuscript.

References

Albright, G.A. (1979). *Anesthesiology* **51**, 285–287.

Altschuld, R.A., Gibb, L. and Kruger, F.A. (1980). *Fed. Proc.* **39**, 1787 (Abstr.).

Anderson, P.A.V. (1987). *J. Exp. Biol.* **133**, 231–248.

Bean, B.P. (1985). *J. Physiol. (London)* **86**, 1–30.

Bean, B.P. (1989). *Annu. Rev. Physiol.* **51**, 367–384.

Bernard, C. (1976). *In* "Development and Physiological Correlates of Cardiac Muscle" (M. Lieberman and T. Sano, eds), pp. 169–184. Raven Press, New York.

Berry, M.N., Friend, D.S. and Scheuer, J. (1970). *Circ. Res.* **26**, 679–687.

Bkaily, G. (1990). *In* "Frontier in Smooth Muscle Research" (N. Sperelakis and J.D. Woods, eds), pp. 507–515. Allan R. Liss Inc., New York.

Bkaily, G. and Sperelakis, N. (1985). *Am. J. Physiol.* **248**, H745–749.

Bkaily, G., Sperelakis, N. and Doane, J. (1984). *Am. J. Physiol.* **247**, H1018–H1026.

Bkaily, G., Sperelakis, N., Renaud, J.-F. and Payet, M.D. (1985). *Am. J. Physiol.* **248**, H961–965.

Bkaily, G., Caillé, J.-P., Payet, M.D., Peyrow, M., Sauvé, R., Renaud, J.-F. and Sperelakis, N. (1988a). *Can. J. Physiol. Pharmacol.* **66**, 731–736.

Bkaily, G., Jacques, D., Yamamoto, T., Sculptoreanu, A., Payet, M.D. and Sperelakis, N. (1988b). *Can. J. Physiol. Pharmacol.* **66**, 1017–1022.

Bkaily, G., Payet, M.D., Benabderrazik, M., Renaud, J.-F., Sauvé, R., Bacaner, M.B. and Sperelakis, N. (1988c). *Can. J. Physiol. Pharmacol.* **66**, 190–196.

Bkaily, G., Peyrow, M., Sculptoreanu, A., Jacques, D., Regoli, D. and Sperelakis, N. (1988d). *Pfluegers Arch.* **412**, 448–450.

Bkaily, G., Peyrow, M., Yamamoto, T., Sculptoreanu, A., Jacques, D. and Sperelakis, N. (1988e). *Mol. Cell. Biochem.* **80**, 59–72.

Bkaily, G., Jasmin, G., Constantin T., Proshek, L., Yamamato, T., Sculptoreanu, A., Peyrow, M. and Jacques, D. (1990). *Muscle and Nerve* **13**, 939–948.

Bkaily, G., Jacques, D., Sculptoreanu, A., Yamamoto, T., Carrier, D., Vigneault, D. and Sperelakis, N. (1991). *J. Mol. Cell. Cardiol.* **23**, 25–39.

Bloom, S., Brady, A.J. and Langer, G.A. (1974). *J. Mol. Cell. Cardiol.* **6**, 137–147.

Bolli, P., Muller, F.B., Linder, L., Raine, A.E.G., Resink, T.J., Erne, P., Kiowski, W., Ritz, R. and Buhler, F.R. (1987). *Circulation* **75**, 221–228.

Bossu, J.-L. and Fletz, A. (1984) *Neurosci. Lett.* **51**, 241–246.

Brenner, G.M. and Wenzel, D.G. (1972). *Toxicol. Appl. Pharmacol.* **23**, 251–262.

Brown, A.M. and Yatani, A. (1986). *In* "The Heart and Cardiovascular Systems" (H.A. Fozzard, E. Haber, R.B. Jennings, A.M. Katz and H.E. Morgan, eds), pp. 627–636. Raven Press, New York.

Brown, A.M., Lee, K.S. and Powell, T. (1981a). *J. Physiol. (London)*, **318**, 479–500.

Brown, A.M., Lee, K.S. and Powell, T. (1981b). *J. Physiol. (London)*, **318**, 455–477.

Buckingham, R.E., Clapham, J.C., Hamilton, T.C., Longman, S.D., Norton, J. and Poyser, R.H. (1986). *J. Cardiovasc. Pharmacol.* **8**, 798–804.

Burrows, M.T. (1912). *J. Med. Assoc.* **55**, 2057–2058.

Callaghan, J.T., Goldberg, M.R. and Brunelle, R. (1988). *Drugs*, **36**, S77–S82.

Carbone, E., Prestipino, G., Spadavecchia, L., Franciolini, F. and Possani, L.D. (1982). *Pfluegers Arch.* **408**, 423–431.

Carlson, E.C., Grosso, D.S., Romero, S.A., Frangakis, C.J., Byus, C.V. and Bressler, R. (1978). *J. Mol. Cell. Cardiol.* **10**, 449–459.

Castle, N.A., Haylett, D.G. and Jenkinson, D.H. (1989). *Trends Neurosci.* **12**, 59–65.

Cauvin, C., Tejerina, M. and Van Breemen, C. (1987). *Am. J. Physiol.* **253**, H1612–H1617.

Clark, M.G., Gannon, B.J., Bodkin, N., Pattern, G.S. and Berry, M.N. (1978). *J. Mol. Cell. Cardiol.* **10**, 1101–1121.

Clarkson, C.W. and Hondeghem, L.M. (1985). *Anesthesiology* **62**, 396–405.

Cohen, M.L. and Colbert, W.E. (1986). *Drug Dev. Res.* **7**, 111–124.

Coyle, D.E. and Sperelakis, N. (1987). *J. Pharmacol. Exp. Ther.* **242**, 1001–1005.

Davis, N.L. and deJong, R.H. (1982). *Anesth. Analog.* **61**, 62–64.

DeHaan, R.L. (1967). *Dev. Biol.* **16**, 216–249.

Delaflotte, S., Auguet, M., Pirotzky, E., Clostre, F. and Braguet, P. (1989). *J. Auton. Pharmacol.* **9**, 211–219.

Earle, W.R., Sandford, K.K., Evans, V.J., Waltz, H.K. and Shannon, J.E., Jr. (1951). *J. Natl. Cancer Inst.* **12**, 133–154.

Enemar, A., Falck, B. and Hakanson, R. (1965). *Dev. Biol.* **11**, 268–283.

Escande, D. (1989). *Pfluegers Arch.* **414**, S93–S98.

Escande, D., Thuringer, D., Leguern, S. and Cavero, I. (1988). *Biochem. Biophys. Res. Commun.* **154**, 620–625.

Farmer, B.B., Harris, R.A., Jolly, W.W., Hathaway, D.R., Hatzberg, A., Watanabe, A.M., Whitlow, A.L. and Besch, H.R., Jr. (1977). *Arch. Biochem. Biophys.* **179**, 545–558.

Farmer, B.B., Mancina, M., Williams, E.S. and Watanabe, A.M. (1983). *Life Sci.* **33**, 1–8.

Follmer, C.H., Tex Eick, R.E. and Yeh, J.Z. (1987). *J. Physiol. (London)* **384**, 169–197.

Fox, A.P., Nowycky, M.C. and Tsien, R.W. (1987a). *J. Physiol. (London)* **394**, 149–172.

Fox, A.P., Nowycky, M.C. and Tsien, R.W. (1987b). *J. Physiol. (London)* **394**, 173–200.

Freeman, S.E., Leake, B., Sadedin, D.R. and Gray, P.J. (1984). *Cardiovasc. Res.* **18**, 233–243.

Freer, R.J., Pappano, A.J., Peach, M.J., Bing, K.T., McLean, M.J., Vogel, S. and Sperelakis, N. (1976). *Circ. Res.* **39**, 178–182.

Garber, S.S. (1988). *Biophys. J.* **54**, 767–776.

Gisbert, M.-P. and Fischmeister, R. (1988). *Circ. Res.* **62**, 660–667.

Glick, M.R., Burns, S.H. and Reddy, W.J. (1974). *Anal. Biochem.* **61**, 32–42.

Goldberg, M.R. (1988). *J. Cardiovasc. Pharmacol.* **12**, Suppl. 2, 541–549.

Gordon, H.P. and Brice, M.C. (1974). *Exp. Cell. Res.* **85**, 311–318.

Goshima, K. (1970). *Exp. Cell. Res.* **63**, 124–130.

Grossett, A. and Hicks, P.E. (1986). *Br. J. Pharmacol.* **89**, 500 p.

Hagiwara, N., Irisawa, H. and Kameyama, M. (1988). *J. Physiol. (London)* **359**, 233–253.

Halbert, S.P., Bruderer, R. and Lin, T.M. (1971). *J. Exp. Med.* **133**, 677–695.

Hamilton, T.C. and Weston, H.J. (1989). *Gen. Pharmacol.* **20**, 1–19.

Hille, B. (1975). *Biophys. J.* **15**, 615–618.

Hollenberg, M. (1971). *Circ. Res.* **28**, 148–157.
Hondeghem, L.M. and Katzung, B.G. (1984). *Annu. Rev. Pharmacol. Toxicol.* **24**, 387–423.
Horackova, M. and Murphy, M.G. (1988). *Pfluegers Arch.* **411**, 564–572.
Horres, C.R., Aiton, F.J. and Lieberman, M. (1979). *Am. J. Physiol.* **236**, C163–C170.
Ikeda, S. and Schofield, G.G. (1987). *J. Physiol. (London)* **389**, 255–270.
Isenberg, G. and Klockner, U. (1980). *Nature* **284**, 358–360.
Isenberg, G. and Klockner, V. (1982). *Pfluegers Arch.* **335**, 6–18.
Ishima, Y. (1968). *Proc. Jpn. Acad.* **44**, 170–177.
Jacobson, S.L. (1977). *Cell. Struct. Funct.* **2**, 1–9.
Jacobson, S.L. and Piper, H.M. (1986). *J. Mol. Cell. Cardiol.* **18**, 661–678.
Jacobson, S.L., Kennedy, C.B. and Mealing, A.R. (1983). *Can. J. Physiol. Pharmacol.* **61**, 1312–1316.
Jasmin, G. and Proschek, L. (1984). *Can. J. Physiol. Pharmacol.* **62**, 891–898.
Jasmin, G., Pasternac, A., Bkaily, G. and Proschek, L. (1991). *In* "The Calcium Channels: their Properties, Functions and Clinical Relevance" (L. Hurwitz, L.D. Partridge and J.K. Leach eds), pp. 295–326. CRC Press, Boston.
Kao, C.Y. and Nishiyama, A. (1986). Action of saxitoxin on peripheral neuromuscular systems. *J. Physiol. (London)* **180**, 50–66.
Karsten, U., Kossler, A., Janiszewski, E. and Wollenberger, A. (1973). *In Vitro* **9**, 139–146.
Kobayashi, M., Ochi, R. and Ohizumi, Y. (1987). *Br. J. Pharmacol.* **92**, 665–671.
Kotelko, D.M., Shnider, S.M., Dailey, P.A., Brizgys, R.V., Levinson, G., Shapiro, W.A., Koike, M. and Rosen, M.A. (1984). *Anesthesiology* **60**, 10–18.
Kuzuya, F., Naito, M., Asai, K.-L., Shibata, K. and Iwata, Y. (1983). *Artery* **12**, 51–59.
LeDouarin, G., Renaud, J.-F., Renaud, D. and Coraboeuf, E. (1974). *J. Mol. Cell. Cardiol.* **6**, 523–529.
Lee, K.S., Weeks, T.A., Kao, R.L., Akaike, N. and Brown, A.M. (1979). *Nature* **278**, 269–271.
Lewis, W.H. (1928). *Carnegie Inst. Wash. Contrib. Embryol. No.* **90**, 18, 1–12.
Lynch, C. (1986). *Anesth. Analg.* **65**, 551–559.
Marty, A. and Neher, E. (1983). *In* "Single Channel Recording" (ed B. Sackmann and E. Neher), pp. 107–172. Plenum Press, New York.
Marx, G.F. (1984). *Anesthesiology* **60**, 3–5.
McCleskey, E.W., Fox, A.P., Feldman, D.H., Cruz, L.J., Olivera, B.M., Tsien, R.W. and Yoshikami, D. (1987). *Proc. Natl. Acad. Sci. U.S.A.* **84**, 4327–4331.
McLean, M.J. and Sperelakis, N. (1974). *Exp. Cell. Res.* **86**, 351–364.
McLean, M.J., Lapsley, R.A., Shigenobu, K., Murad, F. and Sperelakis, N. (1975). *Dev. Biol.* **42**, 196–201.
McLean, M.J., Renaud, J.-F., Sperelakis, N. and Niu, M.C. (1976). *Science* **191**, 297–299.
Mettler, F.A., Grundfest, H., Crain, S.M. and Murray, M.R. (1952). *Trans. Am. Neurol. Assoc.* **77**, 52–53.
Mitra, R. and Morad, M. (1985). *Am. J. Physiol.* **249**, H1056–H1060.
Moore, R.D. (1983). *Biochim. Biophys. Acta* **737**, 1–49.
Nag, A.C., Fischman, D.A., Aumont, M.C. and Zak, R. (1977). *Tissue and Cell* **9**, 419–436.
Nathan, R.D., Pooler, J.P. and DeHaan, R.L. (1976). *J. Gen. Physiol.* **67**, 27–44.

Nishio, M., Muramatsu, I., Kigoshi, S. and Fujiwara, M. (1988). *Naunyn-Schmiedeberg's Arch. Pharmacol.* **337**, 440–446.

Osterrieder, W. (1988). *Naunyn-Schmiedeberg's Arch. Pharmacol.* **337**, 93–97.

Pandey, K.N., Inagami, T., Girard, P.R., Kwo, J.F. and Misono, K.S. (1987). *Biochem. Biophys. Res. Commun.* **148**, 589–595.

Pappano, A.J. (1976). *In* "Developmental and Physiological Correlates of Cardiac Muscle" (M. Lieberman and T. Sano, eds), pp. 235–248. Raven Press, New York.

Patlak, J.B. and Ortiz, M. (1985). *J. Gen. Physiol.* **86**, 89–104.

Patten, B.M. (1956). *U. Mich. Med. Bull.* **22**, 1–21.

Pelhate, M., Laufer, J., Pichon, Y. and Zlotkin, E. (1984). *J. Physiol.* **79**, 309–317.

Poste, G. (1971). *Exp. Cell Res.* **65**, 359–367.

Powell, T. and Twist, V.W. (1976). *Biochem. Biophys. Res. Commun.* **72**, 327–333.

Powell, T., Steen, E.M., Twist, V.W. and Woolf, N. (1978). *J. Mol. Cell. Cardiol.* **10**, 287–292.

Powell, T., Sturridge, M.S., Suvarna, S.K., Terrar, D.A. and Twist, V.W. (1981). *Br. Med. J.* **283**, 1013–1015.

Pretlow, T.E., Glick, M.R. and Reddy, W.J. (1972). *Am. J. Pathol.* **67**, 215–223.

Rajs, J., Sundberg, M., Sundby, G.-B., Danell, N., Tornling, G., Biberfeld, P. and Jakobsson, S.W. (1978). *Exp. Cell. Res.* **115**, 183–189.

Renaud, J.-F., Sperelakis, N. and LeDouarin, G. (1978). *J. Mol. Cell. Cardiol.* **10**, 281–286.

Renaud, J.-F., Bkaily, G., Benabderrazik, M., Jacques, D. and Sperelakis, N. (1988). *Mol. Cell. Biochem.* **80**, 73–78.

Romanoff, A. (1960). *The Avian Embryo: Structure and Functional Development*, pp. 1–1305. Macmillan, New York.

Rosenquist, G. and DeHaan, R.L. (1966). *Contrib. Embryol. Carnegie Inst. Washington* **263**, 113–121.

Rosenthal, M.D. and Warshaw, J.B. (1973). *J. Cell Biol.* **58**, 332–339.

Schanne, O.F. and Bkaily, G. (1981). *Can. J. Physiol.* **59**, 443–467.

Schneider, J.A. and Sperelakis, N. (1975). *J. Mol. Cell. Cardiol.* **7**, 249–273.

Seyama, I., Yamada, K., Kato, R. and Masutani, T. (1988). *Biophys. J.* **53**, 271–274.

Shigenobu, K. and Sperelakis, N. (1971). *J. Mol. Cell. Cardiol.* **3**, 271–286.

Shimada, Y. and Fischman, D.A. (1976). *In* "Developmental and Physiological Correlates of Cardiac Muscle" (M. Lieberman and T. Sano, eds), pp. 81–102. Raven Press, New York.

Shimada, Y., Moscona, A.A. and Fischman, D.A. (1974). *Dev. Biol.* **36**, 428–446.

Sorbera, L.A. and Morad, M. (1989). *Science* **247**, 969–973.

Sperelakis, N. (1967). *In* "Electrophysiology and Ultrastructure of the Heart" (T. Sano, V. Mizuhina and K. Matsuda, eds), pp. 81–108. Bunkodo, Tokyo.

Sperelakis, N. (1972a). *In* "Electrical Phenomena in the Heart" (W.C. DeMello, eds), pp. 1–61. Academic Press, New York.

Sperelakis, N. (1972b). *Biochim. Biophys. Acta* **266**, 230–237.

Sperelakis, N. (1978). Proceedings of the Conference on Cardiovascular Toxicology, *Environ. Health Perspect.* **26**, 243–267.

Sperelakis, N. (1980). *In* "The Slow Inward Current and Cardiac Arrhythmias"

(D.P. Zipes, J.C. Bailey and V. Elharrar, eds), pp. 221–262. Martinus Nijhoff, The Hague.

Sperelakis, N. (1981). *In* "Cardiac Toxicology" (T. Balazs, ed), vol. 1, pp. 39–108. CRC Press, Boca Raton, Florida.

Sperelakis, N. (1982). *In* "Cardiovascular Toxicology" (E.W. VanStee, ed.). Raven Press, New York.

Sperelakis, N. and Bkaily, G. (1987). *In* "*In vitro* Methods in Toxicology" (C.K. Atterwill and C.E. Steele, eds), pp. 58–108. University Press, Cambridge.

Sperelakis, N. and McLean, M.J. (1978a). *In* "Recent Advances in Studies on Cardiac Structure and Metabolism" (T. Kobayashi, Y. Ito and G. Rona, eds), vol. 12, pp. 645–666. University Park Press, Baltimore.

Sperelakis, N. and McLean, M.J. (1978b). *In* "Developmental Aspects – Fetal and Newborn Cardiovascular Physiology" (L.D. Longo, ed.), vol. 1, pp. 191–236. Garland Press, New York.

Sperelakis, N. and Shigenobu, K. (1972). *J. Gen. Physiol.* **60**, 430–453.

Sperelakis, N., Shigenobu, K. and McLean, M.J. (1976). *In* "Developmental and Physiological Correlates of Cardiac Muscle" (M. Lieberman and T. Sano, eds), pp. 209–234. Raven Press, New York.

Sperelakis, N., Bkaily, G., Sada, H. and Kojima, M. (1988). *In* "Fetal and Neonatal Development" (C.T. Jones, ed.), pp. 113–124. Perinatalogy Press, New York.

Steinberg, M.I., Ertel, P., Smallwood, J.K., Wyss, V. and Zimmerman, K. (1988). *J. Cardiovasc. Pharmacol.* **12**, S30–S40.

Strichartz, G. (1984). *J. Gen. Physiol.* **84**, 281–305.

Suignard, G. (1979). *J. Physiol.* **75**, 733–740.

Thakkar, J.K. and Sperelakis, N. (1987). *J. Dev. Physiol.* **9**, 497–505.

Vahouny, G.V., Starkweather, R. and Davis, C. (1970). *Science* **167**, 1616–1618.

Vahouny, G.V., Wei, R.W., Tamboli, A. and Albert, E.N. (1979). *J. Mol. Cell. Cardiol.* **11**, 339–357.

Weiss, L. (1959). *Exp. Cell Res.* **17**, 499–507.

Wenzel, D.G., Wheatley, J.W. and Byrd, G.D. (1970). *Toxicol. Appl. Pharmacol.* **17**, 774–785.

Weston, A.H. and Abbott, A. (1987). *Trends Pharmacol. Sci.* **8**, 283–284.

Wheeler, K.P., Watt, D.D. and Lazdunski, M. (1983). *Pfluegers Arch.* **397**, 164–165.

Wheeler, D.M., Bradley, E.L. and Woods, W.T. (1988). *Anesthesiology* **68**, 201–212.

Yanagisawa, T., Hashimoto, H. and Taira, N. (1988). *Br. J. Pharmacol.* **95**, 393–398.

Yatani, A., Kirsch, G.E., Possani, L.D. and Brown, A.M. (1988a). *Am. J. Physiol.* **254**, H443–H451.

Yatani, A., Kunze, D.L. and Brown, A.M. (1988b). *Am. J. Physiol.* **254**, H140–147.

Discussion

P. Laduron

Dr Bkaily has a beautiful model for this pharmacological dissection, but the problem is that the system is devoid of neuronal control. I think neuronal control is very important in cardiotoxicity.

G. Bkaily
When a drug is tested in our laboratory it is not tested only *in vitro* but also in animals and later in the clinic. The main objective for this meeting is to demonstrate that it is a good model for the study of toxicology *in vitro*. I could also show some *in vivo* or clinical data. We usually go from the channel receptor up to the patient.

R. Ulrich
Cardiac myocytes are notoriously difficult to load with fura-2. The dye tends to load into the mitochondria. Is Dr Bkaily confident that his cytosolic calcium measurements are indeed cytosolic calcium and not rather reflecting total calcium?

G. Bkaily
We do not only use AM fura-2 for this but we also couple the patch clamp with this technique, so that only the acidic form of fura-2 is used. This goes only to the cytoplasm, never to either the mitochondria or to the sarcoplasmic reticulum. We are aware that this is one of the limitations of using the AM fura-2 molecule.

15

Primary Cultures of Rat Cardiac Myocytes as Tools in Assessing Drug-Induced Cardiotoxicity

R.G. ULRICH*, D.K. PETRELLA†,
D.G. BRANSTETTER*, A.E. BERGER‡,
L. PUDDINGTON‡, E. SUN* AND
C.T. CRAMER*

*Investigative Toxicology, †Drug Development Toxicology and
‡Cell Biology Research Units, The Upjohn Company,
Kalamazoo, MI 49001, USA

Introduction

Primary cultures of cardiac cells have been used over the past several decades as an *in vitro* model to study a variety of cardiac functions, including muscle cell growth and differentiation, events related to stimulus-coupled and spontaneous contraction, and regulation of cellular activities such as maintenance of membrane potentials, ion balance and energy metabolism. In addition to studies on normal function, many investigators have explored myocardial cell function associated with the pharmacological activity of drugs and *in vivo* pathologies such as ischaemia and adverse reactions to xenobiotic exposure.

IN VITRO METHODS IN TOXICOLOGY
ISBN 0-12-388175-7

Since the deleterious side effects of drugs are initiated at the cellular level, it is of considerable benefit to understand drug interactions at this level. Cultured heart cells provide a model for investigating these interactions in an environment that is chemically and physically uniform and free from the influence of blood flow, hormonal factors and central nervous system controls. The application of cultured beating heart cells to the investigation of drug toxicity essentially began with the work of Wenzel *et al.* (1970) on nicotine, based on the earlier studies by Kokubu and Pollak (1962) on non-beating cells from rabbit heart. With the utility of cell culture techniques apparent, studies were expanded to include a variety of drugs with known or suspected cardiotoxic effects; for example, compounds representing a multitude of chemical entities including tricyclic antidepressants, caffeine, diazepam, amphotericin B, chlorpromazine and clofibrate have been examined by Acosta and colleagues (reviewed by Acosta *et al.*, 1985) using neonatal rat heart cells. Heart cells for toxicological studies have been derived from several sources, but the most commonly used are neonatal and, to a lesser but increasing extent, adult rat heart. Studies on drug toxicity may be broadly divided into two categories: (1) those for the examination of several compounds within a structural class or with similar activities for comparative toxicity purposes (Acosta and Ramos, 1984; Wenzel and Cosma, 1984a,b) and (2) those for examining mechanisms of toxicity. Perhaps the most widely studied compounds in terms of the latter are the anthracyline antitumour agents studied by several laboratories (for example, see Seraydarian and Artaza, 1979; Lampidis *et al.*, 1980; Combs *et al.*, 1985; Chacon and Acosta, 1991). In the industrial laboratory, the use of cultured cells to examine several drugs for comparative toxicity purposes has the distinct advantages that only milligram amounts are required, thus keeping initial costs to a minimum, and minimizing the numbers of animals needed to make compound selections prior to full-scale drug-safety assessment. Alternatively, mechanistic studies enable us to determine risk more precisely and (ideally) design better drugs by establishing structure–toxicity relationships. As with other *in vitro* assays, the interpretation of data and extrapolation to *in vivo* requires caution.

To a great extent, the value of data obtained from *in vitro* experiments with heart cells is dependent on both the techniques used to isolate and culture cells and the techniques used for examination of cell function (assay end points). This chapter reviews several important considerations in using cultured neonatal heart cells to study drug toxicity *in vitro*, and includes examples from our own experiences as well as those of others found in the literature. The terms myocyte and muscle cell are used synonymously, and refer to cells that contain myofibrils and contract spontaneously. Non-muscle cells include fibroblasts and cells derived from the vasculature (endothelial and smooth muscle cells).

Isolation and Culture Techniques

Neonatal Rat Heart Cell Isolation

Procedures for isolation of neonatal heart cells were first described by Harary and Farley (1960, 1963). Improvements on technique evolved through contributions of several laboratories, particularly work by Mark and Strasser (1966), and Wenzel and Cosma (1984a,b). Hearts are removed from approximately twenty 1–5-day-old rat pups, with younger pups generally producing higher viability yields. Hearts or removed ventricles are minced into small pieces and incubated with gentle agitation in an enzyme solution, usually trypsin (Mark and Strasser, 1966) or trypsin with collagenase (Wenzel and Cosma, 1984a,b). Successive digestions (two or five) are pooled. The resultant digest is subjected to a separation technique (discussed below) and plated in Petri dishes. Plating efficiency of muscle cells can be increased by use of extracellular matrix components; several have been examined, including various collagens, fibronectin and laminin (Borg et al., 1984). In our hands, laminin (0.75 ml; 8 μg/ml; in medium per 35 mm dish) has provided the most satisfactory and consistent results (Ulrich et al., 1988). Additionally, the flattened morphology that myocytes assume on this matrix eases morphological assessments, and helps limit the surface area available for non-muscle cell proliferation. Cells remain in culture for 3–7 days before use; by this time they have established synchronously beating monolayers.

Muscle and Non-Muscle Cells

It is important to evaluate the cell population constituents; the population of cells in culture cannot be assumed to be homogeneous with regard to the muscle cell component. To the contrary, cell cultures that are relatively pure (80–90%) muscle cells on day 1 are generally 40% or more non-muscle cells by day 7 in culture (see Fig. 15.1). Although the myocytes retain potential for cell division (Kasten, 1972), the non-muscle cells proliferate considerably faster. Knowledge and acknowledgement of the non-muscle cell component are of particular importance when assessing compounds with specific toxicities towards the cardiac myocyte as opposed to other cell types, as illustrated in Figs 15.2 and 15.3. In this example, the toxicity of an unknown contaminant in an experimental compound

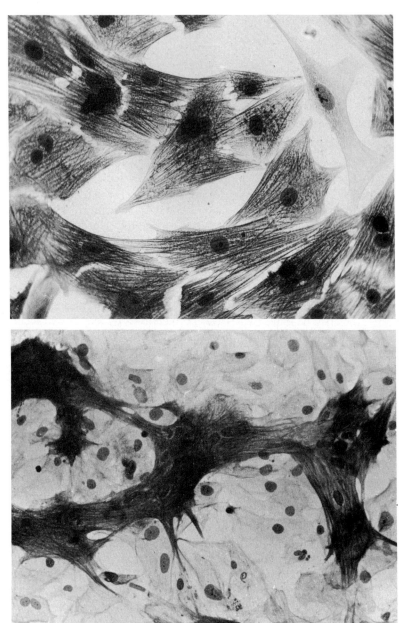

Fig. 15.1 Coomassie Blue R250-stained neonatal rat heart cells (a) purified by centrifugal elutriation and after 5 days in culture, and (b) heart cell cultures prepared by the pour-off technique. The muscle cell component, identified by densely stained myofibrils, is greater in procedure (a). Original magnification = 400×.

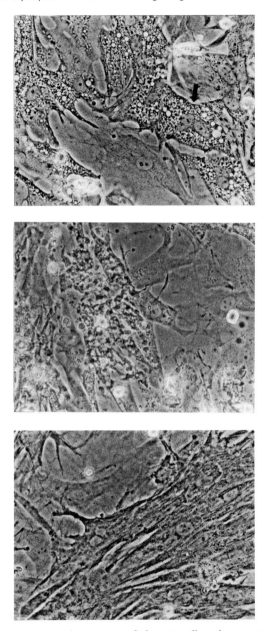

Fig. 15.2 Phase-contrast microscopy of heart cell cultures treated with an experimental compound containing an unknown contaminant indicates the toxicity to be specific for the muscle cell component; (a) low-dose culture shows vacuolation of the muscle cell (arrow); surrounding non-muscle cells are unaffected; (b) high-dose culture shows only non-muscle cells remaining viable in the culture; (c) control culture. Original magnification = 400×.

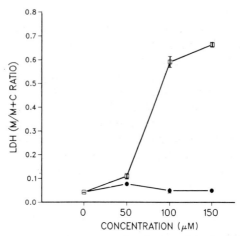

Fig. 15.3 Dose–response curve measuring lactate dehydrogenase (LDH) release from heart cell cultures illustrated in Fig. 15.2. The maximum response was 65%, which approximately coincides with the muscle cell component of these cultures at day 7. Activity for LDH is expressed as the ratio of medium levels to medium plus cell levels (total). □, drug treated; ●, vehicle control.

was assessed by morphology (Fig. 15.2) to be specific for the muscle cell component of 7-day-old cultures. The dose–response curve for enzyme release had a maximum value of 65% (Fig. 15.3), which approximately coincided with the muscle cell component of the culture; the non-muscle cells did not respond to the compound within the concentration range tested. From this it can be extrapolated that if a population of cells were to contain few muscle cells in proportion to non-muscle, the sensitivity of the assay (detection limits) would be greatly reduced. If relatively pure muscle cell populations cannot be obtained, studies can be designed that measure cardiac-specific isozymes (Van Der Laarse *et al.*, 1979) or that compare populations enriched for the various cell types (Wenzel and Cosma, 1984a,b).

Muscle cells can be distinguished from non-muscle cells by light microscopy combined with various staining methods; phase-contrast or similar methods of observing living cultures are not sufficient, since muscle and non-muscle cells are similar in overall morphology. For example, Marvin *et al.* (1979) have used Masson's trichrome to distinguish muscle from non-muscle cells, based on red (muscle cell) versus blue–grey (non-muscle cell) differential coloration. We have used the simple stain, Coomassie Blue R250, to distinguish cells that contain myofibrils (muscle cells) from those that do not (Ulrich *et al.*, 1988; see Fig. 15.1).

To enrich for muscle cells after enzyme digestion, two methods are currently in use. The first, described by Blondel *et al.* (1971), relies on differential attachment of the cell types; non-muscle cells attach quickly to the Petri dish and muscle cells are poured off and replated. This method yields populations that are 70–90% muscle cells. For greater purity, the second method, centrifugal elutriation of the suspension (Ulrich *et al.*, 1988), can be employed; this method yields populations >95% muscle cells. Regardless of which method is used, plating cells at high density (1.5×10^5 cells/cm^2) helps to limit the non-muscle cell growth. It is also possible to limit non-muscle cell growth by nutritional or serum restriction (Clark, 1976; Klein and Daood, 1985) or the use of antimitotics (Freyss-Beguin and Van Brussel, 1980; Libby, 1984); the latter method is generally less attractive when the cardiotoxic potential of drugs is examined because of potential interactions. Since protein binding is important for the solubility and delivery of many drugs, it is important that some serum should remain in the medium. The activity of the myocytes in culture can be enhanced by culture manipulations such as the addition of noradrenaline (Marino *et al.*, 1990) or coculture with autologous neurons (Lloyd and Marvin, 1990).

End Points for Assessing Toxicity

Determining the appropriate end points is perhaps the most difficult and most critical component in the application of heart cell cultures to drug toxicity studies. In order for data obtained from *in vitro* studies to have value in the drug candidate selection process, the end points for determining toxicity should correlate as much as possible with *in vivo* observations. Ideally, the *in vitro* assay end points are both mechanism- and target-organ-based, but this may require an extensive *in vivo* toxicology database on the parent or lead compound. Without meeting these criteria, however, the utility of the assay (*in vivo* relevance) is diminished, as encountered by Dorgelo *et al.* (1986), since compounds that are not cardiotoxic *in vivo* may artifactually inhibit function or produce toxicity *in vitro*.

For comparative studies it is usually necessary to examine many compounds in a given series, thus assays must remain simple and straightforward. For mechanistic studies, usually one one or two compounds are examined, and the complexity and specificity of the end point assay can be increased accordingly.

End Points for Comparative Studies

Comparative studies generally include comparisons of cell viability, light microscopy of cell morphology and contraction rate measurements. The first step in examining cell viability is to establish a dose–response curve for the presence of cytosolic enzymes in the tissue culture medium, usually lactate dehydrogenase (LDH) or creatine phosphokinase (CPK), relative to total enzyme activity or protein per plate and as a function of increasing drug concentration. During these experiments most technical details such as vehicle effects, drug solubility and stability are resolved, and the degree of tolerance (maximum tolerated or no toxic effect level) of cells to the drug is determined. Using the maximum tolerated dose, effects on cell morphology (i.e. bleb formation, vesiculation, loss of myofibrils) and contractile activity (change in rate or arrhythmia) that do not result in cell lysis can be evaluated, and a time–response curve, if appropriate, can be established. Contractile activity is sensitive to a variety of influences, including temperature and exposure to bright light, making quantification difficult» Contraction rates for control cultures can vary considerably from one preparation to another (normal range is 30–180 contractions per minute) and drugs that induce arrhythmias can produce different rates within a culture dish. As a result, values are usually recorded as percentage control or simply +/− to allow for comparison between isolations. To monitor cells with minimal light exposure, we use a SIT camera (Dage-MTI, Inc.) coupled to a Panasonic 6300 video

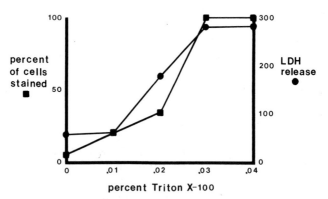

Fig. 15.4 Dose–response curve for myocytes treated with Triton X-100 comparing lactate dehydrogenase (LDH) in tissue culture medium (●) to uptake and staining with fluorescent antibodies against actin as determined by fluorescence microscopy (■). In this injury, cells release cytosolic enzymes through loss of plasma membrane integrity rather than release or rupture of blebs.

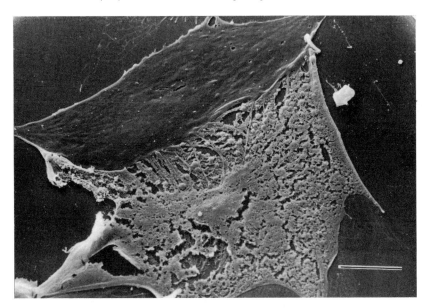

Fig. 15.5 Scanning electron micrograph of rat cardiac myocytes treated with 0.025% Triton X-100 illustrating an intact cell adjacent to a lysed cell. In these cultures, medium levels of cytosolic enzymes result from cell lysis rather than bleb rupture or release; blebs are not formed. Bar = 10 μm.

cassette recorder and time–date generator. This provides for a video tape record of morphological changes and contractile activity. For long-term observations, an incubator stage is required to maintain temperature and atmosphere. Contractile activity can be recorded by several means, such as a television monitor equipped with a photodiode detector (Lampidis *et al.*, 1980), closed-loop tracking of latex microspheres (Schuette *et al.*, 1987), or simply counting for on-screen timed video sequences.

End Points for Mechanistic Studies

For mechanistic studies, end points are selected depending on the *in vivo* effects for the drug. These end points evaluate a variety of cellular components and include closer examination of plasma and organellar membrane integrity, ultrastructural changes, functional and biochemical modifications.

Enzyme leakage alone may serve as a sufficient end point for mechanistic studies, such as those of Persoon-Rothert *et al.* (1989) using α-hydroxybutyrate dehydrogenase leakage to examine the modification of isoproterenol toxicity by various agents. Enzyme leakage methods may not provide an accurate assessment of viability when release of cellular materials is due to reversible cell injury rather than lysis. Such release may occur during the "tying-off" of surface blebs as discussed by Piper *et al.* (1984). For conditions that produce this form of injury, loss of plasma membrane integrity can be quantified using antibodies against muscle proteins. For example, injury produced by oxygen or nutrient deprivation was detected with cardiac myosin adsorbed to fluorescent microspheres, measured by fluorescence-activated cell sorting (FACS) (Khaw *et al.*, 1982). We have produced similar results in studies on oxygen deprivation or membrane-active drugs using fluorescein isothiocyanate (FITC)-labelled rabbit anti-actin antibodies. We have demonstrated a correlation between cell lysis and antibody staining by treating myocytes with the membrane-active detergent Triton X-100 in the presence of FITC–anti-actin. The dose–response curve for LDH release correlates with cell staining as determined by fluorescence microscopy (Fig. 15.4), and examination of cells by scanning electron microscopy (Fig. 15.5) shows that cells release enzyme by cell lysis rather than bleb formation. Having established this correlation, a series of experiments with oxygen-deprived myocytes were performed. Using analysis of fluorescence by FACS (Fig. 15.6), we found an increase in

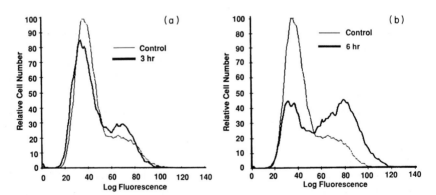

Fig. 15.6 Fluorescence-activated cell sorting of myocytes deprived of oxygen for 3–6 h in the presence of fluorescein isothiocyanate (FITC)-labelled anti-actin antibodies shows a shift in fluorescence from non-specific (left peak) to FITC-specific (right peak) fluorescence at 3 h (a) which is increased further at 6 h (b) as more cells lyse. Significant levels of the cytosolic enzyme lactate dehydrogenase are found in the culture medium earlier than 3 h, indicating a release through some mechanism other than cell lysis.

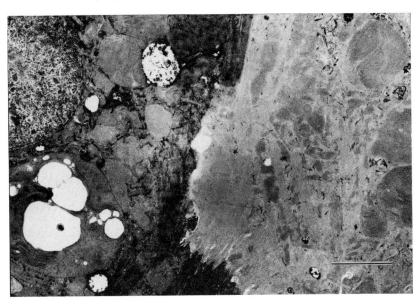

Fig. 15.7 Transmission electron microscopy of cultured heart cells treated with doxorubicin in the presence of horseradish peroxidase (HRP) as a tracer for cell permeability. These cells show mitochondrial vesiculation and myofibrillar disruption, and loss of membrane integrity is indicated by HRP uptake (dark stain). Bar = 2 μm.

FITC-specific fluorescence (corresponding to cell lysis rather than enzyme leakage) as a function of time. These studies produce an accurate assessment of cells that have lost membrane integrity, and provide a method for the rapid evaluation of potential drug intervention therapy or toxicity. It may be necessary to differentiate between release of cytosolic enzymes by blebbing or cell lysis for each new class of compound.

For expanded studies on morphology, electron microscopy is used. For example, transmission electron microscopy provides for a more detailed examination of cell morphology for compounds such as doxorubicin that produce structural modifications. Ultrastructural studies can be enhanced by the use of tracers such as horseradish peroxidase (HRP) or antibodies to examine membrane integrity at dose levels that do not produce significant increases in enzyme leakage (Fig. 15.7). Scanning electron microscopy allows the investigator to differentiate between enzyme release by cell lysis (as illustrated in Fig. 15.5) or formation and release of blebs (Fig. 15.8).

Studies can also be designed to assess modification of specific cellular constituents by covalent binding. For example, in mechanistic studies on

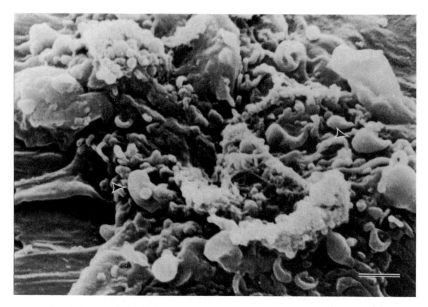

Fig. 15.8 Blebs are a common feature of toxic injury to the myocyte. Larger blebs can be seen by light microscopy, but smaller blebs require scanning electron microscopy, as illustrated here. Release or rupture of blebs can result in increased medium levels of cytosolic enzymes without cell lysis, as in Fig. 15.6. Bar = 1.0 μm.

the antibiotic paldimycin (U-70, 138F), which produces toxic effects on striated muscle (Branstetter *et al.*, 1987) and apparent cardiac death in dogs, we used ^{14}C-labelled drug to identify covalent association of drug-related material to cellular proteins. Cell monolayers were first treated with 0.5% Triton X-100, which extracts cellular membranes and cytoplasm but leaves the cytoskeleton intact. This was followed by extraction with 10 mM deoxycholate, and finally 8 M urea to dissociate any remaining non-covalent bonds. Extracts were resolved by polyacrylamide gel electrophoresis and autoradiography (Fig. 15.9), and covalent associations were observed for most cell proteins and in an apparently dose-dependent manner to actin. This technique allows for the examination of specific protein modifications that may result from toxic drug exposure, but does require radiolabelled drug. Treatment of cells with this compound also produces arrythmias and inhibition of contraction at non-cytotoxic concentrations; more work is required, however, to identify a mechanistic correlation. Specific functions such as ATP production and ion transport can be measured by a variety of techniques (Acosta *et al.*, 1985). Many techniques using fluorescence microscopy of living cells are available to

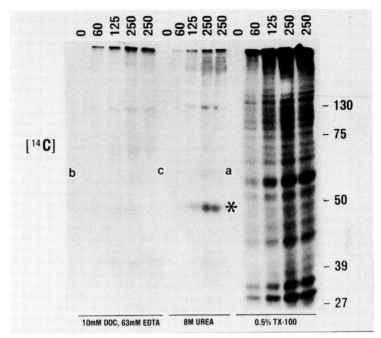

Fig. 15.9 Autoradiogram of a polyacrylamide gel from myocytes treated with ^{14}C-labelled paldimycin (U-70,138F) at levels of 0, 60, 125 or 250 μg/ml (high dose lanes are from two separate experiments. Following drug exposure, cells were serially extracted with 0.5% Triton X-100 (TX-100), which extracted all but cytoskeletal proteins (a), followed by 10 mm deoxycholate (DOC) with 63 mm EDTA (b), and finaly 8 m urea to dissociate remaining non-covalently bound material (c). Drug-related material was observed to be covalently linked to many cell proteins, and in an apparent dose-dependent manner to actin (*).

assess a variety of toxicological end points and organellar activities, including gap junctional integrity with Lucifer Yellow (Burt and Spray, 1989), and calcium homoeostasis with fura-2 (Cobbold and Rink, 1987). These and other approaches can be combined to define the cellular response to injury.

Conclusions

Much information on potential for or mechanism of cardiac toxicity by drugs can be derived from *in vitro* studies using cardiac myocytes. There are limitations to this approach, however, that must be realized. Random screening of compounds with only cell lysis or effect on contractile activity can yield misleading results unless the relevance to *in vivo* activity can be substantiated, and should therefore be avoided. Also, drug toxicities that are dependent on metabolism will generally be missed unless specifically addressed, and there is the potential for age and species variations in response. Most of these potential drawbacks can be included in study design, and such studies can result in the development of better pharmaceuticals with the use of fewer animals.

References

Acosta, D. and Ramos, K.J. (1984). *Toxicol. Environ. Health* **14**, 137–143.

Acosta, D., Sorensen, E.M.B., Anuforo, D.C., Mitchell, D.B., Ramos, K., Santone, K.S. and Smith, M.A. (1985). *In Vitro Cell. Dev. Biol.* **21**, 495–504.

Blondel, R., Roijen, I. and Cheneval, J. (1971). *Experientia* **273**, 356–358.

Borg, T.K., Rubin, K., Lundgren, E., Borg, K. and Obrink, B. (1984). *Dev. Biol.* **104**, 86–96.

Branstetter, D., Stout, C., Parker, A. and Bus, J. (1987). *The Pharmacologist* **29**, 187.

Burt, J.M. and Spray, D.C. (1989). *Circ. Res.* **65**, 829–837.

Chacon, E. and Acosta, D. (1991). *Toxicol. Appl. Pharmacol.* **107**, 117–128.

Clark, W.A. (1976). *Dev. Biol.* **52**, 263–282.

Cobbold, P.H. and Rink, T.J. (1987). *Biochem. J.* **248**, 313–328.

Combs, A.B., Acosta, D. and Ramos, K. (1985). *Biochem. Pharmacol.* **34**, 1115–1116.

Dorgelo, F.O., Biessen, E. and Alin, G.M. (1986). *ATLA* **14**, 14–22.

Freyss-Beguin, M. and Van Brussel, E. (1980). *Biol. Cell* **37**, 111–118.

Harary, I. and Farley, B. (1960). *Science* **131**, 1674.

Harary, I. and Farley, B. (1963). *Exp. Cell Res.* **29**, 451.

Kasten, F.H. (1972). *In Vitro* **8**, 128–149.

Khaw, B.A., Scott, J., Fallon, J.T., Cahill, S.L., Haber, E. and Homcy, C. (1982). *Science* **217**, 1050–1053.

Klein, I. and Daood, M. (1985). *In Vitro Cell. Dev. Biol.* **21**, 693–696.

Kokubu, T. and Pollak, O.J. (1962). *Exp. Mol. Pathol.* **1**, 293–303.

Lampidis, T.J., Henderson, I.C., Israel, M. and Canellos, G.P. (1980). *Cancer Res.* **40**, 3901–3909.

Libby, P. (1984). *J. Mol. Cell. Cardiol.* **16**, 803–811.

Lloyd, T.R. and Marvin, W.J. (1990). *J. Mol. Cell. Cardiol.* **22**, 333–342.

Marino, T.A., Walter, R.A., Cobb, E., Palasiuk, M., Parsons, T. and Mercer, W.E. (1990). *In Vitro Cell Dev. Biol.* **26**, 229–236.

Mark, G.E. and Strasser, F.F. (1966). *Exp. Cell Res.* **44**, 217–233.

Marvin, W., Robinson, R., and Hermsmeyer, K. (1979). *Circ. Res.* **45**, 528–540.

Persoon-Rothert, M., van der Valk-Kokshoorn, E.J.M., Egas-Kenniphaas, J.M., Mauve, I. and van der Laarse, A. (1989). *J. Mol. Cell. Cardiol.* **21**, 1285–1291.

Piper, H.M., Schwartz, P., Spahr, R., Hutter, J.F. and Spieckermann, P.G. (1984). *J. Mol. Cell. Cardiol.* **16**, 385–388.

Seraydarian, M.W. and Artaza, L. (1979). *Cancer Res.* **39**, 2904–2944.

Schuette, W.H., Burch, C., Roach, P.O. and Parrillo, J.E. (1987). *Cytometry* **8**, 101–103.

Ulrich, R.G., Elliget, K.A. and Rosnick, D.K. (1988). *J. Tissue Cult. Methods* **11**, 217–221.

Van Der Laarse, N., Hollaar, L., Kokshoorn, L.J.M. and Witteveen, S.A.G.J. (1979). *J. Mol. Cell. Cardiol.* **11**, 501–510.

Wenzel, D.G. and Cosma, G.N. (1984a). *Toxicology* **33**, 103–115.

Wenzel, D.G. and Cosma, G.N. (1984b). *Toxicology* **33**, 117–128.

Wenzel, D.G., Wheatley, J.W. and Byrd, G.D. (1970). *Toxicol. Appl. Pharmacol.* **17**, 774–785.

F. Oculo- and Oto-toxicity

16

Oculotoxicity *In Vitro*

A. BRUININK

*Institute of Toxicology, ETH and University of Zürich, CH-8603
Schwerzenbach, Switzerland*

Introduction

Although retinopathy induced by chemical substances is of considerable
interest today, *in vitro* oculotoxicity screening for chemicals and drugs is
stil a new field of research. One reason for this may be the interspecies
variability in neuronal organization of the eye as well as its complexity.
Although the histological subdivision of the eye into several layers is
simple and generally the same in all vertebrates, the distribution of the
nerve cell processes is species-specific and the function of each cell type
highly complex (Ehinger and Floren, 1976). This makes it in some
cases more difficult to interpret and extrapolate morphological and
neurochemical findings from one animal species to others and to man.
In the present chapter several *in vitro* oculotoxicity screening systems are
described and the techniques developed in our laboratory are presented.

Targets

Every drug, depletion of certain endogenous compounds, disease or
hereditary disorder primarily affects certain sensitive cells. The degeneration of the neuronal retina can be roughly divided into four types on
the basis of the main target.

IN VITRO METHODS IN TOXICOLOGY
ISBN 0-12-388175-7

The Neuronal Retina

Some drugs cause selective toxic effects on the neuronal retina. For example, lithium, especially in combination with exposure to light, disrupts the organization of the outer segments of the photoreceptor cells (Federspiel-Eisenring *et al.*, 1988). Furthermore, depending on the doses, long-term exposure to lithium can cause irreversible retinal degeneration.

Retinal Pigmented Epithelium (RPE)

Administration of certain drugs leads primarily to malfunction of the RPE and as a consequence the photoreceptor cells degenerate. Sometimes this is associated with increased glial cell phagocytic activity. Disorders of the RPE are not only caused by certain drugs but also occur in the course of inherited or acquired diseases. Examples of such lesions are advanced stages of the delayed amelanotic mutant line of the chick and experimentally induced uveitis (Fite *et al.*, 1985). An example of a selective drug that causes RPE malfunctions is chloroquine (Meier-Ruge and Cerletti; 1966, Ings, 1984). All cases are characterized by progressive alterations of RPE cells, i.e. disorganization, loss of basal folds and gradual detachment of the retina.

Transport Between the Neuronal Retina and RPE

Disruption of transport of endogenous compounds involved in the visual cycle or of outer segments of the rod photoreceptor cells induces malfunction of the photoreceptor cells. The pink-eye RCS rat is an example of an animal with this type of lesion. In this animal the transport of interstitial retinol-binding protein is reduced. This results in accumulation of retinol in the photoreceptor outer segments, leading to photoreceptor cell death (Gonzalez-Fernandez *et al.*, 1985).

Retinal Vascular System

Clinical experience indicates that exposure of premature infants to prolonged hyperoxia causes vasoconstriction, vaso-obliteration and in some cases destruction of the retinal vascular system. After return to ambient air, these lesions often progress to retrolental fibroplasia, the blinding disease of premature infants (James and Lanman, 1976).

In Vitro Systems

A number of experimental procedures can be used for the *in vitro* investigation of oculotoxic chemicals. Each system has its own degree of complexity. As a general rule it can be stated that the similarity of a system to the *in vivo* situation is directly related to the degree of complexity of the *in vitro* model. Of the test systems described here, only a few have been developed for measuring general oculotoxic effects. However, they can all be used for this. The type of *in vitro* assay purpose chosen for measuring oculotoxic effects depends mainly on the test substances or on the disease to be investigated. No existing *in vitro* system is able to measure all the above induced effects, partly because not all target sites are present, and partly because the maximum culture period is too short to allow development of the adverse effects. Furthermore, for most drugs or diseases the main target cell type is unknown. For these reasons it is not advisable to use only one type of *in vitro* culture. At present four *in vitro* retinal systems can be distinguished. They are briefly described in the following paragraphs.

Organ Culture of the Whole Eye

For this assay, the eyes of adult cats are enucleated under anaesthesia. The eyes are then cannulated at the opththalmociliary artery (Dawis *et al.*, 1985; Schneider and Zrenner, 1987) allowing test substances to be introduced or washed out by the perfusion solution. Effects caused by the administration of the chemicals are measured electrophysiologically. The reference electrodes are positioned at the cornea and at the posterior pole of the eye. Standing potential, electroretinogram and light peak recordings are made using a glass pipette placed in the vitreous humor. The advantage of this method is that the *in vivo* situation can be perfectly simulated. The concentration of the test substance at the target cells is comparable with the *in vivo* situation if the concentration in the perfusate is the same as that in the bloodstream. The disadvantage is that, per eye, recordings can be made for only up to 6 h. Therefore only acute effects can be measured, and no conclusions can be reached about whether the reversibility of the induced effects is possible beyond these 6 h. The concentration of the test substance at the target cells remains unknown. Furthermore, a considerable number of animals is needed for these experiments.

One disadvantage, i.e. the short culture period, can be overcome if eyes are taken from embryonic animals. Depending on the age of the animals, the eyes can be kept in culture for 5–6 days (Sidman, 1961). In this model, chemically induced injuries are measured with the help of histopathological techniques.

Neuronal Retina Explants

In this assay, the neuronal retina with or without the RPE is dissected out of embryonic or neonatal eyes. Some researchers make a few short radial incisions in order to culture the flattened whole retina (Liu *et al.*, 1988), whereas others culture thin strips of the eyes. *In vitro*, these retinas develop well in the presence of serum. During culture, the neuronal retina differentiates into several layers (Bird, 1986; Liu *et al.*, 1988; Caffé *et al.*, 1989; Spence and Robson, 1989; Sparrow *et al.*, 1990). Because RPE exerts a specific stimulus on growth and tissue differentiation of the neuronal retina at least *in vitro*, e.g. formation of photoreceptor outer segments, the coculture of neuronal retina with RPE is to be preferred over cultures without (Liu *et al.*, 1988). These explants lend themselves to electron miocroscopic investigation of the the effects of the test substance on the cellular organization of the neuronal retina (Bird, 1986; Caffé *et al.*, 1989). In addition histochemical techniques are also used (Liu *et al.*, 1988; Sparrow *et al.*, 1990). The degree and length of neurite outgrowth out of the explants can also be taken as a differentiation parameter (Lima *et al.*, 1989). The advantage of this culture type is its three-dimensional organization. The disadvantage is, however, that it is very difficult, if not impossible, depending on the parameters measured, to quantify small effects on the degree of differentiation or viability. Furthermore, these tests are very time consuming.

A variation of the second *in vitro* system is the culture of explants and of cells harvested from such explants. This technique was developed by the group of Tripathi in 1984 using freshly excised, pure, immature retinal vascular explants from 8–10-day-old rabbits (Tripathi and Tripathi, 1984). A characteristic of such explants is that, after 24–36 h, cells start to migrate out of the explants to the surface of the culture chamber. With mitotic activity a monolayer of cell growth is established. Using this method, we were able to investigate the direct effects of hyperoxia and/or drugs. The end points we chose were morphological changes detected by light microscopy and electron microscopy.

Reaggregate Cell Cultures

Almost 40 years ago Moscona introduced a procedure for cell aggregation using a rotation technique. From these studies it has now been established that dissociated cells reassemble into multicellular aggregates within which they reconstruct their original tissue patterns and continue to differentiate (see Moscona, 1974). For these cultures serum-containing media were used. Honegger and coworkers found a method to keep differentiating brain reaggregates for several months by culturing under totally serum-free conditions (Honegger *et al.*, 1979). In our laboratory we culture reaggregated retinal cells under serum-free conditions. For this, neuronal retina from embryonic chick (stage 28–29 according to Hamburger and Hamilton, 1951) is dissected out (Fig. 16.1, Bruinink and Reiser, 1991). Rotation-mediated reaggregating cell cultures are prepared from mechanically dissociated retinal cells. It has been found that during culture, cells migrate to form various layers. Figure 16.2 is an electron micrograph of a reaggregate culture after 13 days. The external surface is covered by a layer of Müller cells and some melanosome-containing cells, the so called glia-limitans. These observations confirm the finding that some cells of the neuronal retina can transdifferentiate into pigmented-epithelium-like cells (Pritchard, 1981). The next layer is characterized by

Cell-Cultures

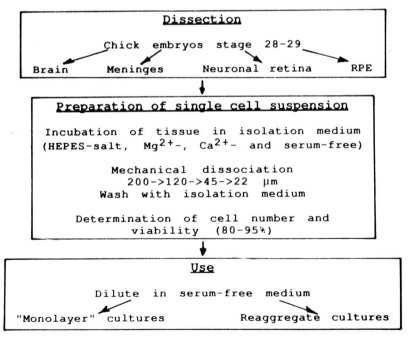

Fig. 16.1 Schematic representation of the cell culture preparation.

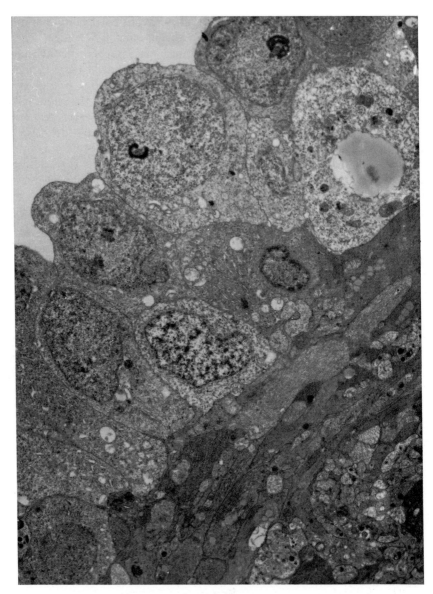

Fig. 16.2 Electron photomicrograph of an embryonic chick neuronal retina reaggregate after 13 days in culture (×4756) (Photo: Dr Ch. Holderegger).

the presence of developing photoreceptor cells. Under this layer other cells, neurites and synapses are seen. No photoreceptor rosettes are present within the reaggregate. This is in contrast to the findings of Linser and Perkins (1987) who used serum-containing culture medium. In the presence of serum, polarity of this type, without rosettes, as described for our system, appears only if neuronal retina cells are cocultured with ciliary pigmented cells (Layer and Willbold, 1989). At present we are characterizing the various layers and cells in these layers in order to detect drug-induced changes in reaggregate organization. For these studies only a small number of reaggregates is needed. Besides electron microscopic and histochemical studies, enzyme activity and receptor density measurements can be made using reaggregate homogenates. The disadvantage of such studies is that many reaggregates are needed to obtain only one reproducible measurement. A further disadvantage is the space requirement per culture. Applying the conventional method as described by Honegger *et al.* (1979), only between 50 and 100 flasks can be placed on one gyratory shaker (Table 16.1). This disadvantage can

Table 16.1
Comparison between reaggregate and "monolayer" cultures

	Monolayer	Reaggregate
Survival	14–20 days	> 42 days
Differentiation	Relatively slow, mostly 2-dimensional	Relatively fast, 3-dimensional
Kind of test	Acute, short term	Acute → long term
Space and cell requirement*	5×10^4 cells/well (96-well plates)	4×10^7 cells/flask (4 ml; 25 ml flask)
Wells/flask per incubator	> 20 000	100 (25 ml flasks), 50 (50 ml flasks) or ⩾ 450 (6-well plates)
Handling of cultures	Easy	Medium has to be changed every second day
Detection of morphological changes during culture	Easy	Difficult or impossible
Measurements of end points	Easy	Complicated; more (other) end points can be measured

* 1 egg → retina, 10×10^6 cells; RPE, 0.25×10^6 cells.

partly be overcome by modifying this procedure as follows: 25 ml Erlenmeyer flasks are seeded with 40×10^6 cells/4 ml, on day 0. The content of each flask is subdivided into two 2 ml portions on day 1. Each portion plus 4 ml of fresh medium is transferred into a 50 ml Erlenmeyer flask. On day 2, 2 ml of supernatant is discarded. The rest is subdivided into four 1 ml portions. Each portion plus 1 ml of medium is transferred into each well (ϕ (diameter) well=3.5 cm) of a 6-well culture plate. throughout the culture period the rotation velocity is 81 r.p.m. With this modification, at least 450 cultures can be placed on a shaker without encroachment on form and size of the reaggregates.

"Monolayer" Cultures

In this type of culture dissociated cells are allowed to attach to and grow on the surface of the culture wells. Reaggregate and monolayer cultures each have their own advantages and disadvantages (Table 16.1). If a prolonged survival and an *in vivo*-like three-dimensional organization is important, the reaggregate culture system should be chosen. However, if low space and cell requirements, easy handling of the cultures, the detection of morphological changes during treatment and quick and sensitive measurement of end points, such as viability and the presence of certain proteins, are key aspects, then monolayer cultures are to be preferred. The monolayer cultures can be subdivided into cultures of the various cell types present in the culture well and thus provide *in vitro* models for the target cells or cell groups under investigation.

Müller Cells

It is hypothesized that the phagocytic activity of retinal glial cells plays a role in the response of the retina to certain pathological conditions. Mano and Puro (1990) have developed a method to measure this phagocytic activity using Müller cells from postmortem human eyes. For this, fluorescein-labelled carboxyl microspheres or polystyrene latex beads are added to the cultures as well as various concentrations of the test substance. After 24 h, uptake is measured by electron microscopy or flow cytometry. The advantage of this test is its simplicity. The disadvantage is that the relevance of the outcome remains to be established.

Retinal Pigmented Epithelium (RPE)

The phagocytosis of outer segments of the rod photoreceptor cells (ROS) by the RPE is a key aspect of retinal physiology. Lentrichia *et al.* (1987)

have developed a method to test how far various drugs can affect association of ROS with RPE. For this, secondary cultures of chick embryo RPE cells are incubated with a bovine ROS preparation together with various concentrations of a test substance. After incubation the rhodopsin content is determined spectrophotometrically and by radioimmunoassay. Until now, only carbohydrates have been tested. The advantage of this kind of test is that an important RPE-specific characteristic is tested. The disadvantage is that other functional effects, e.g. cytotoxicity, are not taken into account.

In our laboratory, drug-induced changes in cell viability are measured using the MTT- and Neutral Red-uptake test, as previously described (Bruinink and Reiser, 1991). The dissociated RPE cells are cultivated in serum-free medium (Fig. 16.1). One day after plating, the various concentrations of the test substance are introduced into the system. Seven days later, viability is measured. An example of a control culture is shown in Plate 16.1. So far the effects of chloroquine and thioridazine have been measured. For choloroquine the pigment epithelium is the predominant site of pathological lesions. Our *in vitro* findings are in agreement with this observation: cytotoxic effects of chloroquine occur at lower concentrations than in cultures of embryonic chick brain, meninges and neuronal retina (cultured in the dark or in a 12/12 h light/dark cycle) (Table 16.2) (Bruinink *et al.*, 1991). Chloroquine concentrations inducing cytotoxic effects on RPE cells are comparable to human blood concentrations leading to chloroquine retinopathy.

Table 16.2
Effect of chloroquine on viability of cell cultures of chick embryonic cells

Tissue	$\log(IC_{50}$ (μM)) $\pm$ s.e.m. (IC_{50} (M))	
	Neutral Red uptake	MTT-dehydrogenase activity
RPE	-0.010 ± 0.097 (0.977)	-0.011 ± 0.064 (0.975)
Meninges	0.594 ± 0.049 (3.924)	0.541 ± 0.045 (3.475)
Retina (D)	0.818 ± 0.071 (6.571)	0.703 ± 0.072 (5.047)
Retina (L)	0.842 ± 0.050 (6.950)	0.816 ± 0.082 (6.546)
Brain	0.437 ± 0.047 (2.738)	0.321 ± 0.047 (2.095)

Data are expressed in log (IC_{50}) values and are the means $\pm$ s.e.m. of three to six experiments. Retina (D), neuronal retina cultured in the dark; retina (L), neuronal retina cultured under a light/dark cycle (12/12 h).

Neuronal Retina

Cultures of neuronal retina are prepared as previously described (Bruinink and Reiser, 1990). In these cultures not only viability but also nerve cell differentiation can be measured. The technique used is to assay the amount of neurofilament 68KD and 160KD and microtubule-associated protein type 5 (MAP5) antigens. MAP2 is present in insufficient concentration to be included in the test system. Furthermore, binding of peanut (*Arachis hypogaea*) agglutinin (PNA) lectin can be studied. The quantity of neurofilament molecules can be taken as an index for neurite outgrowth. MAPs are a group of proteins that are copurified with tubulin during repeated cycles of temperature-dependent polymerization. Some of these proteins such as MAP2 and MAP5 are specifically found in neurons only. MAP2 is usually encountered in dendrites and only rarely in axons, whereas MAP5 (also known as MAP1X) is more or less axon specific. Both proteins have been demonstrated to be developmentally regulated (Tucker and Matus, 1987). No specific binding of MAP5 antibodies was found in cultures of the Müller cells, but only in a defined population of neurites (Plate 16.2A,B).

Carbohydrate moieties of cell surface glycoproteins and glycolipids may play important functional roles in defining the specificity of cellular interactions such as those required in the establishment and maintenance of synaptic junctions. The cellular glycoprotein composition is age dependent. Plant lectins are selective ligands for specific carbohydrates. PNA binds specifically to β-D-galactose (1-3)-D-galactosamine residues. In the retina of neonatal rats, PNA binds to photoreceptor cells, preferentially to the inner and outer segments and synaptic pedicles of cone photoreceptor cells, and to discrete regions within the outer synaptic layer (Blanks and Johnson, 1983). In the retina, an increase in specific PNA lectin binding is present throughout the postnatal development.

In our cultures, cells of the neuronal retina were found to differentiate during the first 10–13 days in culture independently of the cell density at plating, as indicated by the binding of PNA lectin (Fig. 16.3). The maximum level of PNA-lectin binding was directly correlated with the number of cells per well at plating. In contrast, Sparrow et al. (1990) could not detect *de novo* expression of differentiated molecular properties in serum-containing retinal cultures of gestational day 13–14 rats. According to others (see Savage et al., 1988) no cell proliferation is visible by light microscopy. In agreement with this finding, no change in MTT dehydrogenase activity was observed during culture (Fig. 16.3A). Furthermore, the cytostatic drug 1-β-D-arabinofuranosylcytosine (ARA-C) did not affect cultures of the neuronal retina at those concentrations at

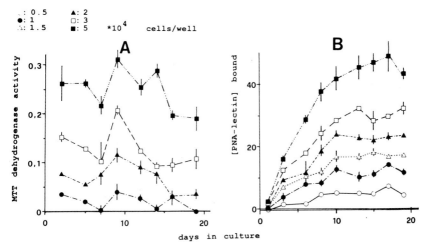

Fig. 16.3 Developmental pattern of MTT dehydrogenase activity (A) and PNA-lectin binding (B) in monolayer cultures of embryonic chick neuronal retina. (For experimental details, see Bruinink and Reiser (1990)). Half of the medium was replaced by fresh medium at day 8, 10, 13 and 15 *in vitro*.

which it inhibits viability (proliferation) and differentiation in embryonic chick brain and meninges cultures (Fig. 16.4). The brain and meninges cultures contain rapidly proliferating cells (astroglia and fibroblast, respectively). In our test system drug effects are measured after 8 days in culture. Drugs are added on day 1. Until now only the effect of bismuth, tretinoin free or bound to bovine serum albumin, thioridazin, chloroquine (Table 16.2) and ARA-C (Fig. 16.4) have been measured (Bruinink *et al.*, 1991 and 1992; Bruinink, 1992).

Final Remarks

Neuronal explants, reaggregate cultures and monolayer cultures have an important advantage over organ culture of the total eye, namely their prolonged *in vitro* survival (between 20 and at least 35 days). Acute as well as effects induced by long-term application of the test substance can be measured. On the other hand the threshold toxic concentration of the test substance at the target cells *in vitro* is, although known, not equivalent to threshold toxic blood concentration *in vivo* because of the difference in organization of the neuronal retinal cells and/or the absence of a blood–retina barrier.

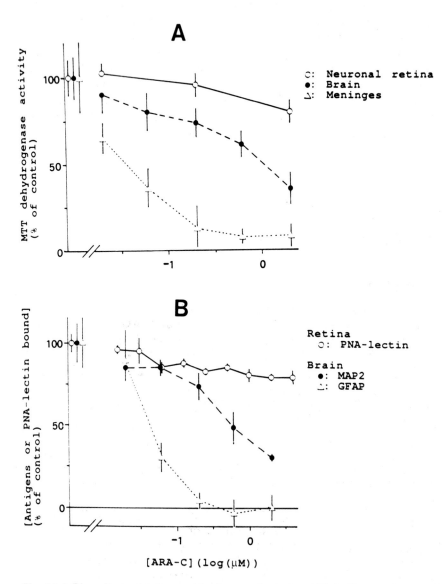

Fig. 16.4 The effect of 1-β-D-arabinofuranosylcytosine (ARA-C) on cultures of embryonic chick neuronal retina, brain and meninges as measured by MTT dehydrogenase activity (A) and expression of glial fibrillary acidic protein (GFAP) and MAP2 (brain), and PNA-lectin binding (retina) (B).

In vitro research using animal retinal tissue may give much information about the target cells and the mechanisms by which the test substance is acting. However, in extrapolating these data to the *in vivo* human situation, it must be taken into account that only direct effects can be measured and that interspecies variability in retinal organization does exist. In order to be sure that there are no drug-induced oculotoxic side effects, it is advisable to conduct *in vivo* toxicology studies with the compounds found to have the least toxic effects in the *in vitro* systems. These animal studies should include simple routine tests of ocular toxicity during treatment (Niemeyer and Früh, 1989).

Acknowledgements

I thank Professor G. Zbinden and Dr C. Maravelias for their critical reading of the manuscript.

References

Bird, M.M. (1986). *Cell Tissue Res.* **245**, 563–577.
Blanks, J. and Johnson, L.V. (1983). *J. Comp. Neurol.* **221**, 31–41.
Bruinink, A. and Reiser, P. (1991). *Int. J. Dev. Neurosci.* **9**, 269–279.
Bruinink, G., Zimmermann, G. and Reisen, F. (1991). *Arch. Toxicol.* **65**, 480–484.
Bruinink, A. (1992). *In* "The Brain in Bits and Pieces" (G. Zbinden ed.), pp. 23–50. MTC Verlag, Zollikon.
Bruinink, A., Reiser, P., Müller, M., Gähwiler, B.H. and Zbinden, G. (1992). *Toxicol. in Vitro*. in press.
Caffé, A.R., Visser, H., Jansen, H.G. and Sanyal, S. (1989). *Curr. Eye Res.* **8**, 1083–1092.
Dawis, S., Hofmann, H. and Niemeyer, G. (1985). *Vision Res.* **25**, 1163–1177.
Ehinger, B. and Floren, I. (1976). *Cell Tissue Res.* **175**, 37–48.
Federspiel-Eisenring, E., Rem, Ch., Pfeilschifter, J. and Dietrich, C. (1988). *Klin. Mbl. Augenheilk.* **192**, 134–140.
Fite, K.V., Bengston, L. and Doran, P. (1985). *J. Comp. Neurol.* **231**, 310–322.
Gonzalez-Fernandez, F., Fong, S.L., Liou, G.I. and Bridges, C.G.B. (1985). *Invest. Ophthalmol. Vis. Sci.* **26**, 1381–1385.
Hamburger, V. and Hamilton, H.L. (1951). *J. Morphol.* **88**, 49–92.
Honegger, P., Lenoir, D. and Favrod, P. (1979). *Nature* **282**, 305–308.
Ings, R.M.J. (1984). *Drug Metab. Rev.* **15**, 1183–1212.
James, S.L. and Lanman, J.T. (1976). *Pediatrics* **67**, (Suppl.), 591–642.
Layer, P.G. and Willbold, E. (1989). *Cell Tissue Res.* **258**, 233–242.
Lentrichia, B.B., Itoh, Y., Plantner, J.J. and Kean, E.L. (1987). *Exp. Eye Res.* **44**, 127–142.
Lima, L., Matus, P. and Drujan, B. (1989). *Int. J. Neurosci.* **7**, 375–382.

Linser, P.J. and Perkins, M.S. (1987). *Cell Diff.* **20**, 189–196.
Liu, L., Cheng, S.H., Jiang, L.Z., Hansmann, G. and Layer, P.G. (1988). *Exp. Eye Res.* **46**, 801–812.
Mano, T. and Puro, D.G. (1990). *Invest. Ophthalmol. Vis. Sci.* **31**, 1047–1055.
Meier-Ruge, W. and Cerletti, A. (1966). *Excerpta Med. Int. Congr. Ser.* **114**, 228.
Moscona, A.A. (1974). *In* "The Cell Surface in Development" (A.A. Moscona, ed.), pp. 67–99. John Wiley and Sons, New York.
Niemeyer, G. and Früh, B. (1989). *Klin. Mbl. Augenheilk.* **194**, 355–358.
Pritchard, D.J. (1981). *J. Embryol. Exp. Morphol.* **62**, 47–62.
Savage, F.J., Day, J.E., Hogg, P. and Grierson, I. (1988). *Eye* **2**, 164–179.
Schneider, T. and Zrenner, E. (1987). *Doc. Ophthalmol.* **65**, 287–296.
Sidman, R.L. (1961). *Dis. Nerv. Syst. Suppl.* **22**, (4th Suppl.), 14–20.
Sparrow, J.R., Hicks, D. and Barnstable, C.J. (1990). *Dev. Brain Res.* **51**, 69–84.
Spence, S.G. and Robson, J.A. (1989). *Neuroscience* **32**, 801–812.
Tripathi, B.J. and Tripathi, R.C. (1984). *Current Eye Res.* **3**, 193–208.
Tucker, R.P. and Matus, A.I. (1987). *Development* **101**, 535–546.

Discussion

A. Vernadakis
Have you detected any effects on the Müller cells, any contact with the neurons? There were some very nice Müller cells in the cultures.

A. Bruinink
We have a coculture, but have not measured the effects on the Müller cells separately. We have not had the monoclonal antibodies until now for measuring the effects of these cells, or separate cultures for the Müller cells. This is the next thing we want to do.

C. Atterwill
Isolated whole retinae can be dark- and light-adapted and show different responses in those situations. Can the same be done with the cultures, and will they show different effects in dark- and light-adapted states?

A. Bruinink
We have two different kinds of cultures, in which the cells are only in the dark or have a 12/12-h light/dark cycle. We have tested the effect of chloroquine on the two systems and find no differences.

17

Drug Ototoxicity Tested on Inner Ear Sensory Hair Cells *In Vitro*

D. DULON, T. SAITO, H. HIEL and J.-M. ARAN

Laboratoire d'Audiologie Expérimentale, INSERM U-229, Université de Bordeaux II, Hôpital Pellegrin, 33076 Bordeaux, France

Introduction

Cochlear outer hair cells have been well established as the primary targets of various ototoxic agents. These sensory cells isolated from the auditory organ and maintained in short-term culture are used as a model for studying the acute effects of these noxious agents. We briefly review here recent results concerning the toxic effects of the aminoglycoside antibiotics and demonstrate that these molecules interfere with the intracellular calcium homoeostasis of the sensory cells.

Ototoxicity

Inner ear sensory hair cells are sensitive to various noxious agents. Irreversible damage to the sensory cells can be observed in conjunction with aminoglycoside antibiotics, diuretics, cisplatin, acoustic trauma and

IN VITRO METHODS IN TOXICOLOGY
ISBN 0-12-388175-7

other agents (Table 17.1). The aminoglycoside antibiotics represent the largest class of ototoxic agents and are also the most important in terms of their extensive clinical use and reported cases of ototoxicity. The toxicity of these agents has been extensively described in both clinical therapy and animal research, but the cellular and molecular mechanisms of their toxicity remain still to be defined. The development of ototoxicity in the guinea pig following treatment with various aminoglycoside antibiotics has been the subject of extensive research in our laboratory (Aran *et al.*, 1982; Dulon *et al.*, 1986, 1988). The intoxication leads to irreversible loss of hair cells which appears after 2 weeks of daily treatment (Fig. 17.1). The outer hair cells of the auditory organ are the cells primarly affected and this is, in general, true whatever the type of noxious agent (Table 17.1 and Fig. 17.2). We recently demonstrated by autoradiography and immunochemistry after *in vivo* exposure that the outer hair cells specifically incorporate and accumulate the aminoglycoside antibiotic in their lysosomal system (Hayashida *et al.*, 1989; Aran, 1990). However, we still do not know why the sensory hair cells and in particular the outer hair cells are the preferential target of these molecules. The lack of information on the molecular mechanisms of ototoxicity results essentially from the technical difficulty of carrying out biochemical

Table 17.1
Drugs implicated in ototoxicity

Analgesic antipyretics	Quinine
	Salicylates
Aminoglycoside antibiotics	Streptomycin
	Neomycin
	Gentamicin
	etc.
Polypeptide antibiotics	Viomycin
	Vancomycin
Antineoplastics	Diaminedichloroplatinum (cis-DDP)
Diuretics	Ethacrynic acid
	Furosemide
Metallo compounds	Arsenicals
	Mercurials
Environment	Noise
	Time

The drugs known to be toxic to the inner ear present a great diversity in their molecular structures and pharmacological actions. Auditory effects range from transient symptoms such as tinnitus to a permanent reduction in auditory acuity which can reach a total and permanent deafness.

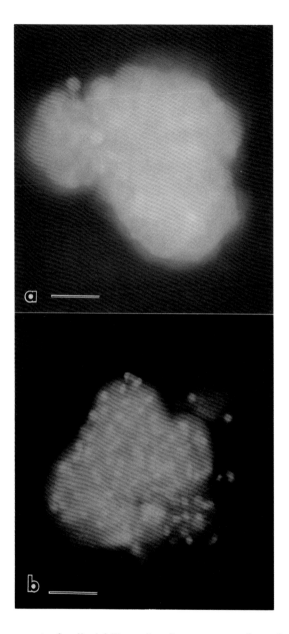

Plate 5.1 Assessment of cell viability using fluorescent probes. Glomeruli cell viability assessed by fluorescein diacetate 100 μg/ml and ethidium bromide 6.25 ng/ml and monitored using an epifluorescence filter combination with a 580 nm dichroic mirror, an excitation barrier filter 390–490 nm and an emission barrier filter of 510–515 nm on a Nikon Diaphot, bar line 20 μm, Ektachrome-400 daylight. Green fluorescein shows viable cells and damaged cells fluoresce red. (a) Freshly isolated glomeruli after 15 min show a few damaged (red) cells. (b) Glomeruli exposed to 5 μM mercuric chloride for 15 min show an extensive number of damaged cells.

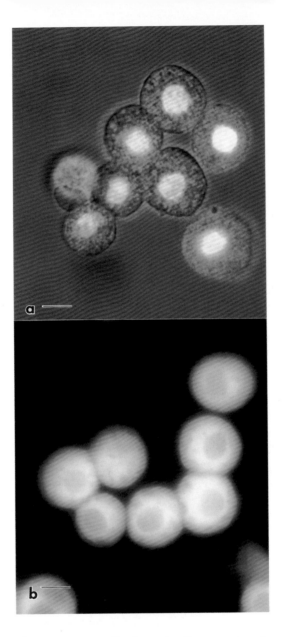

Plate 5.2 Organelle compartmentalization using fluorescent probes. (a) Selective staining of nuclei within isolated hepatocytes using FluoroBora-T. Concentration of probe 5 μg/ml in 140 mM NaCl plus 25 mM 3-[N-tris(hydroxymethyl) methyl-amino]-2-hydroxypropanesulphonic acid buffer, pH 7.4 to complex the probe. Monitored using an epifluorescence filter combination of an excitation barrier filter 470 nm and an emission barrier filter of 535 nm on a Nikon Diaphot, bar length 10 μm, Ektachrome-400 daylight. (b) Selective staining of cytoplasm within isolated hepatocytes using FluoroBora-II thought to highlight the Golgi apparatus. Concentration of probe 5 μg/ml in 140 mM NaCl plus 25 mM 3-[N-tris (hydroxymethyl)methylamino]-2-hydroxypropanesulphonic acid buffer, pH 7.4, to complex the probe. Monitored using an epifluorescence filter combination of an excitation barrier filter 370 nm and an emission barrier filter of 420 nm on a Nikon Diaphot, bar length 10 μm, Ektachrome-400 daylight.

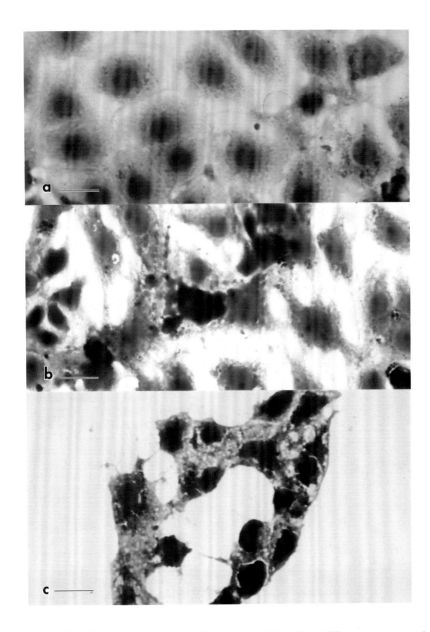

Plate 5.3 Sensitivity of cultured medullary interstitial cells to 100 mM paracetamol (acetaminophen) at (a) 0, (b) 15 and (c) 60 min. These micrographs show the sensitivity to paracetamol, and the heterogeneity of cell response. Formaldehyde-fixed and Giemsa-stained cells, bar length 20 μm.

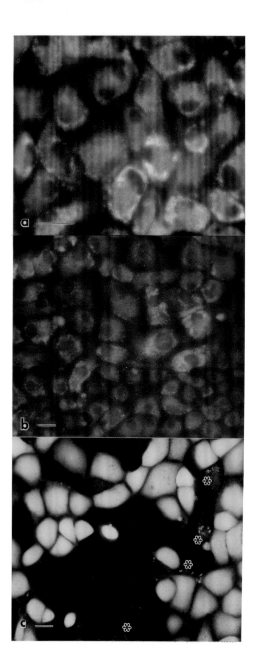

Plate 5.4 The application of fluorescent probes to study the acute sensitivity of cultured rat medullary interstitial cells. The fluorescent probes show significant heterogeneity in the presence of lipid droplets and peroxidase activity, and provide some evidence that the presence of both of these characteristics predispose cells to injury from papillotoxins. (a) Nile Red (Molecular Probes Inc., USA) staining of lipid droplets, seen as gold points in cultured medullary interstitial cells. Note heterogeneity in the amount and distribution of lipid droplets. (b) 2′,7′-Dichlorodihydrofluorescein (Molecular Probes Inc., USA) staining peroxidase activity heterogeneously (the green fluorescence best seen over nuclei, where there is no lipid staining) in medullary interstitial cells also stained with Nile Red. (c) Cultured medullary interstitial cells exposed to 10 μM 2-bromoethanamine for 30 min and stained with both 2′,7′-dichlorodihydrofluorescein and Nile Red. There are only residues of lipid droplets (asterisks), suggesting these cells were the first to undergo degeneration. Rat medullary interstitial cells grown under standard conditions (see Benns *et al.*, 1985), stained with either Nile Red and/or 2′,7′- dichlorodihydrofluorescein 2 μg/ml in buffer, monitored using an epifluorescence filter combination with a 400–440 nm excitation barrier filter and an emission barrier filter of 470 nm on a Nikon Diaphot, bar length 20 μm for a, b and c, Ektachrome-400 ASA-daylight type.

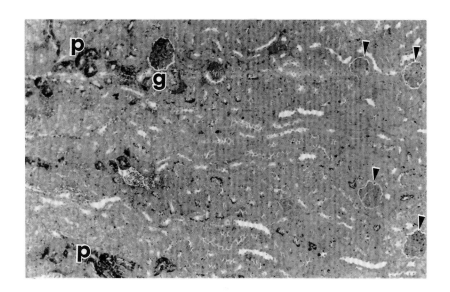

Plate 5.5 Semithin section of male rat kidney cortex 15 min after i.p. administration of 9 mg mercuric chloride/kg. Mercury deposits are visible as black grains after silver enhancement. Whereas cortical glomeruli (arrowheads) are unstained by the silver solution, a juxtamedullary glomerulus (g) and adjacent proximal tubular segments (p) show clear signs of mercury deposition. Silver intensification of the distribution of mercury and haematoxylin and eosin counterstaining, magnification ×98, Nikon Diaphot microscope, Nikon FE2 SLR camera, Kodak Ektachrome 100 ASA, Tungsten.

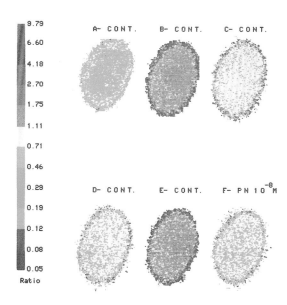

Plate 14.1 Blockade of spontaneous increases of $[Ca]_i$ by PN 200-110 during spontaneous contractions of single heart cells of 3-day-old chick embryo using the fura-2 Ca^{2+} imaging technique. (A) Intracellular free Ca^{2+} distribution before initiation of spontaneous contraction. (B) Increase in $[Ca]_i$ during contraction. (C,D) Decrease in $[Ca]_i$ during cessation of the spontaneous contraction. (D) Reincrease of $[Ca]_i$ during recontraction of the single cells. (F) Addition of 10^{-8}M PN 200-100 immediately inhibits the pacemaker activity of the single cells and no spontaneous increase in $[Ca]_i$ could be seen in the presence of this drug. Cell number CPE08. The experiments were carried out using PTI Imagescan System (Photon Technology International, Princeton, NJ, USA). (Bkaily *et al.*, unpublished results.)

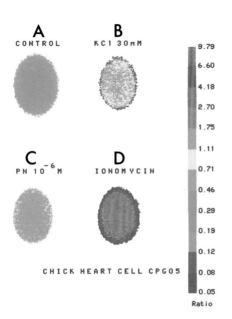

Plate 14.2 PN 200-110 blockade of the sustained increase in $[Ca]_i$ induced by high $[K]_o$. (A) Control (5.4 mM $[K]_o$) digital colour image maps of free Ca^{2+} concentration (ratio image). (B) Sustained increase in $[Ca]_i$ after 5 min in the presence of high $[K]_o$ (30 mM). (C) Addition of 10^{-6} M PN 200-110 decreased the $[Ca]_i$ back towards the control level. (D) Ionomycin and EGTA (not shown) were added subsequently to obtain maximal and minimal fluorescence respectively. The vertical scale at the right gives the numerical value of colour in the ratio images. (Bkaily et al., unpublished results.)

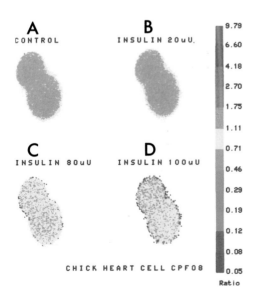

Plate 14.3 Effects of insulin on the distribution of intracellular free Ca^{2+} in two tightly attached single heart cells from a 10-day-old chick embryo. (A) Intracellular distribution of free Ca^{2+} (ratio image) in control Tyrode solution. (B) Absence of effect of 20 μU of insulin on $[Ca]_i$ distribution. (C,D) 1 min after increasing the concentration of insulin up to 80 and 100 μU. Note that the $[Ca]_i$ increased in both single cells. Vertical scale at the right gives the numerical value of colour in the ratio images. (Bkaily et al., unpublished results.)

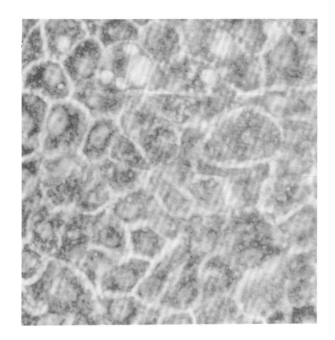

Plate 16.1 Light photomicrograph of an embryonic chick retinal pigment epithelium culture after 8 days *in vitro* (×300).

Plate 16.2 over page

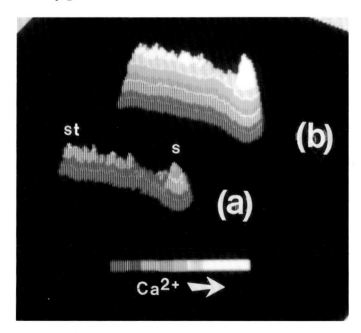

Plate 17.1 Ca^{2+} imaging during depolarization of outer hair cells. Depolarization induces Ca^{2+} entry into isolated outer hair cells. Intracellular free Ca^{2+} is imaged in pseudo-colours and in pseudo-3D using the fluorescent probe fluo-3, before (a) and after (b) K^+-depolarization in the same cell. The area of the stereocilia and the synaptic region of the sensory cell are indicated by ST and S respectively.

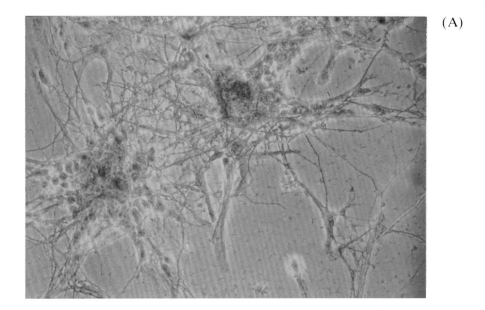

(A)

(B)

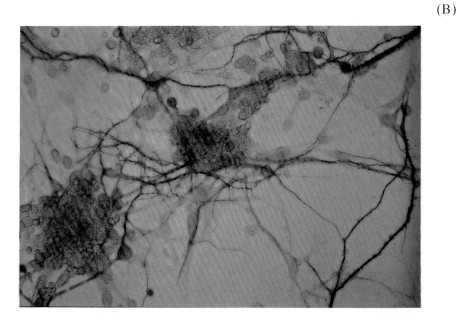

Plate 16.2 Light micrograph of the MAP5 stained cell cultures of embryonic chick neuronal retina cells after 8 days *in vitro* (×126). (A) Phase contrast, (B) brightfield.

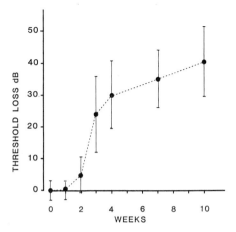

Fig. 17.1 Hearing loss generated by the aminoglycoside antibiotic gentamicin in the guinea pig. Auditory function was monitored from electrodes permanently implanted in the auditory cortex. Guinea pigs were treated daily for 3 weeks with 60 mg of gentamicin/kg body weight. A significant degradation in auditory acuity, expressed as an increase in threshold of response (loss in dB), appeared during the second week of treatment. Note that auditory responses continued to deteriorate irreversibly after the treatment had stopped.

investigations in the sensory inner ear tissues. The mammalian auditory organ is composed of only a few thousand sensory cells (approximately 10 000, one-quarter being inner hair cells and three-quarters being outer hair cells). In this context, the recent ability to maintain these sensory cells in short-term culture has provided a powerful tool for biochemical investigations at the cellular and molecular levels. This technique allows direct access to the sensory structures and makes it possible to study simultaneously their physiology, pharmacology and sensitivity to noxious agents. The present chapter will mainly focus on our recent investigations on the toxicity of the aminoglycoside antibiotics on cochlear outer hair cells *in vitro* (Dulon *et al.*, 1989a,b).

Acute Exposure to Aminoglycoside Antibiotics Does Not Influence Outer Hair Cell Viability and Motility *In Vitro*

The particular physiology of the outer hair cells in the auditory organ may explain their greater sensitivity to noxious stimuli. Unlike the inner hair cells, they do not transfer acoustic information to the nervous system, but generate, under efferent control, an active micromechanical process

D. Dulon *et al.*

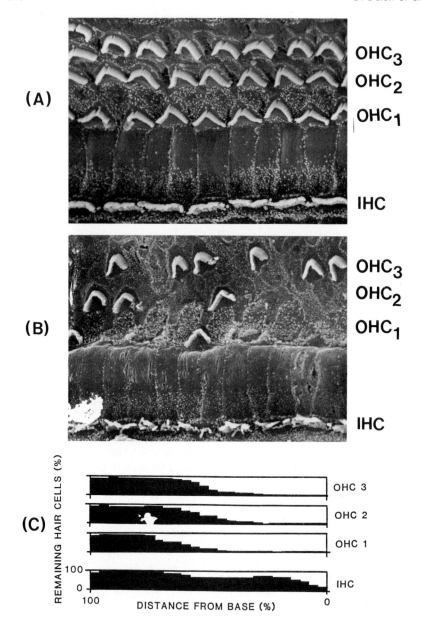

responsible for the extraordinary sensitivity and frequence selectivity of the mammalian auditory system (for review see Dulon and Aran, 1990). The recently demonstrated motile properties or contractions of isolated outer hair cells *in vitro* (Brownell *et al.*, 1985; Dulon et al., 1990) are thought to be the way by which these cells tune the mechano-electrical responses of the inner hair cells. These active motile properties of the outer hair cells could therefore be the specific target of ototoxic agents such as the aminoglycoside antibiotics.

Isolated outer hair cells *in vitro* were used in order to test whether ototoxic agents modify their viability or active motile properties. Incubation of the hair cells with various concentrations of gentamicin up to 1 mM did not significantly alter their viability (Dulon *et al.*, 1989a). The motile properties of the cells tested by K^+ depolarization or electrical stimulation were also unaffected in the presence of gentamicin (Fig. 17.3). These results indicate that short-term exposure of the hair cells to gentamicin appears to be non-toxic regardless of the maintenance of the integrity of their plasma membrane or their contractile properties. Information on long-term exposure to aminoglycoside molecules *in vitro* is now required. However, the currently available dissociation procedure and technique of short-term culture of mammalian hair cells do not permit investigations *in vitro* beyond 6–10 h. This is in part due to the great difficulty in reproducing *in vitro* the complex environment of the cochlear hair cells *in vivo*. *In vivo*, the hair cells are bathed in two different media, the endolymph (rich in K^+) in which the hair bundles are bathed and the perilymph (rich in Na^+), in which the cell body is bathed.

Fig. 17.2 Pattern of cochlear destruction by the aminoglycoside antibiotic gentamicin. (A) Surface view of a normal guinea pig organ of Corti. This view comes from the middle turn of the cochlea and is visualized by scanning electron microscopy (SEM). The three rows of outer hair cells (OHC_1, OHC_2, OHC_3) present ciliary bundles which form a characteristic "W". The single row of inner hair cells (IHC) present stereocilia arranged in a line along the longitudinal axis. (B) Surface view of the organ of Corti of a gentamicin-treated guinea pig. While the IHC are essentially intact, note that the OHC are preferentially affected by the ototoxic treatment. A similar pattern of sensory cell destruction can be observed by other ototoxic molecules such as the anticancer drug cis-DDP. (C) Histocochleogram showing the pattern of destruction of the sensory cells along the cochlea. Note that the hair cells from the base of the cochlea which code for the high auditory frequencies (starting at 0% in the figure) are preferentially damaged by the treatment.

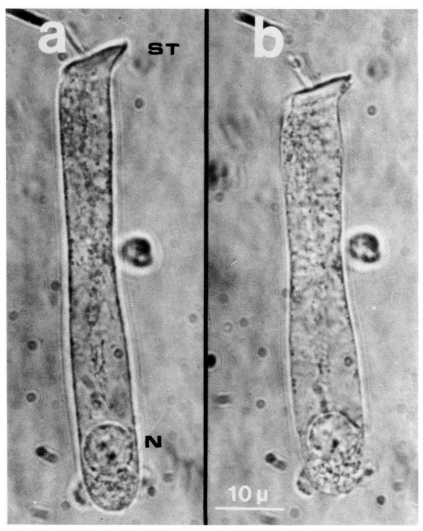

Fig. 17.3 Motile properties of outer hair cells are not affected by acute exposure to gentamicin. Outer hair cells have motile responses that can be elicited *in vitro* by chemical depolarization (high-K⁺ solution) or by electrical stimulation (intracellular current injection through a microelectrode or extracellular exposure to an electrical field). The responses of these cells are imaged here before (a) and after (b) such stimulation. These motile properties of the outer hair cells are not affected after acute exposure to gentamicin. ST indicates the position of the stereocilia and N that of the nucleus.

Uptake and Cellular Localization of Gentamicin in Isolated Hair Cells *In Vitro*

A key aspect in elucidating the molecular mechanism of ototoxicity is to know how the toxic agents penetrate the cells and where the molecules go. As previously mentioned, our recent autoradiographical investigations with [^{3}H]gentamicin and immunochemistry have indicated the lysosomal structure as the site of accumulation in the outer hair cells after treatment *in vivo* (Fig. 17.4). However, it remains to be determined how and where these molecules penetrate the sensory cells, and what are the physiological consequences of this accumulation of gentamicin in the lysosomes. In this context, we have studied the uptake of these molecules *in vitro* in order to know where they bind to the sensory cells and whether they penetrate rapidly after acute exposure. A fluorescent derivative of gentamicin, fluoroisothiocyanate (FITC)–gentamicin, was used to assess the binding and uptake of this molecule in isolated sensory cells. After short exposures (up to 6 h), the fluorescent molecule did not penetrate the outer hair cells *in vitro* but bound externally in the area of the efferent synapse and to a lesser extent in the area of the cuticular plate (Fig. 17.5). These results indicate that gentamicin does not penetrate the sensory cells rapidly. Its incorporation may be by slow endocytosis which is probably linked to the auditory transduction, since it seems to be potentiated by functional depolarization of the cell, as suggested by our previous studies *in vivo* (Hayashida *et al.*, 1989; Aran, 1990). This phenomenon may explain the slow onset of aminoglycoside ototoxicity, even though these molecules rapidly come into contact with the sensory cells (through the perilymph) during treatment *in vivo* (Dulon *et al.*, 1986).

Aminoglycoside Antibiotics Block Ca²⁺ Channels in Isolated Outer Hair Cells

Aminoglycoside antibiotics have also been demonstrated to have neuro-muscular toxicity (for a review see Pittinger and Adamson, 1972) and these drugs were recently shown to impair transmembrane Ca^{2+} flux in isolated nerve terminals, presumably by blocking Ca^{2+} channels (Knaus *et al.*, 1987; Atchison *et al.*, 1988). The aim of our investigation was to determine whether aminoglycoside antibiotics interfere *in vitro* with the homoeostasis of the intracellular Ca^{2+} of the outer hair cells. In response to K^+-depolarization, intracellular Ca^{2+} concentration (monitored by microspectrofluorimetry with fluorescent probes fluo-3 or indo-1) can be rapidly increased from 100 nM to values above 1 μM indicating the

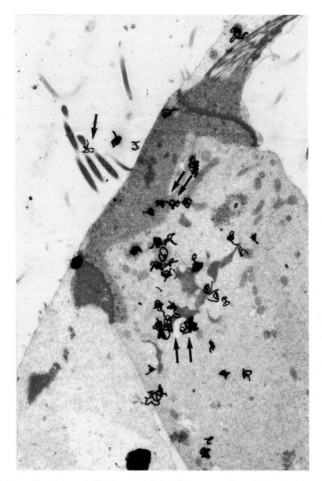

Fig. 17.4 Localization of [³H]gentamicin by autoradiography in the guinea pig cochlea after treatment *in vivo*. The figure shows the apical part of an outer hair cell viewed under transmission electron microscopy. The sensory cells preferentially accumulate the molecule of gentamicin in their lysosomal system predominantly underneath the cuticular plate.

presence of voltage-activated Ca^{2+} channels in these cells (Plate 17.1). The two different aminoglycoside antibiotics tested, gentamicin and neomycin, blocked the Ca^{2+} entry under depolarization with an IC_{50} of 50 μM (Fig. 17.6). Such a block may have several consequences on the physiology of the cells such as alteration of the cell membrane potential which appears to be predominantly determined by a Ca^{2+}-activated K^+ current (Ashmore and Meech, 1986) but may also influence

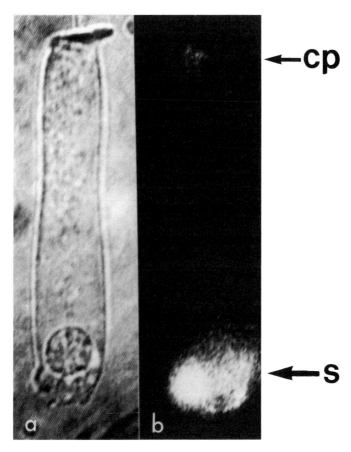

Fig. 17.5 Uptake of FITC–gentamicin in outer hair cells after acute exposure *in vitro*. Hair cells were incubated for 3 h with 0.2 mM FITC–gentamicin. The figure shows the same cell viewed in transmitted light (a) and under fluorescence (b). Note that the fluorescence is associated with the synaptic region (S) and the cuticular plate (CP).

the contractile responses of the outer hair cells by blocking Ca^{2+} influx (Dulon *et al.*, 1990). Furthermore, it should be noted that aminoglycosides have been shown to block the transduction channels in bullfrog hair cells (for a review, see Hudspeth, 1989). It remains to be determined whether and, if so, how this acute channel blockade observed *in vitro* is linked to the toxic process which leads to the death of the sensory cell *in vivo*.

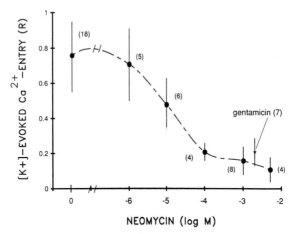

Fig. 17.6 The aminoglycoside antibiotics, neomycin and gentamicin, block K^+-evoked Ca^{2+} entry into isolated outer hair cells. Intracellular Ca^{2+} is monitored with the fluorescent indicator fluo-3 as in Plate 17.1. The value R is the ratio of the relative increase in fluorescence upon depolarization in the presence of various concentrations of drug compared to the fluorescence maximum of the intracellular dye. $R = (F_k - F_0)/(F_{max.} - F_o)$ where F_0 is the radiance value of the cell before stimulation, F_k is the cell radiance after 60 s depolarization and $F_{max.}$ is the cell radiance obtained by the addition of the Ca^{2+} ionophore, ionomycin (10 μM).

Ototoxicity of Other Noxious Agents

Similar investigations to those described for the aminoglycosides can be used to study the ototoxicity of the drugs listed in Table 17.1. Recently, the potential cytotoxic effects of inflammatory mediators (endotoxin and free radicals) which can be generated during otitis media were also evaluated in short-term cultures of outer hair cells (Dulon *et al.* 1989b; Huang *et al.*, 1990). Incubation with endotoxins from two Gram-negative pathogens increased the rate of hair cell death fourfold to sixfold *in vitro*. Free radicals (generated by exposure of the cells to UV light or excitation of intracellular fluorescent dyes) produced morphological damage to hair cells within 60 s. These effects were delayed by addition of free-radical scavengers (Dulon *et al.*, 1989b). These results suggest that inflammatory mediators are rapidly cytotoxic to hair cells and are therefore potentially ototoxic if they permeate the round window membrane during otitis media.

We have also recently started to investigate the ototoxicity of the anticancer drug cis-DDP (diaminedichloroplatinum) *in vitro*. Ototoxicity of this molecule is a well-recognized adverse effect of intensive use in clinical therapy. As observed for the aminoglycosides, our preliminary results indicate that cis-DDP also does not affect cell viability during acute exposure *in vitro*. The possible action of this molecule on the motility and ionic currents of the outer hair cells is currently under investigation (Saito *et al.*, 1991).

Acknowledgements

We gratefully acknowledge J.P. Erre for electrophysiological assessment of auditory function, A. Guilhaume for scanning electron microscopy and C. Aurousseau for drug assays and preparation of figures. We also wish to thank M. Biguerie for his technical assistance.

This research was supported in part by grants from the Conseil d'Aquitaine and the Ligue Nationale Contre le Cancer (Paris).

References

Aran, J.M. (1990). *Adv. Audiol.* **7**, 42–46.
Aran, J.M, Erre, J.P., Guilhaume, A. and Aurousseau, C. (1982). *Acta Otolaryngol.* suppl. 390.
Ashmore, J.F. and Meech, R.W. (1986). *Nature* **322**, 368–371.
Atchison, W.D., Adgate, L. and Beaman, C.M. (1988). *J. Pharmacol. Exp. Ther.* **245**, 394–401.
Brownell, W.E., Bader, C.R., Bertrand, D. and de Ribeaupierre, Y. (1985). *Science* **227**, 194–196.
Dulon, D. and Aran, J.M. (1990). *Médecine/Sciences* **6**, 744–754.
Dulon, D., Aran, J.M., Zajic, G. and Schacht, J. (1986). *Antimicrob. Agents Chemother.* **30**, 96–100.
Dulon, D., Aurousseau, C., Erre, J.P. and Aran, J.M. (1988). *Acta Otolaryngol.* **106**, 219–225.
Dulon, D., Zajic, G., Aran, J.M. and Schacht, J. (1989a). *J. Neurosci. Res.* **24**, 338–346.
Dulon, D., Zajic, G. and Schacht, J. (1989b). *Int. J. Rad. Biol.* **55**, 1007–1014.
Dulon, D., Zajic, G. and Schacht, J. (1990). *J. Neurosci.* **4**, 1388–1497.
Hayashida, T., Hiel, H., Dulon, D., Erre, J.P., Guilhaume, A. and Aran, J.M. (1989). *Acta Otolaryngol.* **108**, 404–413.
Huang, M., Dulon, D. and Schacht, J. (1990). *Ann. Otol. Rhinol. Laryngol.* **99**, (suppl. 148), 35–38.
Hudspeth, A.J. (1989). *Nature* **341**, 397–404.
Knaus, H.G., Streissnig, J., Koza, A. and Glossman, H. (1987). *Naunyn-Schmiedeberg's Arch. Pharmacol.* **336**, 583–586.
Pittinger, C.B. and Adamson, R. (1972). *Annu. Rev. Pharmacol.* **12**, 169–184.
Saito, T., Moataz, R. and Dulon, D. (1991). *Hearing Res.* **56**, 143–147.

Part III

Reproductive Toxicity and Carcinogenesis

A. Reproductive Toxicity

18

Testicular Cell Culture as a Model System for Male Reproduction: Hormone Action and Toxicity Testing

J. MATHER

Genentech Inc., South San Francisco, CA, USA

Introduction

The testis is an enormously complex endocrine organ. In addition to being the site of production of sperm, it secretes the testosterone necessary for the development and maintenance of secondary sex characteristics. The testis is composed of a mass of seminiferous tubules which are limited by a basement membrane and one or more layers of peritubular myoid cells (see schematic representation in Fig. 18.1). Inside the basement membrane are the Sertoli cells and the developing germ cells which give rise to spermatids. Sertoli cells are extremely important because they function to support and regulate the development of the spermatogonia, spermatocytes and spermatids (Jegou *et al.*, 1988). The peritubular cells that form tight junctions with the Sertoli cells divide the interstitial and tubular compartments of the testis; they contribute part of the material which forms the basement membranes surrounding the tubular compartment; furthermore they are androgen responsive and produce substances which influence Sertoli cell function (Skinner, 1987). As isolation and

IN VITRO METHODS IN TOXICOLOGY
ISBN 0-12-388175-7

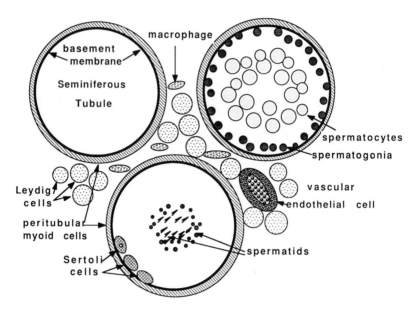

Fig. 18.1 Schematic representation of the cell types making up the testis and their relationships to each other.

culture techniques have been developed for peritubular cells (Mather and Phillips, 1984a), we are beginning to understand more about the very important functions of these cells.

The interstitial tissue between the tubules contains the Leydig cells which produce the androgens necessary for the development and maintenance of all the male secondary sex characteristics. Other cell types in the interstitial space include fibroblasts, interstitial macrophages and the endothelial cells which are part of the microvasculature of the testis (Fig. 18.1). Each of these cells makes a significant contribution to the proper functioning of the testis. It is important, therefore, to be able to study the functions of these cells separately so that we may better understand the contribution of each of them to the production of a mature sperm.

The three-dimensional structure of the testis and the maintenance of the blood–testis barrier is critical to its proper functioning. It might even be said that, unlike some of the other organs, the fourth dimension is also important in the testis. The timing of this developmental process from the first stem cell division to the mature sperm is very precise and very precisely maintained. If it is interrupted, the whole process of spermatogenesis ceases and the developing germ cells degenerate.

What is known about how these various cell types relate to each other is undoubtedly only partially complete and yet is very complicated. There is complex autocrine and paracrine regulation with each of the different cell types producing multiple factors, both soluble and matrix-type, that are important in the regulation of the entire testis (Mather, 1984; Skinner, 1987). Much of our understanding of these interactions has come from using primary cultures enriched for specific cell types (e.g. Leydig, Sertoli or peritubular cells) and established cell lines. Work remains to be done to fit these data into the current view of *in vivo* physiology and endocrinology.

Testicular Cell Lines

Both established cell lines and primary cell and organ cultures can be used for *in vitro* studies of testicular somatic cells (Fig. 18.2). Using several cell culture systems, as well as animals, can lead to more rapid advances in understanding, since each experimental system has unique advantages and disadvantages. Established clonal cell lines are more defined since they contain only one type of cell. If care is taken in the maintenance of the cell lines, the results obtained can be more reproducible in different laboratories and at different times than is possible with primary cultures. Primary cultures may vary as a function of strain, age or hormonal or nutritional status of the animals from which the cultures were derived. On the other hand, cellular physiological responses can be diminished or amplified by prolonged maintenance in the specialized conditions of monolayer culture containing a single cell type. It may thus be difficult to study a desired response using an established cell line because the line is more (or less) sensitive to the test substance than a primary culture would be. The advantages and disadvantages of using primary cultures and established cell lines are listed in Table 18.1.

Cocultures are cultures containing two or more types of cell and may mix established cell lines and primary cultures. Such cultures can be used when it is impossible to maintain a cell type as an isolated cell (e.g. spermatogonia) or when the major purpose of the culture system is to study the interaction of two different cell types. Organ cultures maintain all or part of the three-dimensional structure of the tissue and may therefore be more appropriate for studying cell–cell or cell–matrix interactions.

Rodent testis can be separated rather easily into interstitial and tubular tissue, and then further purified into Leydig cells or macrophages from the interstitium, peritubular cells or Sertoli cells from the tubular tissue

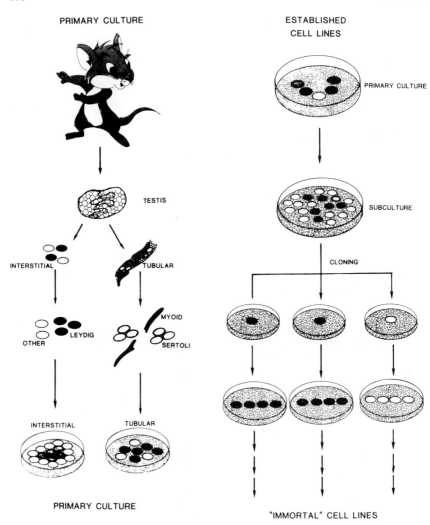

Fig. 18.2 Schematic representation of the derivation and use of primary cultures and established clonal cell lines derived from testicular cell types.

(Mather and Phillips, 1984a; Mather and Bardin, 1988). Some years ago in our laboratory, we used this approach to establish cell lines from primary cultures derived from immature animals enriched for these cell types. These lines represent some of the somatic cell types (Sertoli, Leydig and peritubular myoid) in the testis of rat and mouse and were derived with no overt transformation events (Mather, 1980; Mather and

Table 18.1

Comparison of uses and properties of primary cultures and established cell lines

Primaries	Clonal cell line
Usually several cell types	Single cell type present
Dividing/non-dividing	Cell division
Usually requires high cell density	Can use low density
"Carryover" from *in vivo*	Can control environment
Isolation procedure important	Subculture procedure important

Phillips, 1984b). Other investigators have taken the approach of using testicular somatic cell tumours to establish cell lines (Shin, 1967; Shin *et al.*, 1968; Ascoli, 1982). The currently available established cell lines representative of testicular cell types are listed in Table 18.2.

It is important to keep in mind the differences between test systems when interpreting the results obtained from *in vitro* screening efforts. Some of the differences between *in vitro* and *in vivo* exposure to a drug or hormone include:

1) *The presence of multiple cell types.* As discussed above, the testis contains multiple cell types, only one of which is represented in cultures of clonal cell lines. Even primary cultures and cocultures may alter the cell associations. Thus an effect that requires more than one cell type to be present or the correct association of multiple cell types may not be observable in monoculture *in vitro*.

Table 18.2

Characteristics of established testicular cell lines

Cell line	Cell type	Species	Source	Reference
TM4*	Sertoli	Mouse	Primary 13-day-old testis	Mather (1980)
TR-M	Peritubular	Rat	Tumour	Mather and Phillips (1984b)
TR-1	Endothelial	Rat	Primary 30-day-old testis	Mather *et al.* (1982)
TM3*	Leydig	Mouse	Primary 13-day-old testis	Mather (1980)
R2C*	Leydig	Rat	Tumour	Shin *et al.* (1968)
I10A*	Leydig	Mouse	Tumour	Shin (1967)
MA10	Leydig	Mouse	Tumour	Ascoli (1982)
LC540	Leydig	Rat	Tumour	Steinberger (1970)

* These lines are available through the American Type Culture Collection, Rockville, MD, USA.

2) *Secondary effects from one organ to another.* The pituitary–gonadal axis, for example, is very important in regulating and maintaining testicular function. Testicular damage may occur *in vivo* that results from damage to the pituitary. Of course, such effects would not be seen when an *in vitro* system containing only testicular tissue is used.

3) *The mode of presentation of the hormone, growth factor or drug.* In the body, many of the steroids, vitamins and related compounds are almost immediately bound to carrier proteins and are very seldom seen by any cell as a free agent. These may be quite toxic when not bound to their respective carrier proteins. Thus presentation of a test drug *in vitro* in an unbound form may lead to toxicities at levels that would not occur were the factor bound to a carrier protein.

4) *Inactivation, activation or sequestration in vivo.* The testicular Sertoli cells form junctions between cells which, together with the basement membrane and peritubular cells, form the blood–testis barrier. Thus there are two distinct compartments, the luminal and interstitial, which provide very different microenvironments for the cells they contain. A drug may thus be toxic to spermatocytes *in vitro*, but in fact never reach these cells when delivered *in vivo*.

Selecting the Appropriate Culture System

With the above considerations in mind, one can briefly discuss which culture system should be used for toxicity testing (Bardin *et al.*, 1982) and special considerations in using each type of culture system. We can go back and forth from one type of system to another and learn a great deal in the process of so doing. With primary cultures, the species, strain and age (Rich *et al.*, 1983) of the animal at the time the culture is initiated are important and should be kept constant between laboratories if results are to be compared. The health and nutritional state of the animal at the time of culture may also influence the behaviour of primary cultures so that supplier, method of housing, etc. should be controlled.

When using established cell lines, the passage level of a cell line is important. Certainly cell lines change in culture, but it is a simple matter to establish a frozen cell bank and use the cells for all the tests within a few passages of a given point in time. Thus, these factors are all controllable and should not be seen as an insurmountable barrier to establishing a reproducible and meaningful assay system. The medium, type of culture and configuration are also important parameters, but again all controllable and subject to established quality control procedures.

The question of using transformed versus normal cells can be discussed at greath length, but most frequently there is not much choice and we have to use what is available. The state of transformation of the reported testicular cell lines is shown in Table 18.2.

With regard to serum versus serum-free culture, I am a strong proponent of serum-free culture because of the control it provides over the culture conditions (Mather *et al.*, 1982a). Serum is not a *single* substance but a complex mixture, and it varies from batch to batch and from one country to another. This can cause a great deal of difficulty in trying to establish a reproducible assay system and in the interpretation of results obtained. Testicular cells (with the exception of those residing in the vasculature of the testis) are not exposed to serum but rather to interstitial fluid, lymphatic fluid or tubular fluid, all of which vary considerably in composition from serum (Setchell, 1970). There is thus reason to believe that it is possible to provide an environment more closely related to that seen *in vivo* by omission of serum and provision of appropriate hormones and growth factors. Serum is, in fact, detrimental to the maintenance of Leydig cell function (Mather *et al.*, 1982b) and spermatogenic cell survival *in vitro* (Kierzenbaum and Tres, 1987).

It is important to define carefully what one wishes to measure before selecting the culture system to be used. Stimulation or inhibition of growth can be measured using established cell lines. With primary culture this is not always possible. For example, Sertoli cells derived from a mature animal do not divide. The stimulation or inhibition of cell growth can provide a very effective end point for a screen because it is the end result of a complex set of functions that the cell has to perform. The interruption of any one of these functions would result in a decrease in growth. Such effects might be missed by looking at a more restricted end point (e.g. cAMP production) with a much more defined pathway. Measurement of population growth rates can thus be a very sensitive way of defining whether or not there is an effect of a drug and which cell type is most sensitive to the drug (for example, see Zhuang *et al.*, 1983). Understanding the mechanism of the growth promotion or inhibition is a more complex matter and is not yet completely understood for most known mitogens.

Observation of morphological change as an *in vitro* end point can be another fast easy method for general screening, although somewhat difficult to quantify. It can, however, be a very important indication of an effect, particularly in cell types, such as Sertoli cells, which do not divide in culture (Zhuang *et al.*, 1983). Changes in association of two types of cell can, of course, be looked at in cocultures but not in monoculture (Mather and Phillips, 1984b; Mather *et al.*, 1990).

We can also look for stimulation or inhibition of cell-produced substances such as proteins (Wright *et al.*, 1981), steroids, etc. *In vitro* systems can be used most effectively if we understand the exact physiological system to which the drug is targeted. For example, a screen to detect drugs that interfere with androgen production might be performed using primary Leydig cell cultures (Mather *et al.*, 1981; Morris *et al.*, 1985). Several investigators have monitored the effects of hormones and drugs on Sertoli cell function as measured by the secretion of androgen-binding protein (ABP) or transferrin (for example, see Perez-Infante *et al.*, 1986).

A Special Case: Study of Germ Cells *In Vitro*

This leads us into one of the problems that arise when using *in vitro* systems for studying testicular toxicology. There are cell lines that are derived from most of the somatic cell types in the testis, but 80% of the testis is composed of germ cells. There are no germ-cell-derived cell lines available with the exception of teratoma-derived lines (which seem to resemble embryoid cells more than they do sperm). We may hope eventually to be able to develop a non-transformed stem-cell line, but once these cells enter meiosis they are on a pathway to terminal differentiation.

Although spermatogenic cells cannot be maintained for more than a few hours as monocultures, there are several ways of observing germ cells in primary cultures. Isolated tubules can be cut so that each section contains only certain stages of spermatogenesis. These sections, or small pieces of tubules, can then be cultured as sort of mini organ culture (Parvinen *et al.*, 1983). This model system has the advantage that all the cell associations are maintained. Interestingly, some of the information for these cell–cell associations is contained within the cells which can re-form specific associations *in vitro*. Even with established cell lines, some of these types of cellular interactions can be studied (Mather and Phillips, 1984b). The disadvantage of most organ cultures is that they cannot be maintained for very long *in vitro* and begin to lose function within a few days. More recently systems such as perifusion have been used to maintain cell function for more prolonged periods of time (Kiertzenbaum and Tres, 1987).

We have chosen, however, to study monolayer or bilayer cocultures of Sertoli cells, which comprise the monolayer, and spermatogonia which attach to this monolayer. In such a coculture, the spermatogonia maintain their intracellular bridges and will persist in culture for up to a week. We have used rat Sertoli–germ cell cocultures to look at the effect of various hormones and growth factors on germ cell survival and proliferation *in vitro* (Mather *et al.*, 1990). The distribution of germ cells of different stages of development can be controlled by the method of isolation of the cells and the age of the animals at the time of isolation. We have cultured the cells in hormone-supplemented serum-free medium to provide a more defined background for the cultures.

When these cultures are treated with the testicular hormone, activin, there are two very marked effects. Instead of clusters of one or two germ cells, these clusters now contain 16 to 32 germ cells each, suggesting that the normal development and proliferation of spermatogonial cells has continued *in vitro* (Fig. 18.3). This effect of activin on spermatogonial proliferation was confirmed using thymidine incorporation, autoradiography and fluorescence-activated cell analysis. Secondly, there is a reassociation of the Sertoli cells. This can be seen after only 48 h of treatment, and by 72 h the cells from the monolayer are again forming the tubule-like structures (Mather *et al.*, 1990). This happens in the absence of peritubular cells, therefore the information required for the reassociation must be contained within the Sertoli cell or the Sertoli and germ cells.

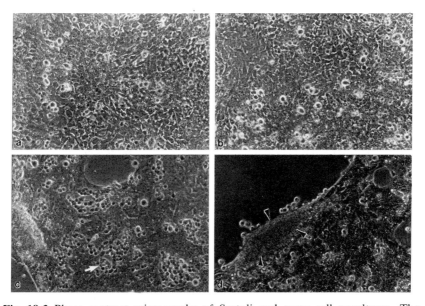

Fig. 18.3 Phase-contrast micrographs of Sertoli and germ cell cocultures. The cultures are shown at 48 h after addition of hormone. Arrows indicate spermatocytes and spermatogonial clusters. The activin-treated cultures (lower panels) are beginning to reaggregate. Cultures shown in (a)–(c) are at 122× magnification. (a) 5F control; (b) 5F + inhibin A (100 ng/ml); (c) 5F + activin A (100 ng/ml); (d) 5F + activin A (61× magnification). Reproduced from Mather *et al.* (1990) with permission.

In this experiment we can thus see an example of an agent (activin) which influences both cell proliferation (spermatogonia) and cell morphology.

Such cocultures can thus help us to look at the early stages of spermatogenesis. However, nothing has been identified so far that would allow us to detect genetic damage to the sperm which could then be transmitted to future generations. The current state of development of *in vitro* systems for testicular cells does not allow full progression of spermatogenesis to mature sperm which could then be used for *in vitro* fertilization and analysis of genetic damage.

In summary, we have a number of options for studying testicular function and drug toxicity *in vitro*. We can use both established cell lines and primary cultures of selected cell types or cocultures of several cell types. These model systems each have their own advantages and disadvantages. The more defined the mode of action of a drug, the more likely it is that we will be able to select the proper *in vitro* test system initially and to apply the knowledge we gain from such experiments to the *in vivo* situation.

References

Ascoli, M. (1982). *J. Biol. Chem.* **257**, 13306–13311.

Bardin, C.W., Taketo, T., Gunsalus, G.L., Koide, S.S. and Mather, J.P. (1982). *In* "Branbury Report II: Environmental Factors in Human Growth and Development" (V.R. Hunt, M.K. Smith and D. Worth, eds), vol. 11, pp. 337–354. Cold Spring Harbor Press, Cold Spring Harbor, New York.

Jegou, B., Le Magueresse, B., Sourdaine, P., Pineau, C., Velez de la Calle, J.F., Garnier, D.H., Guillou, F. and Boisseau, C. (1988). *In* "The Molecular and Cellular Endocrinology of the Testis" (B.A. Cooke and R.M. Sharpe, eds), vol. 50, pp. 21–27. Serrono Symposia Publications, Raven Press, New York.

Kierzenbaum, A.L. and Tres, L.L. (1987). *Ann. N.Y. Acad. Sci.* **513**, 146–157.

Mather, J. (1980). *Biol. Reprod.* **23**, 243–250.

Mather, J.P. (1984). *In* "Mammalian Cell Culture: The Use of Serum-Free and Hormone Supplemented Media" (J.P. Mather, ed.), pp. 167–193. Plenum Press, New York.

Mather, J.P. and Bardin, C.W. (1988). *In* "*In Vitro* Models for Cancer Research V". CRC Press, Boca Raton, Florida.

Mather, J.P. and Phillips, D.M. (1984a). *In* "Methods in Molecular and Cell Biology" (D. Barnes, D. Sirbasku and G. Sato, eds), pp. 29–45. Alan R. Liss, New York.

Mather, J.P. and Phillips, D.M. (1984b). *J. Ultrastruct. Res.* **87**, 263–274.

Mather, J.P., Haour, F. and Saez, J.M. (1981). *Steroids* **38**, 35–44.

Mather, J.P., Perez-Infante, L.Z., Zhuang, V. and Phillips, D.M. (1982a). *Ann. N.Y. Acad. Sci.* **383**, 44–68.

Mather, J.P., Saez, J.M., Dray, F. and Haour, F. (1982b). *In* "Cold Spring

Harbor Conferences on Cell Proliferation" (G. Sato and R. Ross, eds), vol. 9, pp. 1117–1128.

Mather, J.P., Attie, K.A., Woodruff, T.K., Rice, G.L. and Phillips, D.M. (1990). *Endocrinology* **127**, 3206–3214.

Morris, I.D., Bardin, C.W. and Mather, J.P. (1985). *IRCS Med. Sci.* **13**, 1052–1053.

Parvinen, M., Wright, W.W., Phillips, D.M., Mather, J.P., Musto, N.A. and Bardin, C.W. (1983). *Endocrinology* **112**, 1150–1152.

Perez-Infante, V., Bardin, C.W., Gunsalus, G.L., Musto, N.A., Rich, K.A. and Mather, J.P. (1986). *Endocrinology* **118**, 383–392.

Rich, K.A., Bardin, C.W., Gunsalus, G.L. and Mather, J.P. (1983). *Endocrinology* **113**, 2284–2293.

Setchell, B.P. (1970). *In* "The Testis" (A.D. Johnson, W.R. Gomes and N.L. Vandemark, eds), pp. 101–218. Academic Press, New York.

Shin, S. (1967). *Endocrinology* **81**, 440–448.

Shin, S., Yoshihiro, Y. and Sato, G.H. (1968). *Endocrinology*, **82**, 614–616.

Skinner, M.K. (1987). *Ann. N.Y. Acad. Sci.* **513**, 158–171.

Steinberger, A. (1970). *Ann. Meeting Soc. Reprod.*, abstr. p. 4.

Wright, W.W., Musto, N.A., Mather, J.P. and Bardin, C.W. (1981). *Proc. Natl. Acad. Sci. U.S.A.* **78**, 7565–7569.

Zhuang, L.Z., Phillips, D.M., Gunsalus, G.L., Bardin, C.W. and Mather, J.P. (1983). *J. Androl.* **4**, 336–344.

Discussion

Y. Vandenberghe

Is there any explanation for the expanded Leydig cell survival by adding vitamin E?

J. Mather

No. It is interesting that vitamin E will increase the cell survival of mouse cells but is not sufficient to maintain the receptors for gonadotrophins, and in rat cells it does not seem to have much effect. Other antioxidants are effective in porcine cultures, but none of them is as good as vitamin E. However, vitamin E deficiency leads to sterility, so this observation probably reflects a real role for vitamin E in the testis.

H. Brun

What is the mechanism of the toxicity of gossypol on TM_3 and on the production of androgen-binding protein (ABP) by Sertoli cells?

J. Mather

I think with TM_3 the toxicity is entirely non-specific. As other people

have said, if enough of anything is put in, including water, the cells will
be killed, virtually every cell line could be killed by gossypol at that very
high level. It is a steroid-like structure, and steroids will also kill all cells
at high concentrations. We do not know the action on ABP.

F. Marano

Gossypol is known to have some effect on mitochondria *in vivo*. Has Dr
Mather found this kind of effect *in vitro*?

J. Mather

When we observed Sertoli cells using electron microscopy, the mitochondria were not normal in the gossypol-treated cells. Again, I do not know
what the mode of action is, whether it is direct action on the mitochondria
or is related to some of the other phenomena.

P.M. Foster

Do you think that activin is the mitotic factor described by Tony Bellué
about 10 years ago?

J. Mather

That is a good question and an intriguing possibility. I would have to
look at the reported properties of his SGF to see if it looks like the same
compound. We showed that activin is made by Leydig cells. Everyone
assumes it is also made by Sertoli cells but this has not yet been
demonstrated.

X. Pouradier Duteil

I was very impressed by the reorganization into tubules. Does that occur
from a monolayer without any collagen or other proteins?

J. Mather

Yes, and in the case of the activin-induced reaggregation there is no trace
of basement membrane between or beneath cells in that process. It is
also extremely rapid. In the case of the peritubular-cell-induced reaggregation there is basement membrane between the peritubular and Sertoli
cells. This basement membrane is probably produced by the cells and is
certainly involved in the coculture reaggregation.

B. Jegou

Will the very sophisticated technology that you presented be usable soon
by laboratories specializing in toxicology?

J. Mather

The initial investment for a FACS machine is large. For a company that does toxicology testing it is like testing toxicology for one drug. We have six machines and three of them are just used for bioassay. There is no reason why this cannot be done on a routine basis.

Leydig Cell Cultures in the Prediction of Testicular Toxicity

P.-H. BRUN and A. CORDIER

Unité d'Endocrinotoxicologie, Institut de Recherche sur la Sécurité du Médicament, Rhône-Poulenc Rorer, 20 Quai de la Révolution, 94140 Alfortville, France

Introduction

There are many ways in which substances can act on the testis to perturb spermatogenesis, and this variety reflects the complexity of the mechanisms which regulate testicular function. Some agents act directly on one or more of the cell types within the testis, disrupting testicular function. This may involve a toxic phenomenon directly affecting germ cell proliferation (as in the case of anti-cancer drugs) or inhibition of a metabolic process in Sertoli or Leydig cells. Other compounds are centrally active and affect testicular function indirectly by impairing the hypothalamo–pituitary axis. Finally some compounds modify steroid metabolism and thus the endocrine response by altering the capacity of steroid hormones to bind with vectors, or by affecting their catabolism or their excretion (Stockley, 1970; Thomas and Keenan, 1986).

Histology, blood chemistry assays and functional investigations are necessary to detect testicular toxicity, but they are not always sufficient

IN VITRO METHODS IN TOXICOLOGY
ISBN 0-12-388175-7

to explain the mechanism of toxicity and to identify the target, since the same injury may result from direct or indirect impact.

Cell cultures can be used as an adjunct to *in vivo* studies of drug-related toxicology, and Leydig cell cultures provide a complementary method for exploring possible testicular impact. They can be used as:

1) Simple and rapid screening tests
2) Tests with which to investigate the sequence of morphological, biochemical and molecular changes produced by exposure to chemicals and thus to explore the mechanisms underlying toxic injuries.

We will briefly recall the structure of the mammalian testis and of Leydig cells and go on to describe the different types of Leydig cell cultures developed. We will then discuss the possible uses of these cultures in the context of toxicology and define the limits and prospects of this approach.

Structures and Functions of the Testis and Leydig Cell

The mammalian testis has two complementary functions which take place in distinct but interacting areas. Spermatozoa are produced in the seminiferous tubules, whereas androgens are produced by the Leydig cells which are embedded in the interstitial tissue. The seminiferous tubules occupy 65–90% of the testis, depending on the species involved. Each tubule has a diameter of between 200 and 250 μm (Setchell and Pilsworth, 1989) and consists of a peritubular layer of myoid cells which surround the Sertoli and germ cells. The Sertoli cells adhere to the basal membrane of the tubule and extend up to the lumen, surrounding the germ cells. In the basement membrane, the Sertoli cells are interconnected by tight junctions, which constitute part of the blood–testis barrier (Griswold, 1988) which regulates the influx of molecules into the tubule. The Sertoli cells synthesize and secrete proteins (Lacroix and Fritz, 1982; Tindall *et al.*, 1985; Skinner *et al.*, 1989) and fluid (Steinberger *et al.*, 1984; Setchell, 1986) into the tubule and provide the germ cells with the optimum biochemical environment for spermatogenesis. In addition, Sertoli cells interact functionally with the myoid cells (Skinner and Fritz, 1985, 1986) and these interactions seem to be under testosterone control (Skinner and Fritz, 1985); the myoid cells are also involved in the regulation of spermatogenesis. The interstitial tissue contains blood and lymph vessels, nerves and Leydig cells. The anatomical structure of the interstitial tissue varies from one mammalian species to another.

Thus, in rodents, the interstitial tissue is sparse, with large lymphatic spaces, and the Leydig cells are clustered around the blood capillaries. In man and domestic ruminants, the Leydig cells form isolated clumps, whereas in the pig and the horse, the interstitial tissue consists of numerous densely-packed Leydig cells (Fawcett *et al.*, 1973; Setchell, 1978).

Testosterone, which is produced by the Leydig cells, has a major influence on the male reproductive tract, inducing its embryonic differentiation, acting on the maturation of germ cells and playing an important role in the development of the secondary sex gland activities (Waller *et al.*, 1985). All the structures of the testis are closely interrelated by regulatory factors which can modulate their function and morphology in order to provide optimum conditions for spermatogenesis (Tabone *et al.*, 1984; Benhamed *et al.*, 1985a,b; Waller *et al.*, 1985; Le Magueresse *et al.*, 1986; Perrard-Sapori *et al.*, 1986; Pinon-Lataillade *et al.*, 1988; Sharpe *et al.*, 1988; Matsumoto, 1989).

Testicular function is influenced by two major gonadotropic hormones, luteinizing hormone (LH) and follicle-stimulating hormone (FSH) (Phillips *et al.*, 1985). These two hormones are bound to specific receptors on the Leydig cell membrane (LH) and Sertoli cell membrane (FSH) to induce an increase in steroid and protein synthesis via a cyclic AMP(cAMP)-mediated response (Dorrington *et al.*, 1975; Catt *et al.*, 1979; Tindall *et al.*, 1985; Dufau *et al.*, 1987; Means *et al.*, 1976).

The Leydig and Sertoli cells exert negative feedback control on the hypothalamus and anterior pituitary respectively, via blood androgen and inhibin levels. The mechanisms controlling male reproductive tract function are complex and influenced by intra- and extra-testicular factors which ensure appropriate hormone synthesis and initiate and maintain optimum spermatogenesis.

The testis contains several enzyme systems involved in the metabolism of xenobiotics, and these enzymes are principally contained in the Leydig and germ cells. These enzyme systems include alcohol dehydrogenase, glutathione transferases, epoxide hydrolase, aryl hydrocarbon hydroxylase and cytochrome *P*-450 activities (Mukhtar *et al.*, 1978; Lee *et al.*, 1980a; Luketich *et al.*, 1983; Anderson *et al.*, 1985; Yamauchi *et al.*, 1988). These enzymes are not induced by hepatic inducers (Lee *et al.*, 1980b) and are present at a lower level than in the liver. The testis is able to metabolize xenobiotics (especially in the Leydig cells), but the nature and degree of the metabolizing pathways differ from those found in the liver (Chapin and Phelps, 1990), which complicates the prediction of the *in vivo* testicular toxicity from *in vitro* data.

Testosterone Synthesis Pathways

Leydig cells have the typical morphology of hormone-secreting cells, containing high densities of mitochondria, free ribosomes, smooth and rough endoplasmic reticulum and an abundant Golgi apparatus (Keeney *et al.*, 1988). The main function of these cells is to synthesize and secrete androgens, in particular testosterone. Most of the cholesterol within the testis is in an unesterified form (Van der Molen *et al.*, 1972), but in the Leydig cells cholesterol is pooled in lipid droplets in an esterified form. The cholesterol esters have to be hydrolysed before being converted into steroid hormones. The cholesterol is either taken up by the testis from plasma lipoproteins or is synthesized *in situ* from acetate. Within the mitochondria, this cholesterol is then metabolized to form pregnenolone (Pignataro *et al.*, 1983). The cholesterol side-chain is removed by a cholesterol side-chain-cleavage enzyme within the mitochondria: this enzyme requires NADPH, molecular oxygen, flavoprotein and an enzyme complex in order to perform the hydroxylation reaction involved in removing the side chain (Burstein and Gut, 1971). Under the action of 20α- and 22β-hydroxylases, the cholesterol is converted into hydroxycholesterol metabolites, which in turn yield the steroid pregnenolone. The conversion of cholesterol into pregnenolone constitutes the limiting step in steroidogenesis. It is controlled by LH and also depends on the activity and concentration of the cholesterol side-chain-cleavage enzyme.

The pregnenolone formed is then exported into the endoplasmic reticulum, where it is converted into testosterone (Fig. 19.1) via the $\Delta 4$ and $\Delta 5$ pathways, which vary from one species to another. In the rat testis, the $\Delta 4$ pathway appears to be predominant (Bell *et al.*, 1968), whereas the $\Delta 5$ is the most significant pathway in man and some other species (Yanahara and Troen, 1972; Oh and Tamaoki, 1973). A switch from the $\Delta 5$ to the $\Delta 4$ pathway is possible at any stage and so there are many possible pathways by which testosterone can be synthesized from cholesterol. In addition, the reactions involving 17α-hydroxylase and C-17,20-lyase are part of a single cytochrome *P*-450 system (Nakajin and Hall, 1981; Nakajin *et al.*, 1981). Another pathway has been suggested which involves the steroid sulphates. The starting point of this steroidogenesis pathway is pregnenolone sulphate, which is formed as a result of conversion of pregnenolone by a sulphate enzyme (Notation and Ungar, 1969a,b). Pig and horse testis secrete large amounts of steroid sulphates (Setchell and Cox, 1982; Setchell *et al.*, 1983; Orava *et al.*, 1985b), mainly oestrone and dehydroepiandrosterone sulphate.

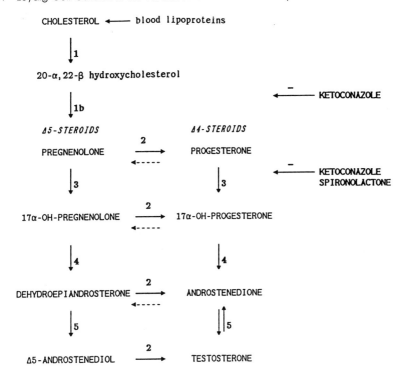

Fig. 19.1 Impact of ketoconazole and spironolactone on steroidogenesis pathways.

Regulation of Leydig Cell Function

Effects of Luteinizing Hormone (LH)

LH is the main trophic hormone which stimulates Leydig cell testosterone production (Dufau *et al.*, 1974; Mendelson *et al.*, 1975; Catt and Dufau, 1976; Chasalow *et al.*, 1979; Catt *et al.*, 1980; Hsueh, 1980; Payne *et al.*, 1980; Ewing *et al.*, 1983). The interaction between LH and its receptors induces a cascade of events: stimulation of adenylate cyclase, cAMP production, activation of protein kinases, increase in the activity of the

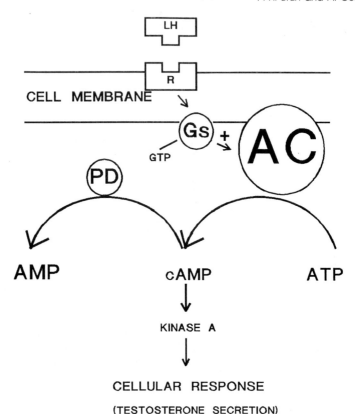

Fig. 19.2 Diagram showing the various stages involved in Leydig cell function from the binding of LH to the response of the cell (synthesis of testosterone), highlighting the possible points of impact of xenobiotics. R= receptor; AC= adenylate cyclase; Gs= stimulatory subunit of protein G; PD= phosphodiesterase.

cytochrome *P*-450 involved in steroidogenesis and androgen production (Mendelson *et al.*, 1975; Catt *et al.*, 1979, 1980; Rommerts and Brinkman, 1981; Rommerts *et al.*, 1983) (Fig. 19.2). After exposure to LH/human chorionic gonadotropin (hCG), there is an initial rise in both cAMP and testosterone levels (Fig. 19.3) with a concomitant down-regulation of the LH receptors and the temporary disappearance of free hCG-binding sites for 120 h after hCG injection (Haour and Saez, 1977; Catt *et al.*, 1979; Nozu *et al.*, 1981a). Steroid synthesis peaks when 1% of the receptors are occupied by hCG molecules (Mombrial *et al.*, 1985) and total occupancy of the sites is obtained with 1×10^{-10} to 3×10^{-10}M hCG, which desensitizes the cells (Mather *et al.*, 1982a; Mombrial *et al.*, 1985),

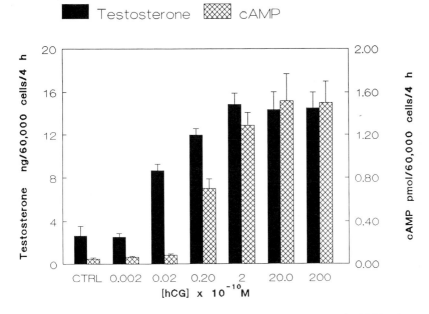

Fig. 19.3 hCG concentration–response curve for testosterone and cAMP release by cultured porcine Leydig cells. On day 3 of the culture, porcine Leydig cells were stimulated by various concentrations of hCG for 4 h incubation periods. The culture medium was analysed for testosterone and cAMP content. Values shown are means ± s.D. of three independent experiments.

so that a second administration of hCG produces no further increase in testosterone. During the desensitization period, there is a decrease in the number of LH receptors, and the coupling system between the receptor and the adenylate cyclase is modified. There is also a blockade of steroidogenesis, which is correlated with a decrease in both lyase and 17α-hydroxylase activities (Saez *et al.*, 1978a,b; Chasalow *et al.*, 1979; Guillou *et al.*, 1985).

LH also plays an important role in the development of Leydig cell function (Chase *et al.*, 1982), both in terms of the total number of cells (Christensen and Peacock, 1980), and in maintaining the integrity of the smooth endoplasmic reticulum (Ewing *et al.*, 1983).

Effects of Other Pituitary Hormones

Treatment of immature rats with FSH increases the number of LH receptors without modifying testosterone production (Chen *et al.*, 1977). In immature hypophysectomized rats, FSH treatment increases both the number of LH receptors and testicular responsiveness to this hormone (Chen *et al.*, 1976, 1977). Using Leydig and Sertoli cell cocultures, it has been shown that FSH does not act directly on Leydig cell function, but interacts with a protein secreted by Sertoli cells (Benhamed *et al.*, 1985a, b; Verhoeven and Cailleau, 1985; Perrard-Sapori *et al.*, 1986).

Prolactin (Prl) acts on specific Leydig cell receptors (Hafiez *et al.*, 1972; Bartke, 1980) to modulate both the LH receptor level and steroid production. Conversely, LH modifies the prolactin receptor level of Leydig cells (Chan *et al.*, 1981). There is a close relationship between the effects of LH and Prl in regulating these two types of receptor, and the regulatory process, which depends on the species and on the concentration of each hormone, also influences Leydig cell responsiveness.

Growth hormone (GH) can also stimulate the steroidogenic response of Leydig cells; however, the mechanism involved remains to be elucidated (Purvis *et al.*, 1981).

Effects of Oestrogens

Oestrogens can influence testicular function. The administration of oestrogens to male rats decreases testosterone synthesis, resulting in a concomitant accumulation of progesterone and 17α-hydroxyprogesterone, due to reduced 17α-hydroxylase and C-17,20-lyase activities (Kremers *et al.*, 1977; Van Beurden *et al.*, 1978; Nozu *et al.*, 1981a,b). The modifications of steroidogenesis pathways caused by oestradiol are the same as those produced by LH during the desensitization period, and oestradiol could be one of the mediators of hCG-induced Leydig cell desensitization. In the male rat, oestrogens modify testicular steroid metabolism, *in vivo* and *in vitro*, but this finding cannot be extrapolated, *in vitro*, to other species, such as pigs and mice (Saez *et al.*, 1983).

Effects of Glucocorticoids

All the situations which induce an elevation of the endogenous adrenal corticosteroids have a direct inhibitory effect on Leydig cell steroidogenesis (Charpenet *et al.*, 1981; Welsh *et al.*, 1982; Bernier *et al.*, 1984). The presence of glucocorticoid receptors in Leydig cells (Evain *et al.*, 1976) may account for the direct effect of cortisol on testicular steroid metabolism. Steroidogenesis is blocked as a result firstly, of decreased gonadotropin stimulation of cAMP production and secondly of reduced 17α-hydroxylase activity (Welsh *et al.*, 1982). This enzyme seems to determine a critical step in the regulation of steroidogenesis by endogenous steroids.

Effects of Various Factors

Other factors such as insulin, somatomedin-c (Bernier *et al.*, 1986; Saez *et al.*, 1988), catecholamines (Renier *et al.*, 1987), fibroblast growth factor (FGF) (Sordoillet *et al.*, 1988), epidermal growth factor (EGF) (Welsh and Hsueh, 1982), transforming growth factor (TGFβ) (Morera *et al.*, 1988), lipoproteins (Quinn *et al.*, 1981; Benahmed *et al.*, 1983), albumin (Melsert *et al.*, 1989), vitamins A and E (Mather *et al.*, 1982b, 1983) and prostaglandins (Haour *et al.*, 1979) also modulate Leydig cell function both *in vivo* and *in vitro*, and act as regulating factors on testicular metabolism.

Leydig Cells in Culture

Leydig cell cultures can be used as a tool with which to investigate certain aspects of the physiology of the testis. Various culture methods are available, and the one chosen will depend on the question under consideration. Leydig cell lines, which do not express all the properties of the normal cell, may sometimes be more appropriate than primary cell culture. Cells in primary culture initially express and conserve many of the specific functions of the *in vivo* cells. There are also various differences between normal Leydig cells and Leydig tumour cells, the most important difference being the type of steroid secreted (Ascoli and Puett, 1978).

In this section, Leydig cell lines and primary culture will be discussed successively, with special attention being paid to the advantages and critical points in each case.

Leydig Cell Lines

Leydig cell lines maintain some of the specific functions of the original cell and can be used to provide important information about these functions. For this reason, Leydig cell lines may be preferred to primary culture when attempts are made to clucidate the processes involved in hormone biosynthesis, hormone action and the regulation of the expression of Leydig cell function.

Most of these cell lines are derived from tumour or non-tumour Leydig cells from either mouse or rat.

Mouse Leydig tumour cell lines

MA-10 cell lines and derivatives
The MA-10 cloned cell line derives from a transplantable murine Leydig tumour (M5480). This clone is characterized by the presence of functional hCG receptors. Under basal conditions, the MA-10 cells produce mainly progesterone and 20α-dihydroprogesterone, but no testosterone, indicating some modification of the steroidogenic pathway. MA-10 cells can be stimulated by hCG, which activates the adenylate cyclase system, resulting in the production of cAMP. Cholera toxin and 8-Br-cAMP can also stimulate steroid production by these cells.

The MA-10 cell clone can be maintained in culture for 100 generations without any changes in the hCG-binding activity (Ascoli, 1981a). This Leydig tumour cell line has been used to study the effect of gonadotropin (Ascoli, 1981b) and regulatory factors (Pereira *et al.*, 1987; Pandey *et al.*, 1985, 1986; Ascoli *et al.*, 1987) on steroidogenesis, cholesterol metabolism (Freeman and Ascoli, 1983; Freeman, 1987a) and the toxic effects of drugs, especially the impact of ketoconazole on steroid production (Chaudhary and Stocco, 1989).

Over time, the MA-10 cells progressively lose their ability to synthesize steroids in culture and constitute a heterogeneous population (Kilgore and Stocco, 1989). Subcloning of the MA-10 line led to the isolation of the MA-10 LP subclone (Kilgore and Stocco, 1989). MA-10 LP cells are stimulated by hCG and $(Bu)_2$-cAMP, producing much lower levels of progesterone than the MA-10 line. The difference results in a lesion located after the production of cAMP and before cholesterol side-chain-cleavage enzyme (Kilgore and Stocco, 1989; Kilgore *et al.*, 1990). This line provides an interesting model for use in investigating a specific step in steroidogenesis.

The K9 cell line derives from a hybridization of freshly isolated mouse Leydig cells and MA-10 cells and secretes testosterone in response to hCG stimulation, although it loses this property after 3 months in culture, while the other functions (hCG-binding activity, cAMP production) are maintained throughout a 6-month culture period. However, testosterone secretion is lower than that observed in mouse Leydig cells in primary culture. The K9 cells express hCG receptors and, as in normal Leydig cells, prolonged exposure to hCG induces a decrease in hCG binding, related to the down-regulation of receptors (Finaz *et al.*, 1987).

The loss of testosterone production after 3 months in culture is explained by the conversion of the K9 cells into the parental phenotype MA-10; this necessitates frequent subclonings to maintain this specific function.

MLTC-1 cell line
The MLTC-1 Leydig cell line derives from the transplantable mouse Leydig tumour, M5480 (Ascoli and Puett, 1978). MLTC-1 cells specifically bind hCG with a high affinity ($K_d = 5.4 \times 10^{-10}$M). Studies of isolated membranes indicate the presence of a single class of receptor ($K_d = 1.0 \times 10^{-10}$M). hCG binding induces the stimulation of adenylate cyclase, resulting in the production of cAMP in a time- and concentration-dependent fashion.

Adenylate cyclase activity can also be stimulated by cholera toxin. When the MLTC-1 cells are exposed to hCG, they produce progesterone but not testosterone (Rebois, 1982). Under basal conditions, these cells do not produce progesterone, but small amounts of testosterone can be detected (Ascoli and Puett, 1978). This cell line has been used to study the mechanism of action of hCG on LH receptors and on the adenylate cyclase system (Rebois *et al.*, 1983), as well as the fate of the hCG receptor after hCG binding. These studies have shown that the internalization and degradation of the bound hCG occurs rapidly and mainly inside the cell (Kellokumpu, 1987). These cells have also been used to study the process of desensitization (down-regulation) after hCG exposure (Rebois and Fishman, 1983, 1984, 1986; Rebois *et al.*, 1987; Inoue and Rebois, 1989) and the toxic effects of drugs, especially the interactions of taxol with steroid production and microtubule polymerization (Rainey *et al.*, 1985).

The B-1 mouse Leydig tumour cell line
B-1 cells are derived from a mouse Leydig cell tumour (T 124958-R). The growth of these cells is markedly dependent on oestrogen (Sato *et al.*, 1987; Nishizawa *et al.*, 1988) and androgen (Nishizawa *et al.*, 1989). This cell line has been used to study the effect of compounds, such as vanadate (Sata *et al.*, 1987), hydroxytamoxifen (Nishizawa *et al.*, 1988) and arachidonic acid (Nishizawa *et al.*, 1990) as well as the metabolism of oestrogen receptor (Miyashita *et al.*, 1990).

The TM3 mouse clonal cell line of non-tumorigenic testicular cells

The TM3 cell line was isolated from an immature mouse testicular primary culture (Mather, 1980). After plating, initially, in serum-free medium, and later with increasing concentrations of foetal calf serum, the cells were morphologically selected and then cloned. The TM3 clone was isolated one year after plating. TM3 cells have an epithelial morphology and do not induce any tumours after inoculation in nude mice. TM3 cells express specific LH receptors on their membrane, produce cAMP in basal conditions and, after hCG exposure, can metabolize cholesterol and progesterone (Mather, 1980).

This cell line has been used to study specific receptors, such as arginine vasopressin (Maggi *et al.*, 1989) and calcitonin receptors (Nakhla *et al.*, 1989). Calcitonin stimulates the basal production of testosterone via an increase in cAMP concentration and also increases the number of oestrogen and androgen receptors in TM3 cells. TM3 cells have also been used to study the hormonal regulation of enzymes in the testis (Vanha-Perttula *et al.*, 1986; Osterman and Terracio, 1987), cell interactions (Mather and Phillips, 1984), the toxic effects of chemical compounds, such as gossypol, on testosterone production (Zhuang *et al.*, 1983) and the regulation of the expression of Leydig cell function (Mather, 1982; Lee *et al.*, 1989).

The R2C rat Leydig tumour cell line

The R2C cell line was obtained from a rat tumour. It is characterized by steroid hormone synthesis which is independent of trophic hormone control (Freeman, 1987b). Indeed, R2C cell membranes have few hCG receptors, and the intracellular level of cAMP in these cells is too low to induce a steroidogenic response. Steroid hormones, particularly progesterone, are secreted by a cAMP-independent mechanism, under the control of an extramitochondrial factor which is cycloheximide-sensitive and identical with that synthesized by normal Leydig cells. R2C cells are also characterized by a high level of cytochrome *P*-450 aromatase activity (Lephart *et al.*, 1990).

This cell line has been used to study the hormonal and neurohormonal control of gonadal function (Gonzalez-Manchon and Vale, 1989; McMurray *et al.*, 1989).

Table 19.1 summarizes the media and supplements used in Leydig cell line cultures.

Primary Cultures of Leydig Cells

When cells are seeded, they lose part of their environment, in particular, their position in the source organ, complex cell–cell and tissue–cell interactions, some of the factors required for cell viability and function, and the fluids (lymph or blood) in which they are bathed *in vivo*. In addition, culturing of cells requires a detailed knowledge of the physiology of the cell cultured in order to control the culture conditions and to

Table 19.1

Media and supplements used for Leydig cell culture-cell lines

Species	Clone	Media	Supplements	Examples
Mouse	MA-10	Waymouth MB752/1 Waymouth MB752/1 Waymouth MB752/1	10% FBS BSA 15% HS	Ascoli (1981) Freeman (1987b) Chaudhary *et al.* (1989) Ascoli (1981b) Pandey *et al.* (1986)
	MA-10 LP	Waymouth MB752/1	15% HS	Kilgore *et al.* (1989, 1990)
	K9	DMEM	15% FCS	Finaz *et al.* (1987)
	MLTC-1	RPMI 1640	10% FCS	Rebois (1982) Kellokumpu (1987)
	MLTC-1	DMEM: HAMF12		Rainey *et al.* (1985)
	B1	MEM	10% FBS, Ins, E2	Nishizawa *et al.* (1988) Miyashita *et al.* (1990)
	TM3 TM3	DMEM: HAMF12 DMEM: HAMF12	5% FCS, Ins, Tr, EGF 5% HS, 2.5 NBBS Ins, Tr, EGF	Mather (1980) Zhuang *et al.* (1983)
Rat	R2C R2C R2C	Waymouth MB752/1 HAMF10 HAMF12	BSA 15% HS, 2.5% FCS 15% HS, 2.5% FCS	Freeman (1987a) Gonzalez-Manchon and Vale (1989) Lephart *et al.* (1990)

Abbreviations: BSA = bovine serum albumin, FBS = foetal bovine serum, FCS = foetal calf serum, NBBS = new-born bovine serum, HS = horse serum, Tr = transferrin, Ins = insulin, EGF = epidermal growth factor, DMEM: HAMF12 = Dulbecco's modified Eagle's medium and Ham's nutrient mixture F12 (1:1), HAMF10 = Ham's nutrient mixture F10, MEM = Eagle's minimum essential medium.

define the most appropriate composition of the culture medium for the cell type, and the most significant parameters for follow-up during culture.

Leydig cells from different species do not express the same properties in culture in terms of steroid secretion, maintenance of LH receptors and cell responsiveness.

The age of the source animals is also a critical factor: far fewer Leydig cells can be recovered from the testes of mature animals than from the testes of immature animals. The lower the germ cell content of the testis, the higher the yield and quality of the Leydig cells. Accordingly, testes of immature animals (2–4 weeks old) are usually used (Mather et al., 1981; Rommerts et al., 1982).

Three species are commonly used for Leydig cell culture: rats, mice and pigs. However, some studies have been performed using cells from other species, including dog, rabbit, hamster and guinea-pig (Oh and Tamaoki, 1973; Boyden et al., 1980; Zirkin et al., 1980).

Dispersal of the tissue: preparation of crude interstitial cells

The first step in the dispersal of the testis involves mechanical, thermic and/or enzymic techniques.

Disaggregation of mouse testis cells can be performed either by a non-enzymic procedure involving slow and careful aspiration into a syringe fitted with 6 mm diameter silicone tubing (Schumacher et al., 1978, 1979), or by a procedure using a dispase enzyme (Merkel et al., 1990).

Rat, pig and human Leydig cells are dispersed using both mechanical and enzymatic dispersal techniques, with varying shaking rates, duration of incubation, rinsing buffer, filter type and temperature (Dufau et al., 1974; Klinefelter et al., 1987; Mather et al., 1981, 1982a; Simpson et al., 1987). Rat, pig and human Leydig cells are sensitive to mechanical forces, whereas enzymic dispersal alone is not sufficient for cell isolation.

The dispersal protocol varies according to the amount of testis to be dispersed and the sensitivity of the tissue to mechanical and enzymic techniques.

Purification of crude interstitial cells

After dispersal, the cells for collection are separated by centrifuging, then filtered through nylon gauze to eliminate any pieces of undigested tissue and finally washed. The cell suspension is then purified by density gradient centrifugation using metrizimide (Dufau et al., 1978; Payne et al., 1982), Ficoll (Janszen et al., 1976) or Percoll (Lefevre et al., 1983) to separate the Leydig cells from the germ and myoid cells, erythrocytes and cell debris. A Percoll gradient can also be used to separate different subpopulations of Leydig cells (Lefevre et al., 1983): this procedure yields a population containing 80–90% Leydig cells.

After gradient centrifugation, the purity of the Leydig cell preparation is determined by using an histochemical staining for 3β-hydroxysteroid dehydrogenase (Wiebe, 1976), which is a specific enzyme present in Leydig cells, and the viability is determined by the Trypan Blue exclusion test.

Leydig cell cultures

Culture medium and supplemented factors (Table 19.2)
The culture medium must promote the Leydig cell population by preventing the survival of other cell types. The addition of factors to the medium can also help to select a specific cell population; and these added factors may be species specific.

MEM (Dufau *et al.*, 1974), Dulbecco's Eagle's MEM supplemented with 1–10% foetal calf serum (Hunter *et al.*, 1982), RPMI 1640 (Lefevre *et al.*, 1983) and HAMF12/DMEM (Mather *et al.*, 1981, 1982a) have been used for Leydig cell culture. These culture media can be supplemented by hormones, such as insulin, human transferrin, α-tocopherol, EGF and lipoproteins. In some cases, serum is added to the culture medium to provide the cells with supplementary growth factors and hormones. Foetal calf serum (0.1%), in the presence of α-tocopherol, enhances steroid production by porcine Leydig cells (Haour *et al.*, 1983).

Culture conditions
As for other cell types, temperature, pH, pCO_2, humidity, culture substrate and cell density are critical parameters. Temperature must approximate to that of the testis *in vivo* (32–34°C). Cells are usually plated on uncoated plates appropriate for tissue culture. In some cases, plates coated with collagen, laminin or fibronectin are used to facilitate cell attachment.

The cell density varies according to the parameters measured. Leydig cells are seeded at a concentration of about 2×10^5 to 3×10^5 cells per cm^2.

The Leydig Cell: A Potential Target of Chemical Compounds

Drug Impact on the Testis and Place of Leydig Cell Cultures in the Prediction of the Testicular Toxicity of Chemical Compounds

The testis is a target organ for a variety of chemicals (Setchell, 1978; Waller *et al.*, 1985; Thomas and Keenan, 1986). Numerous drugs affecting the testis or extratesticular sites may cause testicular injuries, which generally result in inhibition of spermatogenesis.

Blood flow, an important factor in the transport of oxygen, nutrients

Table 19.2
Media and supplements used for Leydig cell culture-primary culture

Species	Media	Supplements	Purification	Examples
Rat	KRBG	BSA	Ficoll-met-rizoate	Janszen et al. (1976)
	McCoy's 5a			Hsueh (1980)
	M199	BSA, 0.5% FCS	Percoll	Browning et al. (1981, 1983)
	DMEM: HAMF12	Tr, Ins, EGF	Ficoll	Rommerts et al. (1982)
	MEM	1% FCS	Ficoll	Rommerts et al. (1982)
	DMEM: HAMF12	Tr, Ins, EGF	Percoll	Browning et al. (1983)
	DMEM	0.1% BSA	Percoll	Cooke et al. (1983)
	RPMI 1640	Tr, Ins, Vit E, 0.1%FCS	Percoll	Lefevre et al. (1983)
	MEM	5% FCS	Percoll	Janecki et al. (1984)
	DMEM		Percoll	Yee and Hutson (1985)
	M199		Percoll	Klinefelter and Ewing (1987)
	DMEM: HAMF12	4% FCS, LP	Cytodex 3 bead	Klinefelter and Ewing (1988)
Mouse	DMEM: HAMF12	Tr, Ins, EGF, 0.02% and 10% FCS		Mather and Sato (1979)
	MEM		Percoll	Schumacher et al. (1979)
	DMEM	10% FCS		Hunter et al. (1982)
	M199	Tr, Ins, EGF		Murphy and Moger (1982)
	DMEM	0.1% BSA, 1% FCS	Percoll	Cooke et al. (1983)
	M199	BSA	Percoll	Merkel et al. (1990)
Pig	DMEM: HAMF12	Tr, Ins, EGF, Vit E, 0.1 and 0.5% FCS	Percoll	Mather et al. (1981, 1982a) Bernier et al. (1983) Mombrial et al. (1985)
Human	M199	BSA	Percoll	Simpson et al. (1987)

Abbreviations: KRBG = Krebs–Ringer bicarbonate buffer, BSA = bovine serum albumin, FCS = foetal calf serum, Tr = transferrin, Ins = insulin, EGF = epidermal growth factor, Vit E = vitamin E, LP = lipoprotein, DMEM: HAMF12 = Dulbecco's Modified Eagle's Medium and Ham's nutrient mixture F12 (1:1), M199 = medium 199, MEM = Eagle's minimum essential medium.

and regulatory hormones to and from the testis (Setchell, 1990), can be modified by compounds and thus may induce testis injury (Vermeulen, 1982). Indeed, vasoconstrictors, such as histamine (O'Steen, 1963) or epinephrine (Chatterjee and Paul, 1968), glucose deficiency and a diabetic state (Faerman *et al.*, 1972) can all lead to testicular disorders.

Several agents may interfere with the production of spermatozoa by acting either directly on germ cells, e.g. anticancer drugs (Mecklenburg *et al.*, 1975; Thachil *et al.*, 1981; Meistrich *et al.*, 1982; Russell *et al.*, 1983; Velez de la Calle *et al.*, 1988), or indirectly, either by impairing the function of Sertoli cells, e.g. phthalates (Gray and Gangolli, 1986; Chapin *et al.*, 1988; Lloyd and Foster, 1988) and cisplatin (Pogach *et al.*, 1989a,b), or that of Leydig cells (Morris *et al.*, 1988; Azouri *et al.*, 1989; Cavallini *et al.*, 1990).

Other drugs may induce testicular disorders by acting on the hypothalamo–pituitary axis. These agents interfere with gonadotropin release by a neuronal mechanism and/or by increasing prolactin secretion (Wood and Lyengar, 1988). Antihypertensive drugs (reserpine), tranquillizers, barbiturates, opiates, antiadrenergic agents, serotonin and dopamine antagonists can all induce impotence and alterations in gonadal activity by such mechanisms (Horowitz and Goble, 1979; Thomas and Keenan, 1986). Ethanol is also a gonadal toxin, and inhibits testosterone secretion via a direct mechanism on Leydig cells, but can also affect testicular function by inhibiting gonadotropin release (Cicero and Bell, 1982; Van Thiel, 1983; Santucci *et al.*, 1983).

In addition, some drugs which provoke the induction or inhibition of hepatic enzymes, in particular cytochrome *P*-450, can influence the metabolism of steroids in the testis and the adrenals.

Finally, the overproduction of glucocorticosteroids by the adrenals may also influence testicular function by inhibiting Leydig cell steroidogenesis (Welsh *et al.*, 1982).

In vivo, drug-induced testicular damage is common and the mechanisms responsible are varied. Interference with or blocking of any link in the chain of biological events which control the testis function may result in testicular injury. Histological examinations, blood hormone assays and functional investigations can detect testicular toxicity, but are not always sufficient to explain the mechanism of toxicity and to identify the site of impact, since direct or indirect impact can lead to the same injury. The development of a cell culture model is therefore required to elucidate the toxic effects of drugs and to complement conventional hormone studies.

Leydig cells in primary culture have been used in toxicological studies, which have been performed by the authors listed below using the cell cultures indicated:

1) Rat Leydig cells, the most commonly used cells (Cooke *et al.*, 1975; Janszen *et al.*, 1977; Sairam and Berman, 1979; Pont *et al.*, 1982; Van Thiel *et al.*, 1983; Kan *et al.*, 1985; Sikka *et al.*, 1985, 1988; Rommerts *et al.*, 1988; Orpana *et al.*, 1989; Ng and Liu, 1990);
2) Mouse Leydig cells (Schurmeyer and Nieschlag, 1984; Pearce *et al.*, 1986; Johansson, 1989a,b);
3) Porcine Leydig cells (Bernier *et al.*, 1984; Orava *et al.*, 1985a, 1989; Albertson *et al.*, 1988; Penhoat *et al.*, 1988; Orava, 1989; French and Welsh, 1990);
4) Human Leydig cells (Albertson *et al.*, 1988).

Several studies have also been performed using rodent Leydig cell lines (Dix and Cooke, 1981; Zhuang *et al.*, 1983; Rainey *et al.*, 1985).

Primary Culture of Porcine Leydig Cells as a Model for Predicting the Testicular Toxicity of Compounds

Methods

Isolation of Leydig cells

Table 19.3 shows an example of a protocol adapted from Mather *et al.* (1981, 1982a) used to isolate and culture Leydig cells from 2–4-week-old pigs. This procedure yields 1×10^7 to 1.5×10^7 interstitial cells per testis, with 75–90% Leydig cells.

Table 19.3
Isolation and culture of Leydig cells from 2–4-week-old pigs (Mather *et al.*, 1981, 1982a)

---

(1) Collect the testes in RPMI 1640
(2) Remove the capsule and mince the testes
(3) Expose minced testes to collagenase–dipase 0.3% + trypsin inhibitor 0.03% at 34°C for 10 min with gentle magnetic stirring
(4) Collect and centrifuge the supernatant
(5) Repeat enzymic dispersal of the tubules two to three times
(6) Wash the pellets and pool all of them
(7) Filter through Nitex (150 and 60 μm opening)
(8) Layer the filtered cell suspension over the top of a discontinuous Percoll gradient and centrifuge at 2500 *g* for 20 min at 4°C
(9) Remove the band corresponding to Leydig cells and wash it twice
(10) Assess the purity of the Leydig cell preparation by histochemical staining for 3β-hydroxysteroid dehydrogenase, and the cell viability by the Trypan Blue exclusion test
(11) Plate in HAMF12: DMEM (1:1) supplemented with transferrin (5 μg/ml), vitamin E (10 μg/ml), insulin (5 μg/ml) and foetal calf serum (0.1%)

Justification of this primary Leydig cell culture procedure

In these conditions, Leydig cells in culture maintain the specific functions of the *in vivo* cell, for various lengths of time, depending on the source species. The use of a medium with a low serum concentration but supplemented with hormones gives a better selection of Leydig cells, enhanced viability and cell function, decreased fibroblastic proliferation and easy follow up of the specific parameters of the cultured cells (Mather and Sato, 1979). However, under these culture conditions, there is almost no cell multiplication (Benhamed *et al.*, 1983).

Collagenase treatment does not induce extensive cellular damage. It provides a satisfactory method for establishing long-term culture, for studying LH membrane receptors and for measuring androgen secretion.

Cultures of interstitial tissues from immature pigs present many advantages over rodent Leydig cell cultures (Mather *et al.*, 1981). The immature pig testis contains a high percentage of Leydig cells (40–60%), compared with only 3% in rat testis (Mori and Christensen, 1980), which facilitates isolation and results in the expression of more hCG receptors (Mather *et al.*, 1981). Unlike rat and mouse Leydig cells (Hunter *et al.*, 1982; Klinefelter and Ewing, 1988, 1989), porcine Leydig cells can be maintained in a chemically defined medium without losing the specific properties required for *in vitro* studies: indeed, porcine Leydig cells maintain the hCG receptors and the entire steroidogenesis pathway including testosterone production throughout the cell's lifespan in culture (Mather *et al.*, 1981).

The principal steroidogenesis pathway in the pig testis is the $\Delta 5$ pathway (which is the same as in human testis), whereas in the rat it is the $\Delta 4$ pathway (Phillips *et al.*, 1985).

Leydig cells in culture usually progressively lose their specific functions and undergo dedifferentiation (Steinberger, 1975). However, porcine Leydig cells maintain their specific functions in culture (Fig. 19.4). After 4 days in culture, testosterone and cAMP production begin to decrease, and this can be attributed to impairment of several enzymatic complexes and, in particular, to a fall in 17α-hydroxylase (Verhoeven *et al.*, 1982). In opposition, progesterone levels begin to rise after 5 days in culture. All these observations clearly indicate a progressive loss of the constitutive enzymes with increasing culture time, particularly 17α-hydroxylase.

Effect of compounds on porcine Leydig cells in primary culture

A compound may affect the cell at various levels (Fig. 19.2). Primary cultures of Leydig cells maintain many of the *in vivo* functions of the cells, and this distinguishes them from Leydig cell lines. In addition,

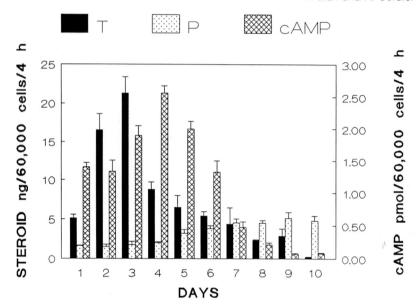

Fig. 19.4 Influence of the duration of culture on testosterone (T), progesterone (P) and cAMP secretion. On 10 consecutive days, cells were stimulated by hCG (2×10^{-10} M) for 4 h. Testosterone, progesterone and cAMP were assayed in the incubation media. Values shown are means $\pm$ s.d. of three independent experiments.

primary cultures of porcine Leydig cells, which present the advantages previously described, also provide a model suitable for studying the impact of compounds on the main functional steps of the cell:

1) hCG binding at membrane receptors
2) Message transduction and amplification
3) Second messenger synthesis (cAMP)
4) Steroid synthesis and more particularly testosterone synthesis

For these reasons, piglet Leydig cells in primary culture were used to evaluate the *in vitro* effects of chemicals on steroid synthesis.

Methods
Leydig cell function was assessed from steroid production, cAMP biosynthesis and binding of ^{125}I-labelled hCG to Leydig cells. A cytotoxicity test was also performed to differentiate between non-specific cell toxicity and specific interactions with cell functions.

Three compounds, chosen for their known effects on Leydig cells in man and animals, were tested in the culture model (Brun *et al.*, 1991):

ketoconazole and *spironolactone* are known to modify steroid metabolism in Leydig cells (Fraser, 1979; Pont *et al.*, 1982); *chlorpromazine* does not act directly on Leydig cells, but interferes with the secretion of gonadotropins.

Results and discussion
As shown in Fig. 19.5, ketoconazole induced a rapid fall of testosterone level, with an $IC_{50} = 0.1$ μM. In contrast, progesterone assays revealed a significant increase in production at 0.2 μM (130% of control) and a decrease at higher concentrations, with an $IC_{50} = 13$ μM. This drug induced a decrease in steroid secretion without significant cytotoxicity. At 72 h after removal of the drug, complete restoration of testosterone secretion was observed at concentrations of 0.2 and 2 μM ketoconazole; at higher concentrations, testosterone production remained depressed (Table 19.4).

Ketoconazole inhibits microsomal cytochrome *P*-450 (Kan *et al.*, 1985;

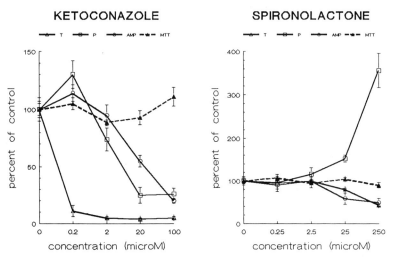

Fig. 19.5 Influence of ketoconazole and spironolactone on steroid and cAMP production by cultured porcine Leydig cells. On day 3 of the culture, Leydig cells were treated with various concentrations of drugs and stimulated by hCG (2 × 10^{-10} M) for 4 h. Testosterone (T), progesterone (P) and cAMP (AMP) were assayed in the incubation media and the cell viability (MTT) was evaluated by MTT staining. The results were expressed as a percentage of the vehicle control, which was taken as 100% (control values = 15.5 ± 2.2 ng of testosterone/60 000 cells per 4 h, 1.94 ± 0.28 ng progesterone/60 000 cells per 4 h, 1.26 ± 0.18 pmol cAMP/60 000 cells per 4 h and 0.620 ± 0.035 optical density for cytotoxicity evaluation). Values shown are means ± s.d. (*n* = 9).

Table 19.4
Reversibility of testosterone inhibition after drug removal

Ketoconazole

Concentration (μM)	0	0.2	2	20	100
% of control	100 ± 14	120 ± 15	111 ± 5	33 ± 7***	5 ± 1***

Spironolactone

Concentration (μM)	0	0.25	2.5	25	250
% of control	100 ± 18	110 ± 5	119 ± 16	120 ± 10	107 ± 8

Chlorpromazine

Concentration (μM)	0	0.3	3	30	300
% of control	100 ± 18	110 ± 7	120 ± 9	59 ± 5**	18 ± 5***

After treatment and stimulation of Leydig cells with drugs and hCG for 4 h, the medium was removed and replaced by fresh culture medium. The reversibility of the inhibition produced by the drugs was assessed from the response to hCG stimulation 24 h (in the case of spironolactone and chlorpromazine: control value = 12.8 ± 1.4 ng testosterone/60 000 cells per 4 h) and 72 h (for ketoconazole: control value = 8.5 ± 0.8 ng testosterone/60 000 cells per 4 h) after the drugs had been washed out. Each value corresponds to the mean ± s.d. of three independent experiments. Asterisks denote significant difference from the control values (** $P < 0,01$; *** $P < 0.001$).

Albertson et al., 1988) in the testis, but also in other tissues containing cytochrome P-450, such as the adrenal gland (Kowal, 1983), ovary, kidney and liver (Kan et al., 1985). It preferentially inhibits 17α-hydroxylase, C-17, 20-lyase (Albertson et al., 1988; Sikka et al., 1985) and the cholesterol-side-chain-cleavage enzyme (Kan et al., 1985) (Fig 19.1). The type of enzyme which is inhibited in the steroidogenesis chain depends on the concentration of drug present (Albertson et al., 1988).

In our studies, ketoconazole did not modify the hCG binding to its receptors. However, ketoconazole did impair the cAMP response of Leydig cells to hCG (IC_{50} = 30 μM), indicating that the drug may act at membrane level, in particular on the adenylate cyclase system (Brun et al., unpublished work). The absence of cytotoxicity confirms that ketoconazole has a specific impact on the steroidogenesis pathway. These results can be related to the in vivo situation where routine ketoconazole treatment, corresponding to peak blood levels of 5–80 μM drug (Brass et al., 1982), results in a decrease in the testosterone level. In both man and animal species, the administration of low doses of ketoconazole (200 mg/day) leads to transient, but rapidly reversible, decrease in the testosterone level (Santen et al., 1983; Sonino, 1987; De Coster et al., 1984). After higher daily doses in man (800–1200 mg/day), testosterone serum concentrations fall markedly, with functional hypogonadism (Sonino, 1987).

Spironolactone caused a 40% reduction in testosterone secretion at 250 μM (IC_{50} = 200 μM) (Fig. 19.5). It concomitantly increased progesterone secretion at concentrations from 25 μM, with an increase to nearly 400% of the control value at 250 μM. The effects of spironolactone on testosterone production were completely reversible after drug elimination and did not cause cell mortality. Spironolactone did not change the hCG binding to its receptors, but did induce a slight inhibition of cAMP release (IC_{50} = 140 μM). The main effect of spironolactone on testicular steroidogenesis is an interaction with the 17α-hydroxylase enzyme (Fig. 19.1), by interaction with the heme component of cytochrome *P*-450 (Fraser, 1979; Menard *et al.*, 1979). The limited effect of spironolactone observed on testosterone secretion can be explained by its slight inhibitory potential towards 17α-hydroxylase activity (Penhoat *et al.*, 1988). These *in vitro* findings are in agreement with the *in vivo* effects of spironolactone, which may induce gynaecomastia and reduction of libido by interacting with testosterone receptors in target organs rather than by impairing testicular function (Fraser, 1979). In addition, spironolactone may modify the cAMP release by acting on the adenylate cyclase system (Brun *et al.*, unpublished work). This drug is an interesting compound for testicular toxicology studies because it blocks a specific enzyme (17α-hydroxylase) in the testicular steroidogenesis pathway.

Chlorpromazine impaired steroid production by the Leydig cells from 30 μM (Fig. 19.6). Chlorpromazine was cytotoxic towards the Leydig cell in primary culture at concentrations from 3 μM, and the steroid inhibition induced by this compound was correlated to its cytotoxicity. This inhibition was not reversible (Table 19.4).

Chlorpromazine is known to block the release of pituitary gonadotropins and to induce hyperprolactinaemia (Chatterjee, 1965; Apter *et al.*, 1983). The alteration in steroid production observed *in vitro* was correlated with progressive cell necrosis, confirming that the drug does not act specifically on steroid metabolism.

This example clearly demonstrates the importance of evaluating cell viability when interpreting changes in steroid levels. The effect of chlorpromazine on steroidogenesis is related to some extent to its cell toxicity, whereas the two other compounds studied have a specific inhibitory effect on steroidogenesis which does not result from general cell damage.

The results for the compounds tested in the porcine Leydig cell culture are in accordance with the corresponding effects observed *in vivo*. Therefore, porcine Leydig cells in primary culture constitute a good model for the detection of Leydig cell injuries induced by compounds. The model was shown to be specific and able to discriminate between

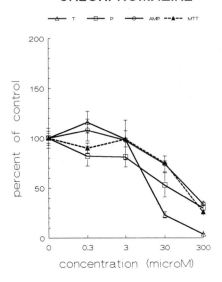

Fig. 19.6 Influence of chlorpromazine on steroid and cAMP production by cultured porcine Leydig cells. On day 3 of the culture, Leydig cells were treated with various concentrations of drug and stimulated by hCG (2×10^{-10} M) for 4 h. Testosterone (T), progesterone (P) and cAMP (AMP) were assayed in the incubation media and the cell viability (MTT) was evaluated by MTT staining. The results were expressed as a percentage of the vehicle control, which was taken as 100% (control values = 15.5 ± 2.2 ng testosterone/60 000 cells per 4 h, 1.94 ± 0.28 ng progesterone/60 000 cells per 4 h, 1.26 ± 0.18 pmol cAMP/60 000 cells per 4 h and 0.620 ± 0.035 optical density for cytotoxicity evaluation). Values shown are means ± S.D. ($n = 9$).

steroidogenesis inhibitors and cytotoxic chemicals. The miniaturization of the culture model makes it suitable for screening large numbers of compounds for inhibitory effects on steroid synthesis. Finally, this model provides an appropriate method for the initial investigation of potential testicular toxicity of endocrine origin.

Discussion and Conclusion

There are many target cells for chemical compounds within the testis, and interference with, or blocking of, any link in the system can affect the reproductive process. The central nervous system, hepatic and adrenal glands all influence testicular function. Toxicity studies on Leydig cells are one way of investigating reproductive toxicity. Histological examinations, blood hormone assays, functional investigations and sperm studies are necessary to detect testicular toxicity, and Leydig cell cultures complement conventional hormone studies for investigating the mechanism of toxicity and identifying the site of toxicity, since direct or indirect impacts can lead to the same injury. In addition, the numerous interactions that occur between the different cell types that constitute the testis make the study of the testicular toxicity of a compound highly complex (Chapin and Phelps, 1990).

Models in which several types of cell co-exist in the same culture offer interesting perspectives on the field of testicular toxicology. These techniques allow more accurate assessment of the testicular toxicity of a molecule through the study of the restoration of cell–cell relationships and the metabolic structures that exist *in vivo*. One of the possibilities is a system of coculture in two independent compartments within a single well (Byers *et al.*, 1986; Janecki and Steinberger, 1986); this system can be used for the combined culture of Sertoli and germ cells (Janecki *et al.*, 1988), of Leydig and Sertoli cells (Chapin *et al.*, 1990), or of Sertoli and peritubular cells (Ailenberg and Fritz, 1988). This system of coculture, which is technically difficult and costly, makes it possible to reconstitute some of the events found *in vivo*. However, it must be reserved for particular applications.

The contribution of mammalian cell culture methods to the elucidation of the mechanisms of chemical-induced toxicity is important. Validation must be the first step in the development of these methods. The reliability of the culture procedure and the interpretability of the results are the two main aspects of validation and they are not the same for culture models used for screening molecules and those used to elucidate the mechanisms of the toxicity. It is necessary to characterize the cells *in vitro* in order to evaluate how the cells have maintained their specific functions; the age of the culture, the loss of cellular interactions and the addition of serum to the culture medium are all factors that can accelerate the loss of specific cell functions (Bottenstein *et al.*, 1979; Orly *et al.*, 1980; Taub, 1990). Cell culture conditions, the factors influencing the cells in culture and the parameters chosen for evaluating cell functions must be checked. The use of defined media for the development of cell cultures has helped to improve culture conditions, by facilitating the identification of the substances required for the expression of the differentiated cell functions, the purification of the biological compounds secreted by the cells and the action of exogenous molecules on the cells. The exposure to the test chemicals and the evaluation of the cytotoxicity must also be optimized and standardized. The use of several specific parameters to measure the impact of a toxin on the cells and the mechanism of toxicity is preferable to using a single assessment system (Frazier, 1990). The better a model assesses the different mechanisms of toxicity of a compound on cells, the lower the number of false positive and false negative responses.

In vitro models are devoid of factors that relate to pharmacokinetic mechanisms, tissue repair and cell–cell interactions, and this, together with their limited metabolic activity, makes it necessary to interpret *in vitro* results in the light of *in vivo* data (LD_{50}, plasma concentrations, etc.). It is obvious that the toxic impact of a compound on the genital sphere can be studied in detail only in the whole animal (or man). However, under optimum conditions, a validated cell culture model used in a well-defined field can provide the toxicologist with data that can be extrapolated to predict the probable toxicity of the test compound in the *in vivo* situation.

Acknowledgements

The authors thank Mss Ghosh and Reibaud for their help in the preparation of the manuscript.

References

Ailenberg, M. and Fritz, I.B. (1988). *Endocrinology* **122**, 2613–2618.
Albertson, B.D., Frederick, K.L., Maronian, N.C., Feuillan, P., Schorer, S., Dunn, J.F. and Loriaux, D.L. (1988). *Res. Commun. Chem. Pathol. Pharmacol.* **61**, 17–26.
Anderson, R.A.J., Quigg, J.M., Oswald, C. and Zaneveld, L.J.D. (1985). *Biochem. Pharmacol.* **34**, 685–695.
Apter, A., Dickerman, Z., Gonen, N., Assa, S., Prager-Lewin, R., Kaufman, H., Tyano, S. and Laron, Z. (1983). *Am. J. Psychiat.* **140**, 1588–1591.
Ascoli, M. (1981a). *Endocrinology* **108**, 88–95.
Ascoli, M. (1981b). *J. Biol. Chem.* **256**, 179–183.
Ascoli, M. and Puett, D. (1978). *Biochemistry* **75**, 99–102.
Ascoli, M., Euffa, J. and Segaloff, D.L. (1987). *J. Biol. Chem.* **262**, 9196–9203.
Azouri, H., Bidart, J.M. and Bohuon, C. (1989). *Biochem. Pharmacol.* **38**, 567–571.
Bartke, A. (1980). *Fed. Proc.* **39**, 2577–2581.
Bell, J.B.G., Vinson, G.P., Hopkin, D.J. and Lacy, D. (1968). *Biochim. Biophys. Acta* **164**, 412–420.
Benahmed, M., Reventos, J. and Saez, J.M. (1983). *Endocrinology* **112**, 1952–1957.
Benahmed, M., Grenot, C., Tabone, E., Sanchez, P. and Morera, A.M. (1985a). *Biochem. Biophys. Res. Commun.* **132**, 729–734.

Benahmed, M., Reventos, J., Tabone, E. and Saez, J.M. (1985b). *Am. J. Physiol.* **248**, E176–E181.

Bernier, M., Gibb, W., Haour, F., Collu, R., Saez, J.M. and Ducharme, J.R. (1983). *Biol. Reprod.* **29**, 1172–1178.

Bernier, M., Gibb, W., Collu, R. and Ducharme, J.R. (1984). *Can. J. Physiol. Pharmacol.* **62**, 1166–1169.

Bernier, M., Chatelain, J.P., Mather, J.P. and Saez, J.M. (1986). *J. Cell. Physiol.* **129**, 257–263.

Bottenstein, J.E., Skaper, S.D., Varon, S.S. and Sato, G.H. (1979). *Exp. Cell Res.* **125**, 183–189.

Boyden, T.W., Pamenter, R.W. and Silvert, M.A. (1980). *J. Reprod. Fertil.* **59**, 25–30.

Brass, C., Galgiani, J.N., Blaschke, T.F., Defelice, R., O'Reill, R.A. and Stevens, D.A. (1982). *Antimicrob. Agents Chemother.* **21**, 151–158.

Browning, J.Y., D'Agata, R. and Grotjan, H.E. (1981). *Endocrinology* **109**, 667–669.

Browning, J.Y., Heindel, J.J. and Grotjan, H.E. (1983). *Endocrinology* **112**, 543–549.

Brun, P.H., Leonard, J.F., Moronvalle, V., Caillaud, J.M., Melcion, C. and Cordier, A. (1991). *Toxicol. Appl. Pharmacol.* **108**, 307–320.

Burstein, S. and Gut, M. (1971). *Recent Prog. Horm. Res.* **27**, 303–349.

Byers, S.W., Hadley, M.A., Djakiew, D. and Dym, M. (1986). *J. Androl.* **7**, 59–68.

Catt, K.J. and Dufau, M. (1976). *Biol. Reprod.* **14**, 1–15.

Catt, K.J., Harwood, J.P., Aguilera, G. and Dufau, M.L. (1979). *Nature*, **280**, 109–116.

Catt, K.J., Harwood, J.P., Clayton, R.N., Davies, T.F., Chan, V., Katikineni, M., Nozu, K. and Dufau, M. (1980). *Recent Prog. Horm. Res.* **36**, 557–622.

Cavallini, L., Malendowicz, L.K., Mazzocchi, G., Belloni, A.S. and Nussdorfer, G.G. (1990). *Virchows Arch. [B]* **58**, 215–220.

Chan, V., Katikinemi, M., Davies, T.F. and Catt, K.J. (1981). *Endocrinology*, **108**, 1607–1612.

Chapin, R.E. and Phelps, J.L. (1990). *Toxicol. In Vitro* **4**, 543–559.

Chapin, R.E., Gray, T.J.B., Phelps, J.L. and Dutton, S.L. (1988). *Toxicol. Appl. Pharmacol.* **92**, 467–479.

Chapin, R.E., Phelps, J.L., Somkuti, S.G., Heindel, J.J. and Burka, L.T. (1990). *Toxicol. Appl. Pharmacol.* **104**, 483–495.

Charpenet, G., Tache, Y., Forest, M.G., Haour, F., Saez, J.M., Bernier, M., Ducharme, J.R. and Collu, R. (1981). *Endocrinology* **109**, 1254–1258.

Chasalow, F., Marr, H., Haour, F. and Saez, J.M. (1979). *J. Biol. Chem.* **254**, 5613–5617.

Chase, D.J., Dixon, G.E.K. and Payne, A.H. (1982). *Prog. Clin. Biol. Res.* **112**, 209–219.

Chatterjee, A. (1965). *Experientia* **21**, 545–546.

Chatterjee, A. and Paul, B.S. (1968). *Endocrinology* **52**, 406–407.

Chaudhary, L.R. and Stocco, D.M. (1989). *Biochem. Int.* **18**, 251–262.

Chen, Y.I., Payne, A.H. and Kelch, R.P. (1976). *Proc. Soc. Exp. Biol. Med.* **153**, 473–475.

Chen, Y.I., Shaw, M.J. and Payne, A.H. (1977). *Mol. Cell. Endocrinol.* **8**, 291–299.

Christensen, A.K. and Peacock, K.C. (1980). *Biol. Reprod.* **22**, 383–391.
Cicero, T.J. and Bell, R.D. (1982). *Steroids* **40**, 561–568.
Cooke, B.A., Janszen, F.H.A., Clotscher, W.F. and van der Molen, H.J. (1975). *Biochem. J.* **150**, 413–418.
Cooke, B.A., Hunter, A.M.G., Sullivan, M.H.F. and Dix, C.J. (1983). *J. Steroid Biochem.* **19**, 359–366.
De Coster, R., Beerens, D., Dom J. and Willemsens, G. (1984). *Acta Endocrinol.* **107**, 275–281.
Dix, C.J. and Cooke, B.A. (1981). *Biochem. J.* **196**, 713–719.
Dorrington, J.H., Roller, N.F. and Fritz, I.B. (1975). *Mol. Cell. Endocrinol.* **3**, 57–70.
Dufau, M.L., Mendelson, C.R. and Catt, K.J. (1974). *J. Clin. Endocrinol. Metab.* **39**, 610–613.
Dufau, M.L., Horner, K.A., Hayashi, K., Tsuruhara, T., Conn, P.M. and Catt, K.J. (1978). *J. Biol. Chem.* **253**, 3721–3729.
Dufau, M.L., Khanum, A., Winters, C.A. and Tsai-Morris, C.H. (1987). *J. Steroid Biochem.* **27**, 343–350.
Evain, D., Morera, A.M. and Saez, J.M. (1976). *J. Steroid Biochem.* **7**, 1135–1139.
Ewing, L.L., Wing, T.Y., Cochran, R.C., Kromann, N. and Zirkin, B.R. (1983). *Endocrinology* **112**, 1763–1769.
Faerman, I., Vilar, O., Rivarola, M.A., Rosner, J.M., Jadzinski, M.N., Fox, D., Perez-Lloret, A., Bernstein-Hahn, L. and Saraceni, D. (1972). *Diabetes* **21**, 23–30.
Fawcett, D.W., Neaves, W.B. and Flores, M.N. (1973). *Biol. Reprod.* **9**, 500–532.
Finaz, C., Lefèvre, A. and Dampfhoffer, D. (1987). *Cell Biol.* **84**, 5750–5753.
Fraser, R. (1979). *Biochem. Soc. Trans.* **7**, 559–562.
Frazier, J.M. (1990). *J. Am. Coll. Toxicol.* **9**, 355–359.
Freeman, D.A. (1987a). *Endocrinology* **120**, 124–132.
Freeman, D.A. (1987b). *J. Biol. Chem.* **262**, 13061–13068.
Freeman, D.A. and Ascoli, M. (1983). *Biochim. Biophys. Acta* **754**, 72–81.
French, J.T. and Welsh, T.H.Jr. (1990). *Acta Endocrinol. Copenh.* **122**, 101–106.
Gonzalez-Manchon, C. and Vale, W. (1989). *Endocrinology* **125**, 1666–1672.
Gray, T.J.B. and Gangolli, S.D. (1986). *Environ. Health Perspect.* **65**, 229–235.
Griswold, M.D. (1988). *Int. Rev. Cytol.* **110**, 133–156.
Guillou, F., Martinat, N. and Combarnous, Y. (1985). *FEBS Lett.* **184**, 6–9.
Hafiez, A.A., Bartke, A. and Lloyd, C.W. (1972). *J. Endocrinol.* **53**, 223–230.
Haour, F. and Saez, J.M. (1977). *Mol. Cell. Endocrinol.* **7**, 17–24.
Haour, F., Kouznetzova, B., Dray, F. and Saez, J.M. (1979). *Life Sci.* **24**, 2151–2158.
Haour, F., Bommelaer, M.C., Bernier, M., Sanchez, P., Saez, J.M. and Mather, J.P. (1983). *Mol. Cell. Endocrinol.* **30**, 73–84.
Horowitz, J.D. and Goble, A.J. (1979). *Drugs* **18**, 206–217.
Hsueh, J.W. (1980). *Biochem. Biophys. Res. Commun.* **97**, 506–512.
Hunter, M.G., Magee-Brown, R., Dix, C.J. and Cooke, B.A. (1982). *Mol. Cell. Endocrinol.* **25**, 35–47.
Inoue, Y. and Rebois, R.V. (1989). *J. Biol. Chem.* **264**, 8504–8508.
Janecki, A. and Steinberger, A. (1986). *J. Androl.* **7**, 69–71.
Janecki, A., Pawlowski, T., Lukaszyk, A. and Kozak, W. (1984). *Folia Histochem. Cytobiol.* **22**, 179–186.
Janecki, A., Jakubowiak, A. and Steinberger, A. (1988). *J. Androl.* **9**, 126–132.

Janszen, F.H.A., Cooke, B.A., van Driel, M.J.A. and van der Molen, H.J. (1976). *J. Endocrinol.* **70**, 345–359.

Janszen, F.H.A., Cooke, B.A. and van der Molen, H.J. (1977). *Biochem. J.* **162**, 341–346.

Johansson, B. (1989a). *Toxicol. In Vitro* **3**, 33–35.

Johansson, B. (1989b). *Bull. Environ. Contam. Toxicol.* **42**, 9–14.

Kan, P.B., Hirst, M.A. and Feldman, D. (1985). *J. Steroid Biochem.* **23**, 1023–1029.

Kellokumpu, S. (1987). *Exp. Cell Res.* **168**, 299–308.

Keeney, D.S., Mendis-Handagama, S.M.L.C., Zirkin, B.R. and Ewing, L.L. (1988). *Endocrinology* **123**, 2906–2915.

Kilgore, M.W. and Stocco, D.M. (1989). *Endocrinology* **124**, 1210–1216.

Kilgore, M.W., Rommerts, F.F.G., Wirtz, K.W.A. and Stocco, D.M. (1990). *Mol. Cell. Endocrinol.* **69**, 9–16.

Klinefelter, G.R. and Ewing, L.L. (1988). *In Vitro Cell Dev. Biol.* **24**, 545–549.

Klinefelter, G.R. and Ewing, L.L. (1989). *In Vitro Cell. Dev. Biol.* **25**, 283–288.

Klinefelter, G.R., Hall, P.F. and Ewing, L.L. (1987). *Biol. Reprod.* **36**, 769–783.

Kowal, J. (1983). *Endocrinology* **112**, 1541–1543.

Kremers, P., Tixhon, Ch. and Gielen, J. (1977). *J. Steroid. Biochem.* **8**, 873–877.

Lacroix, M. and Fritz, I.B. (1982). *Mol. Cell. Endocrinol.* **26**, 247–258.

Lee, I.P., Suzuki, K., Mukhtar, H. and Bend, J.R. (1980a). *Cancer Res.* **40**, 2486–2492.

Lee, I.P., Suzuki, K., Lee, S.D. and Dixon, R.L. (1980b). *Toxicol. Appl. Pharmacol.* **52**, 181–184.

Lee, W., Mason, A.J., Schwall, R., Szonyi, E. and Mather, J.P. (1989). *Science* **243**, 396–398.

Lefevre, A., Saez, J.M. and Finaz, C. (1983). *Horm. Res.* **17**, 114–120.

Le Magueresse, B., Le Gac, F., Loir, M. and Jegou, B. (1986). *J. Reprod. Fertil.* **77**, 489–498.

Lephart, E.D., Peterson, K.G., Noble, J.F., George, F.W. and McPhaul, M.J. (1990). *Mol. Cell. Endocrinol.* **70**, 31–40.

Lloyd, S.C. and Foster, P.M.D. (1988). *Toxicol. Appl. Pharmacol.* **95**, 484–489.

Luketich, J.D., Melner, M.H., Guengerich, F.P. and Puett, D. (1983). *Biochem. Biophys. Res. Commun.* **111**, 424–429.

Maggi, M., Morris, P.L., Kassis, S. and Rodbard, D. (1989). *Int. J. Androl.* **12**, 65–71.

Mather, J.P. (1980). *Biol. Reprod.* **23**, 243–252.

Mather, J.P. (1982). *In Vitro* **18**, 990–996.

Mather, J.P. and Phillips, D.M. (1984). *J. Ultrastruct. Mol. Struct. Res.* **87**, 263–274.

Mather, J.P. and Sato, G.H. (1979). *Exp. Cell Res.* **124**, 215–221.

Mather, J.P., Saez, J.M. and Haour, F. (1981). *Steroids* **38**, 35–44.

Mather, J.P., Saez, J.M. and Haour, F. (1982a). *Endocrinology* **110**, 933–940.

Mather, J.P., Saez, J.M., Haour, F. and Dray, F. (1982b). *In* "Cold Spring Harbor Conference on Cell Proliferation", Vol. 9, pp. 1117–1128. Cold Spring Harbor Laboratory, Cold Spring Harbor, NY.

Mather, J.P., Saez, J.M., Dray, F. and Haour, F. (1983). *Acta Endocrinol.* **102**, 470–475.

Matsumoto, A.M. (1989). *In* "The Testis", Second Edition (H. Burger and D. de Kretser, eds), pp. 181–196. Raven Press, New York.

McMurray, C.T., Devi, L., Calavetta, L. and Douglass, J.O. (1989). *Endocrinology* **124**, 49–59.

Means, A.R., Fakunding, J.L., Huckins, C., Tindall, D.J. and Vitale, R. (1976). *Recent Prog. Horm. Res.* **32**, 477–527.

Mecklenburg, R.S., Hetzel, W.D., Gulyas, B.J. and Lipsett, M.B. (1975). *Endocrinology* **96**, 564–570.

Meistrich, M.L., Finch, M., da Cunha, M.F., Hacker, U. and Au, W.W. (1982). *Cancer Res.* **42**, 122–131.

Melsert, R., Hoogerbrugge, J.W. and Rommerts, F.F.G. (1989). *Mol. Cell. Endocrinol.* **64**, 35–44.

Menard, R.H., Guenthner, T.M., Kon, H. and Gillette, J.R. (1979). *J. Biol. Chem.* **254**, 1726–1733.

Mendelson, C., Dufau, M. and Catt, K. (1975). *J. Biol. Chem.* **250**, 8818—8823.

Merkel, U., Angermuller, S. and Merz, W.E. (1990). *Cell. Mol. Biol.* **36**, 213–224.

Miyashita, Y., Hirose, T., Kouhara, H., Kishimoto, S., Matsumoto, K. and Sato, B. (1990). *J. Steroid Biochem.* **35**, 561–567.

Mombrial, F.C., Bommelaer, M.C., Sanchez, P. and Haour, F. (1985). *J. Recept. Res.* **5**, 45–57.

Morera, A.M., Cochet, C., Keramidas, M., Chauvin, M.A., de Peretti, E. and Benahmed, M. (1988). *J. Steroid Biochem.* **30**, 443–447.

Mori, H. and Christensen, A.K. (1980). *J. Cell Biol.* **84**, 340–354.

Morris, I.D., Lendon, R.G. and Zaidi, A. (1988). *J. Endocrinol.* **119**, 467–474.

Mukhtar, H., Lee, I.P. and Bend, J.R. (1978). *Biochem. Biophys. Res. Commun.* **83**, 1093–1098.

Murphy, P.R. and Moger, W.H. (1982). *Biol. Reprod.* **27**, 38–47.

Nakajin, S. and Hall, P.F. (1981). *J. Biol. Chem.* **256**, 3871–3876.

Nakajin, S., Hall, P.F. and Onoda, M. (1981). *J. Biol. Chem.* **256**, 6134–6139.

Nakhla, A.M., Bardin, C.W., Salomon, Y., Mather, J.P. and Janne, O.A. (1989). *J. Androl.* **10**, 311–320.

Ng, T.B. and Liu, W.K. (1990). *In Vitro Cell. Dev. Biol.* **26**, 24–28.

Nishizawa, Y., Sato, B., Miyashita, Y., Tsukada, S., Hirose, T., Kishimoto, S. and Matsumoto, K. (1988). *Endocrinology* **122**, 227–235.

Nishizawa, Y., Sato, B., Nishii, K., Kishimoto, S. and Matsumoto, K. (1989). *Cancer Res.* **49**, 1377–1382.

Nishizawa, Y., Nishii, K., Kishimoto, S., Matsumoto, K. and Sato, B. (1990). *Anticancer Res.* **10**, 317–322.

Notation, A.D. and Ungar, F. (1969a). *Biochemistry* **8**, 501–506.

Notation, A.D. and Ungar, F. (1969b). *Steroids* **14**, 151–159.

Nozu, K., Dehejia, L., Zawistowich, L., Catt, K.J. and Dufau, M.L. (1981a). *J. Biol. Chem.* **256**, 12875–12882.

Nozu, K., Matsuura, S., Catt, K.J. and Dufau, M.L. (1981b). *J. Biol. Chem.* **256**, 10012–10017.

Oh, R. and Tamaoki, B. (1973). *Acta Endocrinol.* **74**, 615–624.

Orava, M. (1989). *J. Interferon Res.* **9**, 135–141.

Orava, M., Cantell, K. and Vihko, R. (1985a). *Biochem. Biophys. Res. Commun.* **127**, 809–815.

Orava, M., Haour, F., Leinonen, P., Ruokonen, A. and Vihko, R. (1985b). *J. Steroid Biochem.* **22**, 507–512.

Orly, J., Sato, G. and Erickson, G.F. (1980). *Cell* **20**, 817–827.

Orpana, A.K., Eriksson, C.J.P. and Harkonen, M. (1989). *J. Steroid Biochem.* **33**, 1243–1248.

O'Steen, W.K. (1963). *Proc. Soc. Exp. Biol. Med.* **113**, 161–163.

Osterman, J. and Terracio, L. (1987). *Ann. New York Acad. Sci.* **513**, 370–372.

Pandey, K.N., Kowacs, W.J. and Inagami, T. (1985). *Biochem. Biophys. Res. Commun.* **133**, 800–806.

Pandey, K.N., Inagami, T. and Misono, K.S. (1986). *Biochemistry* **25**, 8467–8472.

Payne, A.H., Downing, J.R. and Wong, K.L. (1980). *Endocrinology* **106**, 1424–1429.

Payne, A.H., Wong, K.L. and Vega, M.M. (1982). *J. Biol. Chem.* **255**, 7118–7122.

Pearce, S., Sufi, S.B., O'Shaughnessy, P.J., Donaldson, A. and Jeffcoate, S.L. (1986). *Contraception* **34**, 639–646.

Penhoat, A., Darbeida, H., Bernier, M., Saez, J.M. and Durand, Ph. (1988). *Mol. Cell. Endocrinol.* **60**, 55–60.

Pereira, M.E., Segaloff, D.L., Ascoli, M. and Eckstein, F. (1987). *J. Biol. Chem.* **262**, 6093–6100.

Perrard-Sapori, M.H., Chatelain, P., Vallier, P. and Saez, J.M. (1986). *Biochem. Biophys. Res. Commun.* **134**, 957–962.

Phillips, J.C., Foster, P.M.D. and Gangolli, S.D. (1985). *In* "Endocrine Toxicology" (J.A. Thomas, S. Korach and J.A. McLachlan, eds), pp. 117–134. Raven Press, New York.

Pignataro, O.P., Radicella, J.P., Calvo, J.C. and Charreau, E.H. (1983). *Mol. Cell. Endocrinol.* **33**, 53–67.

Pinion-Lataillade, G., Velez de la Calle, J.F., Viguier-Martinez, M.C., Garnier, D.H., Folliot, R., Maas, J. and Jegou, B. (1988). *Mol. Cell. Endocrinol.* **58**, 51–63.

Pogach, L.M., Lee, Y., Giglio, W., Naumoff, M. and Huang, H.F.S. (1989a). *Cancer Chemother. Pharmacol.* **24**, 177–180.

Pogach, L.M., Lee, Y., Gould, S., Giglio, W., Meyenhofer, M. and Huang, H.F.S. (1989b). *Toxicol. Appl. Pharmacol.* **98**, 350–361.

Pont, A., Williams, P.L., Azhar, S., Reitz, R.E., Bochra, C., Smith, E.R. and Stevens, D.A. (1982). *Arch. Intern. Med.* **142**, 2137–2140.

Purvis, K., Cusan, L. and Hansson, V. (1981). *J. Steroid Biochem.* **15**, 77–86.

Quinn, P.G., Dombrausky, L.J., Chen, Y.I. and Payne, A. (1981). *Endocrinology* **109**, 1790–1792.

Rainey, W.E., Kramer, R.E., Mason, J.I. and Shay, J.W. (1985). *J. Cell. Physiol.* **123**, 17–24.

Rebois, R.V. (1982). *J. Cell Biol.* **94**, 70–76.

Rebois, R.V. and Fishman, P.H. (1983). *J. Biol. Chem.* **258**, 12775–12778.

Rebois, R.V. and Fishman, P.H. (1984). *J. Biol. Chem.* **259**, 3096–3101.

Rebois, R.V. and Fishman, P.H. (1986). *Endocrinology* **118**, 2340–2348.

Rebois, R.V., Beckner, S.K., Brady, R.O. and Fishman, P.H. (1983). *Proc. Natl. Acad. Sci. U.S.A.* **80**, 1275–1279.

Rebois, R.V., Bradley, R.M. and Titlow, C.C. (1987). *Biochemistry* **26**, 6422–6428.

Renier, G., Gaulin, J., Gibb, W., Gollu, R. and Ducharme, J.R. (1987). *Can. J. Physiol. Pharmacol.* **65**, 2053–2058.

Rommerts, F.F.G. and Brinkman, A.O. (1981). *Mol. Cell. Endocrinol.* **21**, 15–28.

Rommerts, F.F.G., van Roemburg, M.J.A., Lindh, L.M., Hegge, J.A.J. and van der Molen, H.J. (1982). *J. Reprod. Fertil.* **65**, 289–297.

Rommerts, F.F.G., Bakker, G.H. and Van der Molen, H.J. (1983). *J. Steroid Biochem.* **19**, 367–373.

Rommerts, F.F.G., Teerds, K.J. and Hoogerbrugge, J.W. (1988). *Mol. Cell. Endocrinol.* **55**, 87–94.

Russell, L.D., Lee, I.P., Ettlin, R. and Malone, J.P. (1983). *Tissue Cell.* **15**, 391–404.

Saez, J.M., Haour, F. and Cathiard, A.M. (1978a). *Biochem. Biophys. Res. Commun.* **81**, 552–558.

Saez, J.M., Haour, F., Tell, G.P.E., Gallet, D. and Sanchez, P. (1978b). *Mol. Pharmacol.* **14**, 1054–1062.

Saez, J.M., Benhamed, M., Reventos, J., Bommelaer, M.C., Monbrial, C. and Haour, F. (1983). *J. Steroid Biochem.* **19**, 375–384.

Saez, J.M., Chatelain, P.G., Perrard-Sapori, M.H., Jaillard, C. and Naville, D. (1988). *Reprod. Nutr. Develop.* **28**, 989–1008.

Sairam, M. and Berman, M.I. (1979). *Steroids* **33**, 233–242.

Santen, R.J., Van Den Bossche, H., Symoens, J., Brugmans, J. and Decoster, R. (1983). *J. Clin. Endocrinol. Metab.* **57**, 732–736.

Santucci, L., Graham, T.J. and Van Theil, D.H. (1983). *Alcoholism* **7**, 135–139.

Sato, B., Miyashita, Y., Maeda, Y., Noma, K., Kishimoto, S. and Matsumoto, K. (1987). *Endocrinology* **120**, 1112–1120.

Schumacher, M., Schafer, G., Holstein, A.F. and Hilz, H. (1978). *FEBS Lett.* **91**, 333–338.

Schumacher, M., Schafer, G., Lichtenberg, V. and Hilz, H. (1979). *FEBS Lett.* **107**, 398–402.

Schurmeyer, Th. and Nieschlag, E. (1984). *Acta Endocrinol.* **105**, 275–280.

Setchell, B.P. (1978) "The Mammalian Testis". Cornell University, New York.

Setchell, B.P. (1986). *Aust. J. Biol. Sci.* **39**, 193–207.

Setchell, B.P. (1990). PIO. "6th European Workshop on Molecular and Cellular Endocrinology of the Testis". Mariehamn, Aland Islands.

Setchell, B.P. and Cox, J.E. (1982). *J. Reprod. Fertil. (Suppl).* **32**, 123–127.

Setchell, B.P. and Pilsworth, L.M. (1989). *In* "The Testis" Second Edition (H. Burger and D. de Kretser, eds), pp. 1–66. Raven Press, New York.

Setchell, B.P., Laurie, M.S., Flint, A.P.F. and Heap, R.B. (1983). *J. Endocrinol.* **96**, 127–136.

Sharpe, R.M., Kerr, J.B. and Maddocks, S. (1988). *Mol. Cell. Endocrinol.* **60**, 243–247.

Sikka, S.C., Swerdloff, R.S. and Rajfer, J. (1985). *Endocrinology* **116**, 1920–1925.

Sikka, S.C., Coy, D.C., Lemmi, C.A.E. and Rajfer, J. (1988). *Transplantation* **46**, 886–890.

Simpson, B.J.B., Wu, F.C.W. and Sharpe, R.M. (1987). *J. Clin. Endocrinol. Metab.* **65**, 415–422.

Skinner, M.K. and Fritz, B. (1985). *Mol. Cell. Endocrinol.* **40**, 115–122.

Skinner, M.K. and Fritz, B. (1986). *Mol. Cell. Endocrinol.* **44**, 85–97.

Skinner, M.K., Schlitz, S.M. and Anthony, C.T. (1989). *Endocrinology* **124**, 3015–3024.

Sonino, N. (1987). *N. Engl. J. Med.* **317**, 812–818.

Sordoillet, C., Chauvin, M.A., Revol, A., Morera, A.M. and Benahmed, M. (1988). *Mol. Cell. Endocrinol.* **58**, 283–286.

Steinberger, A. (1975). *Am. Zool.* **15**, 272–278.

Steinberger, A., Dighe, R.R. and Diaz, J. (1984). *Arch. Biol. Med. Exp. (Santiago)* **17**, 267–271.

Stockley, I.H. (1970). *Am. J. Hosp. Pharm.* **27**, 977–985.

Tabone, E., Benahmed, M., Reventos, J. and Saez, J.M. (1984). *Cell. Tissue Res.* **237**, 357–362.

Taub, M. (1990). *Toxicol. In Vitro* **4**, 213–225.

Thachil, J.V., Jewett, M.A.S. and Rider, W.D. (1981). *J. Urol.* **126**, 141–145.

Thomas, J.A. and Keenan, E.J. (1986). *In* "Principles of Endocrine Pharmacology" (J.A. Thomas and E.J. Keenan, eds), pp. 257–290. Plenum, New York.

Tindall, D.J., Rowley, D.R., Murthy, L., Lipshultz, L.I. and Chang, C.H. (1985). *Int. Rev. Cytol.* **94**, 127–149.

Van Beurden, W.M.O., Roodnat, B. and van der Molen, H.J. (1978). *Int. J. Androl.* Suppl.2, 374–383.

Van der Molen, H.J., Bijleveld, M.J., Van der Vusse, G.J. and Cooke, B.A. (1972). *J. Endocrinol.* **57**, vi—vii.

Van Thiel, D.H. (1983). *J. Lab. Clin. Med.* **101**, 21–33.

Van Thiel, D.H., Gavaler, J.S., Cobb, C.F., Santucci, L. and Graham, T.O. (1983). *Pharmacol. Biochem. Behav.* **18**, 317–323.

Vanha-Perttula, T., Mather, J.P., Bardin, C.W., Moss, S.B. and Bellve, A.R. (1986). *Biol. Reprod.* **35**, 1–9.

Velez de la Calle, J.F., Soufir, J.Cl., Chodorge, F., Boisseau, Cl. Kercret, H. and Jegou, B. (1988). *J. Reprod. Fertil.* **84**, 51–61.

Verhoeven, G. and Cailleau, J. (1985). *Mol. Cell. Endocrinol.* **40**, 57–68.

Verhoeven, G., Koninckx, P. and De Moor, P. (1982). *J. Steroid Biochem.* **17**, 319–330.

Vermeulen, A. (1982). *Int. J. Androl.* **5**, 163–182.

Waller, D.P., Killinger, J.M. and Zaneveld, L.J.D. (1985). *In* "Endocrine Toxicology" (J.A. Thomas, S. Korach and J.A. McLachlan, eds), pp. 269–333. Raven Press, New York.

Welsh, T.H. and Hsueh, A.J.W. (1982). *Endocrinology* **110**, 1498–1506.

Welsh, T.H., Bambino, T.H. and Hsueh, A.J.W. (1982). *Biol. Reprod.* **27**, 1138–1146.

Wiebe, J.P. (1976). *Endocrinology* **98**, 505–508.

Wood, P.L. and Lyengar, S. (1988). *In* "The Opioate Receptors" (Pasternak, G.W., ed.), pp. 307–356. Humana Press, Clifton, New Jersey.

Yamauchi, M., Potter, J.J. and Mezey, E. (1988). *Clin. Exp. Res.* **12**, 143–146.

Yanahara, T. and Troen, P. (1972). *J. Clin. Endocrinol. Metab.* **34**, 783–792.

Yee, J.B. and Hutson, J.C. (1985). *Endocrinology* **116**, 2682–2684.

Zhuang, L.Z., Phillips, D.M., Gunsalus, G.L., Bardin, C.W. and Mather, J.P. (1983). *J. Androl.* **4**, 336–344.

Zirkin, B.R., Ewing, L.L., Kromann, N. and Cochran, R.C. (1980). *Endocrinology* **107**, 1867–1874.

Whole Embryo Culture

D.A.T. NEW

*Physiological Laboratory, University of Cambridge, Cambridge
CB2 3EG, UK*

Introduction – Culture Methods

Although the embryos of a wide variety of animals, vertebrate and
invertebrate, have been used at one time or another in toxicological work
(Vouk and Sheehan, 1983), those of birds and mammals have usually
been regarded as having the most relevance to man. A large volume of
literature exists on the response of the chick embryo to various teratogens,
and the work of Jelinek (1979) and of Jelinek and Rychter (1980) has
been particularly important in establishing the chick embryo as a
potentially valuable test organism in teratogenic screening. My own work
has been concerned with cultured mammalian embryos, and particularly
with embryos undergoing organogenesis, since this stage is known to be
the most sensitive to teratogenic agents.

The decision to work with mammalian embryos *in vitro* instead of *in
vivo* was initially made on practical rather than ethical grounds. It was
clear that there were severe limits to the experimental possibilities,
toxicological or otherwise, of the embryo in the pregnant animal. It was
also clear that teratogen screening tests based on the pregnant animal
were very unreliable, and that at least part of this unreliability resulted
from the large variations in the *maternal* metabolism between one species
and another, and even between one individual and another. It was felt
that cultured embryos, isolated from the mother and available for close

IN VITRO METHODS IN TOXICOLOGY
ISBN 0-12-388175-7

observation and manipulation, would offer many research advantages. But a culture system would need to be developed which would reliably support embryonic growth and differentiation during organogenesis, i.e. would support development of the postimplantation embryo. We began culturing postimplantation embryos in the 1960s, using methods based on the pioneer studies of Nicholas (1938) in America and Jolly and Lieure (1938) in France, but it was not until we had made a number of improvements in the 1970s that the techniques became generally acceptable. Now they are used in many different laboratories and have been the subject of several reviews (e.g. New, 1978, 1990; Shepard *et al.*, 1987; Cockroft and Steele, 1987).

Technical details for explanting postimplantation embryos, preparing media and setting up cultures may be found in New (1971) and Cockroft (1990). Several variants of the culture systems are available (New, 1983, 1990) and the choice of system must depend on the requirements of a particular investigation. For the best results, the embryos must be grown in flowing or circulating medium, which can be provided adequately by incubating them in cylindrical bottles rotated on rollers or attached to a rotating drum. Preparation of the culture medium and provision of the optimum oxygen levels at different stages of embryonic development require special care.

In this paper I shall attempt to answer three questions: (1) How good is development of the postimplantation embryo in culture? (2) Do the culture methods provide a practicable method for use in toxicological studies? (3) What reliance can be placed on the results of toxicological tests with cultured embryos?

How Good is Development of Postimplantation Embryos in Culture?

Of the embryos tested so far for postimplantation culture, by far the best are those of rats and mice, and at present these are almost the only species used. Available culture methods can support growth and differentiation of rat and mouse embryos over any part of the second week of gestation, i.e. during the period of organogenesis. The kind of growth obtained falls into three main categories according to the stage of the embryos at explantation.

Embryos Explanted before the Egg Cylinder Stage

These are embryos taken from the mother at preimplantation stages. Most studies aimed at obtaining advanced development have been made with mouse blastocysts and, under appropriate culture conditions, these can develop into egg cylinders showing differentiation of the germ layers and rudimentary embryonic membranes (Wiley and Pederson, 1977), sometimes even somites and a beating heart (Chen and Hsu, 1982). The microstructure of the cultured embryo is often very similar to that *in vivo* but development is much slower, the failure rate is high and few develop beyond the earlier stages of organogenesis.

Embryos Explanted between the Egg Cylinder Stage and the Formation of the Allantoic Placenta

These embryos are very successful in culture. Rat egg cylinders, explanted as early as 8 days of gestation, often develop to well-formed embryos with 30–40 somites; 50–80% of these embryos develop a functioning blood circulation and the rate of organ differentiation is similar to that *in vivo* (Buckley *et al.*, 1978). But the best results are obtained with embryos explanted at head fold or early somite stage (Fig. 20.1). When rat embryos are cultured from the head fold stage (9–10 days gestation), over 95% develop a blood circulation and the average rates of protein synthesis and differentiation over 48 h are indistinguishable from those *in vivo* (New *et al.*, 1976a). Such cultured embryos appear identical in overall growth and development to littermates that have grown for the same period in the uterus. Rates of glucose uptake after 24–36 h in culture are the same as those of freshly explanted embryos of equivalent age (Ellington, 1987, and Fig. 20.2) but other aspects of embryonic metabolism *in vitro* may show differences from *in vivo* (Huber and Brown, 1982). The same embryos continue to differentiate well beyond 48 h but the rate of protein synthesis then falls behind that *in vivo*; after 72 h, the blood circulation has usually failed in many of the embryos and few if any survive to 96 h (New *et al.*, 1976b).

Embryos Explanted after the Formation of the Allantoic Placenta

The allantoic placenta is usually explanted with the embryo but, even when it has a blood circulation in the foetal vessels, there is no flow of culture medium through the placenta equivalent to a maternal blood circulation. This greatly reduces the capacity of the placenta as a

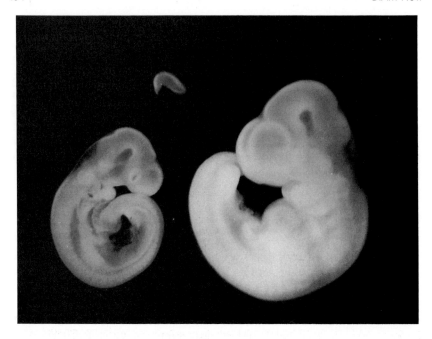

Fig. 20.1 Three embryos from the same rat, explanted at 9.5 days of gestation. Above: at explantation. Left: after 48 h in culture. Right: after 72 h in culture. Amnion and yolk sac (cultured with the embryos) have been removed before photography. Enlargement: 11×.

respiratory and nutritive organ in support of the embryo. The placenta *in vivo* probably begins to contribute to embryonic metabolism from the time of formation of its blood circulation (at about the 17-somite stage, i.e. 11 days of gestation in the rat) and it is noticeable that embryos cultured beyond this time often show a reduced growth rate. Differentiation is usually less affected than the rate of protein synthesis, resulting in embryos or foetuses that are well formed but somewhat smaller than normal (Cockroft, 1973, 1976; Eto and Takakubo, 1985). However, development can be supported up to the stage of digit formation on the limbs (fifteenth day of gestation in the rat).

The characteristic pattern of development of rat and mouse postimplantation embryos in culture is continuous growth and differentiation of a high proportion of the embryos up to a certain stage of development, followed by a rapid decline. The periods of development that can be supported are summarized in Fig. 20.3. Each black area in the figure indicates the extent of development attained by the majority of rat

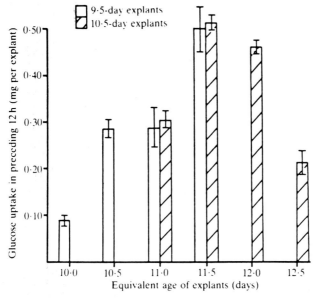

Fig. 20.2 Glucose uptake in culture of rat embryos cultured from 9.5 days gestation and from 10.5 days gestation. (Reprinted, with permission, from Ellington (1987).)

embryos cultured from a particular stage. Embryos explanted at around egg cylinder stage develop in culture for the equivalent of 4–5 days *in vivo*, those explanted at later stages, for progressively shorter periods. Development of mouse embryos is similar at somite stages but somewhat less reliable at presomite stages (Sadler and New, 1981).

Is Whole Embryo Culture a Practicable Method for Toxicology?

Doubts have sometimes been expressed as to whether whole embryo culture, despite its merits, is a practicable method for use in toxicological work. The preparation of embryo cultures for testing toxic agents clearly involves more complex procedures than administering the same agents to whole animals. And this difference is exacerbated by the frequent demand of toxicological studies, particularly screening procedures, for test organisms in large numbers. Are the costs, either in time or money, of producing sufficient numbers of embryos prohibitive?

In my view, the practical difficulties of whole embryo culture have

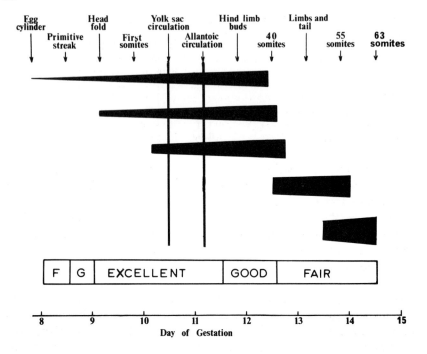

Fig. 20.3 Development in culture obtainable from rat embryos explanted at different stages of organogenesis. The length of each black area indicates the extent of differentiation in culture. The increasing height of the black areas from left to right symbolizes the growth in size of the embryos (not drawn to scale).

often been exaggerated. The animals, materials and apparatus required are all relatively inexpensive. Some parts of the culture procedures need to be carried out meticulously but none presents serious problems. To obtain the best results, the essential requirements are:

1) Careful selection of the stage of development of the embryos. For maximum growth and development, closely comparable with that *in vivo*, it is best to begin with embryos of head-fold or early somite stage (rat, 9–10 days).
2) Embryos must be explanted into culture with the yolk sac attached, so that the yolk sac with its developing blood circulation continues to provide 'placental' support for the embryo. For embryos up to about the 35-somite stage (rat, 12–13 days) the yolk sac is usually left intact; for older embryos, the yolk sac is best opened to expose the developing foetus (Cockroft, 1973).
3) Best results are obtained from embryos cultured in flowing, rather than static, medium. For embryos of more than about 25 somites (rat, 11–12 days), flowing medium is essential.
4) The culture medium must contain at least 50% serum, and rat serum is the most commonly used. The serum must be prepared from blood centrifuged

immediately after extraction from the rat, and must be heat-inactivated before use (Steele, 1972; Steele and New, 1974).

5) The oxygen content of the gas phase of the culture must be adjusted according to the stage of development of the embryos. For embryos of less than 10 somites, best results are obtained with 5–10% oxygen; this is raised to 20–40% for embryos of 10–25 somites, and to 95% for those of more than 25 somites (all the gas mixtures contain 5% CO_2 with the balance in nitrogen).

6) Temperature should be kept within the range 37.0–39.0 °C. Below this, growth is slowed and at 40.0 °C or above serious abnormalities of development appear (Cockroft and New, 1978; Mirkes, 1985).

Of the requirements listed above, only the provision and explantation of the embryos and the provision of culture serum need further consideration as to practicability.

Caging batches of females with males overnight, and selecting those that are sperm positive the following morning, is usually adequate for dating pregnancies to provide large numbers of embryos of a required stage. The tendency of most of the animals to mate within a few hours, and the fairly uniform rate of development of the embryos, ensures that after a specified time most of the embryos are at a closely similar stage of development in comparison both with their littermates and with other litters. This is particularly true of the rat. Explanting postimplantation embryos for culturing requires care but is not difficult. In Cambridge we run a class each year now in which our third-year physiology undergraduates successfully learn the technique in one afternoon. A practised operator can easily explant 50 or more embryos in a day.

The rat serum required for the culture medium is expensive to buy commercially and is better produced in one's own laboratory. Fortunately, it seems to make little difference which age, sex or strain of rat is used to provide the serum and any redundant but healthy rats in the laboratory can be used for the purpose. Costs can be reduced still further by taking blood for serum from the same females killed to provide the embryos. Only 0.5 ml of serum (made up to 1.0 ml of culture medium with DMEM or other synthetic medium) is required to grow an embryo to the early limb bud stage, so a pregnant female can often provide sufficient serum for culturing most or all of her own embryos.

Most workers to date have found rat serum better than that from any other species for culturing rat and mouse postimplantation embryos. However, some recent studies (e.g. Coelho *et al.*, 1989; Klug *et al.*, 1990) have indicated that, suitably prepared, bovine serum can also give satisfactory results. If these findings are generally confirmed, there may be advantages in replacing rat serum by bovine serum where large quantities are required.

In summary, it may be concluded that whole embryo culture is an entirely practicable method for use in toxicological studies.

What Reliance Can Be Placed on the Results of Toxicological Tests with Cultured Embryos?

A large number of toxicological studies, in many different laboratories, have now been made with cultured embryos. Shepard *et al.* (1987) listed 106 agents that had been tested by this method and many more have been examined since. How do such tests compare with those *in vivo*?

One limitation of culture methods is that they are not at present capable of supporting development of the late foetus. Nor is it practicable yet to return cultured postimplantation embryos to the uterus for continued development and examination of long-term effects of treatments (though an interesting preliminary study of such 'reimplantation' has been made by Beddington (1985)). The toxicological applications of the culture techniques are therefore usually restricted to those where the required observations can be made during the 2–4 days of the culture period. Fortunately, the very rapid organogenesis that occurs in rats and mice (about five times the rate in man), and its sensitivity to toxic agents, allows many useful studies to be made within this relatively short period. Any abnormalities of development are often clearly definable and closely correlated with known birth defects (Fig. 20.4). Furthermore, the greater accessibility of the embryo in culture and increased opportunity for precise control of the experimental conditions often confer important advantages over studies *in vivo* (Brown and Fabro, 1982; Cockroft and Steele, 1987; New, 1990; Steele, 1991). It is also possible to remove organs from the cultured embryo for prolonged development *in vitro* (Agnish and Kochhar, 1976).

When there is confusion about which of many possible factors *in vivo* is the source of an abnormality, studies on cultured embryos can often be particularly effective in obtaining a clear-cut answer. An example from our own laboratory may illustrate this. We received a request from one of the drug companies to examine certain of their newly developed hypolipidaemic agents. The company had found from their own *in vivo* tests that these agents were teratogenic when administered to pregnant rats. But they were unable to establish whether it was the drug itself that affected the embryos or – more worrying – whether it was the reduced lipid levels that were harmful. Our tests in culture (Steele *et al.*, 1983)

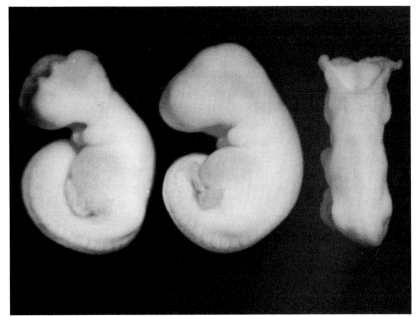

Fig. 20.4 Failure of closure of the head folds in 9.5-day rat embryos grown in culture for 48 h in excess oxygen. The middle embryo is normal. Photographed after removal of the embryonic membranes. Enlargement: 14×.

quickly answered this question. Rat embryos grown in normal serum with the drug developed abnormalities, whilst those grown in hypolipidaemic serum without the drug did not.

An important study by Webster *et al.* (1986) has illustrated how the value of *in vitro* studies may be enhanced by knowledge of the pharmacokinetics of an agent. These workers found that when isotretinoin was added to cultures of rat embryos, the critical level for teratogenesis was between 250 and 500 ng/ml, similar to the critical blood concentration associated with teratogenesis in the human. This is initially a surprising result because the dosage needed to induce teratogenesis in the pregnant rat is more than a hundred times that in the human. But an explanation can be provided by pharmacokinetic data, which suggest that metabolism of the drug is much more rapid in the adult rat than in the adult human.

Addition of liver microsomes to the embryo culture may also provide valuable additional information. This was first demonstrated by Fantel *et al.* (1979) who found that cyclophosphamide was teratogenic in culture only in combination with liver microsomes, indicating that a metabolite of cyclophosphamide rather than the parent compound is the main agent causing abnormalities.

Particularly relevant to human toxicology is the culture of (rat) embryos in human serum. If the serum is taken from hospital patients undergoing chemotherapy, or from alcoholics, smokers, etc., information can be obtained about the effects on embryos of the products of interaction of agents with the human metabolism. This technique was first used with dramatic results by Klein and his colleagues (Chatot *et al.*, 1980). It has to be admitted that rat embryos often grow subnormally in whole human serum and that this sometimes caused problems with the controls in these earlier experiments. But subsequent work (Beck *et al.*, 1985) has shown that the development of rat embryos in human serum can be much improved by the addition of as little as 10% rat serum. As a result this approach would now seem to have considerable promise.

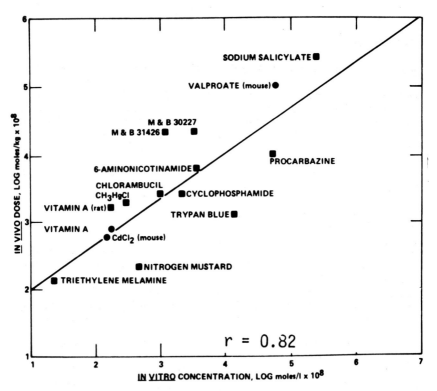

Fig. 20.5 Correlation of minimum effective teratogenic concentrations of various agents *in vivo* and *in vitro*. (Reprinted, with permission, from Kitchin *et al.* (1986).)

Perhaps the most controversial of the possible uses of whole embryo culture has been as a screening procedure for teratogenic agents. Until a few years ago, the balance of the arguments appeared to be heavily against mammalian embryo culture as a practicable screening method (Wilson, 1978). But recently the picture has changed. Several studies, such as those of Schmid *et al.* (1983) and Kitchin *et al.* (1986), have shown cultured embryos to have an impressively high predictive capacity for teratogens (Fig. 20.5). Some commercial laboratories are now developing embryo culture as a screening procedure (Bechter and Schön, 1988; Tesh, 1988). A major collaborative study to assess the potential of embryo culture for teratogen screening is currently being made by five European research laboratories, headed by R. Bechter, P.W.J. Peters, J.J. Picard, B.P. Schmid and J. Stadler. The preliminary results of this study seem very promising and, if confirmed, will greatly strengthen the arguments for the routine use of embryo culture in screening procedures.

References

Agnish, N.D. and Kochhar, D.M. (1976). *J. Embryol. Exp. Morphol.* **36**, 623–638.
Bechter, R. and Schön, H. (1988). *Toxicol. In Vitro* **2**, 1195–1203.
Beck, F., Gulamhusein, A.P. and Huxham, I.M. (1985). *In* "Prevention of Physical and Mental Congenital Defects Part C: Basic and Medical Science, Education, and Future Strategies", pp. 265–270. Alan R Liss, Inc., New York.
Beddington, R.S.P. (1985). *J. Embryol. Exp. Morphol.* **88**, 281–291.
Brown, N.A. and Fabro, S.E. (1982). *In* "Developmental Toxicology" (K. Snell, ed.), pp. 31–57. Praeger, New York.
Buckley, S.K.L., Steele, C.E. and New, D.A.T. (1978). *Dev. Biol.* **65**, 396–403.
Chatot, C.L., Klein, N.W., Piatek, J. and Pierro, L.J. (1980). *Science* **207**, 1471–1473.
Chen, L.T. and Hsu, Y.C. (1982). *Science* **218**, 66–68.
Cockroft, D.L. (1973). *J. Embryol. Exp. Morphol.* **29**, 473–483.
Cockroft, D.L. (1976). *Dev. Biol.* **48**, 163–172.
Cockroft, D.L. (1990). *In* "Postimplantation Mammalian Embryos – A Practical Approach" (A.J. Copp and D.L. Cockroft, eds), pp. 15–40. IRL Press, Oxford.
Cockroft, D.L. and New, D.A.T. (1978). *Teratology* **17**, 277–284.
Cockroft, D.L. and Steele, D.E. (1987). *In* "*In Vitro* Methods in Toxicology" (C.K. Atterwill and C.E. Steele, eds), pp. 365–389. Cambridge University Press, Cambridge.
Coelho, C.N.D., Weber, J.A., Klein, N.W., Daniels, W.G. and Hoagland, T.A. (1989). *J. Nutr.* **119**, 1716–1725.
Ellington, S.K.L. (1987). *Development* **100**, 431–439.
Eto, K. and Takakubo, F. (1985). *J. Craniofac Genet. Dev. Biol.* **5**, 357–361.
Fantel, A.G., Greenaway, J.C., Juchau, M.E. and Shepard, T.H. (1979). *Life Sci.* **25**, 67–72.
Huber, B.E. and Brown, N.A. (1982). *In Vitro* **18**, 599–605.

Jelinek, R. (1979). *In* "Evaluation of Embryotoxicity, Mutagenicity and Carcino-genicity Risks in New Drugs" (O. Benesova, Z. Rychter and R. Jelinek, eds), pp. 195–205. Univerzita Karlova, Praha.

Jelinek, R. and Rychter, Z. (1980). *Arch. Toxicol. Suppl.* **4**, 267–273.

Jolly, J. and Lieure, C. (1938). *Arch. Anat. Micr.* **34**, 307–374.

Kitchin, K.T., Schmid, B.P. and Sanyal, M.K. (1986). *Methods Find. Exp. Clin. Pharmacol.* **8**, 291–301.

Klug, S., Lewandowski, C., Wildi, L. and Neubert, D. (1990). *Toxicol. In Vitro*, **4**, 598–601.

Mirkes, P.E. (1985). *Teratology*, **32**, 259–266.

New, D.A.T. (1971). *In* "Methods in Mammalian Embryology" (J.C. Daniel, ed.), pp. 305–319. W.H. Freeman and Co., San Francisco.

New, D.A.T. (1978). *Biol. Rev.* **53**, 81–122.

New, D.A.T. (1983). *In* "Methods for Assessing the Effects of Chemicals on Reproductive Functions" (V.B. Vouk and P.J. Sheehan, eds), pp. 277–297. John Wiley and Sons Ltd., New York.

New, D.A.T. (1990). *In* "Postimplantation Mammalian Embryos – A Practical Approach" (A.J. Copp and D.L. Cockroft, eds), pp. 1–14. IRL Press, Oxford.

New, D.A.T., Coppola, P.T. and Cockroft, D.L. (1976a). *J. Embryol. Exp. Morphol.* **36**, 133–144.

New, D.A.T., Coppola, P.T. and Cockroft, D.L. (1976b). *J. Reprod. Fertil.* **48**, 219–222.

Nicholas, J.S. (1938). *Anat. Rec.* **70**, 199–210.

Sadler, T.W. and New, D.A.T. (1981). *J. Embryol. Exp. Morphol.* **66**, 109–116.

Schmid, B.P., Trippmacher, A. and Bianchi, A. (1983). *In* "Developments in the Science and Practice of Toxicology" (A.W. Hayes, R.C. Schnell and T.S. Miya, eds), pp. 563–566. Elsevier Science, Amsterdam.

Shepard, T.H., Fantel, A.G. and Mirkes, P.E. (1987). *Banbury Report (Cold Spring Harbor Laboratory)* **26**, 29–44.

Steele, C.E. (1972). *Nature New Biol.* **237**, 150–151.

Steele, C.E. (1991). *Hum. Reprod.* **6**, 144–147.

Steele, C.E. and New, D.A.T. (1974). *J. Embryol. Exp. Morphol.* **31**, 707–719.

Steele, C.E., New, D.A.T., Ashford, A. and Copping, G.P. (1983). *Teratology* **28**, 229–236.

Tesh, J.M. (1988). *Toxicol. In Vitro* **2**, 189–194.

Vouk, V.B. and Sheehan, P.J. (1983). "Methods for Assessing the Effects of Chemicals on Reproductive Functions" (V.B. Vouk and P.J. Sheehan, eds). John Wiley and Sons, New York.

Webster, W.S., Johnston, M.C., Lammer, E.J. and Sulik, K.K. (1986). *J. Craniofac. Genet. Dev. Biol.* **6**, 211–222.

Wiley, L.M. and Pedersen, R.A. (1977). *J. Exp. Zool.* **200**, 389–402.

Wilson, J.G. (1978). *In* "Handbook of Teratology" (J.G. Wilson and F.C. Fraser, eds), vol. 4, pp. 135–154. Plenum Press, New York.

Discussion

C. Roux

We should be very grateful to Dr New for having taught us this interesting technique which is now quite indispensable for everyone involved in teratological studies. It provides a lot of information about the mechanisms of teratogenesis and is very important.

However, as Dr New said, there are some limitations in the technique, mostly arising from its short duration in time, which means that it does not give any information about foetal toxicity or even about some true malformations. In our experience, it appears very important to add histological examination to microscopic examination. This is quite essential in order not to avoid detecting malformation.

From a toxicological point of view, as he said, whole embryo culture can produce a lot of information, but it is only *a* source of information which cannot be used for the whole question of teratology. Whole embryo culture must be considered as something *more*, not as something *instead of*.

I. Purchase
Dr New showed the similarity of rate of development of *in vivo* and *ex vivo* embryos over about 72 h. Can an *ex vivo* embryo be implanted back into a mother and develop normally, or is that period out of the body lethal to it?

D. New
Reimplantation has been done by Beddington, at Oxford, with the earliest embryos; that is, embryos at the head-fold stage, the beginning of organogenesis. She has succeeded in very carefully reintroducing the embryos into the decidua, and a proportion of them have developed to quite late stages of gestation.

The practical objection is that the success rate was only of the order of 7–10%. A great deal of work is necessary to do this, and the reward is only 7–10%. I think the technique is not yet adequate for toxicological work but reimplantation is an interesting possibility if it can be developed further.

N.G. Carmichael
In the end these sorts of techniques have to be applied to interpreting *in vivo* situations. What principles are used in selecting doses for using this as an *in vitro* teratology test?

D. New
When we have made teratological tests *in vitro*, doses have usually been based on such information as could be obtained about the plasma concentrations found *in vivo*.

J.J. Picard

We have done some experiments trying to devise a methodology to screen drugs. I must confess that I am slightly reluctant to place too much weight on lists like the one that has been published, first, because it does not take into account a very great number of factors that are tremendously important for an effect *in vivo* as compared to *in vitro*. One such factor about which I am concerned at the moment is that if we start with two embryos, one displaying one or two somites and the other embryo displaying 15 somites, the concentration may have to be increased 5 or even 10 times to get similar effects. Everything depends upon how the test is done.

My second concern about publishing such lists is what criteria are used to decide that one compound has to be classified as a teratogen and another has not to be so classified? There is a lot of discussion about this, and I am not convinced there is a satisfactory answer.

B. Bkaily

I agree with Dr Roux about the short time there is *in vitro*, which does not permit us to go far in using this preparation. Secondly, a decision cannot be taken just by seeing what the embryo looks like, in terms of volume, size or whatever, to say that it is really the same as *in vivo*. I have seen no functional studies showing that the embryo behaves the same *in vitro* as *in vivo*. I think we must look at all the functions of these embryos before saying whether or not we can use them.

D. New

May I just briefly repeat that it does appear to be identical in morphology, in total protein and DNA contents. I think it is fair to say that it is identical as regards growth.

As regards metabolism, I entirely agree with Dr Bkaily that it is not correct to say it is necessarily identical. Very close parallels have been shown in some things; for example, the rate of glucose uptake is very similar in embryos that have been grown for periods of 24 h previously in culture and in those that are explanted and grown from that point on. In other words, the culture itself has not altered the rate of glucose uptake.

As I mentioned, there are other aspects of the embryo where, as Nigel Brown has shown, there may well be differences in the enzyme patterns within the *in vitro* embryo. This has to be taken into account.

X. Pouradier Duteil

Taking Dr Picard's comment further, does Dr New consider that a drug which is proved not to pass through the placenta in *in vitro* systems is not teratogenic?

D. New

For me, a drug is teratogenic if toxicologists tell me that it is teratogenic!

J.J. Picard

I think a drug can be teratogenic even if it does not pass through the placenta, for example, by changing the maternal metabolism and the hormonal balance.

21

Micromass Limb Bud Cell Cultures: A Model for the Study and Detection of Teratogens

J.-Y. RENAULT and A. CORDIER

Institut de Recherche sur la Sécurité du Médicament, Rhône-Poulenc Rorer, 20 Quai de la Révolution, 94140 Alfortville, France

Introduction

A large number of *in vitro* tests have been proposed for the assessment of teratogenicity. Interest in the development and application of these tests is evident from numerous reviews and commentaries which have appeared (Kimmel *et al.*, 1982; Neubert, 1982; Brown and Freeman, 1984; Faustman, 1988).

These methods have been developed not only in response to increasing pressure to reduce animal experimentation, but also in order to reduce the cost and length of toxicological studies. They also provide a tool with which teratogenic mechanisms can be explored (Palmer, 1978). Standard segment II *in vivo* protocols require high levels of technical expertise, over 100 animals per test compound, and take several weeks to perform (Palmer, 1978; Brown and Freeman, 1984). *In vitro* tests could help in selecting compounds for *in vivo* testing. It has also been suggested that

IN VITRO METHODS IN TOXICOLOGY
ISBN 0-12-388175-7

in vitro assays could predict human teratogenic potential more accurately, since specific human metabolic systems could be added *in vitro*. Furthermore, *in vitro* tests can be used to test biological samples (urine, serum) from exposed humans (Chatot *et al.*, 1980).

In vitro teratogenicity assays have several limitations. It must be remembered that teratogenicity is only one aspect of reproductive toxicology. There are virtually no methods yet available for assessing drug effects on fertility, foetal and postnatal mortality, prenatally induced dysfunctions or the effects of maternal toxicity, although these are important aspects. There are four manifestations of abnormal prenatal development: death, malformation, retardation and functional impairment. Teratogenicity assays detect only the first three.

Designing *in vitro* teratogenicity tests is difficult for two reasons: (1) mammalian embryonic development includes a very complex sequence of proliferation and differentiation processes and (2) mechanisms leading to congenital malformations are generally poorly understood. There is no unifying "somatic mutation theory" for the teratogenesis process as there is for carcinogenesis. *In vitro* models have, therefore, been developed which allow the study of a variety of end points thought to be involved in normal and abnormal development. Such end points include cell death, altered cell–cell interactions, cell migration, reduced biosynthesis, altered cellular, biochemical and morphological differentiation and growth inhibition. However, it should be made clear that we do not know the consequences of these changes *in vivo*. These tests should therefore be considered as a "warning light", suggesting a potential developmental toxicity. This does not restrict their use in screening, since a chemical may induce different manifestations of embryotoxicity in different species. It should also be kept in mind that a given compound may have differing impacts on the embryo, the placenta and the maternal system. The toxicity induced may result from impairment of intracellular interactions, cell–cell communication or cell–matrix interactions or from disturbances of the metabolism or haemodynamics. It is, therefore, possible that as models are reduced in complexity from the pregnant animal to the cell, some teratogens could be missed. This appears to be an unavoidable consequence of simplifying the assays.

The *in vitro* techniques developed by teratologists include whole embryo systems, organ culture systems and primary and established cell culture systems. These systems may be divided into two categories. In the first there is an attempt to reproduce a limited period of embryogenesis. Examples of such methods include the postimplantation whole embryo culture system and differentiating embryonic organ culture systems (Neubert, 1982). In the second category, cells or non-vertebrate organisms are used to assess processes, such as regeneration, cell proliferation or cell–cell communication, which have characteristics similar to the *in vivo* developmental process. Examples of these types of assay include the mouse ovarian tumour cell assay (Braun *et al.*, 1979), the hydra assay (Johnson, 1980), the HEPM proliferation assay (Pratt and Willis, 1985) and the metabolic cooperation assay (Trosko *et al.*, 1982).

Many of the systems in the second category use embryonic or foetal cells maintained in culture. Primary cultures of embryonic cells may undergo differentiation *in vitro*. These systems usually reproduce cellular and biochemical differentiation, not organ morphogenesis. Examples include myoblasts and chondroblasts, which differentiate into muscle cells and chondrocytes respectively. The latter differentiation process may be studied using high-density limb bud cell cultures, also known as micromass or spot cultures. This system will be the subject of this review.

Rationale for Using Chondrogenesis in Limb Bud Cell Cultures as a Teratogenicity Assay

Organogenesis of the Vertebrate Embryonic Limb

The vertebrate embryonic limb is an established model in embryology and teratology. It has been used as a model of developmental processes involving multiple highly interdependent events. It is also able to detect and measure slight deviations in development. (See the extensive reviews of Kochhar (1977) and Kelley *et al.* (1984).)

Limb organogenesis is the result of several developmental mechanisms: polarized outgrowth of the limb bud, cell proliferation, cell death, cell locomotion, biosynthesis of extracellular macromolecules and interactions between the ectoderm and the mesoderm. The latter are of considerable importance. The ectoderm, which is also called the apical ectodermal ridge, is a distinct ridge at the distal tip of the growing limb. The mesoderm is responsible for thickening and maintaining the ridge, which in turn contributes to limb development by specifying limb parts. Normal mesoderm and ectoderm are both required for the successful morphogenesis of the normal limb. Multiple levels of control and regulation exist in the mesoderm and the ectoderm to facilitate the requisite interactions. For instance, cell communication may involve gap junctions, whereas longer-range tissue interactions are mediated through the extracellular matrix. Interference at different stages of development will induce different types of anomalies (amelia, phocomelia, hemimelia). The aetiology of these limb malformations includes genetic factors, environmental factors and combinations of both. Most teratogen-induced defects appear to result mainly from cell necrosis or degeneration.

Chondrogenesis in Limb Bud Cell Culture

The evolution from a small outgrowth from the embryonic flank to the formation of a pentadactyl appendage approximating the adult spatial pattern results mainly from organized chondrogenesis. This morphological differentiation can easily be observed by using the organ limb bud culture technique (Neubert, 1982).

In addition to growing intact limb buds *in vitro*, dissociated limb bud cells have long been used in culture systems (Umansky, 1966). Limb buds can be trypsinized and dispersed into high-density cell cultures, which are also known as micromass or spot cultures. After a few days incubation, these cultures display foci of cartilaginous tissue. This system, which is one of the most commonly used models of *in vitro* tissue differentiation, has been widely used to investigate the biochemical and cellular transformations and regulatory processes involved in tissue differentiation.

Cultures from birds or rodents follow the same pattern of development, which resembles that of chondrogenesis *in vivo*. The first event is a cellular aggregation, which leads to the formation of the blastema. The cells of the aggregated area then express their cartilage phenotype.

A technical point which has long been known is that in order to achieve chondrogenesis, cells have to be inoculated at densities greater than confluency after trypsinization (Umansky, 1966). This demonstrates the importance of cell–cell interactions in initiating chondrogenesis (Solursh, 1983).

Another important consideration is the stage of explantation. Ahrens *et al.* (1977), using chick embryo wing bud cells, have shown that chondrogenesis is highly dependent on the stage of explantation. Only cells from stage 21–24 embryos will condense and form cartilage nodules, whereas cells from earlier stage embryos will aggregate, but not differentiate to form cartilage, and cells from later stages produce cartilage, but without forming aggregates or nodules.

During the first 2 days of incubation, the key event is a cellular condensation (or aggregation) process, which leads to the formation of a blastema. During this aggregation, cells acquire the ability to respond to their environment. The cellular and biochemical events which occur during this process have been extensively studied.

Aulthouse and Solursh (1987) have shown that the galactose-specific lectin, peanut agglutinin, is a specific marker of the blastema, and George-Weinstein *et al.* (1988) have produced monoclonal antibodies which can be used to distinguish mesenchymal myogenic cells from chondrogenic precursor cells. It has been shown by George *et al.* (1983), using tritiated thymidine incorporation, and by Hadhazy and Szollosi (1983), using flow cytometry, that this condensation results from active cell division.

The role of cAMP in chondrogenesis has been extensively studied (Solursh, 1983; Hattori and Ide, 1984, 1985). Endogenous prostaglandins may regulate limb cartilage differentiation (Kosher and Walker, 1983) by acting as local regulators of cAMP (Biddulph *et al.*, 1984). Accordingly, Chepenik *et al.* (1984) have shown that cells undergoing chondrogenesis are able to metabolize endogenous arachidonic acid to prostaglandins and that prostaglandin-like compounds are a prerequisite for chondrogenesis *in vitro*.

It has also been suggested that intracellular Ca^{2+} may also play a role during this cellular condensation (San-Antonio and Tuan, 1986; Bee and Jeffries, 1987).

Another suggestion is that cell shape may be linked to cell differentiation (Solursh, 1983; Zanetti and Solursh, 1986). The possibility that actin microfilaments may play a role in modulating cell shape and subsequently the chondrogenic differentation has also been suggested (Zanetti and Solursh, 1984). Interactions between the actin skeleton and the extracellular matrix components may be crucial in this process.

The final step is the expression of a chondrocyte phenotype by the cultured cells. The differentiation of mesenchyme to form cartilage involves the cessation of type I collagen synthesis and the synthesis of at least two cartilage-specific gene products, type II collagen and chondroitin sulphate proteoglycans. These proteoglycans have been characterized *in vivo* and *in vitro* by De Luca *et al.* (1977) and their sequential appearance has been demonstrated by Franzen *et al.* (1987).

Swalla *et al.* (1983, 1988) have shown that low levels of type II collagen mRNA are present in the mesenchyme bud and increase significantly during condensation. Kosher *et al.* (1986) have studied the changes in the cytoplasmic levels of mRNA coding for the core protein of the major sulphated proteoglycans of cartilage and type II collagen during *in vitro* chondrogenesis. They have shown that there is a marked increase of both types of mRNA during the condensation phase, suggesting that regulation of these two genes is coordinated, although there are quantitative differences in their expression.

The matrix components can be characterized by biochemical or immunological assays or by histochemical staining (Alcian Blue staining at pH 1, Toluidine Blue metachromatic staining at pH 7.4) or [^{35}S]sulphate incorporation into glycosaminoglycans. These assays can be used to assess the differentiation process.

The cell-to-extracellular matrix interactions appear to play an important role in chondrogenesis. Knudson and Toole (1985) have observed a reduction in size of hyaluronate-dependent pericellular coats and a dramatic change in the relative proportion of hyaluronate and chondroitin sulphate produced by mesodermal cells at the time of cellular condensation. San Antonio et al. (1987) have demonstrated that, after cell condensation, heparan sulphate proteoglycans play a role, in initiating the expression of the chondrocyte phenotype or the growth of cartilage nodules.

Hitherto, this model was used exclusively to study chondrogenesis, but recently, Zimmerman et al. (1990) have shown that it may also be used to study endochondral mineralization. Mineralization was obtained by adding β-glycerophosphate to the culture medium, on day 6 of culture, when the nodules had been formed.

This primary culture of mammalian origin reproduces cartilage histogenesis, a fundamental step in the morphogenesis of the skeleton. Various functions, including cell proliferation, cell differentiation, cell-to-cell communication and cell-to-extracellular matrix interactions are implicated in this developmental process. Interference with these basic cell developmental functions may provide primordial teratogenic end points, and so this simple cell culture system appears to be a good model with which to study the teratogenic potential of chemical compounds.

Applicability of the Micromass Test for Studying Chemical Teratogenicity

Mechanistic Studies

Micromass limb bud cell cultures have been used to study the mechanisms responsible for malformations of the structures that are initially modelled in cartilage. Experiments have been performed to investigate mechanisms of malformation induced by inborn mutation or by xenobiotics.

Nanomelia, for instance, is an avian mutation that results in the absence of the cartilage proteoglycan core protein. Using cDNA probes in micromass cultures, Stirpe et al. (1987) have shown that nanomelic chondrocytes synthesize greatly reduced levels of this core protein mRNA and concluded that this mutation affects the regulation of the transcription of the corresponding gene. Another example may be given by brachypodism, which is a murine mutation. Owens and Solursh (1982) isolated limb bud cells from brachypod and wild-type mouse embryos at different stages of development. They compared their ability to form aggregates and cartilaginous nodules in pure and mixed micromass cultures, and concluded that this mutation results in a reduced ability of a specific mesenchyme cell subpopulation to provide an inductive stimulus for chondrogenesis.

Many chemical agents induce chondrogenesis impairment: cytochalasin B (Parker *et al.*, 1978), thiabendazole (Tsuchiya and Tanaka, 1986), jervine (Campbell *et al.*, 1985, 1987), bromodeoxyuridine (Levitt and Dorfman, 1972), cytosine arabinoside (Manson *et al.*, 1977) and even the OH⁻ radicals (Zsupan *et al.*, 1987). The compound most extensively studied is retinoic acid and its derivatives (Pennypacker *et al.*, 1978; Lewis *et al.*, 1978; Hassel *et al.*, 1978; Zimmermann and Tsambaos, 1985; Campbell *et al.*, 1987). This compound is present at low concentrations in the embryonic tissues (5–50 ng/ml), where it promotes proliferation and chondrogenesis in the distal mesodermal cells of the limb bud (Ide and Aono, 1988). However, at higher concentrations (0.5–5 µg/ml), it strongly inhibits chondrogenesis (Renault *et al.*, 1989).

Primary Screening

Methods and results

Wilk *et al.* (1980) and Hassel and Horigan (1982) were the first to use the micromass system as an assay to determine the teratogenic potential of chemicals. They studied the effect of 20 teratogenic and non-teratogenic compounds on the extent of chondrogenesis on micromass limb bud cells. Recently, four groups (Guntakatta *et al.*, 1984; Flint and Orton, 1984; Renault *et al.*, 1989; Wise *et al.*, 1990) have published the results of complete validation studies. These studies were done by testing the impact, in standardized conditions, of a number of structurally unrelated compounds (28, 46, 51 and 23 compounds respectively) on limb bud cells from mouse (Guntakatta *et al.*, 1984; Wise *et al.*, 1990) or rat (Flint and Orton, 1984; Renault *et al.*, 1989). Compounds were classified as teratogens or non-teratogens on the basis of animal studies. Chondrogenesis was measured by a variety of techniques, e.g. [³⁵S]sulphate incorporation (Guntakatta *et al.*, 1984; Wise *et al.*, 1990), or by Alcian Blue staining of the cultures in order to determine the number of cartilaginous nodules (Flint and Orton, 1984) or their total area (Renault *et al.*, 1989). In most studies, cell growth was simultaneously assessed by either tritiated thymidine incorporation (Guntakatta *et al.*, 1984 and Wise *et al.*, 1990) or spectrophotometric measurement of Crystal Violet bound to the cells in the micromass (Renault *et al.*, 1989). There was no assessment of cell growth in Flint's study; however, this author has recently developed a modified assay (Flint, 1987). The modification includes an evaluation based on Neutral Red incorporation by living cells. In all these studies, a range of concentrations was tested to determine the concentration inducing 50% inhibition (IC_{50}). Compounds were then ranked on the basis of their IC_{50} values and the ratio between the IC_{50} for differentiation and IC_{50} for proliferation. They were then classified as either positive or negative according to thresholds defined by each author. In the studies reported, the micromass assay correctly identified 86% (Guntakatta *et al.*, 1984), 82% (Flint and Orton, 1984) or 61% (Renault *et al.*, 1989) of the teratogens and 100% (Guntakatta *et al.*, 1984), 89% (Flint and Orton, 1984), 100% (Renault *et al.*, 1989) or 100% (Wise *et al.*, 1990) of the non-teratogens. Sensitivity was not reported in the Wise study because the compounds tested were mainly non-teratogens.

Discussion

Teratogenicity tests can be validated by selecting a number of compounds which have definitely established mammalian teratogenic potential *in vivo* and testing them *in vitro* using a standardized protocol. The findings of these validation studies can then be discussed using three general approaches (Brown, 1987) based on dichotomous classification, potency and developmental hazard, respectively.

The first approach is the simplest and by far the most common. It is based upon the dichotomous classification of test compounds as teratogens or non-teratogens, and the test result as positive or negative. All the validation studies cited ultimately classify the tested chemicals in this way. Evaluation of the effectiveness of each method is then based on a contingency table analysis, which is used to calculate the sensitivity of the test (percentage of teratogens found to be positive in the assay), the specificity (percentage of the non-teratogens found to be negative in the assay) and the overall accuracy (percentage of compounds correctly classified by the assay). The selection and classification of compounds is critically important in this approach. A proper interpretation of validation performances requires that teratogens and non-teratogens are rigidly defined. This was not the case for the cited studies, in which six compounds were classified differently by the different authors. It would be better to use a reference list of compounds, such as that proposed by a panel of teratologists (Smith *et al.*, 1983) which provides a reasonable starting point (Brown, 1987). For this purpose, the panel defined teratogens as compounds which, in the absence of maternal toxicity, induce embryolethality, growth retardation, structural anomalies or peri- or post-natal dysfunctions in two mammalian species. However, this definition applies to any developmentally toxic substance and not only to teratogens.

The results of the four reported validation studies were remarkably consistent, given the variety of compounds tested, assay conditions and assessment techniques. It should be emphasized that the specificity of the test is critical when attempting to detect the teratogenic potential. Only two of these studies (Renault *et al.*, 1989; Wise *et al.*, 1990) included a sufficiently high number of non-teratogens to allow assessment of specificity and, in both, it was excellent.

It is also interesting to compare these results with those obtained with other tests systems, such as the *Drosophila* embryo (Bournias-Vardiabasis *et al.*, 1982), the attachment test (Braun *et al.*, 1979), the neuroblastoma assay (Mummery *et al.*, 1984) and the HEPM assay (Pratt and Willis, 1985). These assays, which assess a single cell process, performed poorly for both sensitivity and specificity, giving approximately 35% false-positive and false-negative rates. This suggests that the effectiveness of a test depends on the biological complexity of the system used; the more complex the system, the more effective the test is (Brown, 1987).

Another approach to validation is potency correlation, which can be performed by comparing the IC_{50} with the lowest teratogenic dose *in vivo*. This has been performed successfully with the attachment test (Braun *et al.*, 1982). Although a good correlation has been found for some compounds in the micromass test validation reports, further studies are needed to establish the validity of this method. However, the main interest of this approach is that it provides an order of magnitude of the biologically toxic concentration.

The third approach is based on the "developmental hazard" concept. Teratogenicity tests are designed to identify substances that impair development at levels of exposure that are not toxic to the adult. Such substances are described as "developmentally hazardous" and the level of hazard is evaluated as the ratio of the adult toxic dose to the embryotoxic dose. Fabro *et al.* (1982) have proposed a method for calculating this ratio, which they have called the "Relative Teratogenic Index". This approach to *in vitro* test validation involves the comparison of ratio estimates obtained *in vivo* and *in vitro*. The only method specifically designed to estimate this ratio *in vitro* is the hydra test (Johnson, 1980). However, the ratio between the concentration inhibiting chondrogenesis and that inhibiting proliferation in the micromass test has also been proposed as a way of estimating this hazard (Renault *et al.*, 1989; *Wise et al.*, 1990). The higher this ratio, the more likely that the compound will selectively affect development. When this parameter was taken into account, the specificity of the micromass test was found to be excellent (Renault *et al.*, 1989; *Wise et al.*, 1990).

Secondary Screening

From the above discussion, it is clear that it will be difficult to replace current segment II studies by the micromass system or any other *in vitro* system. However, another application of *in vitro* tests is evaluation of the teratogenic potential within a group of chemically related substances, some of which are proven teratogens. When such studies are performed with large series of molecules, the test can be used to establish relationships between their activity and their physicochemical properties (Brown *et al.*, 1989). Compounds selected on the basis of a negative effect *in vitro* must subsequently be tested *in vivo*.

This approach has been attempted using the micromass system in several laboratories. Flint and Boyle (1985) tested a series of 16 triazole antifungals with this assay. They showed that *in vitro* chondrogenesis inhibition was correlated with the lipophilicity of the molecule (characterized by the logP), but was not correlated with the antifungal activity. Using this method, they were able to select non-teratogenic antifungals. Retinoids have also been tested by this method (Kistler, 1987). Friesson *et al.* (1990), using a computer-assisted structure evaluation (CASE), showed that changes in the hydrophobic region of the molecules had the greatest impact on the IC_{50}. Furthermore, they showed that compounds with a logP below a certain value are non-teratogenic *in vivo*.

Future Prospects

Xenobiotic metabolism

Limb bud cell cultures are devoid of any xenobiotic metabolization component. An extrinsic metabolic activation system was added by Wilk *et al.* (1980) when they first attempted to validate the system as a teratogen screening test. Addition to the culture medium of a liver homogenate (S9 fraction) from pretreated rats (usually by Aroclor 1254 or PCB) and metabolic cofactors is probably the method most commonly used. Wiger *et al.* (1989) have cocultivated limb bud cells with rat hepatocytes. The teratogenicity of cyclophosphamide was demonstrated using both systems. Other novel approaches have been proposed.

Flint *et al.* (1984) have developed a technique in which compounds are administered *in vivo* by a single intraperitoneal injection 16 h before laparotomy of pregnant rats. Despite high sensitivity (92%) and specificity (94%), the prediction accuracy was only slightly better than that obtained with the standard *in vitro* treatment. This method could be used to screen compounds for which no *in vitro* metabolic activation system is available.

Brown *et al.* (1986) were able to induce metabolic activity in embryonic limb bud cells. They showed that treatment of pregnant rat with β-naphthoflavone and phenobarbital induced several cytochrome *P*-450 isozymes. They showed that, under these conditions, the cells obtained were able to convert cyclophosphamide into toxic reactive metabolites.

Pharmacokinetics

The micromass test cannot integrate pharmacokinetic constraints. Test concentrations do not vary significantly over time. *In vivo*, tissue distribution, maternal metabolism and elimination are all known to determine embryo exposure. Exposure may be further modified by maternal toxicity. For all these reasons, it is often very difficult to determine whether *in vitro* concentrations are relevant to the *in vivo* situation.

The occurrence of congenital defects is usually considered to be a threshold phenomenon, and many substances induce effects *in vitro* at the concentrations tested, but are not in fact embryotoxic or teratogenic *in vivo* (Brown, 1987). These factors must be considered for each test compound and they highlight the need for pharmacokinetic data. However, in spite of these limitations, the micromass test provides valuable information, particularly in determining the highest concentrations which have no effect on cell growth or differentiation. These concentrations were estimated in three of the four validation papers discussed above (Guntakatta *et al.*, 1984; Flint and Orton, 1984; Renault *et al.*, 1989). Comparison of the *in vitro* No Effect Concentrations with plasma concentrations in man or animals can provide interesting information. For example, retinoic acid inhibits chondrogenesis at concentrations below 1 μg/ml (Renault *et al.*, 1989), which are comparable with serum concentrations observed in man (Nau *et al.*, 1987), whereas aspirin, which has not been reported as a teratogen in man, was toxic *in vitro* only at concentrations in excess of 100 μg/ml (Flint and Orton, 1984; Renault *et al.*, 1989), which are considerably higher than therapeutic levels (Goodman and Gilman, 1975). However, as mentioned above, such comparisons may be invalid if pharmacokinetic, metabolic or physicochemical factors affect the exposure of the embryo to the compound *in vivo* (Brown *et al.*, 1982).

Conclusion

An overview of the recent literature relating to the limb bud cell micromass culture has been presented. The great number of experimental studies cited suggests that this system is a very useful tool for studying normal and abnormal development. It is sufficiently complex and yet easy to perform and this makes it a good system for *in vitro* teratogenicity testing.

Acknowledgements

We would like to thank Roselyne Reibaud for her invaluable assistance with the documentary aspects of this review and François Ballet for his helpful discussion.

References

Ahrens, P.B., Solursh, M. and Reiter, R.S. (1977). *Dev. Biol.* **60**, 69–82.

Aulthouse, A.L. and Solursh, M. (1987). *Dev. Biol.* **120**, 377–384.

Bee, J.A. and Jeffries, R. (1987). *Development* **100**, 73–81.

Biddulph, D.M., Sayer, L.M. and Smales, W.P. (1984). *Exp. Cell Res.* **153**, 270–274.

Bournias-Vardiabasis, N., Teplitz, R.L., Chernoff, G.F. and Seecof, R.L. (1982). *Teratology* **28**, 109–122.

Braun, A.G., Emerson, D.J. and Nichinson, B.B. (1979). *Nature* **282**, 507–509.

Braun, A.G., Buckner, C.A., Emerson, D.J. and Nichinson, B.B. (1982). *Proc. Natl. Acad. Sci. U.S.A.* **79**, 2056–2060.

Brown, L.P., Flint, O.P., Orton, T.C. and Gibson, G.G. (1986). *Fd. Chem. Toxic.* **24**, 737–742.

Brown, L.P., Lewis, D.F., Flint, O.P., Orton, T.C. and Gibson, G.G. (1989). *Xenobiotica* **19**, 1471–1481.

Brown, N.A. (1987). *Arch. Toxicol. Suppl.* **11**, 105–114.

Brown, N.A. and Freeman, S.J. (1984). *Alt. Lab. Anim.* **12**, 7–23.

Brown, N.A., Shull, G., Kao, J., Goulding, E.H. and Fabro, S. (1982). *Toxicol. Appl. Pharmacol.* **64**, 271–288.

Campbell, M., Brown, K.S., Hassel, J.R., Horigan, E.A. and Keeler, R. (1985). *Dev. Biol.* **111**, 464–470.

Campbell, M., Horton, W. and Keeler, R. (1987). *Teratology* **36**, 235–245.

Chatot, C.L., Klein, N.W., Platek, J. and Pierro, L.J. (1980). *Science* **207**, 1471–1473.

Chepenik, K.P., Ho, W.C., Waite, B.M. and Parker, C.L. (1984). *Calcif. Tissue Int.* **36**, 175–181.

De Luca, S., Heinegard, D. and Hascall, V.C. (1977). *J. Biol. Chem.* **252**, 6600–6608.

Fabro, S., Shull, G. and Brown, N.A. (1982). *Terat. Carcin. Mut.* **2**, 61–76.

Faustman, E.M. (1988). *Mutat. Res.* **205**, 355–384.

Flint, O.P. (1987). *In "In Vitro* Methods in Toxicology" (C.K. Atterwill and C.E. Steele, eds), pp. 339–363. Cambridge University Press, New York.

Flint, O.P. and Boyle, F.T. (1985). *Concepts Toxicol.* **3**, 29–35.

Flint, O.P. and Orton, T.C. (1984). *Toxicol. Appl. Pharmacol.* **76**, 383–395.

Flint, O.P., Orton, T.C. and Ferguson, R.A. (1984). *J. Appl. Toxicol.* **4**, 109–116.

Franzen, A., Heinegard, D. and Solursh, M. (1987). *Differentiation* **36**, 199–210.

Frierson, M.R., Mielach, F.A. and Kochhar, D.M. (1990). *Fund. Appl. Toxicol.* **14**, 408–428.

George, M., Chepenik, K.P. and Schneiderman, M.H. (1983). *Differentiation* **24**, 245–249.

George-Weinstein, M., Decker, C. and Horwitz, A. (1988). *Dev. Biol.* **125**, 34–50.

Goodman, L.S. and Gilman, A. (1975). "The Pharmacological Basis of Therapeutics", 5th edition. Macmillan, New York.

Guntakatta, M., Matthews, E.J. and Rundell, J.O. (1984). *Terat. Carcin. Mut.* **4**, 349–56.

Hadhazy, C. and Szollosi, J. (1983). *Acta Biol. Hung.* **34**, 407–414.

Hassel, J.R. and Horigan, E.A. (1982). *Terat. Carcin. Mut.* **2**, 325–331.

Hassel, J.R., Pennypacker, J.P. and Lewis, C.A. (1978). *Exp. Cell Res.* **112**, 409–417.

Hattori, T. and Ide, H. (1984). *Exp. Cell Res.* **150**, 338–346.

Hattori, T. and Ide, H. (1985). *Exp. Cell Res.* **157**, 371–378.

Ide, H. and Aono, H. (1988). *Dev. Biol.* **130**, 767–773.

Johnson, E.M. (1980). *J. Environ. Pathol. Toxicol.* **4**, 153–156.

Kelley, R.O., Fallon, J.F. and Kelly Jr., R.E. (1984). *In* "Issues and Reviews in Teratology" (H. Kalter, ed.), pp. 219–266. Plenum Press, New York.

Kimmel, G.L., Smith, K., Kochhar, D.M. and Pratt, R.M. (1982). *Terat. Carcin. Mut.* **2**, 221–229.

Kistler, A. (1987). *Arch. Toxicol.* **60**, 403–414.

Knudson, C.B. and Toole, B.P. (1985). *Dev. Biol.* **112**, 308–318.

Kochhar, D.M. (1977). *In* "Handbook of Teratology" (J.G. Wilson and F.C. Fraser, eds), vol. 2, pp. 453–480. Plenum Press, New York.

Kosher, R.A. and Walker, K.H. (1983). *Exp. Cell Res.* **15**, 145–153.

Kosher, R.A., Gay, S.W., Kamanitz, J.R., Kulyk, W.M., Rodgers, B.J., Sai, S., Tanaka, T. and Tanzer, M.L. (1986). *Dev. Biol.* **118**, 112–117.

Levitt, D. and Dorfman, A. (1972). *Proc. Natl. Acad. Sci. U.S.A.* **69**, 1253–1257.

Lewis, C.A., Pratt, R.M., Pennypacker, J.P. and Hassel, J.R. (1978). *Dev. Biol.* **64**, 31–47.

Manson, J.M., Dourson, M.L. and Smith, C.C. (1977). *In Vitro* **13**, 434–442.

Mummery, C.L., Van den Brink, C.E., Van den Saag, P.T. and De Laat, S.W. (1984). *Teratology*, **29**, 271–279.

Nau, H., Kochhar, D.M., Creech Kraft, J.M., Loefberg, B., Reiners, J. and Sparenberg, T. (1987). *In* "Approaches to Elucidate Mechanisms in Teratogenesis" (F. Welsh, ed.), pp. 1–16. Hemisphere Publishing Corporation, Cambridge.

Neubert, D. (1982). *Pharmacol. Ther.* **18**, 397–434.

Owens, E.M. and Solursh, M. (1982). *Dev. Biol.* **91**, 376–388.

Palmer, A.K. (1978). *In* "Handbook of Teratology" (J.G. Wilson and F.C. Fraser, eds), vol. 4, pp. 215–253. Plenum Press, New York.

Parker, C.L., Finch, R.A. and Hooper, W.C. (1978). *In Vitro* **14**, 606–615.

Pennypacker, J.P., Lewis, C.A. and Hassel, J.R. (1978). *Arch. Biochem. Biophys.* **236**, 351–358.

Pratt, R.M. and Willis, W.D. (1985). *Proc. Natl. Acad. Sci. U.S.A.* **82**, 5791–5794.

Renault, J.-Y., Melcion, C. and Cordier, A. (1989). *Terat. Carcin. Mut.* **9**, 83–96.
San Antonio, J.D. and Tuan, R.S. (1986). *Dev. Biol.* **115**, 313–324.
San Antonio, J.D., Winston, B.M. and Tuan, R.S. (1987). *Dev. Biol.* **123**, 17–24.
Smith, M.K., Kimmel, G.L., Kochhar, D.M., Shepard, T.H., Spielberg, S.P. and Wilson, J.G. (1983). *Terat. Carcin. Mut.* **3**, 461–480.
Solursh, M. (1983). *In* "Cartilage: Volume 2, Development, Differentiation and Growth", pp. 121–141. Academic Press, London.
Stirpe, N.S., Scott Argraves, W. and Goetinck, P.F. (1987). *Dev. Biol.* **124**, 77–81.
Swalla, B.J., Owens, E.M., Linsenmayer, T.F. and Solursh, M. (1983). *Dev. Biol.* **97**, 59–69.
Swalla, B.J., Upholt, W.B. and Solursh, M. (1988). *Dev. Biol.* **125**, 51–58.
Trosko, J.E., Chang, C.C. and Netzloff, M. (1982). *Terat. Carcin. Mut.* **2**, 31–45.
Tsuchiya, T. and Tanaka, A. (1986). *Toxicol. Lett.* **30**, 19–26.
Umansky, R. (1966). *Dev. Biol.* **13**, 31–56.
Wiger, R., Trygg, B. and Holme, J.A. (1989). *Teratology* **40**, 603–613.
Wilk, A.L., Greenberg, J.H., Horigan, E.A., Pratt, J.H. and Martin, G.R. (1980). *In Vitro* **16**, 269–276.
Wise, L.D., Clark, R.L., Rundell, J.O. and Robertson, R.T. (1990). *Teratology* **41**, 341–351.
Zanetti, N.C. and Solursh, M. (1984). *J. Cell Biol.* **99**, 115–123.
Zanetti, N.C. and Solursh, M. (1986). *Dev. Biol.* **113**, 110–118.
Zimmerman, B. and Tsambaos, D. (1985). *Cell Differ.* **17**, 95–103.
Zimmerman, B., Wachtel, H.C., Noppe, C. and Bernimoulin, J.P. (1990). *Teratology* **42**, 29A.
Zsupan, I., Hadhazy, C., Nagy, C., Jeney, F. and Nagy, I. (1987). *J. Submicrosc. Cytol.* **19**, 445–454.

Discussion

B. Vannier

Could Dr Renault confirm and comment on the response obtained with thalidomide in this micromass test system?

J.-Y. Renault

Thalidomide is considered as a non-teratogen in the rat, and this model makes use of cells from rat embryos; that is probably why this compound does not inhibit chondrogenesis in this culture. However, Dr. Flint obtained positive results with thalidomide, but by using modified culture conditions. For this, he used micromass cultures seeded with a lower cell density.

J.E. Trosko

In the next two presentations both Dr Yamasaki and I will state that gap junctional intercellular communication is strongly linked to regulatory control of cell proliferation and differentiation. Have Dr Renault and his colleagues, who are using this micromass assay, thought of integrating now, measuring what happens when a chemical causes abnormal proliferation and differentiation, and whether there is also abnormal gap junctional communication?

J.-Y. Renault
Yes, the presence of intercellular gap junctions is now well established, and their role in chondrogenesis was studied in this model. Inhibition of this kind of intercellular communication as a teratogenic mechanism has also been investigated, particularly by David Welsh.

P.J.J.M. Weterings
Dr Renault will be aware of an international ring trial that is being performed, organized and initiated by Oliver Flint, in which approximately 70 chemicals are being tested both in the limb bud model and also in the midbrain cell cultures of the same embryos. Midbrain cells were not mentioned in his presentation. Is there some reason for using only the limb bud micromass techniques?

J.-Y. Renault
We have compared limb bud and midbrain micromass cultures as teratogen screening assays and found no real advantages of doubling the workload. This is the reason why we chose to use only limb bud cell cultures for screening purposes. However, midbrain cell cultures are certainly a good model to study teratogens which are specific for the brain development.

P.J.J.M. Weterings
This system is really presented as a screening assay, so is metabolic activation included on a regular basis?

J.-Y. Renault
We are just studying and trying to develop a routine technique for metabolic activation in this system.

J.-J. Picard
Do you think this micromass assay would detect under screening conditions a chemical that would induce spina bifida? There are such nice results, with beautiful correlation, that we would expect to be able to detect that.

J.-Y. Renault
The best way to find out is probably to test teratogens which give only spina bifida.

J.-J. Picard

What is the relevance to development and processes of using cell attachment to lectins fixed on plastic as a complementary test? Would any kind of test do the same? I have some problems in seeing any relevance of this test in that regard.

J.-Y. Renault

Andrew Braun's lectin attachment test is very interesting, particularly because of the positive results obtained with thalidomide. We are now trying to reproduce these results.

J.-R. Claude

For all the *in vitro* methods for teratogenicity and embryotoxicity, one has to consider that the conditions are not the same as for mutagenicity testing. In mutagenicity testing, there is the possibility of preparing activation systems and we know that S9, for example, makes it easier to mimic somehow the *in vivo* situation. In the teratogenicity assays, including the whole embryo cultures, the situation is difficult for different reasons.

First, although direct biological samples can be used, the concentration of metabolites in blood is probably not relevant to the exposure of the foetus to metabolites, if there are active intermediate metabolites. Second, it is difficult to find both good activation systems and adequate concentrations, and it is a very important problem.

Third, biomimetic chemicals or biomimetic catalysts could be used to mimic the production of metabolites directly *in situ* in the medium. This would be very difficult, but it has been studied, especially in Sweden. I think the limitation of this testing, well emphasized by the impossibility of detecting *in vitro* a positive response for thalidomide, is this problem of metabolism and of an active intermediate metabolite as the effective agent in teratogenicity and embryotoxicity.

B. Carcinogenesis

22

Chemical Modulation of Gap Junctional Intercellular Communication *In Vitro*: An *In Vitro* Biomarker of Epigenetic Toxicology

J.E. TROSKO, C.C. CHANG, E. DUPONT, B.V. MADHUKAR and G. KALIMI

Department of Pediatrics/Human Development, Center for Environmental Toxicology, Michigan State University, East Lansing, MI 48824, USA

Introduction

Because of the pervasive use, persistence and known toxic effects of many human-made chemicals in experimental animals and exposed human beings, legitimate concern is raised about the potential health risk to human beings. The challenge – to develop a biologically based risk-assessment model for exposure to these toxic chemicals and to develop meaningful biomarkers – is to understand the molecular/biochemical/cellular mechanisms by which these chemicals work in human beings.

To achieve this goal, experiments on microorganisms, non-human animals, *in vitro* mammalian, including human, cell systems and

IN VITRO METHODS IN TOXICOLOGY
ISBN 0-12-388175-7

epidemiological studies on human beings must be integrated. To date, a plethora of toxicological data exists on many classes of chemicals. However, in spite of all this information, the mechanisms by which any of these chemicals cause birth defects, cancer, neurological effects, reproductive dysfunction or immunological modulations are not understood.

One of the major concerns is the possibility that many toxic chemicals might cause mutations in human beings, either in the somatic or germinal cells (Trosko and Chang, 1978). Consequently, one of the first objectives in testing chemicals is to determine their potential "genotoxicity". This legitimate concern, together with the prevailing paradigm, "carcinogens are mutagens" (Ames *et al.*, 1973), has shaped the nature of a number of studies and their interpretation. Herein lies, in our opinion, one of the problems of understanding how chemicals act in a toxicological manner.

Many chemicals have been shown in bioassay systems to induce cancers in experimental animals ("ergo", within the aforementioned paradigm, "they *must* be genotoxic"). Yet, in several *in vitro* short tests for genotoxicity, many have proved to be negative, or possibly weakly genotoxic (Clive, 1987; Tennant *et al.*, 1987). Without reiterating the major limitations of the animal bioassays (Clayson, 1987), as well as of all short-term *in vitro* tests for genotoxicity (Trosko, 1984; 1989a, b; Douglas *et al.*, 1988; Trosko *et al.*, 1990a,c), the problem is how to interpret these studies. Are animal bioassays good surrogates for human cancers? Can the protocols used in animal bioassay give clues to the mechanisms of action of these chemicals? Do weakly positive or strongly positive results in short-term assays for genotoxicity always mean that the chemical causes mutations? Even if chemicals did cause mutations in these short-term genotoxicity assays, would they cause mutations *in vivo* in humans? What do the negative results in these genotoxicity short-term tests mean? Even if mutations are found in genes (oncogenes) of cancers induced by chemicals, were they caused by the chemicals (Brookes, 1989; Mass and Austin, 1989; Chen *et al.*, 1990; Fox *et al.*, 1990; Mass *et al.*, 1990; Trosko *et al.*, 1990b)?

These and many questions like them must be resolved before a realistic risk assessment can be made for chemicals. Our objective is to examine the possibility that the toxicities induced by many, if not most, chemicals are mediated in experimental animal systems and possibly in exposed human beings via epigenetic mechanisms.

Epigenetic Toxicology

The definition of epigenetic is best understood against the definition of genetic toxicology (Fig. 22.1). A mutation or genotoxic event is one in which the *quality* or *quantity* of genetic *information* of a cell is changed (ostensibly for that cell) irreversibly. On the other hand, an epigenetic event is one in which the *expression* of the genetic information is altered at the transcriptional, translational or posttranslational level. In the former case, to increase, change or delete a base in the DNA would lead to a point mutation, whereas to increase or decrease a single or whole set of chromosomes is indicated by aneuploidy and polyploid induction respectively.

Altered methylation of genes, altered degradation or stabilization of specific mRNAs, or phosphorylation of proteins would represent epigenetic events. These events are all potentially reversible, although the biological sequelae which result from some of them might not be (see later discussion). It should be pointed out that the mechanisms leading to point mutations are probably very different from those leading to changes in

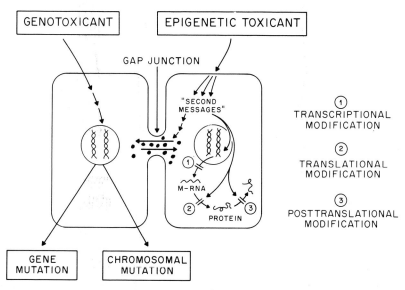

Fig. 22.1 Diagram illustrating the difference between genotoxic and epigenetic chemicals. Those that alter the *quality* or *quantity* of genetic information are *genotoxic*, while those that affect the *expression* of the genetic information, at the transcriptional, translational or posttranslational levels, are *epigenetic* chemicals.

chromosome numbers (non-dysjunctions, polyploid induction), in that the former are most probably induced by errors in DNA replication or the repair of damaged DNA, while the latter might be caused by agents affecting the membrane, spindle fibres and other non-DNA targets. In fact, it might be reasonable to speculate that agents that cause chromosomal mutations are, in many cases, epigenetic agents, in that they do not damage DNA nor do they induce gene mutations. Consequently, it might be very misleading to lump gene-mutation-causing chemicals with those inducing chromosomal mutations.

Another important point to keep in mind is the fact that many assays, presumably designed to measure genotoxicity (e.g. unscheduled DNA synthesis (UDS), drug-resistance mutation markers, single-strand break assays, sister chromatid exchanges (SCE), etc.) are indirect markers for genetic damage. Each of these types of *in vitro* assay used to detect genotoxicants has severe limitations which could mislead one in the interpretation of presumed positive results. These would include chemicals that would:

a) alter nucleotide uptake and nucleotide pools, or stimulate mitogenesis (which then alters labelled precursor specific activities used to study UDS or SCEs);
b) alter gene expression (demethylate/methylate genes, phosphorylate enzymes), thereby repressing or derepressing genes/gene products to cause phenocopies (e.g. thioguanine-resistant (TG^r) and thymidine kinase$^-$ (TK^-); the fast-growing TK^--resistant colonies could represent drug-resistant cells whose genes were repressed by the chemical treatment).

Lastly, DNA strand breaks, chromosome aberrations or micronuclei found after chemical treatment might simply be the secondary (tertiary?) consequence of a non-genotoxic chemical lysing the cytoplasmic compartmentalized hydrolytic nucleases and these, in turn, cause the DNA damage (Bradley *et al.*, 1987).

Finally, the demonstration of mutated oncogenes in chemically induced tumours of rodents has been interpreted as indicating that the chemical is a carcinogen and that the carcinogen is mutagenic. An alternative explanation can be given in at least two cases: that of the furan/furfural-induced tumours in rodents having mutated H-*ras* oncogenes and in 7,12-dimethylbenz[a]anthracene (DMBA)-induced mouse bladder transformed colonies having a mutated Ki-*ras* gene (Brookes, 1989; Mass and Austin, 1989; Chen *et al.*, 1990; Fox *et al.*, 1990; Mass *et al.*, 1990; Trosko *et al.*, 1990b; Wilson *et al.*, 1990). Since there is virtually no evidence that furan/furfural are mutagenic *in vitro*, it could be that these chemicals acted as tumour promoters and promoted spontaneously initiated cells. If the mutation spectrum in the H-*ras* oncogene of the treated rodents is different from that in the non-treated rodent spontaneous tumours, this could be due to a selective growth advantage for specific H-*ras* mutations in the furan/furfural-treated liver environment compared with spontaneously initiated H-*ras* mutations at different sites. In the DMBA-induced transformation example (Brookes, 1989), DMBA only induced transformation in bladder cell cultures of old, but not young, mice and the mutations found in the spontaneous and induced transformants were all in the same Ki-*ras* gene (codon 12, GGT-AGT). The data are best explained by the hypothesis that DMBA acted as a promoter of spontaneously initiated cells.

In summary, it is clear that chemicals can be toxic to cells and organisms by mechanisms that do not cause DNA damage or lead to mutations (Trosko and Chang, 1984, 1985, 1988, 1989). Many chemicals, including pesticides and herbicides, have not been shown to be very mutagenic, and we must ask how these chemicals act to make them toxic. If they are epigenetic toxicants, how do they work and how can one detect their toxicities prior to development, use and exposure (Trosko *et al.*, 1990a)?

Modulated Gap Junctional Intercellular Communication: The Cellular Basis for Epigenetic Toxicology

All multicellular organisms are composites of many cell types, all interacting among and between each other by means of extra-, intra- and inter-cellular communication mechanisms (Trosko *et al.*, 1988) (Fig. 22.2). Homoeostatic control of cell proliferation, cell differentiation and synchronized differentiated functions are mediated by these interconnected communication processes. Growth factors, hormones and neurotransmitters, as molecular signals travelling over space from one cell/tissue to another type of cell/tissue (extracommunication), trigger a finite number of intracellular communication systems (e.g. intracellular modulations of inositol trisphosphate (IP_3), Ca^{2+}, pH and cAMP, phosphorylation of inactive proteins, generation of free radicals, etc.), which in turn, have the potential of up- or down-regulation of gap junctional communication (intercellular communication).

Gap junctions are membrane-associated protein channels which allow ions and small molecules to pass between contiguous cells (Loewenstein, 1979). Most normal cells of solid tissues have these gap junctions. They appear to be highly conserved in all metazoans, with slight variations which appear to be associated with either developmental or differentiated functions within an organism (Saez *et al.*, 1990). These gap junctions can be regulated at the developmental level or transcriptional, translational

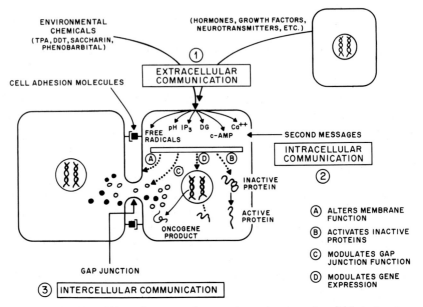

Fig. 22.2 The heuristic schemata characterizes the postulated link between extracellular communication and intercellular communication via various intracellular transmembrane signalling mechanisms. It provides an integrating view of how the neuroendocrine–immune system (mind or brain/body connection) and other multisystem coordinations could occur. While not shown here, activation or altered expression of various oncogenes (and anti-oncogenes) could also contribute to the regulation of gap junction function.

and posttranslational levels by endogenous factors (Spray *et al.*, 1988) and exogenous chemicals (Trosko and Chang, 1988).

Potentially mitogenic cells, when coupled (e.g. contact inhibited), have their regulatory second messages in equilibrium. These coupled cells presumably use gap junctions to regulate growth by keeping important mitogenic triggers *below* a "critical mass" (Sheridan, 1987). If a growth factor (Maldonado *et al.*, 1988; Madhukar *et al.*, 1989; Shiba *et al.*, 1989) or chemical mitogen (Yotti *et al.*, 1979) could down-regulate gap junctional intercellular communication, the second messages also induced by this mitogen could increase within the cell to trigger mitogenesis. In this case, gap junctions serve to couple cells "metabolically".

In postmitotic cells, such as heart muscle cells, the gap junction appears to act as a means to couple cells "electrotonically", in order to ensure synchronization of functions (e.g. tissue contraction). Down-regulation of the gap junction in heart tissue might be responsible for arrhythmia (DeMello, 1982; Manjunath and Page, 1985; Trosko *et al.*, 1990c).

With the cloning of several gap junction genes and the sequencing of protein structure, it seems that the differences seen (e.g. 43 kDa heart connexin versus the 32 kDa liver connexin) might represent sites on the protein for adaptive and differential regulation. Moreover, as a point of speculation, this might also be the reason for differential responses of cell types to exogenous chemicals which could modulate gap junctions (Bombick, 1990). It might well explain species, tissue and cell type effects of many epigenetic toxicants.

If gap junctions are needed to regulate growth and differentiation in the developing organism and to maintain metabolic and electrotonic coupling in the developed organism, chronic or unscheduled modulation of gap junction function could lead to dysfunctional homoeostatic control of growth, differentiation or critical differentiated-synchronized functions. For example, if gap junction intercellular communication (GJIC) is inhibited during a critical period of organogenesis, teratogenesis (Trosko *et al.*, 1982) might be the consequence. If in a carcinogenic-initiated tissue GJIC is down-regulated, the suppressive effect of surrounding normal cells is overcome, and the initiated cell can be promoted (Yotti *et al.*, 1979; Trosko *et al.*, 1983).

If during the maturation of germ cells in the gonad the GJIC is disrupted between the nurse cells (e.g. granulosa or Sertoli cells), differentiation of the germ cells could be affected (Gilula *et al.*, 1976; Larsen *et al.*, 1986). Gossypol, an extract from cotton seed, which has been used as an oral male contraceptive in China, has been shown to inhibit gap junction function in rat Leydig cells (Ye *et al.*, 1990). The function of the nerve cells, which is dependent on coupled glial cells, could also be disrupted if the gap junction function is inhibited, thereby leading to neurotoxicity (Trosko *et al.*, 1987). Uterine contraction (Cole and Garfield, 1986) or heart muscle tissue synchronized contraction (DeMello, 1982) could lead to severe or lethal end points if GJIC was chemically inhibited.

In summary, gap junctional communication exists and appears to be involved in important homoeostatic functions to regulate cell growth and differentiation. Modulation of the various gap junction genes and proteins can be induced by endogenous and exogenous chemicals which trigger a number of intracellular second messages. This modulation can be either adaptive or maladaptive, depending on circumstances (Trosko *et al.*, 1983).

Establishment of *In Vitro* Cellular Communication Processes for
Accurate Extrapolation of Potential Toxicities *In Vivo*

On the basis of the fact that all organs of an organism have interacting
heterologous and homologous cell types within and between tissues in
order to maintain homoeostasis, it can be hypothesized that chemical
disruption of extra-, intra- or inter-cellular communication *in vitro* would
lead to disruption of the regulation of cell growth, cell differentiation
and the functioning of various differentiated processes (Trosko *et al.*,
1990a). Therefore, if one is to use *in vitro* assays to predict a chemical's
ability to function as a toxicant *in vivo* via this mechanism, one must
ensure that the *in vitro* system reflects the complex cellular interactions
found *in vivo*. While, clearly, re-creation of all the *in vivo* extracellular
communicating signals (hormones, growth regulators, dietary components,
neurotransmitters, etc.) would seem to be impossible, the common
practice of using single-cell-type cultures grown on plastic or in liquid
suspension with complex undefined serum-containing media is definitely
not going to provide a close approximation to the *in vivo* state. This
common practice makes the situation even worse when the concept of
cellular interaction, as an important aspect of toxicity, is not even
considered when the results of a chemical's effects on *in vitro* cells are
interpreted (Trosko and Chang, 1989).

In recent years, complex homologous or heterologous cell–cell interactions and cell–matrix interactions have been recognized as being important
in maintaining normal cellular function, both *in vitro* and *in vivo* (Reid
and Jefferson, 1984; Edelman and Thiery, 1985), although it was well
known to be important years ago (Eagle, 1965; Potter, 1983). As an
example, the liver, which is a major organ involved in chemical toxicity,
is composed of multiple interacting cell types (Olson *et al.*, 1990). The
previous practice of using freshly prepared and purified hepatocytes as a
means of studying the metabolism and toxicity of many liver hepatotoxicants was based on the assumption that the metabolism/toxicity of the
chemicals in these cells reflects what goes on *in vivo*. Work on cocultures
of hepatocytes with liver epithelial cells and on various substrates in
serum-free medium has demonstrated dramatic effects, not only on the
survival capacity of the hepatocytes (Guillouzo, 1986), but also on their
phenotypes (Reid *et al.*, 1988).

In any *in vitro* system designed to reflect the liver (or any other organ),
one must try to re-create most of the interactions in order to provide a
more realistic extrapolation of the possible *in vivo* toxicities of chemicals.
The problem is to determine how to assess, easily, the *in vitro* conditions
that reflect an approximation of the hepatocytes *in vivo*. Our approach

is to use gap junction function as a "biomarker" of the *in vivo* phenotype of the hepatocyte. The hepatocyte, *in vivo*, is known to contain many gap junctions (Yancey *et al.*, 1979; Traub *et al.*, 1983) which are presumably necessary for maintaining metabolic homoeostasis and the intracellular physiology of the normal hepatocyte phenotype. Gap junction communication, as well as expression of the main gap junction (connexin 32) message of the rat liver, decreases rapidly when hepatocytes are isolated and placed in traditional tissue culture conditions (Reid *et al.*, 1988). On the other hand, when these hepatocytes are placed in culture with particular substrates and growth factors, gap junction message, function and many normal *in vivo* phenotypic markers are seen *in vitro* (Reid *et al.*, 1988).

Recently, various rat liver epithelial and "oval" cells have been shown to have gap junctional communication with each other (Jone *et al.*, 1987), but under one set of culture conditions, they were unable to communicate with the hepatocytes (Mesnil *et al.*, 1987). In addition, we noted that even though the coculturing of hepatocytes with the epithelial cells kept the hepatocytes alive and morphologically "normal" (at the light microscope level), the hepatocytes did not couple with each other via gap junctions. This indicates that the *in vitro* conditions were not reflecting the *in vivo* conditions. The ability to couple via gap junctions could be viewed as a biomarker for normal conditions. However, after treatment of the cells with dexamethasone, hepatocytes regained some of their ability to couple via gap junctions.

Experiments must now be performed in coculture under conditions where hepatocytes are and are not coupled via gap junctions to determine if, after exposure to hepatotoxicants, the metabolites and biological effects reflect *in vivo* observations.

If it is shown that heterologous cocultures with gap junction function as a biomarker are necessary for accurate extrapolation to the *in vivo* situation for the liver, then additional studies must be done for other organs (e.g. lung, breast, gonads, kidney, brain) to achieve organ-specific prediction of toxic chemicals.

Acknowledgements

We wish to express our appreciation to Mrs Beth Lockwood, Ms Heather Rupp, Mr William Paradee and Ms Helen Xu for their technical assistance for the work on which this manuscript is based. The research was supported, in part, by grants to J.E.T. from the US Air Force Office of Scientific Research [AFOSR-89-0325], the NIEHS [1P42ES04911] and the National Cancer Institute [CA21104]. We also wish to acknowledge the excellent word-processing skills of Mrs Jeanne McHugh.

References

Ames, B.N., Durston, W.E., Yamasaki, E. and Lee, F.D. (1973). *Proc. Natl. Acad. Sci. U.S.A.* **70**, 2281–2285.

Bombick, D.W. (1990). *In Vitro Toxicol.* **3**, 27–39.

Bradley, M.O., Taylor, V.I., Armstrong, M.J. and Galloway, S.M. (1987). *Mutat. Res.* **189**, 69–79.

Brookes, P. (1989). *Carcinogenesis* **2**, 305–307.

Chen, A.C., Brankow, D.W. and Herschman, H.R. (1990). *Carcinogenesis* **11**, 817–822.

Clayson, D.B. (1987). *Mutat. Res.* **185**, 243–269.

Clive, D. (1987). *J. Clin. Res. Drug Dev.* **1**, 11–41.

Cole, W.C. and Garfield, R.E. (1986). *Am. J. Physiol.* **251**, 411–420.

DeMello, W.C. (1982). *Prog. Biophys. Mol. Biol.* **39**, 147–182.

Douglas, G.R., Blakey, D.H. and Clayson, D.B. (1988). *Mutat. Res.* **196**, 83–93.

Eagle, H. (1965). *J. Med. Sci.* **1**, 1220–1228.

Edelman, G.M. and Thiery, J.P. (1985). *In* "The Cell in Contact". John Wiley and Sons, New York.

Fox, T.R., Schumann, A.M., Watanabe, P.G., Yano, B.L., Maher, V.M. and McCormick, J.J. (1990). *Cancer Res.* **50**, 4014–4019.

Gilula, N.B., Faucett, D.W. and Aoki, A. (1976). *Dev. Biol.* **50**, 142–168.

Guillouzo, A. (1986). *In* "Isolated and Culture Hepatocytes" (eds A. Guillouzo and C. Guguen-Guillouzo), pp. 313–331. Les Editions INSERM, Paris.

Jone, C., Trosko, J.E. and Chang, C.C. (1987). *In Vitro Cell. Dev. Biol.* **23**, 214–220.

Larsen, W.J., Wert, S.E. and Brunner, G.D. (1986). *Dev. Biol.* **113**, 517–521.

Loewenstein, W.R. (1979). *Biochim. Biophys. Acta* **560**, 1–65.

Madhukar, B.V., Oh, S.Y., Chang, C.C., Wade, M.H. and Trosko, J.E. (1989). *Carcinogenesis* **10**, 13–20.

Maldonado, P.E., Rose, B. and Loewenstein, W.R. (1988). *J. Membr. Biol.* **106**, 203–210.

Manjunath, C.K. and Page, E. (1985). *Am. J. Physiol.* **254**, 170–180.

Mass, M.J. and Austin, S.J. (1989). *Biochem. Biophys. Res. Commun.* **165**, 1319–1323.

Mass, M.J., Schorschinsky, N.S., Lasley, J.A., Beeman, D.K. and Austin, S.J. (1990). *Mutat. Res.* **243**, 291–298.

Mesnil, M., Fraslin, J.M., Piccoli, C., Yamasaki, H. and Guguen-Guillouzo, C. (1987). *Exp. Cell Res.* **173**, 524–533.

Olson, M.J., Mancini, M.A., Venkatachalam, M.A. and Roy, A.K. (1990). *In* "Cell Intercommunication" (W.C. DeMello, ed.), pp. 71–92. CRC Press, Boca Raton.

Potter, V.R. (1983). *In* "Nucleic Acid Research and Molecular Biology" (W.E. Cohn, ed.), p. 161. Academic Press, New York.

Reid, L.M. and Jefferson, D.M. (1984). *In* "Mammalian Cell Culture" (J.P. Mather, ed.), pp. 239–280. Plenum Publishing, New York.

Reid, L.M., Abreu, S.L. and Montgomery, K. (1988). *In* "The Liver: Biology and Pathobiology" (I.M. Arias, W.B. Jakoby, H. Popper, D. Schachter and D.A. Shafritz, eds), pp. 717–737. Raven Press, New York.

Saez, J.C., Spray, D.C. and Hertzberg, E.L. (1990). *In Vitro Toxicol.* **3**, 69–86.

Sheridan, J.D. (1987). *In* "Cell to Cell Communication" (W.C. DeMello, ed.), pp. 187–222. Plenum Press, New York.

Shiba, Y., Sasaki, Y., Hirono, C. and Kanno, Y. (1989). *Exp. Cell Res.* **185**, 535–540.

Spray, D.C., Saez, J.C., Burt, J.M., Watanabe, T., Reid, L.M., Hertzberg, E.L. and Bennett, M.V.L. (1988). *In* "Gap Junctions" (E. Hertzberg and R. Johnson, eds), pp. 227–244. Alan R. Liss, Inc., New York.

Tennant, R.W., Margolin, B.H., Shelby, M.D., Zeiger, E., Haseman, J.K., Spalding, J., Caspary, W., Resnick, M., Stasiewicz, S., Anderson, B. and Minor, R. (1987). *Science* **236**, 933–941.

Traub, O., Druge, P.M. and Willecke, K. (1983). *Proc. Natl. Acad. Sci. U.S.A.* **80**, 733–739.

Trosko, J.E. (1984). *Environ. Mutagen.* **6**, 767–769.

Trosko, J.E. (1989a). *Mutagenesis* **3**, 363–366.

Trosko, J.E. (1989b). *J. Am. Coll. Toxicol.* **8**, 1121–1132.

Trosko, J.E. and Chang, C.C. (1978). *In* "Photochemical Photobiological Reviews" (K.C. Smith, ed.), pp. 135–162. Plenum Press, New York.

Trosko, E.J. and Chang, C.C. (1984). *Pharmacol. Rev.* **36**, 137.

Trosko, J.E. and Chang, C.C. (1985). *In* "Methods for Estimating Risk of Chemical Injury: Human and Non-Human Biota Ecosystems" (V.B. Vouk, G.C. Butler, D.G. Hoel and D.B. Peakall, eds), p. 181. John Wiley and Sons, Chichester.

Trosko, J.E. and Chang, C.C. (1988). *In* "Banbury Report 31: Carcinogen Risk Assessment: New Directions in the Qualitative and Quantitative Aspects" (R.W. Hart and F.G. Hoerger, eds), pp. 139–170. Cold Spring Harbor Laboratory, Cold Spring Harbor, NY.

Trosko, J.E. and Chang, C.C. (1989). *In* "Biologically Based Methods for Cancer Risk Assessment" (C.C. Travis, ed.), pp. 165–179. Plenum Press, New York.

Trosko, J.E., Chang, C.C. and Medcalf, A. (1983). *Cancer Invest.* **1**, 511–526.

Trosko, J.E., Jone, C. and Chang, C.C. (1987). *Mol. Toxicol.* **1**, 83–93.

Trosko, J.E., Chang, C.C., Madhukar, B.V., Oh, S.Y., Bombick, D. and El-Fouly, M.H. (1988). *In* "Gap Junctions" (E.L. Hertzberg and R.G. Johnson, eds), pp. 435–448. Alan R. Liss Inc., New York.

Trosko, J.E., Chang, C.C., Madhukar, B.V. and Oh, S.Y. (1990a). *In Vitro Toxicol.* **3**, 9–26.

Trosko, J.E., Chang, C.C. and Madhukar, B.V. (1990b). *In* "Mouse Liver Carcinogenesis: Mechanisms and Species Comparisons" (D.E. Stevenson, J.A. Popp, J.M. Ward, R.M. McClain, T.J. Slaga and H.C. Pitot, eds), pp. 259–276. Alan R. Liss Inc., New York.

Trosko, J.E., Chang, C.C. and Madhukar, B.V. (1990c). *Toxicol. In Vitro* **4**, 635–643.

Trosko, J.E., Chang, C.C. and Netzloff, M. (1982). *Teratog. Carcinog. Mutagen.* **2**, 31–45.

Wilson, D.M., Goldsworthy, T.L., Popp, J.A. and Butterworth, B.E. (1990). *Proc. Am. Assoc. Cancer Res.* **31**, 103.

Yancey, S.B., Easter, D. and Revel, J.P. (1979). *J. Ultrastruct. Res.* **67**, 229–242.

Ye, Y.X., Bombick, D., Hirst, K., Zhang, G., Chang, C.C., Trosko, J.E. and Akera, T. (1990). *Fundam. Appl. Toxicol.* **14**, 817–832.
Yotti, L.P., Chang, C.C. and Trosko, J.E. (1979). *Science* **206**, 1089–1091.

Discussion

B. Bkaily

I am glad that somebody has talked about gap junctions. It reminded me how important they used to be and why we have forgotten them and their role in cardiac pathology. Does Dr Trosko have any idea about the nature of the channels in the gap junction, if the heart cells are electrically coupled via this gap junction, and how this is good for other cell types?

J.E. Trosko

There are experts here who have studied the physical chemistry of the gap junction structures. I think Dr Yamasaki will describe how they know the exact stereochemistry of the three major types of gap junctions. Another question is why there are three different types almost throughout evolution.

At the present time we speculate that the differences between these different genes are due to the need to regulate, for example, the heart differently from the hepatocyte. Changes of calcium in the heart will be very important, and the heart gap junction gene will probably be very sensitive to intracellular calcium changes; whereas, for the hepatocyte it probably does not matter whether the calcium level increases 4-, 5- or 20-fold until it reaches the point of cytotoxicity.

I suspect this is also one reason why many chemicals are tumour promoting in one organ by blocking gap junctions, but are not so in other organs, because they cannot block those gap junctions. An example is phorbol ester, which blocks gap junctions in almost every cell that has been studied. It presumably works by activating pK_c, phosphorylating the gap junction protein which somehow makes it lipophobic, and then it goes out of the membrane. This happens in the hepatocyte as well as in the keratinocyte, but in the latter it is down-regulated for almost 4 days, whereas the gap junction protein in the hepatocyte is dephosphorylated within 1 h and communication is restored.

It would therefore be predicted that TPA, the phorbol ester, is a tumour promoter of the skin. This is known at least in the mouse skin. Although no-one has tried, or can try, 12-tetradecanoylphorbol-13-acetate (TPA) *in vivo* in the liver, we would predict from *in vitro* results that it would not be a tumour promoter of the liver.

I cannot answer the question, in that using the molecular probes we are only now able to start making some predictions of how these gap junction genes are regulated in the role of either electrotonic stimulation or normal metabolic synchronization.

B. Bkaily
What do you think about the surface charge regulation?

J.E. Trosko
I am not an electrophysiologist and know nothing about that area, but David Spray has shown that there are conditions of electrical potential modulation of gap junctions.

G. Moonen
At a functional level is a given gap junction either open or closed or is it a graded phenomenon?

J.E. Trosko
This is a hotly debated issue today. There is evidence from some groups that modulators of communication do so by gating mechanisms, but there are several competing theories about how it works. Frankly, I am not in that area and am not able to pronounce on any of the current hypotheses.

A. Woolley
You seem to have an excellent test for screening for carcinogenic potential in this system. How soon will it be capable of being used in tests similar to the way in which the Ames test has been used? How many years will it survive and how soon will another test be needed?

J.E. Trosko
It does not escape my attention that Bruce Ames created a monster in 1973 which left his laboratory and has now come back to haunt him. I am convinced that *in vitro* assays to study the phenomenon of chemical modulation of gap junctions is a valid area of research to study mechanisms. I have been telling people who want to make a Trosko assay out of this for tumour promoters or other things not to put my name on it. I do not want what happened to Ames to happen to me.

As every previous speaker has said, no one *in vitro* assay can predict *in vivo* what will happen. There is no question that we know enough about gap junctional communication *in vivo* and *in vitro* to know that there are many modulators. While I can control them in culture, for example, with serum-free media, I cannot in man let alone in a rat. Too many things are going on developmentally, between sexes, because of the wine we drink, the food we eat, and so on. The net effect of all these mixtures can be synergistic, antagonistic, additive or nil. All these effects have now been demonstrated by the Ahlborg Swedish group.

Therefore we can study it *in vitro*, utilize it to understand mechanisms, make some tentative guesses about what might be happening *in vivo*, but we can go no further than that – or give the information to a regulator.

Role of Intercellular Communication in Carcinogenesis and Tumour Suppression

H. YAMASAKI, V. KRUTOVSKIKH, M. OYAMADA*, H. NAKAZAWA AND D.J. FITZGERALD[†]

International Agency for Research on Cancer, 150 Cours Albert Thomas, 69372 Lyon Cedex 08, France
*Present address: Department of Pathology, Sapporo Medical College, Sapporo 060, Japan
†Present address: The Flinders University of South Australia School of Biological Sciences, Bedford Park, S.A. 5042, Australia

Introduction

In multicellular organisms, cell–cell interaction plays a pivotal role in maintenance of homeostasis or control of the cellular society. Cancer cells deviate from the orderly behaviour of the normal cellular society and therefore it has been postulated that intercellular communication is altered during multistage carcinogenesis (Trosko and Chang, 1983; Pitts *et al.*, 1987; Yamasaki, 1990a). For example, growth-factor-mediated

IN VITRO METHODS IN TOXICOLOGY
ISBN 0-12-388175-7

intercellular communication has been strongly implicated in multistage carcinogenesis, as many cellular oncogenes have been identified to code for growth factors or growth factor receptors (Bradshaw and Prentis, 1987). Gap junctional intercellular communication (GJIC) mediates the direct transfer of small molecules and ions from the interior of one cell into adjacent cells, thus keeping connected cells in harmony (Loewenstein, 1979). In fact, most, if not all, tumours or transformed cells show reduced levels of GJIC and there is also evidence that intact GJIC plays an important role in tumour suppression (Yamasaki, 1990b). Here, we briefly review the evidence which suggests a role for intercellular communication in carcinogenesis and in tumour suppression.

Molecular Biology of Intercellular Communication

Our current view of the structure of gap junctions is presented schematically in Fig. 23.1. Gap junction hemi-channels are considered to be composed of six subunit proteins, named connexins. Hemi-channels from plasma membrane of one cell join with those of adjacent cells to form complete channels (Loewenstein, 1979). The complete cDNAs corresponding to at least three different connexin proteins have been cloned and antibodies have been raised (Kumar and Gilula, 1986; Paul, 1986; Beyer *et al.*, 1988; Zhang and Nicholson, 1989). These connexins have both conserved and variable sequences. The study of connexin membrane topology suggests that the *N*- and *C*-terminals of connexins are located in the cytoplasm; the protein is folded into the membrane twice to form an M structure with two extracellular regions and one cytoplasmic region (Goodenough *et al.*, 1988; Milks *et al.*, 1988). The cytoplasmic region contains sequences which can be phosphorylated by tyrosine kinases, cAMP-dependent protein kinase and protein kinase C (Hertzberg and Johnson, 1988).

GIJC can be modulated at various levels. In addition to the usual regulation at the levels of transcription, mRNA stability, translation and posttranslational processing, gap junction functions may be regulated at the level of hemi-channel alignment and gating of mature channels (Hertzberg and Johnson, 1988). For the control of hemi-channel alignment, there is evidence that expression of cellular recognition proteins such as cadherin molecules is essential for the function of GJIC (Mege *et al.*, 1988). As to the gating of mature channels, it is proposed that under certain circumstances the channel can be twisted or closed (Zampighi and Unwin, 1979). When genomic DNA of gap junction proteins is sequenced more completely, we may be able to establish other points of regulation

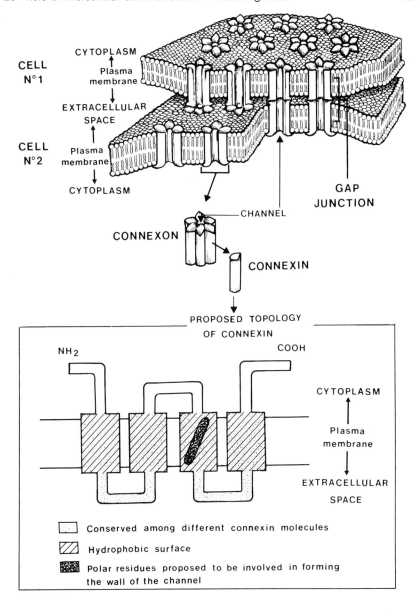

Fig. 23.1 Schematic view of gap junctions in membrane lipid bilayers and topology of connexins. While the structure and topology are generally considered common to various connexin molecules, there are important differences among them which may be related to the regulation of their function (see text and references cited for details).

such as *cis*-element and *trans*-acting factors. The existence of such a variety of modulating mechanisms is relevant to the involvement of gap junctions in carcinogenesis. Thus, it appears that GJIC can be modulated by numerous chemicals or by different physiological conditions which are thought to have roles in mechanisms of carcinogenesis (see Chapter 22). Various types of tumour-promoting agent may act at different points of GJIC regulation.

Another interesting finding regarding the mechanisms of cell–cell contact-mediated control of cell proliferation is a suggested relationship between growth factors and cell–cell adhesion. Masague's group (Anklesaria *et al.*, 1990) has demonstrated that cell–cell adhesion mediated by binding of membrane-anchored transforming growth factor α to epidermal growth factor receptors stimulates cell proliferation. It appears that such a 'juxtacrine' mode of intercellular communication is distinct from the usual humoral (endocrine, paracrine and autocrine) or cell-adhesion molecule (CAM) or gap-junction-mediated intercellular communication. Much more work is needed to elucidate the mechanism of juxtacrine intercellular communication and its possible role in carcinogenesis.

Aberrant Gap Junctional Intercellular Communication in Tumours or Transformed Cells

Extensive studies of GJIC of tumorigenic cells or transformed cells have been carried out (Weinstein and Pauli, 1987). Almost all tumour or transformed cells have reduced GJIC either among themselves (homologous communication) or with surrounding normal cells (heterologous communication). For example, a series of rat liver epithelial cell lines with different degrees of malignant phenotype expression showed a progressive decrease in the level of GJIC as they expressed more malignant phenotypes (Mesnil *et al.*, 1986). On the other hand, Balb/c 3T3 cells transformed by various carcinogens showed a normal level of GJIC. However, regardless of the carcinogen used for induction of transformation, the transformed Balb/c 3T3 cells did not communicate with surrounding normal cells (Enomoto and Yamasaki, 1984; Yamasaki *et al.*, 1987). Such a selective lack of GJIC is believed to be an important feature for the maintenance of transformed phenotypes. We have proposed that, if there is communication between transformed and normal cells, growth-controlling factors may be transferred from normal cells and thus transformed phenotype may reverse (Yamasaki, 1990b). In support of this hypothesis, cAMP, retinoic acid and glucocorticoids caused a resumption of GJIC between transformed and surrounding normal Balb/c 3T3 cells, which was followed by disappearance of certain transformed foci (Yamasaki and Katoh, 1988).

While the above information has come mostly from studies using cultured cells, further results suggest that a progressive decrease in GJIC is also associated with progression of tumours *in vivo*. For example, mouse epidermal cells were established from various stages of mouse skin carcinogenesis. There was a progressive decrease in GJIC from normal to initiated papilloma and carcinoma cells (Klann *et al.*, 1989). The levels of mRNA and protein expression of connexin 32 have been examined during multistage rat liver carcinogenesis. There was a clear decrease in the expression of connexin 32 mRNA and protein in all hepatocellular carcinomas examined (Janssen-Timmen *et al.*, 1986; Beer *et al.*, 1988; Fitzgerald *et al.*, 1989). Most nodules and preneoplastic foci also showed decreased levels of gap junction mRNA and protein, suggesting a progressive loss of GJIC during tumour progression (Fitzgerald *et al.*, 1989; Krutovskikh *et al.*, 1991). Recently, we have developed a method by which we can study the function of gap junctions in liver slices freshly isolated from the liver at various stages of induced carcinogenesis. Such studies have confirmed that hepatocellular carcinoma cells have much less GJIC than normal liver cells. In addition, we found that many preneoplastic foci and nodules showed selective lack of GJIC with surrounding normal cells (Krutovskikh *et al.*, 1991).

Very few studies have been carried out to characterize primary human tumours in terms of their GJIC. We have recently analysed several surgically removed primary hepatocellular carcinomas and found that connexin 32 mRNA level was not decreased in any of these tumours. However, there was increased expression of heart-type connexin, connexin 43, in all of the tumours tested (Oyamada *et al.*, 1990). These results are in contrast with decreased levels of connexin 32 mRNA found in rat hepatocellular carcinomas and suggest that there exist various regulatory mechanisms of GJIC which may be affected during carcinogenesis.

Carcinogens, Oncogenes and Gap Junctional Intercellular Communication

While it is clear that tumours or transformed cells have aberrant GJIC, it is not yet understood how and when such aberrant GJIC occurs during multistage carcinogenesis. Since the pioneering work of the groups of Trosko (Yotti *et al.*, 1979) and Murray and Fitzgerald (1979), it has become clear that certain types of tumour-promoting agent block GJIC.

Such studies suggested a role of blocked GJIC in the tumour-promotion stage (Trosko and Chang, 1983). However, it is also possible that initiating agents affect the gene structure of connexins, leading to loss of functional GJIC. Readers interested in interactions of chemicals with gap junctions are referred to reviews by Trosko *et al.* (1984, 1990a,b).

There is little doubt that activated cellular oncogenes and inactivated cellular tumour suppressor genes are critically involved in carcinogenesis. The relationship between GJIC and oncogenes has been studied extensively (Table 23.1). Here again, we must emphasize the importance of heterologous GJIC. Our own results suggest that heterologous communication can regulate the expression of oncogenes (Bignami *et al.*, 1988). For example, when NIH 3T3 cells were transfected with v-*myc*, v-*fos* or polyoma large T genes, heterologous communication with non-transfected

Table 23.1

Effect of oncogenes on homologous and heterologous gap junctional intercellular communication[a]

Oncogene	Cells	Homologous communication[b]	Heterologous communication[c]
v-*src*	NRK	↓	NT
	NIH 3T3	↓	NT
	Quail and chick embryo fibroblasts	↓	NT
	NIH 3T3	→	−
c-*src*	NIH 3T3	↓	NT
v-*ras*	NIH 3T3	→	−
EJ-*ras*[H]	Balb/c 3T3	→	−
	Rat liver epithelial cell line IAR20	→	+
	Rat liver epithelial cell line	↓	NT
v-*myc*	NIH 3T3	→	+
v-*fos*	NIH 3T3	→	+
v-*mos*	C3H10T1/2	→ or ↑	NT
PyMT	Rat F cells	↓	NT
	NIH 3T3	→	−
PyLT	NIH 3T3	→	+
SV40T	Human hepatocytes	↓	NT
	Human keratinocytes	↓	NT
	Human fibroblasts	↓	↓

[a] Individual references can be found in Yamasaki (1990a)
[b] Homologous communication is the communication among oncogene-containing cells and their communication capacity was compared with that of normal counterparts.
[c] Heterologous communication is the presence (+), absence (−) or decrease (↓) of communication between oncogene-containing cells and normal cells measured in coculture of these two types of cells.
↓, decreased; →, no change; ↑, enhanced; NT, not tested.

cells was unchanged. However, v-*src*, v-*ras* and polyoma middle T gene-containing cells did not communicate with surrounding normal cells although they did communicate between themselves. In addition, only those that did not have heterologous communication clonally expanded to form morphologically distinct foci over normal cells, suggesting a good correlation between the lack of heterologous communication and the appearance of transformed foci (Bignami *et al.*, 1988).

Role of Gap Junctional Intercellular Communication in Tumour Suppression

If a lack of GJIC between tumour cells and surrounding normal cells is essential for the maintenance of transformed phenotypes, we may further postulate that resumption of intercellular communication between tumour cells and normal cells could act as a tumour suppressor and thereby eliminate transformed phenotypes. In fact, in the existing literature, there are reports that cell–cell contact between tumour cells and normal cells can suppress transformed phenotypes. Our own results as well as those of others suggest that gap junctional intercellular communication *per se* may be responsible (Table 23.2).

Tumour suppression is usually studied in the context of genetic damage, and several tumour-suppressor genes have been identified (Knudson, 1985; Baker *et al.*, 1989). Few studies have examined whether mechanisms of action of any tumour-suppressor genes involve intercellular communication, in particular GJIC. However, interesting recent results have been reported in relation to allelic deletions involving chromosome 18q that occur in more than 70% of human colorectal cancers (Vogelstein *et al.*, 1988). The DCC gene which resides in this region has been cloned and the predicted amino acid sequence of cDNA showed a sequence homology to a cell-adhesion molecule N-CAM (Fearon *et al.*, 1990). As CAM proteins are apparently involved directly in the regulation of GJIC (Mege *et al.*, 1988; Jongen *et al.*, 1990), the loss of a DCC gene on chromosome 18q may lead to decreased GJIC. More recently, Frixen *et al.* (1991) have reported a close correlation between a lack of E-cadherin expression and increased invasiveness of human carcinoma cell lines. These results suggest that intercellular-communication-related genes may form a family of tumour-suppressor genes.

Table 23.2
Suppression of transformed phenotypes by contact with normal counterparts (see
Yamasaki 1990b, for details and individual references)

Cell type	Evidence of GJ communication involved in the suppression[a]
Polyoma virus-BHK21 cells	—[b]
SV40-Swiss 3T3	Rescue of transformed foci by croton oil
Chemically transformed C3H10T1/2	—
UV+TPA transformed C3H10T1/2	Rescue of transformed foci by TPA
Tumorigenic rat tracheal epithelial cells (*in vivo* transplant)	—
Harvey sarcoma virus-transformed mouse epidermal cells (+ dermal fibroblast *in vivo* grafting)	—
Chemically transformed mouse epidermal cells	—
Chemically and virally transformed C3H10T1/2 cells	Dye transfer
Chemically transformed Balb/c 3T3 cells (with dbcAMP, retinoic acid, glucocorticoids)	Dye transfer
C-*myc*- or N-*myc*-transformed 3T3 cells	—
v-*myc*-transformed NIH 3T3 cells	—
v-*myc*, v-*fos*, PL-LT-transformed Balb/c 3T3 cells	Dye transfer

[a] This was obtained either by adding GJIC blocking agents (croton oil or 12-O-tetradecanoylphorbol 13 acetate (TPA)) to rescue transformed foci, or by direct measurement of GJIC between transformed and normal cells.
[b] No attempt was made to relate the suppression to GJIC.

Acknowledgements

We thank Dr J. Cheney for editing the manuscript and Ms C. Fuchez for skillful secretarial help. Part of the work carried out in our laboratory was supported by grants from NCI (R01 CA40534) and from the Commission of the European Communities (EV4V-0040-F).

References

Anklesaria, P., Teixido, J., Laiho, M., Pierce, J.H., Greenberger, J.S. and Massagué, J. (1990). *Proc. Natl. Acad. Sci. U.S.A.* **87**, 3289–3293.
Baker, S.J., Fearon, E.R., Nigro, J.M., Hamilton, S.R., Preisinger, A.C., Jessup,

J.M., van Tuinen, P., Ledbetter, D.H., Barker, D.F., Nakamura, Y., White, R. and Vogelstein, B. (1989). *Science* **244**, 217–221.
Beer, D.C., Neveu, M.J., Paul, D.L., Rapp, U.R. and Pitot, H.C. (1988). *Cancer Res.* **48**, 1610–1617.
Beyer, E.C., Goodenough, D.A. and Paul, D.L. (1988). *In* "Gap Junctions" (E.L. Hertzberg and R.G. Johnson, eds), pp. 165–175, Alan R. Liss, New York.
Bignami, M., Rosa, S., Falcone, G., Tato, F., Katoh, F. and Yamasaki, H. (1988). *Mol. Carcinogen.* **1**, 67–75.
Bradshaw, R.A. and Prentis, S. (1987). *In* "Oncogenes and Growth Factors". Elsevier, Amsterdam.
Enomoto, T. and Yamasaki, H. (1984). *Cancer Res.* **44**, 5200–5203.
Fearon, E.R., Cho, K.R., Nigro, J.M., Kern, S.E., Simons, J.W., Ruppert, J.M., Hamilton, S.R., Preisinger, A.C., Thomas, G., Kinzler, K.W. and Vogelstein, B. (1990). *Science* **247**, 49–56.
Fitzgerald, D.J., Mesnil, M., Oyamada, M., Tsuda, H., Ito, N. and Yamasaki, H. (1989). *J. Cell. Biochem.* **41**, 97–102.
Frixen, U.H., Behrens, J., Sachs, M., Eberle, G., Voss, B., Warda, A., Löchner, D. and Birchmeier, W. (1991). *J. Cell Biol.*, in press.
Goodenough, D.A., Paul, D.L. and Jesaitis, L. (1988). *J. Cell Biol.* **107**, 1817–1824.
Hertzberg, E.L. and Johnson, R.G. (1988). *In* "Gap Junctions". Alan R. Liss, New York.
Janssen-Timmen, U., Traub, O., Dermietzel, R., Rabes, H.M. and Willecke, K. (1986). *Carcinogenesis* **7**, 1475–1482.
Jongen, W.M.F., Fitzgerald, D.J., Piccoli, C., Takeichi, M. and Yamasaki, H. (1990). *Proc. Am. Assoc. Cancer Res.* **31**, 139.
Klann, R.C., Fitzgerald, D.J., Piccoli, C., Slaga, T.J. and Yamasaki, H. (1989). *Cancer Res.* **49**, 699–705.
Knudson, A.G., Jr (1985). *Cancer Res.* **45**, 1437–1443.
Krutovskikh, V.A., Oyamada, M. and Yamasaki, H. (1991). *Carcinogenesis* **12**, 1701–1706.
Kumar, N.M. and Gilula, N.B. (1986). *J. Cell Biol.* **103**, 767–776.
Loewenstein, W.R. (1979). *Biochim. Biophys. Acta* **560**, 1–65.
Mege, R.M., Matsuzaki, F., Gallin, W.J., Goldberg, J.I., Cunningham, B.A. and Edelman, G.M. (1988). *Proc. Natl. Acad. Sci. U.S.A.* **85**, 7274–7278.
Mesnil, M., Montesano, R. and Yamasaki, H. (1986). *Exp. Cell Res.* **165**, 391–402.
Milks, L.C., Mukar, N.M., Houghten, R., Unwin, N. and Gilula, N.B. (1988). *EMBO J.* **7**, 2967–2975.
Murray, A.W. and Fitzgerald, D.J. (1979). *Biochem. Biophys. Res. Commun.* **91**, 395–401.
Oyamada, M., Krutovskikh, V.A., Mesnil, M., Partensky, C. and Yamasaki, H. (1990). *Mol. Carcinogen.* **3**, 273–278.
Paul, D.L. (1986). *J. Cell Biol.* **103**, 123–134.
Pitts, J.D., Kam, E. and Morgan, D. (1987). *In* "Gap Junctions" (E.L. Hertzberg and R.G. Johnson, eds), pp. 397–409. Alan R. Liss, New York.
Trosko, J.E. and Chang, C.C. (1983). *J. Am. Coll. Toxicol.* **2**, 5–22.
Trosko, J.E., Jone, C. and Chang, C.C. (1984). *In* "Models, Mechanisms and Etiology of Tumour Promotion" (M. Börzsönyi, N.E. Day, K. Lapis and H.

Yamasaki, eds), pp. 239–252. (IARC Scientific Publ. No. 56), International Agency for Research on Cancer, Lyon.

Trosko, J.E., Chang, C.C. and Madhukar, B.V. (1990a). *Toxicol. In Vitro* **4**, 635–643.

Trosko, J.E., Chang, C.C., Madhukar, B.V. and Klaunig, J.E. (1990b). *Pathobiology* **58**, 265–278.

Vogelstein, B., Fearon, E.R., Hamilton, S.R., Kern, S.E., Preisinger, A.C., Leppert, M., Nakamura, Y., White, R., Smits, A.M.M. and Bos, J.L. (1988). *New Engl. J. Med.* **319**, 525–532.

Weinstein, R.S. and Pauli, B.U. (1987). *CIBA Found. Symp.* **125**, 240–260.

Yamasaki, H. (1990a). *Carcinogenesis* **11**, 1051–1058.

Yamasaki, H. (1990b). *In* "Tumor Suppressor Genes" (G. Klein, ed.), pp. 245–266. Marcel Dekker, New York.

Yamasaki, H. and Katoh, F. (1988). *Cancer Res.* **48**, 3490–3495.

Yamasaki, H., Hollstein, M., Mesnil, M., Martel, N. and Aguelon, A.-M. (1987). *Cancer Res.* **47**, 5658–5664.

Yotti, L.P., Chang, C.C. and Trosko, J.E. (1979). *Science* **206**, 1089–1091.

Zampighi, G. and Unwin, P.N.T. (1979). *J. Mol. Biol.* **135**, 451–464.

Zhang, J.L. and Nicholson, B.J. (1989). *J. Cell Biol.* **109**, 3391–3401.

Discussion

B. Bkaily

It was mentioned in Dr Trosko's talk that a single cell does not have gap junctions, so how can the reappearance of gap junctions after cell communication (which means that two cells come together) be explained?

J.E. Trosko

We obviously do not understand the dynamic processes of regulating gap junctions. Bill Larsen has done a lot of freeze fracture and electron microscopy on the dynamics of gap junctions. He has shown that when some cells are treated with chemicals that down-regulate gap junctions they can be invaginated into vesicles into the cytoplasm where they sit until they are needed. If single cells have gap junctions which are open, of course that will be lethal to the cells. When cells are going to divide or be disrupted it is critical for those gap junctions to be closed or removed from the membrane. When two cells then reattach, the membranes by touching must send some signal to the cell to have those vesicles with gap junction re-emerge in the membrane.

This is exactly what Larsen sees: these vesicles going back to the membrane. There can be protein and RNA synthesis inhibitors present, and the gap junctions that appear were previously synthesized gap junctions.

B. Bkaily
Are there gap junctions in early embryonic states?

J.E. Trosko
It has been shown that in the early stages, the fertilized egg to the blastocyst stage, apparently the gap junction genes are not expressed or the protein is not made. They start to appear at the glioblastic stage or when the differentiation starts.

B. Bkaily
What is the explanation for this: that there is no coupling between cells, no communication?

J.E. Trosko
There is no gap junctional communication. The primary function of the fertilized egg is to proliferate. When it reaches a certain mass the physical environment changes, which must be a signal to induce gap junctions. Certain cells start to communicate and there is partition.

I. Purchase
Dr Yamasaki showed quite elegantly how some of the genotoxic carcinogens perhaps alter genes which code for gap junctions. I think this work started originally by it being shown that many of the chemicals like TPA which affect gap junctional activity in contiguous cells are not genotoxic. It is therefore difficult to understand how they could create such an effect by interacting with a genome. It must be a direct effect on the membrane in some way or on some message between the DNA and the membrane.

This leaves me feeling uncomfortable that what is being observed is a consequence of carcinogenesis rather than a cause. I am not yet convinced that these effects of non-genotoxic chemicals interacting with gap junctions are causative rather than just a phenomenon which happens to occur at the same time. Can Dr Yamasaki convince me otherwise?

H. Yamasaki
I have not shown that the structure of a gap junction gene is altered by carcinogenesis, only the oncogenes are altered. We want to show that expression of the altered oncogenes may be modulated by non-genotoxic carcinogens. Looking at many tumours, I do not think that the gap junction gene itself is completely mutated or functionally lost because there is always some communication, although there is still a possibility which we are working on. This means that if there is a mutation it is not

a structural gene but perhaps some regulatory gene. So far there is no evidence that the gap junction gene is mutated or affected by genotoxic carcinogens.

J.E. Trosko
I think Lowenstein's paper in *Science* (1989) finally answered the question of chicken or egg relationship between transformation and gap junctions. He used a temperature-sensitive src gene which, when expressed, blocks gap junctions. Under non-permissive conditions no src gene was expressed, the cells communicated and were not transformed. He then changed the temperature, and showed the message that the src gene made, the protein's appearance, the blockage of communication, the onset of DNA synthesis, the change of morphology and the transformation.

In other words, the blockage in communication followed the protein of the sarcogene product, which preceded DNA synthesis and the morphological change and transformation. Thus, in terms of this one system, the blockage of communication occurred prior to the morphological transformation.

B. Jegou
Do you think that modulation of gap junctions plays a role only in carcinogenesis or may such modulation interfere in normal cell–to–cell communication in normal tissue?

H. Yamasaki
I think the carcinogenesis process is essentially the defects in cell growth and in differentiation. Therefore a communication defect may lead to the imbalance in normal tissue.

B. Jegou
How does the cell distinguish between a blockage of gap junctions that leads, for example, to carcinogenesis and one that leads to, say, induction of mitosis?

J.E. Trosko
Growth, wound healing – all these things. We have to be very careful, which is why I do not want my name put on an assay. If a chemical modulates gap junctions, this proves to a regulator that the chemical is bad. If it was a regulatory test now, phenobarbital would not pass it. Phenobarbital blocks gap junctions, which is pharmacologically good. Unfortunately for rats, high levels of phenobarbital given chronically lead to tumour promotion, and apparently it can lead to teratogenicity in

pregnant women. Here is a case where there is good news and bad news, adaptability as well as non-adaptability of modulation of gap junctions.

Retinoic acid is another classic case. At present, retinol A is used for psoriasis. It induces differentiation of the keratinocytes of highly proliferating cells. If the person being treated is a pregnant woman, the retinol A, which is very lipophilic, is systematically taken to the foetus where it induces differentiation in foetal cells that normally would not be communicating, leading to teratogenesis. Again, there is both good and bad news in the one individual by the same compound by the same mechanism.

We have to be very selective in interpreting what a chemical does by modulating gap junctions. I have said repeatedly that many people representing drug and chemical companies throw out potentially valuable chemicals because of the Ames assay. They should not do this. If these chemicals were tested for modulation of gap junctions many of them could possibly be pharmacologically useful because they modulate gap junctions if the chemicals are used properly. Phenobarbital is a classic example.

24

Current Status of Cell Transformation Assays for the *In Vitro* Detection of Carcinogens

V.C. DUNKEL

U.S. Food and Drug Administration, 200 C Street, S.W. Washington, DC 20204, USA

Introduction

Approximately 15 years ago, the National Cancer Institute (NCI) initiated a programme to determine the usefulness and reliability of cell transformation assays for testing chemicals for carcinogenic potential (Dunkel, 1976). Initially, studies focused on the standardization and definition of methodology. The evaluation of a large number of carcinogenic and non-carcinogenic chemicals was then undertaken. The cell culture systems selected for this evaluation included both fibroblast and epithelial cells. As is evident from the model systems listed in Table 24.1, this was a sizeable undertaking, and considerable effort was expended in the evaluation of the methods selected (Dunkel *et al.*, 1977, 1981; Pienta *et al.*, 1977; Traul *et al.*, 1979, 1981; Pienta, 1980; Sivak *et al.*, 1980); subsequently an evaluation of the C3H 10T1/2 assay was added (Dunkel *et al.*, 1988). It was recognized at the time that *in vitro* transformation tests would probably be of "most immediate value" in

IN VITRO METHODS IN TOXICOLOGY
ISBN 0-12-388175-7

Table 24.1
Mammalian cell transformation model systems for identifying carcinogens

---

I. Fibroblasts
    Early-passage diploid cell strains
        1. Syrian hamster embryo clonal assay
        2. Syrian hamster embryo transplacental assay
    Cell lines
        1. Balb/3T3 focus assay
        2. Fischer rat embryo focus or clonal assay
        3. Fischer rat embryo/C-type virus assay
II. Epithelial cells
        1. Rat liver
        2. Rat mammary gland
        3. Mammalian skin

---

screening for direct-acting chemicals; therefore, additional effort would have to be given to the development of activation systems for those chemicals requiring metabolism to their reactive form.

Approximately a decade after initiation of the NCI programme, a report was published by an IARC/NCI/EPA Working Group (1985) in which it was stated that cell transformation had not been "fully exploited" for screening chemicals for carcinogenic potential. This failure to use these assays adequately was attributed by the working group to several factors including (1) limited knowledge about molecular and cellular mechanisms of carcinogenesis, (2) the more technically demanding nature of the transformation assays compared with other *in vitro* screening methods, (3) the subjectivity in scoring morphologically transformed foci, and (4) a lack of international validation of the methods. Nevertheless, the working group produced guidelines for transformation assays with C3H/10T1/2 and Balb/3T3 cells.

More recently, a survey, sponsored by Health and Welfare Canada, queried investigators working in research and testing laboratories about the cell transformation methods they were currently using (Dunkel *et al.*, 1990). The responses indicated that the methods described in specific primary published references were generally used and that few significant changes had been incorporated into the procedures. In fact, 36% of the respondents indicated that no modifications had been incorporated into the protocol described in the primary published reference. The publications identified as primary references were those of Reznikoff *et al.* (1973a,b) for the C3H/10T1/2 assay, Kakunaga (1973) for the Balb/3T3 assay and Pienta (1980) for the Syrian hamster embryo (SHE) assay. Additionally, the information obtained in this survey on current laboratory practices together with information in various publications was used to develop composite protocols and guidelines for these three assays.

Because *in vitro* cell transformation is generally considered to be highly relevant to the *in vivo* process, it has been widely used for examining mechanistic aspects of chemical carcinogenesis that would be difficult to carry out with available animal models. Some of the areas that have been investigated include: initiation/promotion; the role of cell cycle in carcinogen sensitivity; inhibition of transformation; the relationship between transformation, gene mutation and other genetic events; the induction of biochemical markers; activation of oncogenes; intercellular communication; and viral/carcinogen interactions. In most instances, such studies utilize carcinogens that are well characterized with respect to chemical class and type and magnitude of response obtained in the transformation assay.

In contrast, when *in vitro* transformation assays are used for evaluating chemicals for carcinogenic potential, the systems, in theory, are expected to respond to compounds in a wide variety of chemical classes, including chemicals classified as both genotoxic and non-genotoxic. Essentially, the need is for the assay(s) to meet a level of reliability that would provide confidence in the data generated. Such reliability is dependent upon several factors. These include (1) the interlaboratory reproducibility and intralaboratory repeatability, (2) the sensitivity of the method, that is, the ability of chemical carcinogens to induce morphological transformation in the test system, (3) the specificity of the method or the lack of a transformation response for non-carcinogens and (4) the accuracy of the test, that is, the degree of correspondence with *in vivo* carcinogenesis test results. Examination of these factors will provide an indication of the current status of cell transformation assays.

Interlaboratory Reproducibility

In general, studies on the intra- and inter-laboratory variability of cell transformation assays have been limited. One of the first reported evaluations was carried out with the SHE assay (Tu *et al.*, 1986). Three laboratories participated in this study and tested a total of 13 chemicals, of which eight were identified as model compounds and five as "tested under code". To eliminate some variables, each laboratory used similar protocols, target cells from the same preparation, and the same lot of foetal bovine serum (either 10% or 20%). A graded scoring system was also established and colonies were classified as transformed (T), morphologically altered (MA) or normal. A T colony was characterized by loss of contact inhibition with cells growing over adjacent cells and over feeder-layer cells. These colonies could consist of either fibroblastic or epithelial-like cells, and at least 50% of the periphery of the multilayered colony had to show this random growth pattern. An MA colony was stated to differ from a T colony only 'by the degree of aberrancy' and was characterized by having less than 50% but generally more than 10% of the periphery with an aberrant growth pattern. Normal colonies displayed a clearly defined orientation. The model compounds used in this study were benzo[a]pyrene (B(a)P), 7,12-dimethylbenz[a]anthracene (DMBA), N-methyl-N'-nitro-N-nitrosoguanidine (MNNG), nitroquino-line-N-oxide (NQO), lead chromate (PbCrO$_4$), N-2-fluorenylacetamide (FAA), pyrene (PYR) and anthracene (ANTH). Because clear dose responses in the induction of T and MA colonies were not frequently observed, the results for all dose levels tested were pooled, and positive or negative responses were based on pooled data. The authors concluded that the data for these model compounds showed agreement on activity, that is, all chemicals were either positive or negative in all repeat tests in the individual laboratories as well as between laboratories. The coded chemicals tested were 2,6-dichloro-p-phenylenediamine, 4,4'-oxydianiline, cinnamyl anthranilate, dichlorvos and reserpine, which were considered to be representative of environmental chemical classes. The responses with these chemicals varied between the participating laboratories as well as within any one laboratory. It was concluded that the assay required modification before it could become a routine tool for screening.

At the same time that this report appeared on the interlaboratory evaluation of the SHE assay, LeBoeuf and Kerckaert (1986) published their initial work on the growth of SHE cells in medium containing reduced sodium bicarbonate concentration, which produced a lower pH (6.65 to 6.75) under 10% CO$_2$ gassing conditions. For cells not treated with carcinogens, they reported enhanced cell growth and an increase in the number of colonies having a transformed-like morphology. Subsequently, they reported that morphological transformation of SHE cells by B(a)P was increased when the transformation assay was performed with such modified medium (LeBoeuf and Kerckaert, 1987). Still later, a comparison of test results from two laboratories was published (LeBoeuf et al., 1989). In this study, four carcinogens (3-methylcholanthrene (MCA), B(a)P, MNNG and FAA) and one non-carcinogen (ANTH) were tested in the assay using medium at pH 6.70 and pH 7.35. In contrast with the previous interlaboratory evaluation (Tu et al., 1986), each laboratory prepared its own pool of SHE cells and obtained its own lot of foetal bovine serum. Positive responses were obtained in both laboratories with all four carcinogens and a negative response with the non-carcinogen when the assay was performed in medium at pH 6.70. In contrast, only B(a)P produced a positive response in both laboratories when medium at pH 7.35 was used; the other three carcinogens were negative. The non-carcinogen, anthracene, was positive in one laboratory and was not tested in the other laboratory at this pH. It is noteworthy that neither MCA nor MNNG induced positive responses with medium at pH 7.35, since both chemicals have been previously reported as positive in the SHE cell assay (Heidelberger et al., 1983). In addition, Przygoda et al. (1985) reported positive transformation responses with SHE cells from a number of different pools by MCA and MNNG under 10% and 20% CO_2 gassing conditions (this produced a pH of the medium of approximately 7.4 and 7.1 respectively). When the cultures were incubated at 10% CO_2 in air, 6/11 or 55% of the pools were transformed by MCA; when the cells were incubated at 20% CO_2, 6/7 or 86% of cells in the individual pools were transformed. A similar enhancement was obtained with MNNG; 5/11 or 45% of the cell pools were transformed when incubated in 10% CO_2 and 6/7 or 86% of the pools were transformed when 20% CO_2 was used.

In 1988 Dunkel et al. reported results for an interlaboratory evaluation of the C3H/10T1/2 assay. In this study, two laboratories tested a total of 46 chemicals, the majority of which were tested under code. Seven chemicals were active in both laboratories and 14 were inactive. When the total number of chemicals was adjusted for assays considered "no test" ("no test" was defined as a negative response that did not reach a level of 25% toxicity at the highest dose) in either one or both laboratories, as well as for tests of chemicals yielding positive results in only one laboratory, comparable responses were obtained for 21/35, or 60%, of the chemicals tested. In this study, no effort was made to standardize the testing procedure rigorously. There were differences in the number of target cells plated by the two laboratories (10^4 vs 10^3), and in the medium used (Eagle's minimal essential medium (MEM) vs Eagle's basal medium (BME)), and each laboratory independently identified and selected lots of foetal bovine serum for the ability to support optimal growth, cloning of the cells and transformation by MCA. It is debatable whether greater reproducibility would have been attained if there were not these variations.

No studies on interlaboratory reproducibility have been carried out with the Balb/3T3 transformation asssay. The US EPA Gene-tox report (Heidelberger et al., 1983) lists five chemicals (B(a)P, benzo[e]pyrene (B(e)P), MCA, NQO and phenanthrene) as having been tested with Balb/3T3 in more than one laboratory. The data show that responses with these chemicals were reproducible among laboratories. Table 24.2 lists test results from a number of different publications for another small

Table 24.2
Interlaboratory comparison of *in vitro* transformation test results with Balb/3T3
cells

Chemical	Response	References
Aflatoxin B₁	+	Cortesi *et al.* (1983)
	+	Friedrich *et al.* (1985)
	+	Lubet *et al.* (1990)
Methyl-*N'*-nitro-*N*-nitrosoguanidine	+	Dunkel *et al.* (1981)
	+	Cortesi *et al.* (1983)
	+	Friedrich *et al.* (1985)
	+	Lubet *et al.* (1990)
Urethane	+	Friedrich *et al.* (1985)
	+	Casto (1990)
Diethylstilboestrol	−	Dunkel *et al.* (1981)
	+	Friedrich *et al.* (1985)
	+	Fitzgerald *et al.* (1989)
4-Dimethylaminoazobenzene	−	Dunkel *et al.* (1981)
	−	Friedrich *et al.* (1985)

group of chemicals of wider diversity. Positive transformation test results
were obtained by all laboratories with aflatoxin B₁, MNNG and urethane;
diethylstilboestrol was negative in one laboratory and positive in two.
4-Dimethylaminoazobenzene was negative in both laboratories. In one of
the laboratories obtaining a positive response with diethylstilboestrol, a
modified transformation protocol was used (Fitzgerald *et al.*, 1989).
Although the data from such an evaluation are not equivalent to data
obtained when multiple laboratories are testing the same chemicals under
code, they do provide some indication of what the assay may be capable
of doing.

Sensitivity, Specificity, Predictive Value and Accuracy

A final objective in the evaluation of any *in vitro* test system has been
to determine its overall reliability. The factors assessed to determine such
reliability, as previously indicated, are sensitivity (number of carcinogens
inducing transformation/total carcinogens tested), specificity (number
of non-carcinogens not inducing transformation/total non-carcinogens),
predictive value (number of transforming carcinogens/total number of
chemicals inducing transformation), and the accuracy of the test (number

of chemicals with "correct" results/total chemicals tested). One problem encountered in doing such evaluations is the reliability of the data and interpretation of the results from long-term *in vivo* carcinogenicity assays. This is especialy true for chemicals classified as non-carcinogens and has the potential to lead to compromised conclusions. Prival and Dunkel (1989) highlighted this problem in a publication in which they re-evaluated the mutagenicity and *in vivo* carcinogenicity data for 25 chemicals classified as giving "false positive" mutagenic responses in *Salmonella typhimurium*. They concluded that only two of the chemicals categorized as non-carcinogens could be classified as definitively non-carcinogenic. For the other 23 chemicals, either the data were inadequate to draw a conclusion or there was an indication that the chemical or structurally related chemicals might be carcinogenic. A number of different evaluations have been made of the reliability of *in vitro* transformation assays; the results should be viewed as providing only an indication of the effectiveness of an assay, since the *in vivo* carcinogenicity data in some cases should have been analysed more critically.

Pienta (1979) reported the results for 106 chemicals tested in the SHE clonal assay. When the assays were performed without exogenous metabolic activation, 89% (64/72) of the carcinogens induced transformation. As summarized in Table 24.3, when exogenous metabolic activation was incorporated into the assay, all carcinogens that were initially negative transformed the cells, giving an assay sensitivity of 100%. Similarly, the absence of response for the non-carcinogens was 100% (34/34). According to this publication, the assay had an accuracy of 100%.

In the subsequent evaluation of transformation data with SHE cells carried out by the EPA Gene-tox Program, the results were considerably different (Heidelberger *et al.*, 1983). In this review, data were compiled from reports published by a number of different laboratories. Data for 156 chemicals were analysed; 52 of the chemicals were classified as carcinogens (data on carcinogenicity derived from the EPA Gene-tox report or updated by comparison with information in the IARC Monographs (IARC, 1987)); two were classified as non-carcinogens, and the remaining 102 chemicals could not be classified. As shown in Table 24.3, the sensitivity for this group of carcinogens was 61% (32/52). One non-carcinogen gave a positive response and the other was negative. Although few data are given for non-carcinogens, the accuracy (accuracy = correct test results/total carcinogens and non-carcinogens tested) for these data is 6.1.% (33/54).

Kuroki and Sasaki (1985) reported a similar evaluation for the transformation assays using C3H 10T1/2 and Balb 3T3 cells. The data they used were derived from the EPA Gene-tox report (Heidelberger

Table 24.3
Reliability of *in vitro* transformation assays

| Parameter[a] | SHE (%) | | Balb/3T3 (%) | | C3H 10T1/2 (%) | |
	Pienta (1979)	Gene-Tox (1983)	Kuroki and Sasaki (1985)	Dunkel *et al.* (1990)	Kuroki and Sasaki (1985)	Dunkel *et al.* (1990)
Sensitivity	100	61.1	67.8	72.2	80.8	50
Specificity	100	ND	66.7	33.3	60.0	100
Predictive value	100	60.3	95.0	76.4	91.3	100
Accuracy	100	61.1	67.8	62.5	77.4	62.5

[a] Sensitivity = number of carcinogens positive/total carcinogens tested; specificity = number of non-carcinogens negative/total carcinogens tested; predictive value = number of positive carcinogens/total number of positive chemicals; accuracy = number of chemicals with correct results/total chemicals tested.
ND, not determined.

et al., 1983) with an update of results reported since that paper was published. The total number of chemicals tested with one or both cell systems was 104; 67 with 10T1/2 cells, 55 with 3T3 cells and 17 with both cell types. Of the known carcinogens, 26 were tested with 10T1/2 cells and 28 with 3T3 cells. As observed previously with the SHE cell assay, few of the chemicals tested were non-carcinogens: five with 10T1/2 and three with 3T3 cells. As shown in Table 24.3, the sensitivity was 80.8% (21/26) with 10T1/2 cells and 67.8% (19/28) with 3T3 cells; the specificity was 60.0% (3/5) and 66.7% (2/3) respectively. The predictive value was calculated to be over 90% for each cell system and the overall accuracy of these assays was 77.4% (24/31) with 10T1/2 and 67.8% (21/31) with 3T3 cells.

More recently, Dunkel *et al.* (1988) published a study on the comparative evaluation in two laboratories of 46 chemicals tested in the 10T1/2 assay. A large number of the chemicals used in this study had been tested for carcinogenicity in the NCI/NTP bioassay programme, and a diverse group of chemicals was represented. One of the laboratories also tested a subset of the same 37 chemicals, using the Balb/3T3 transformation assay (Dunkel *et al.*, 1981; Sivak and Tu, 1983; Sivak, 1990). A list of the 37 chemicals tested and their responses in each transformation assay is presented in Table 24.4. The carcinogenicity for this data set is taken from the NTP Chemical Status Report (7/3/90) or from the IARC Monographs (1987). As shown, 18 of the chemicals were carcinogens, and seven were non-carcinogens; for 12 chemicals there were insufficient data to classify the compounds. From these test results, the sensitivity, specificity, predictive value and accuracy were calculated (Table 24.3). For this evaluation, chemicals giving a questionable transformation response were considered negative. Thus, the sensitivity for this group of chemicals was 72.2% (13/18) with 3T3 cells and 50.0% (9/18) with 10T1/2 cells, and the specificity was 33.3% (2/6) and 100% (6/6) respectively. The predictive value was 76.4% (13/17) for 3T3 cells and 100% (9/9) for 10T1/2 cells. The overall accuracy for both of these assays was 62.5% (15/24 correct responses).

A comparison of the results with these two cell systems shows that some of the strongest responses in both assays were obtained with polycyclic aromatic hydrocarbons. In addition, 3T3 cells responded to a wide range of chemicals including aromatic amines and metal derivatives. Seven chemicals (aniline, beryllium sulphate, cinnamyl anthranilate, dibenz[*a*,*h*]anthracene, diphenylnitrosamine, lead acetate and tris(2,3-dibromopropyl) phosphate) induced positive responses in 3T3 cells but were not detected with 10T1/2 cells. Three carcinogens (4-amino-2-nitrophenol, 5-nitro-*o*-toluidine and nitrilotriacetic acid) were negative with 3T3 cells but were positive in the 10T1/2 assay. Only two carcinogens (benzo[*e*]pyrene and diethylstilboestrol) were negative in both transformation assays. In contrast with previous reports indicating that transformation of 10T1/2 cells by MNNG required the use of synchronous cultures (Bertram and Heidelberger, 1974; Grisham *et al.*, 1979), it was observed in this study that MNNG would induce a positive response using an asynchronous cell population.

Conclusion

Cell transformation *in vitro* has been defined as the induction of heritable premalignant or malignant changes in cells that do not express these characteristics under controlled conditions of cell cultivation (Freeman, 1981). This definition encompasses a number of different cellular changes including anchorage-independent growth, decreased requirement for serum, oncogene activation, loss of contact inhibition, alterations in cellular morphology and, probably the most important, the ability of the transformed cells to give rise to tumours on implantation into an appropriate host. Because cells transformed *in vitro* and cells from tumours share some of these same characteristics, *in vitro* transformation provides a model system useful not only for studying cellular and molecular mechanisms but also for the determination of the carcinogenic potential of chemicals.

Table 24.4

Comparison of *in vitro* transformation test results with Balb/c 3T3 and C3H 10T1/2 cells

Chemical	*In vivo* carcinogenicity[a]	*In vitro* transformation Balb/3T3[b]	C3H 10T1/2[c]
Benzo[*a*]pyrene	+	+	+
Ethyl methanesulphonate	+	+	+
3-Methylcholanthrene	+	+	+
4,4′-Methylenebis(*NN*-dimethylaniline)	+	+*	+
Michler's ketone	+	+*	+
N-Methyl *N*′-nitro-*N*-nitrosoguanidine	+	+	+
Aniline	+	+	−
Beryllium sulphate	+	+	?
Cinnamyl anthranilate	+	+*	?
Dibenz[*a,h*]anthracene	+	+*	−
Diphenylnitrosamine	+	+	−
Lead acetate	+	+	−
Tris(2,3-dibromopropyl) phosphate	+	+*	?
4-Amino-2-nitrophenol	+	?*	+
Nitrilotriacetic acid trisodium salt	+	?*	+
5-Nitro-*o*-toluidine	+	−*	+
Benzo[*e*]pyrene	+	−	−
Diethylstilboestrol	+	−	−
3-Chloromethylpyridine HCl	−	−	−
Lithocholic acid	−	−*	−
NN-Dicyclohexylthiourea	−	+*	−
Methoxychlor	−	+	−
4-Nitro-*o*-phenylenediamine	−	+*	−
p-Phenylenediamine	−	+*	−
7,12-Dimethylbenz[*a*]anthracene	I	+	+
N-Acetoxyacetylaminofluorene	I	+*	?
2-Nitro-*p*-phenylenediamine	I	+*	?
2-Acetylaminofluorene	I	−	?
Anthracene	I	−	−
7-Bromomethyl-12-methylbenz[*a*]-anthracene	I	−	?
p-Chloroaniline	I	−	+
3-Nitropropionic acid	I	−*	?
Phenanthrene	I	−	−
Pyrene	I	−*	−
p-Quinone dioxime	I	−*	−

[a] Carcinogenicity results: + = positive; − = negative; I = insufficient data.
[b] The data are from Dunkel *et al.* (1981) or were provided by Drs. Sivak and Tu; the latter are identified by an asterisk.
[c] The data for all studies with C3H 10T1/2 cells are from Dunkel *et al.* (1988).

The data summarized in this review would, at first, appear to indicate that *in vitro* transformation methods might not be satisfactory for screening chemicals of unknown activity since the accuracy of these test systems was in the 60–70% range. However, when these data are compared with the results obtained with *in vitro* mutagenicity tests, they appear to be as good as or possibly better than such methods. Tennant *et al.* (1987), in a study comparing results from four short-term mutagenicity tests with those obtained in carcinogenicity assays, reported the following correlations: gene mutation in bacteria (*Salmonella typhimurium*), 62%; chromosomal aberrations in mammalian cells in culture, 60%; sister chromatid exchange in mammalian cells in culture, 62%; and gene mutation in mammalian cells in culture (mouse lymphoma), 60%. In addition, except for the *Salmonella* assay, the predictive value for the mutagenicity tests was not as good as that obtained with the transformation assays. It could be argued that the number of chemicals used for the current analyses were insufficient and that the analyses reported by Tennant *et al.* provided a more stringent test of the methodology, but this was unlikely to be the case.

The survey supported by Health and Welfare Canada provided ample evidence that transformation assays are being used essentially as described in the original publications (Dunkel *et al.*, 1990). Several areas, however, require further work that could result in the development of testing procedures or schemes with greater potential than that currently provided by *in vitro* mutagenicity tests. These include the development of more readily usable exogenous metabolic activation, amplification of the transformation phenotype, development of biochemical end points to replace or to complement the morphological change and the advancement of methods for evaluation of chemicals for promoting activity.

References

Bertram, J.S. and Heidelberger, C. (1974). *Cancer Res.* **34**, 526–537.
Casto, B. (1990). Personal Communication.
Cortesi, E., Saffiotti, U., Donovan, P.J., Rice, J.M. and Kakunaga, T. (1983). *Teratogen. Carcinogen. Mutagen.* **3**, 101–110.
Dunkel, V.C. (1976). *In* "Screening Tests in Chemical Carcinogenesis" (R. Montesano, H. Bartsch and L. Tomatis, eds), pp. 25–28. IARC Scientific Publications No. 12, Lyon, France.
Dunkel, V.C., Wolff, III, J.S. and Pienta, R.J. (1977). *Cancer Bull.* **29**, 167–174.
Dunkel, V.C., Pienta, R.J., Sivak, A. and Traul, K.A. (1981). *J. Natl. Cancer Inst.* **67**, 1303–1315.
Dunkel, V.C., Schechtman, L.M., Tu, A.S., Sivak, A., Lubet, R.A. and Cameron, T.P. (1988). *Environ. Mol. Mutagen.* **12**, 21–31.

Dunkel, V.C., Rogers, C., Swierenga, S.H.H., Brillinger, R.L., Gilman, J.P.W. and Nestman, E.R. (1991). *Mutat. Res.* **246**, 285–300.

Fitzgerald, D.J., Piccoli, C. and Yamasaki, H. (1989). *Mutagenesis* **4**, 286–291.

Freeman, A.E. (1981). *In* "Mammalian Cell Transformation by Chemical Carcinogens" (N. Mishra, V. Dunkel and M. Mehlman, eds), pp. 37–45. Senate Press Inc., Princeton Junction, NJ.

Friedrich, U., Thomale, J. and Nass, G. (1985). *Mutat. Res.* **152**, 113–121.

Grisham, J.W., Greenberg, D.S., Smith, G.J. and Kaufman, D.G. (1979). *Biochem. Biophys. Res. Commun.* **87**, 969–975.

Heidelberger, C., Freeman, A.E., Pienta, R.J., Sivak, A., Bertram, J.S., Dunkel, V.C., Francis, M.W., Kakunaga, T., Little, J.B. and Schechtman, L.M. (1983). *Mutat. Res.* **114**, 283–385.

IARC (1987). IARC Monographs on the Evaluation of Carcinogenic Risks to Humans. Overall Evaluation of Carcinogenicity: An Updating of *IARC Monographs* Volumes 1 to 42. Supplement 7. Lyon, France.

IARC/NCI/EPA Working Group (1985). *Cancer Res.* **45**, 2395–2399.

Kakunaga, T. (1973). *Int. J. Cancer* **12**, 463–473.

Kuroki, T. and Sasaki, K. (1985). *In* "Transformation Assay of Established Cell Lines: Mechanisms and Applications" (T. Kakunaga and H. Yamasaki, eds), pp. 93–118. IARC Scientific Publications No. 67, Lyon, France.

LeBoeuf, R.A. and Kerckaert, G.A. (1986). *Carcinogenesis* **7**, 1431–1440.

LeBoeuf, R.A. and Kerckaert, G.A. (1987). *Carcinogenesis* **8**, 689–697.

LeBoeuf, R.A., Kerckaert, G.A., Poiley, J.A. and Raineri, R. (1989). *Mutat. Res.* **222**, 205–218.

Lubet, R.A., Kouri, R.E., Curren, R.A., Putman, D.L. and Schechtman, L.M. (1990). *Environ. Mol. Mutagen.* **16**, 13–20.

Pienta, R.J. (1979). *In* "Carcinogens: Identification and Mechanisms of Action" (A.C. Griffin and C.R. Shaw, eds), pp. 121–141. Raven Press, New York.

Pienta, R.J. (1980). *In* "Mammalian Cell Transformation by Chemical Carcinogens" (N. Mishra, V. Dunkel and M. Mehlman, eds), pp. 47–83. Senate Press Inc., Princeton Junction, NJ.

Pienta, R.J., Poiley, J.A. and Lebherz, III, W.B. (1977). *Int. J. Cancer* **19**, 642–655.

Prival, M.J. and Dunkel, V.C. (1989). *Environ. Mol. Mutagen.* **13**, 1–24.

Przygoda, R.T., Takayama, K., Traul, K.A. and Tummey, A. (1985). *In Vitro Cell. Dev. Biol.* **21**, 32–38.

Reznikoff, C.A., Brankow, D.W. and Heidelberger, C. (1973a). *Cancer Res.* **33**, 3231–3238.

Reznikoff, C.A., Bertram, J.S., Brankow, D.W. and Heidelberger, C. (1973b). *Cancer Res.* **33**, 3239–3249.

Sivak, A. (1990). Personal Communication.

Sivak, A. and Tu, A.S. (1983). *Toxicologist* **3**, 142.

Sivak, A., Charest, M.C., Rudenko, L., Silveira, D.M., Simons, I. and Wood, A.M. (1980). *In* "Mammalian Cell Transformation by Chemical Carcinogens" (N. Mishra, V. Dunkel and M. Mehlman, eds), pp. 133–180. Senate Press Inc., Princeton Junction, NJ.

Tennant, R.W., Marlogin, B.H., Shelby, M.D., Zeiger, E., Haseman, J.K., Spalding, J., Caspary, W., Resnick, M., Stasiewicz, S., Anderson, B. and Minor, R. (1987). *Science* **236**, 933–941.

Traul, K.A., Kachevsky, V. and Wolff, J.S. (1979). *Int. J. Cancer* **23**, 193–196.

Traul, K.A., Hink, R.J., Wolff, J.S. and Korof, W. (1981). *J. Appl. Toxicol.* **1**, 32–37.

Tu, A., Hallowell, W., Pallotta, S., Sivak, A., Lubet, R.A., Curren, R.D., Avery, M.D., Jones, C., Sedita, B.A., Huberman, E., Tennant, R., Spalding, J. and Kouri, R.E. (1986). *Environ. Mutagen.* **8**, 77–98.

Part IV

Present Status of *In Vitro* Toxicity

Can *in vitro* toxicology at present provide an alternative to animal testing? An answer to this question has been requested from experts in different fields and the following articles offer their views on:

1) The validation and acceptance of *in vitro* tests
2) The scientific perspectives of *in vitro* testing
3) The position of
   - registration authorities
   - industry
   - the Commission of the European Communities
   - academic and government-funded organizations

These opinions have been submitted to a general discussion which is reported in detail following the statements. Dr Michael Balls, Chairman of the Trustees of the Fund for the Replacement of Animals in Medical Experiments (FRAME) acted as the moderator; the affiliation of the participants is indicated in the list of contributors.

25

The Validation and Acceptance of *In Vitro* Toxicity Tests

M. BALLS

FRAME (Fund for the Replacement of Animals in Medical Experiments), 34 Stoney Street, Nottingham NG1 1NB and Department of Human Morphology, University of Nottingham Medical School, Nottingham NG7 2UH, UK

Introduction

It is now widely agreed that, if *in vitro* toxicity tests are to replace any of the animal test procedures currently recognized by regulatory authorities, they must first be shown to be no less relevant, reproducible or useful for identifying the potential hazard represented by chemicals and products to man, other animals or the environment in general, under given conditions of exposure, as a contribution to risk assessment and as a basis for risk limitation and risk management.

Demonstration of the relevance and reliability of a procedure for a given purpose is known as *validation*, and validation should follow the completion of test development (the definition and establishment of a new procedure) and should precede promotion of acceptance for incorporation into regulatory toxicology for a particular purpose.

Except in relation to genotoxicity, little formal attention had been paid to how validation studies should be planned and conducted, until an

IN VITRO METHODS IN TOXICOLOGY
ISBN 0-12-388175-7

international workshop was held at Amden in Switzerland, early in 1990. This workshop was followed a few months later by a second international workshop, on the regulatory acceptance of validated non-animal tests, which was held at Vouliagmeni, in Greece. The full reports of both these workshops were published in volume 18 of *ATLA – Alternatives to Laboratory Animals* (Balls *et al.*, 1990a,b).

I shall refer to the main conclusions and recommendations of these two workshops, while adding some further personal comments on scientific, political and strategic aspects of the validation process and on the regulatory acceptance of *in vitro* tests.

Validation

The purpose of a validation study should be fully defined at the outset, especially in relation to level of toxicity assessment (toxic potential, toxic potency, hazard or risk), the type of test involved (screening, adjunct or replacement), the type of toxicity to be evaluated (e.g. ocular irritancy, hepatotoxicity, neurotoxicity), and the chemical spectrum of interest (e.g. all known chemicals or surfactants).

Tests should only be included in a validation study after they have been adequately developed and documented, and if their purposes are well defined and consistent with the overall objective of the validation study.

Validation consists of four main stages (in addition to advance planning): intralaboratory assessment, interlaboratory assessment (including a blind trial), test database development and evaluation.

The selection of appropriate sets of chemicals for use in validation studies is a matter of crucial importance and great difficulty. The relevance and reliability of data from animal tests, even when they are available, is questionable. Animal data should not be used uncritically to establish the "truth" against which the results of *in vitro* tests are judged to be "true" or "false", negatives or positives (Balls and Clothier, 1989). Thus, wherever possible, since the welfare of human beings is the principal concern in toxicity testing, evaluation of the relevance of *in vitro* test results should be based on human toxicology data.

Both the Amden and Vouliagmeni workshops recommended that the establishment of an International Reference Chemical Data Bank was a matter of the highest priority (see also, Purchase, 1990), to provide open-access listings of scientifically selected chemicals, backed by toxicological data reviews, safety advice and a source of chemicals of known purity and stability.

The Amden report also provides some suggested definitions of terms used in the context of validation, plus detailed guidelines on validation programme design and on practical aspects of intralaboratory assessment, interlaboratory assessment and test database development, and a discussion of criteria for the evaluation of validation studies (e.g. test performance, relevance, logistical considerations and battery selection). Finally, attention was paid to integration of the stages of the validation process and implementation of the outcomes of validation studies.

The authors of the Amden report hope that it will provide useful guidance for researchers, regulators and others, and that it will stimulate discussion among all concerned.

Scientific Validation Versus Political Validation

Validation should primarily be a scientific process, in that relevance and reliability should be evaluated strictly on the basis of scientific criteria and of the standard of conduct and reporting of the study in question. Hence, the Amden report recommends that the ideal number of laboratories to be involved at the interlaboratory assessment stage is *four* – on the grounds that any scientific advantages to be gained by having five, six or more participating laboratories would be outweighed by disadvantages, such as extra cost and greater complexity of management.

There is, however, another view – that the acceptance of new methods will be facilitated and speeded up if the validation process involves as many laboratories as possible and in as many countries as possible. The 1988–89 validation study on the Fixed Dose Procedure (FDP) is a classic example of a politically motivated validation exercise (van den Heuvel, 1990). This study, largely funded by the EEC, involved 31 laboratories in 12 countries, and 20 chemicals were tested (Table 25.1). Meanwhile the LD_{50} test was conducted in one laboratory.

I am strongly in favour of the recommendation in the Amden report that only four laboratories should normally be involved in a validation study, for the following reasons. Firstly, studies involving many laboratories tend to result in the testing of only a small number of chemicals, e.g. ten groups of four laboratories each testing 20 chemicals (i.e. 40 laboratories, 200 chemicals) would be a more profitable investment of resources than having 40 laboratories all test the same 20 chemicals. Secondly, the more validation studies that take place, the better will be the selection of non-animal tests from which some will survive to later stages of evaluation for acceptability, e.g. ten groups of four laboratories each comparing three methods (i.e. 30 methods in all) would be preferable

Table 25.1
Scientific validation versus political validation

	Scientific	Political
Ideal number of laboratories	4	> 30
Cost	Relatively low	Very high
Time taken	Usually less	Usually more
Complexity of organization	Much less	Much greater
Number of chemicals tested	Much more	Much less
Expectancy of a positive outcome	Much lower	Much higher
Current acceptability of outcome	Much lower	Much higher

to having 40 laboratories all comparing the same three methods. Thirdly, the bigger the study, the greater is the desire for a positive outcome as a return on the funds, time and effort invested, *and* the greater is the likelihood that a new method will have been developed while the study was under way, which promises to be better than any of those included in it! This could be said to have happened with two lengthy trials on alternatives to the Draize eye irritancy test, currently being run in Europe. Both these trials have concentrated on the Neutral Red uptake (NRU) cytotoxicity test and chick chorioallantoic membrane (CAM) tests, while a later trial undertaken by the US CTFA has selected the FRAME Neutral Red release and EYTEX™ (Gordon and Bergman, 1987) methods as being of particular promise. Thus, it could also be argued that, the bigger the trial, the *less* likely it is that a positive scientific outcome will be achieved!

Therefore, if the overwhelming reason for the multilaboratory multinational trial is political, another solution must be found to overcome resistance to change based on nationalism, bureaucracy or vested interests among toxicologists or members of national regulatory bodies. That solution ought also to be achieved on a scientific basis, but, if necessary, it, too, will have to be political.

Regulatory Acceptance

The concluding recommendation of the Amden workshop was that: "*The regulatory and legislative authorities should be encouraged to welcome scientifically-validated methods and to accept their incorporation into toxicity testing practices*". The promotion of such acceptance was the aim of the Vouliagmeni workshop, at which nine of the 17 participants were associated with European regulatory agencies. It was agreed that: *"Reduction, refinement and replacement of the use of animal toxicity test procedures are desirable objectives, and the replacement of some current procedures should be achievable in the foreseeable future"*.

Central to the Vouliagmeni report is a recommendation that, before the formal acceptance of a new method and its incorporation into regulatory practice are considered, the results of the validation study should be evaluated by one or more independent panels (i.e. independent of the trial in question). Such panels would consider the quality and conduct of the validation trial itself, and the quality of reporting and analysis of results and of the conclusions drawn. They would then assess the value of an adequately validated method in competition with others already validated or in the course of validation, the need for such a method, and the practicability of its use as part of the regulatory process.

When it is concluded that a test (or battery of tests) should be recommended for incorporation into regulatory practice, it should be brought to the attention of an appropriate national agency, which would, in turn, take it to an appropriate international agency. International agencies, such as the OECD and EEC, already have procedures for the notification, consideration and adoption of new test methods. Some harmonization and rationalization of such procedures is necessary, and the principle of mutual acceptance of data should also be promoted.

The great potential value of the independent assessment recommendation is that it could be used to obviate the need for "political" validation, by, in effect, performing the same function of facilitating the widespread acceptance of a well-validated procedure.

The Vouliagmeni report also recommends that it may sometimes be appropriate for *in vitro* tests to be performed in parallel with required animal tests, as an aspect of the validation process.

Finally, the report concludes that: *"All conceivable and practicable steps should be taken to make the formal acceptance and incorporation of non-animal toxicity test procedures into regulatory practice as smooth and rapid a process as possible"*.

Scientific Reasons for Acceptance

There is a great need for an objective reappraisal of the basis and value of regulatory practice centred on animal test procedures. Most, if not all, the tests in current use would not meet either the standards set for validation at Amden or convince the kind of independent assessment panels envisaged at Vouliagmeni of their value in terms of reliability and relevance. Toxicity testing as currently practised is scientifically questionable (Heywood, 1990; Parke *et al.*, 1990; Roberfroid and Goethals, 1990). Those who support its continuation along present lines seem to say that both the value of the tests themselves and the interpretation of the meaning in terms of human safety of the results they provide are based on their own knowledge and experience. Yet they would not countenance the acceptance and incorporation into practice of an *in vitro* test solely on the basis of the knowledge and experience of *in vitro* toxicologists! And only when a drug has to be withdrawn because of unexpected adverse reactions in man do they suddenly bring species differences to the fore and remind us that we cannot expect *total* safety!

It must be recognized that the laboratory animal will always be only that – it will never be a truly adequate model for man. Non-animal test procedures, however, are only in their infancy, and there is undoubtedly great scope for further technical developments, which in the future will transform the relevance and reliability of prospective assessments of the toxicity of new drugs and other chemicals.

One major strategic question is whether reform of attitudes toward the current dependence of toxicity testing on animal procedures is a prerequisite for the proper validation and rational incorporation of non-animal tests into regulatory practice. Should *in vitro* toxicologists permit validation to be based on comparisons between *in vitro* data and *animal* data? Should they even try to provide regulators with the same kinds of predictions and classification criteria that they currently get from animal tests? The problem with that approach is that the predictions based on *in vitro* data closely tailored to an animal test will be as limited in value as predictions based on the animal test itself.

We must beware of suggestions that the proper place for *in vitro* studies is as prescreens or adjuncts to be run before or alongside the "definitive" (i.e. animal) studies (van den Heuvel and Fielder, 1990). What is the point of seeing a quantitative mechanistically-based, scientifically-defensible, fully-validated and independently-recommended test merely as a prelude or sideline to studies based on empirically-based, unvalidated, qualitative animal procedures of doubtful relevance and reliability?

Ideally, where humans are the primary subject of interest, human toxicological data should be used in the validation process. But reliable human data are not easily obtained. This problem is being confronted in the MEIC (Multi-centre Evaluation of *In Vitro* Cytotoxicity) study being run by the Scandinavian Society for Cell Toxicology, which has provided very promising early results (Ekwall *et al.*, 1989). Ultimately, computer-based predictions and *in vitro* studies on human cells and tissues, followed by carefully planned and tightly controlled human volunteer studies, should become the basis of assessment of many types of chemicals and products, including drugs and cosmetics. Only when both animal tests *and* animal cells are replaced will the problem of species differences have been truly overcome.

Nevertheless, despite the logic of this line of argument, *in vitro* toxicologists must also be realistic. So, provided that there is due awareness of what is being done, and why, the use of animal data during validation assessments may be advisable, both on practical grounds and as a means of encouraging recognition and regulatory acceptance.

Legislative Reasons for Acceptance

It is often stated that animal tests are carried out in order to comply with legal requirements, so changes to the laws concerned must be made before the accepted animal tests can be replaced. Happily, a number of these laws are now being modified, partly in order to allow for the incorporation of validated non-animal tests into regulatory practice.

However, it must also be remembered that the 1980s have seen the passage of *other* laws specifically aimed at improving the protection of animals used for scientific purposes. The British *Animals (Scientific Procedures) Act 1986* (Anon, 1986a) is based on a Government statement that: "*All experiments that are unnecessary, use unnecessarily large numbers of animals, or are unnecessarily painful are indefensible*". The Government minister responsible for the administration of the Act is required to weigh the benefits likely to accrue from a particular programme of work against the adverse effects likely to be caused to the animals to be used, before granting a project licence. He must also ensure that the project licence applicant has fully considered the feasibility of achieving the purpose of the work without using protected animals.

The 12 Member States of the European Communities must comply with Directive 86/609/EEC (Anon, 1986b), which states, *inter alia*, that: "*An experiment shall not be performed if another scientifically satisfactory method of obtaining the result sought, not entailing the use of an animal, is reasonably and practicably available*", and that: "*All experiments shall be designed to avoid distress and unnecessary pain and suffering to the experimental animals*".

It is doubtful whether much of current regulatory toxicity testing in animals could meet these various criteria – in terms of scientific necessity, of specific likelihood of benefit, or of design to minimize adverse effects. That these laws will be used to force a reassessment and rationalization of regulatory toxicology has been foreseen by Zbinden (1988):

"A common feature of many new animal protection laws is the requirement to demonstrate the advisability, in some countries even the unconditional necessity, of all proposed animal experiments. It is probable that the reviewing applications for toxicological studies will expect more justification for an animal experiment than the simple statement that the proposed test is necessary because it is required by a regulatory guideline".

In addition, the clauses requiring the use of non-animal methods, wherever possible, provide a legislative requirement that regulatory agencies accept into regulatory practice non-animal tests which have been properly validated and shown to be relevant and reliable. Again, the role of the independent assessment panels recommended by the Vouliagmeni workshop could be crucial here. It is to be hoped that endorsement of a non-animal procedure by such a panel would come to be seen as a legal requirement that the method be accepted and incorporated into practice.

Conclusions

The undoubted potential of *in vitro* methods, not only as a basis for a more modern, more scientifically based toxicology (Roberfroid and Goethals, 1990), but also as a basis for the more scientific application of toxicity tests, represents a great challenge to *in vitro* toxicologists, whose contribution to the development, validation and assessment of new methods and procedures will be crucial. It is very important that regulatory incorporation should be a *permissive* process, rather than a restrictive one. Any well-designed and scientifically defensible study incorporating any properly validated and independently recommended test procedures should be acceptable.

Finally, the practice of regulatory toxicology as some sort of pseudo-scientific art (Dayan, 1986), performable only by members of some kind of exclusive magic circle, should be overthrown. A much greater investment in *in vitro* toxicology will rescue toxicology as a whole from the decline in its reputation and status. The result will be better science, greater protection of human beings and the environment as a whole, greater efficiency in developing new compounds and products, and greater humanity, as the animal suffering that inevitably results from current practices steadily declines toward extinction.

References

Anon. (1986a). *Animals (Scientific Procedures) Act 1986*. HMSO, London.
Anon. (1986b). *Off. J. Eur. Communities* **29** (L358), 1–29.

Balls, M., Blaauboer, B., Brusick, D., Frazier, J., Lamb, D., Pemberton, M., Reinhardt, C., Roberfroid, M., Rosenkranz, H., Schmid, B., Spielmann, H., Stammati, A.-L. and Walum, E. (1990a). *ATLA* **18**, 313–337.

Balls, M., Botham, P., Cordier, A., Fumero, S., Kayser, D., Koëter, H., Koundakjian, P., Gunnar Lindquist, N., Meyer, O., Pioda, L., Reinhardt, C., Rozemond, H., Smyrniotis, T., Spielmann, H., Van Looy, H., van der Venne, M.-T. and Walum, E. (1990b). *ATLA* **18**, 339–344.

Balls, M. and Clothier, R.H. (1989). *Mol. Toxicol.* **1**, 547–559.

Dayan, A. (1986). *In* "Chemical Testing and Animal Welfare", pp. 91–109. National Chemicals Inspectorate, Solva, Sweden.

Ekwall, B., Bondesson, I., Castell, J.V., Gómez-Lechón, M.J., Hellberg, S., Högberg, J., Jover, R., Pondosa, X., Romert, L., Stenberg, K. and Walum, E. (1989). *ATLA* **17**, 83–100.

Gordon, V.C. and Bergman, H.C. (1987). *In* "*In Vitro* Toxicology: Approaches to Validation" (A.M. Goldberg, ed.), pp. 293–302. Mary Ann Liebert, New York.

Heywood, R. (1990). *ATLA* **18**, 354–355.

Parke, D.V., Ioannides, C. and Lewis, D. (1990). *ATLA* **18**, 91–102.

Purchase, I.F.H. (1990). *ATLA* **18**, 345–348.

Roberfroid, M.B. and Goethals, F. (1990). *ATLA* **18**, 19–22.

van den Heuvel, M.J. (1990). *In* "LD50 Testing and Classification Schemes: the Possibilities for Change", pp. 71–82. CEC, Brussels.

van den Heuvel, M.J. and Fielder, R.J. (1990). *Toxicol. In Vitro* **4**, 675–679.

Zbinden, G. (1988). *In* "National and International Drug Safety Guidelines" (S. Adler and G. Zbinden, eds), pp. 7–19. MTC Verlag, Zollikon.

Scientific Perspectives on the Role of *In Vitro* Toxicity Testing in Chemical Safety Evaluation

J.M. FRAZIER

The Johns Hopkins University, 615 North Wolfe Street, Baltimore, MD 21205, USA

Introduction

The application of *in vitro* technologies to the problems of chemical safety evaluation is a current topic of interest to academia, industry and government. The development of these technologies has progressed rapidly in the 1980s and many applications can be foreseen for the 1990s. Societal pressures have helped to catalyse events which were already in progress as a result of scientific and economic imperatives. However, expectations for change must be realistic in the context of scientific capabilities and the areas in which progress can be made must be clearly defined. To improve communications on these issues it is essential to make a clear distinction between toxicological research, on the one hand, and toxicity testing, on the other (Frazier and Goldberg, 1990).

Research is the process by which new knowledge is obtained. This process is characterized by the application of the scientific method to hypothesis testing. The optimum experimental system which is required

IN VITRO METHODS IN TOXICOLOGY
ISBN 0-12-388175-7

to attain the goals of research successfully is defined by the particular hypothesis to be tested. In some cases the experimental question will require whole animal models, in others *in vitro* models are most appropriate. The point is, *a priori* the best experimental model cannot be legislated but must be selected by the researcher who is familiar with both the research hypothesis and the biological nuances of the model systems.

In the case of toxicity testing, the scientific question is always the same – will the chemical or product formulation be safe under the expected conditions of use? In many cases, the converse question is equally important – what are the restrictions which must be placed on the use of a new chemical or product formulation which will ensure the protection of health and welfare of the user and the environment? Since the scientific question to be answered by toxicity testing is basically the same, the overall procedure to answer this question is well defined, and testing guidelines have been promulgated to attain this goal. The currently accepted procedures for toxicity testing are based on whole animal models which are utilized to provide the dataset for regulatory decision making. Decisions on the acceptability of a new product or on the restriction of use of new materials involves a complex evaluation of this *in vivo* toxicity dataset which includes various extrapolation processes and the application of safety factors. This integrated procedure – development of animal toxicity data, extrapolation to man and application of safety factors – which has evolved over the past 50–60 years, is highly successful in the protection of human and environmental health and welfare. The issue at hand is not whether we should replace a flawed system but whether we can continue to evolve the existing system to include the technological breakthroughs which have occurred in cell culture and bioanalytical methodologies. In this sense, evolution should imply improvements in predicting and controlling toxicological risks associated with the development of new products. *In vitro* toxicological testing systems have the potential to impact significantly on toxicity testing and safety evaluation. Successful application of these new technologies requires appropriate validation of the proposed methods as well as the development of new capabilities to extrapolate these data to the toxicological situation under consideration (Frazier, 1990a; OECD, 1990).

With these comments in mind, the major focus of this discussion will concern several scientific issues which must be appreciated in order to develop fully the potential of *in vitro* systems for the purpose of toxicity testing (Goldberg and Frazier, 1989). In particular, the correspondence between *in vitro* and *in vivo* dose–response relationships will be appraised and the role of *in vitro* toxicity testing systems in the safety evaluation process explored.

Dose–Response Relationships

The cornerstone of any toxicological evaluation is the establishment of the dose–response relationship which is used to predict the degree of biological response expected under various levels of exposure. The objective is to identify the most sensitive adverse biological response expected and determine a safe level of exposure at which the probability of experiencing any adverse effects is low enough to be acceptable to society. It is very important to emphasize that it is not possible to guarantee that there will be no toxicity; the best that one can do is establish a certain level of confidence that the safety margin is adequate and that there is very little probability of detrimental effects being observed.

The objectives of this process can be illustrated graphically (Fig. 26.1).

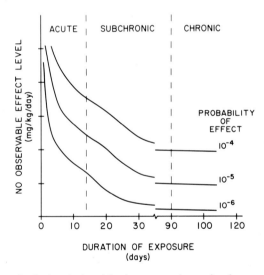

Fig. 26.1 A hypothetical relationship between the safe dose rate for a new chemical and the duration of exposure where hepatotoxicity is the end point under consideration. Each curve represents a different probability for observing an hepatotoxic effect (i.e. the curve designated 10^{-6} represents the curve where there is a one in a million chance of observing human hepatotoxicity when an individual is exposed to the given agent at the dose rate and duration indicated).

In this hypothetical graph, the safe level of exposure (expressed in mg/kg per day) is plotted versus the duration of exposure. For argument's sake, this graph was created to represent the safe level of human exposure to a particular chemical which will not result in observable hepatotoxicity. Similar graphs could be constructed for each feasible target organ toxicity (e.g. nephrotoxicity, neurotoxicity, haematopoietic toxicity). In general, higher doses can be tolerated for short times, therefore the limiting rate at short durations of exposures is such that the product of the dose rate and duration time gives the single acute dose which can be tolerated without observing hepatotoxicity, i.e. the acute no observable effect level (NOEL). For long durations of exposure, the asymptotic value of exposure rate will be the chronic NOEL. Given such relationships for all possible toxicities, the goal of the safety evaluation process is to select the safe level of exposure under both acute and chronic conditions which will prevent toxicity in the most sensitive target tissue. Thus, the acute NOEL may be based on nephrotoxicity, while the chronic NOEL may be dictated by pulmonary toxicity. In Fig. 26.1, the NOEL for various levels of probability of effect is illustrated. The appropriate probability curve selected for a particular safety decision will depend on the expected size of the population to be exposed and other mitigating circumstances. For example, greater risks can be tolerated for antineoplastic agents since the lifesaving benefits are paramount.

To this point, this discussion has been somewhat theoretical. The practical side becomes apparent when it is realized that the data needed to generate such NOEL relationships is provided by animal testing. Testing guidelines are established to provide three types of data relevant to this problem – acute, subchronic and chronic toxicity testing data. These data are utilized to construct three separate dose–response curves for the three time frames of importance. Because whole animals are used in these studies, dose–response curves are obtained simultaneously for all tissues, as well as integrated biological systems, which are actually evaluated at the termination of the study. Figure 26.2 illustrates hypothetical dose–response relationships for data collected from three tissues, liver, kidney and lung. If no toxicity is observed for any other tissues evaluated during the study, then it is assumed that the dose–response curves for those tissues must fall to the right of the highest doses tested for the particular chemical under investigation. Whole animal toxicity testing protocols thus provide information which can be used to identify the most sensitive end points at the three specific time points (usually 14 days, 90 days or 2 years) relating to acute, subchronic and chronic toxicity. Before potential human toxicity can be predicted, these animal data must be extrapolated to low doses. This is a consequence of the fact that

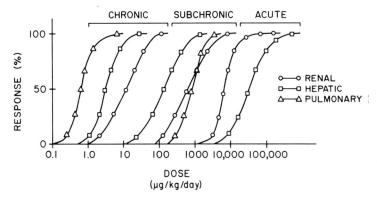

Fig. 26.2 Hypothetical dose–response data for renal, hepatic and pulmonary toxicity obtained from a complete toxicological evaluation including acute, subchronic and chronic toxicity studies. Note, in this hypothetical case, there is no observed pulmonary toxicity in the acute toxicity studies.

limited animal numbers per test group restricts the statistical sensitivity of the tests such that higher doses must be utilized to observe statistically significant effects. In addition, the animal data must be extrapolated to man (species extrapolation) by various scaling algorithms. Given the uncertainties in these extrapolations and the uncertainty in genetic variability among human populations, various safety factors are applied to predict the acute and chronic NOEL in man. The process as described is basically how chemical safety evaluations are conducted.

The critical component of this evaluation is the dose–response relationship. It is important to understand the nature of this relationship and the factors which control it to appreciate the relationship between *in vitro* and *in vivo* toxicity testing. The basic components of the toxicological process which influence the dose–response relationship are illustrated in Fig. 26.3. The dose–response relationship results from the integration of all the processes which fall between exposure on the left side of the diagram and the response measured, which falls somewhere within the sequence of events depicted on the right side of the diagram. The major components in the relationship are toxicokinetics, initiation and toxicodynamics. Toxicokinetics includes all the kinetic processes which determine the relationship between the exposure dose (the nominal dose in the dose–response relationship) and the delivered dose (the actual dose of the active form of the toxicant at the site of the molecular targets). Initiation is the molecular reaction between the active form of the toxicant and the molecular target. This reaction can be a reversible

The Toxicological Process

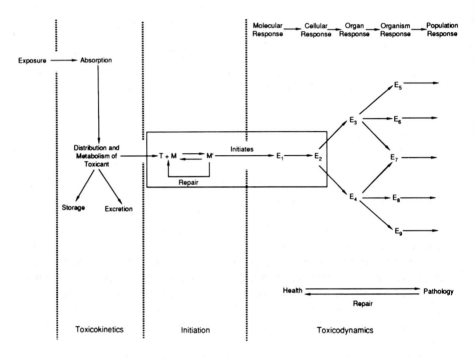

Fig. 26.3 The toxicological process includes three components: toxicokinetics, initiation and toxicodynamics. In the initiation process, the toxicant (T), or its metabolites, interacts with a molecular target (M) resulting in a perturbation (M'). This alteration initiates a sequence of events (E_1, E_2, etc.) which propagates the effect to higher levels of biological organization. (Reprinted from Frazier, (1990b) with permission of Mary Ann Liebert, Inc., Publishers.)

reaction, as in the case of competitive inhibition of an enzyme, or irreversible, as in the case of the formation of a covalent adduct. The initiation reactions set off a sequence of events, beginning at the molecular level and cascading to higher levels of biological organization, which ultimately culminates in measurable effects at the level of the chosen response measurement. This sequence of events is referred to as toxicodynamics.

It must be kept in mind that target organ toxicity can be observed as a consequence of both toxicokinetic factors and/or tissue-specific factors. The process of species extrapolation must critically consider whether the mechanisms observed in animal models are operative in man, and if they are operative, what is the quantitative relationship (the scaling factors). The better the mechanistic basis of the observed effects is understood, the more reliability there is in the predictions of the extrapolative process. For therapeutic drugs, much more mechanistic information is usually known, often as a consequence of *in vitro* mechanistic studies, than for most commercial chemicals or household products. Thus, when setting safe levels of exposure, larger safety factors are utilized for the latter materials to compensate for the lack of mechanistic understanding.

Chemical Safety Evaluation

Given the complexities of the *in vivo* dose–response relationship and the necessity to conduct various extrapolations (high dose to low dose, animal to man), the question arises as to the role of *in vitro* systems in this process. As mentioned above, *in vitro* systems already play a significant role in the current practice of safety evaluation. This role is mainly in investigative toxicology which is more closely related to a research role than a testing procedure. *In vitro* systems are used to answer specific questions about metabolic pathways, mechanisms of action and identification of the most appropriate animal model to predict human toxicology. In these roles, the *in vitro* experimental models are not defined by standard testing guidelines, but are selected as the most appropriate model to answer the question at hand.

In contrast, the role of *in vitro* systems in the standardized, toxicological testing strategy must be defined. The basic question is, what can *in vitro* toxicity testing systems tell us about the toxicological process and how can this information be used in the testing strategy and safety evaluation. Referring to Fig. 26.3, it can be argued that *in vitro* testing systems are models for the central core of the toxicological process (indicated by the box in Fig. 26.3) and thus have potential for providing important toxicological information concerning the initiation process and various aspects of the molecular and cellular components of the toxicodynamics phase. It is obvious that if target organ toxicity is a consequence of systemic toxicokinetic processes, then it would not be possible to predict such effects solely on the basis of *in vitro* toxicity testing methods. The development of the scientific basis of predictive toxicokinetics focused on physical–chemical properties, quantum mechanical calculations and *in vitro* measurements of metabolism, tissue partitioning and plasma protein binding is a research priority for the 1990s. Successful development of predictive toxicokinetic techniques will provide an important component of the *in vitro–in vivo* extrapolation process. This objective will be strongly supported by advances in physiologically-based toxicokinetic (PBTK) modelling.

Returning to the issue of what *in vitro* toxicity testing systems can tell us about the toxicological characteristics of new products, there are three major areas for consideration. First, is the issue of "intrinsic cellular toxicity". It seems feasible that a small battery of *in vitro* tests, i.e. several biological systems combined with several end point measurements, can be designed to evaluate the basic toxicological response of cells to test chemicals. If the test battery is properly designed, the *in vitro* dataset provided can be used to: (1) rank chemicals on the basis of their ability to affect cells adversely, (2) identify which cellular processes are most sensitive to the effects of the test chemical, and (3) determine whether metabolic activation will be a likely factor in *in vivo* toxicological effects. Because of the limitation on our ability to make *in vitro* to *in vivo* extrapolations, the information developed in this *in vitro* evaluation cannot be directly utilized to predict *in vivo* toxicity. However, the information provided by this "intrinsic cellular toxicity" evaluation could be invaluable for the efficient design of *in vivo* toxicity studies. Furthermore, chemicals which proved to be exceptionally toxic in the cellular systems whould be carefully scrutinized before further development or *in vivo* testing was considered.

The second issue for *in vitro* toxicity testing is hazard identification. Biological components of test systems derived from various tissues can be used to provide information as to the potential for target organ toxicity. Hazard potential for hepatotoxicity, neurotoxicity, etc. can be obtained by inspecting dose–response relationships using hepatocytes, neurons, proximal tubular cells, etc. as biological components of test systems. Again, these data cannot be used to definitively establish the probability of the corresponding *in vivo* target organ toxicity, but any cell type which exhibits an unusual sensitivity to the test chemical could signal the possibility of a target organ effect which could be monitored in *in vivo* studies.

Finally, *in vitro* testing systems can be used to determine mechanisms of action. The test battery for evaluating intrinsic cellular toxicity of test chemicals could be expanded to include a larger set of end point measurements which would be used in a diagnostic sense to evaluate the most likely mechanisms of toxicity. Such an enlarged test battery would include measurements of specific cellular functions, such as mitochondrial membrane potential and ATP measurements to identify disruption of energy metabolism or chemiluminescent measurements to evaluate lipid peroxidation. Such information is often obtained late in the product safety evaluation process when investigative studies are undertaken. However, if this information was developed early on, it could prove invaluable in decision making.

These three uses for *in vitro* toxicity testing systems are indicative of the valuable role they can play in the safety evaluation process. Properly developed, utilizing advances in basic toxicological research and biotechnology, the role of *in vitro* toxicity tests in chemical safety evaluation will continue to expand. With development of reliable techniques to extrapolate from *in vitro* to *in vivo*, particularly with respect to the toxicokinetic contribution to target organ toxicity, reliance on *in vitro* toxicity testing systems could play a major role in safety evaluation. Whether full replacement of *in vivo* toxicity testing protocols will ever come to pass can only be determined in the future. In the meantime, *in vitro* toxicity testing methods will make a significant scientific contribution to the process as well as reduce the use of animals in toxicity testing.

References

Frazier, J.M. (1990a). *J. Am. Coll. Toxicol.* **9**, 355–359.
Frazier, J.M. (1990b). *In Vitro Toxicol.* **3(4)**, 349–357.
Frazier, J.M. and Goldberg, A.M. (1990). *Cancer Bull.* **42**, 238–244.
Goldberg, A.M. and Frazier, J.M. (1989). *Sci. Am.* **260**, 24–30.
OECD (1990). *Environ. Monogr.* **36**, 62.

Perspectives for *In Vitro* Toxicology in the Regulatory Requirements Related to Safety Evaluation

J.R. CLAUDE
(Member of the EEC Safety Group for Drug Evaluation)

Laboratoire de Toxicologie, Faculté de Pharmacie, 4, Avenue de l'Observatoire, 75006 Paris, France

Safety evaluation is a scientific and ethical necessity if man and his environment are to be preserved in the face of the growing impact of xenobiotics. Safety evaluation comprises several aspects:

1) For chemicals and pesticides: evaluation of the maximum tolerated concentration (MTC) in the context of occupational toxicology and the threat to ecosystems

2) For food additives: estimation of the allowable daily intake (ADI) for consumers

3) For drugs for human or veterinary use: evaluation of the risk/benefit ratio in the subjects treated

4) For cosmetics: evaluation of local tolerance and prediction of possible side effects

In most cases, these basic evaluations are carried out after determining the No Observable Effect Level (NOEL) on the basis of data obtained

IN VITRO METHODS IN TOXICOLOGY
ISBN 0-12-388175-7

from animal studies (acute and repeated-dose toxicity, reproductive toxicity, carcinogenicity, etc.). In consequence, the number of animal studies and laboratory animals used in performing the safety evaluations demanded by regulatory requirements is constantly on the increase. The response from public opinion has been to react against the "cruelty" of the experiments and against the numbers of animals killed in this way each year (estimated at 15 million rodents alone per annum).

Animal models have been in use from the earliest days of the development of modern biology, as codified by Claude Bernard, and were used in the research work involved in 54 out of the 76 Nobel Prizes for Medicine or Physiology awarded since 1901. Their use cannot be avoided, but toxicologists and the public authorities have an obligation to consider four basic questions:

> 1) Is the inflation in the use of laboratory animals due to an excessive number of regulatory requirements?
> 2) Are the studies required by the regulations relevant to safety evaluation in man?
> 3) Is it possible to reduce or eliminate experiments involving pain or injury to animals?
> 4) Can any other relevant models be proposed which could limit or suppress the need for laboratory animals?

In this regard, the approaches proposed by *in vitro* toxicology could offer an alternative to animal studies, but two main difficulties must be taken into account:

> i) The scientific difficulty of obtaining relevant models for long-term toxicity studies or reproductive studies because of the impossibility of simulating organ–organ and mother–embryo relationships
> ii) The technical problem of validation of the alternative methods in practice.

This situation justifies the EEC's attitude to alternative methods: "Conventional methods should be used as long as it has not been demonstrated that alternative methods are able to provide an equivalent safety level for Man and his Environment". Consequently, the attitude of international authorities (EEC, OECD, etc.) and of national agencies (e.g. the French drug safety agency) should be to promote a general policy along three axes:

> 1) A decrease in the regulatory requirements for laboratory animals in two main ways:
>
> > a) international harmonization of the toxicology guidelines to avoid duplicating studies;
> > b) greater flexibility in the guidelines, in order to preserve the freedom of the expert toxicologists and eliminate the "check list" approach to regulatory toxicology.

2) Continued vigilance for the welfare of laboratory animals by increasing the implementation of good laboratory practice standards and by developing a new discipline of ethical considerations, which we could term "ethology".

3) Reconsideration of the strategy of safety evaluation in terms of three complementary stages:

    a) The "screening" phase: intended to screen out and discard any high-risk compounds by making extensive use of (true) alternative methods, under the sole liability of the company (e.g. alternatives to reproductive toxicology studies).

    b) The "regulatory" phase: prior to registration of the compound, during which the data are assembled, notably those obtained from animal experiments. This phase should be restricted to compounds that have demonstrated genuine innovative potential.

    c) The "mechanistic" phase: intended to explain – whenever possible – the mechanism of any toxic or side effects or adverse reactions produced by the new compound in order to provide a relevant evaluation of the benefit/risk ratio and avoid unjustified rejection due to erroneous model-to-man extrapolation. The use of *in vitro* or *ex vivo* methods (not alternative methods, but new methods) should be extensively promoted for this purpose.

These three axes should be incorporated into a rational international charter concerning regulatory requirements relating to safety evaluation. This charter should clearly define the complementary situation of *in vitro* toxicology relative to *in vivo* toxicology on the basis of the state-of-the-art methods available.

Industry's Needs for *In Vitro* Toxicology: A Personal View

I.F.H. PURCHASE

*ICI Central Toxicology Laboratory, Alderley Park, Macclesfield,
Cheshire SK10 4TJ, UK*

Toxicology is an applied science which is becoming increasingly important in terms of its socioeconomic impact on society. With increasing public awareness of issues related to environmental safety, the only practical way of identifying the toxic hazards of natural or synthetic chemicals is by the appropriate toxicological testing. This is particularly so for environmental toxicants, where the human exposure is likely to be so low that the adverse effects on human health will be difficult to discern against the background burden of disease. Within this context, toxicology has an important impact on human hazard assessment, which, when taken in conjunction with exposure, allows estimates of likely human risk. In terms of industrial development, toxicology continues to play a leading role in identifying safe chemicals for incorporation into products for sale and, via appropriate hazard and risk assessment, defining the safe circumstances of use.

Academic research has used the study of the mechanism of action of toxic chemicals as a means of deepening the understanding of normal physiological processes. While this is an extremely important branch of toxicology, and relies heavily on *in vitro* techniques, it is not the subject of this discussion.

IN VITRO METHODS IN TOXICOLOGY
ISBN 0-12-388175-7

Primary Purposes of Industrial Toxicology

Industrial organizations have a legal and ethical responsibility to ensure that their products are safe. International regulations now lay down the toxicological testing required for the development of new chemical entities. Virtually all of the tests required by regulatory authorities are based on animal studies. In addition to the final regulatory testing, industry is involved in selecting from candidate development compounds those that are likely to represent the least toxic hazard. In this respect, the testing regimes can be considered as testing for non-toxicity, for the ideal outcome is for a non-toxic chemical which has significant use potential.

Regulations also require that new formulations, manufactured by blending existing chemicals of known toxicity, should be safe. This may sometimes require toxicological testing.

Regulations are now being developed to ensure that existing chemicals already on the market are tested to modern standards. In this case the purpose of the testing is to define the toxicological hazard so that an appropriate risk assessment can be carried out. In some cases, where the toxicological results are contradictory, detailed mechanistic studies may be required in order for appropriate extrapolation from animal toxicological results to human hazard to be carried out.

Against this regulatory background and history of industrial use of toxicology, it is worth examining what role *in vitro* methods may play in the armamentarium of the industrial toxicologist. His primary concern is in the protection of human health; other factors including particularly the ethical issues surrounding animal experiments, must also be taken into account. Thus, any testing system which aims to replace traditional animal studies must have its utility demonstrated. In fact, there is only one *in vitro* test system currently incorporated into regulatory guidelines and that is the testing for mutagencity. All other toxicological work to define toxic hazard is based on the regulations requiring animal tests. Nevertheless, *in vitro* tests have found an important role in industrial toxicology. Of particular importance is the development of *in vitro* tests as screening tests for new chemicals, allowing the selection of the most appropriate chemical for development (Rhodes *et al.*, 1986). In this case standard *in vivo* toxicology is carried out in order to confirm the likely toxic hazard. These same tests can be used for screening existing chemicals in order that suitable prioritization for further testing can take place.

Where mixtures of chemicals of known toxicity are required to be evaluated, *in vitro* screening tests which are targeted on specific end points (such as irritation) are useful in confirming the predictions of the absence of toxicity.

Finally, *in vitro* methods contribute substantially to mechanistic studies which help to identify the reasons for species differences in toxic response. Within this general framework of comparative mechanistic studies, specific work can be done *in vitro* to estimate the likely transdermal absorption using human tissue. This has been shown to be superior to *in vivo* animal work.

Advantages of *In Vitro* Methods

The *in vitro* methods with the greatest utility have the advantage of specific end points allowing determination of the toxic effects with great precision. The simplicity of many *in vitro* tests and the standardization of cell lines and culture conditions provide the opportunity of much more reproducible results than are normally available from *in vivo* tests. Thus, from a scientific point of view, precision and reproducibility are great advantages for *in vitro* tests.

In vitro tests will, of course, reduce animal suffering if they are used in a way which replaces the use of animals. They may also be less expensive than traditional animal studies. For example, an Ames test providing information on potential carcinogenicity, is 200–400 times less expensive than a long-term animal study (although it does not provide equivalent information). However *in vitro* tests may not prove to be cheaper than some of the simpler *in vivo* test methods such as skin irritation testing.

The major disadvantage of *in vitro* testing systems, is the difficulty of extrapolating the results to human hazard assessment. In particular, metabolism, physiological interactions and organ architecture are too complex to model reliably in *in vitro* systems.

Criteria for Selecting Tests for Industrial Use

Progress has already been made in developing *in vitro* tests which are extensively used in industry. There appear to be four criteria which determine the likelihood that particular regulatory toxicological tests can be replaced by *in vitro* methods. These are (Table 28.1):

a) Specificity of end point: End points in toxicological studies vary from the non-specific acute toxicity to the highly specific observations made on some

Table 28.1

Criteria which may be used to identify toxicological end points with the greatest likelihood of successful *in vitro* replacement

	Criteria				
Test Type	Specificity of end point	Specificity of mechanism	No. of doses	Prediction	Likely success
Acute oral	Multiple	Low	1	Quantitative	Poor
Acute dermal	Multiple	Low	1	Quantitative	Poor
Skin irritation	Specific?	Medium	1	Qualitative	Good
Skin corrosion	Specific	High	1	Qualitative	V. Good
Skin sensitivity	Specific?	High	1	Qualitative	V. Good
Eye irritation	Specific?	Medium	1	Qualitative	Good
28-day repeat dose	Multiple	Low	28	Quantitative	V. Poor
Teratology	Specific?	Medium	± 10	Quantitative	Poor
				Qualitative	Good
Multigen	Multiple	Low	$> 10^2$	Quantitative	V. Poor
				Qualitative	Poor
90 day	Multiple	Low	90	Quantitative	V. Poor
Chronic	Multiple	Low	6×10^2	Quantitative	V. Poor
Carcinogenicity	Specific	Medium	6×10^2	Quantitative	V. Poor
				Qualitative	Good
Transdermal absorption	Specific	High	1	Quantitative	V. Good
Mechanistic studies	Specific	V. high	—	—	V. Good

acute studies (such as skin corrosivity). The more specific the end point, the more likely it is that a viable *in vitro* test will be developed.

b) Specificity of mechanism: One of the great advantages of *in vitro* methods is that many are based on a clear understanding of the mechanism of toxic action. Thus, the *Salmonella* mutation assay (Ames test) is based on clearly defined genetic criteria. The more specific the knowledge of the mechanism of action on which the test is based, the more likely it is that a viable *in vitro* method will be developed.

c) Number of doses: The complexity of metabolism and toxicokinetics from multiple dose studies makes it difficult to design an *in vitro* system which mimics the *in vivo* tests. Thus, the fewer the number of doses required to produce a particular toxicological end point, the more likely it is the *in vitro* method will be successful.

d) The required prediction: Where the purpose of the toxicity testing is merely to classify the chemical's toxicity into one of several classes (that is a qualitative test) the *in vitro* test is more likely to be successful. Thus, a test which is aimed at identifying a chemical carcinogen is easier to develop than one which will predict carcinogenic potency.

In Table 28.1 these criteria are used to classify different test types in terms of the likely success for the development of *in vitro* replacements. Mechanistic studies and transdermal absorption studies have a very high likelihood of success. Skin corrosivity and skin sensitivity appear to have a high likelihood of success with skin irritation, eye irritation and qualitative prediction of carcinogenicity and teratogenicity as the next most likely areas for the development of successful *in vitro* tests.

The Importance of Validation

Toxicological testing methods, whether they are for regulatory purposes or for screening, must be capable of predicting the toxic hazard with great precision. In addition, they should be robust and reproducible, they must be capable of being carried out correctly in a wide variety of laboratories and they should be recognized internationally.

There is no shortage of ideas for developing *in vitro* toxicity tests. For any of the end points discussed in Table 28.1 there are numerous *in vitro* methods that have been proposed on the basis of varying degrees of understanding of the toxic mechanisms involved. The practical industrial toxicologist has substantial difficulty in deciding which of these test systems can be used for screening purposes and the regulatory agencies have difficulty in identifying *in vitro* methods which are suitable for regulatory purposes. This problem was identified clearly in the early days of the development of short-term tests for carcinogenicity which were based on *in vitro* methods.

In a paper prepared for the International Commission for Protection Against Environmental Mutagens and Carcinogens (ICPEMC), Purchase (1982) reported on a method of assessing predictive tests for carcinogenicity. The same approach can be used more widely in the appraisal of *in vitro* tests in toxicology. All *in vitro* tests, whether they are based on a clear understanding of mechanism or simply on empirical correlations, require to be validated before a judgement can be made of their likely utility. Validation studies are designed to compare the performance of *in vitro* tests in identifying toxic hazards with those of standard regulatory toxicological tests. Thus, the *in vitro* test system is subjected to validation with a variable number of chemicals with known toxic properties.

Typically, a new test system will be developed by a researcher who believes that a method has something to contribute to the assessment of toxic hazard. It may be one of several hundred tests available and initially it will be developed in a single laboratory. Ultimately, it will be compared in a variety of laboratories using a large number of chemicals so that its robustness, reproducibility and accuracy can be assessed.

As the test system is developed it evolves from a research stage to being a fully established predictive test. This development can be divided into three stages:

a) Stage 1: A developing test: at this stage the researcher believes that his *in vitro* test system is of some value and has developed it on the basis of an understanding of the likely mechanism of toxic action. Generally speaking, during this stage relatively few chemicals will have been tested, often as few as 10 and usually less than 100.

b) Stage 2: A developed test: at this stage the test will have been submitted to a formal validation study where the *in vitro* test will have been used to assess the toxicity of more than 100 chemicals of diverse chemical class. The test may already be in use in some laboratories as a predictive test, particularly in those laboratories who have been involved in the validation studies. A successful test will have been demonstrated to have substantial advantages over existing *in vitro* tests or to complement *in vivo* or *in vitro* test systems.

c) Stage 3: An established predictive test: by the time a test has been fully established, it is in use in a number of laboratories internationally and a large number of chemicals, ideally more than 1000, have been tested. As a consequence, the test system has been shown to be of value by a variety of different organizations and an understanding of its utility in extrapolation is beginning to develop. By this stage also, an understanding of the limitations of the test system in its various uses will have been developed.

It will be extremely helpful if new tests were assessed against these guidelines so that practical toxicologists could select the most reliable test for their studies.

Design of Validation Studies

Experience in the conduct of validation studies has suggested that there are various features which are important in the design and interpretation of validation study results (Purchase, 1982). These include,

a) The collection and classification of chemicals: the chemicals used for validation should be selected from as many chemical classes as possible and should be classified according to their toxicity. Different sets of chemicals will require to be used for different end points and their selection is a key to the successful outcome of a validation study. The classification of the chemicals should be carried out prior to the validation study so that there is no uncertainty as to the status of their toxicological classification.

b) The chemicals should be coded so that the experimental toxicologist is faced with assessing chemicals without knowledge of the preferred outcome of the test result.

c) The experimentalist should be required to provide a clear interpretation of the results for each chemical tested. Equivocal results cannot be used easily in validation studies and they detract from the performance of the predictive tests.

d) The chemicals used should be of a high and known purity.

e) The number of chemicals used in validation studies will determine the likely utility of the test system.

f) Collaboration between laboratories is essential to ensure that the tests are robust and reproducible.

g) Information from *in vitro* systems which provide an indication of the mechanism of action, including metabolism, are an advantage.

Reference Chemical Data Bank

Nowadays there are a large number of validation studies being carried out on *in vitro* test systems. It is not unusual to find that a single chemical will be assigned a different toxic classification in the different validation studies. It has been proposed, therefore, that an international database should be set up so that research toxicologists can have a selection of chemicals available for their validation studies (Purchase, 1990).

The development of a reference data bank would require the identification of the appropriate toxicological end point (e.g. skin sensitization or eye irritation). Once this has been achieved an expert group would have to select a number of chemicals based on the structure and chemical class and toxicological properties. A comprehensive literature review would then be needed in order to allow a careful classification of the chemicals into the appropriate classes for validation purposes. It would then be possible to publish a list of chemicals with the expert evaluations and classifications for use by research toxicologists as has been done previously (Purchase *et al.*, 1981, 1987).

It would also be of considerable value to have a central "bank" in which chemicals of known and high purity could be made available to individual researchers for their validation studies. If properly organized, these chemicals could be provided to the researcher as coded samples, thus encouraging him to report back his results. That would allow the reference data bank to accumulate further information on the toxic properties of the chemical so that the toxicological classification could be continually updated.

Conclusion

The principal purpose of toxicity testing to the industrial toxicologist is for the assessment of human hazard so that safe products can be developed and placed on the market. The concern for animal welfare is, however, also important and this is encouraging toxicologists to seek *in vitro* methods to complement or act as alternative methods to the current regulatory *in vivo* methods. However, it would be unwise for industrial toxicologists to comprise their primary mission of protecting human health.

The key to the development of reliable *in vitro* methods is in the appropriate validation of these methods for the assessment of toxic hazard. A critical feature of validation studies is the selection and classification of chemicals for validation. This is an area in which international collaboration could help set up an international reference chemical data bank for use by researchers interested in developing *in vitro* methods. It is likely that the development of such a chemical data bank would provide a signficant acceleration in the development, validation and regulatory acceptance of *in vitro* toxicology tests.

Practical toxicologists may also require to have a rough method of classifying *in vitro* test systems in terms of their utility for practical screening and testing. Such a system is described which divides test systems into developing, developed or established predictive tests.

References

Purchase, I.F.H. (1982). *Mut. Res.* **99**, 51–52.
Purchase, I.F.H. (1990). *ATLA* **18**, 345–348.
Purchase, I.F.H., Clayson, D.B., Preussmann, R. and Tomatis, L. (1981). *In* "Report of the International Collaborative Program on Evaluation of Short-Term Tests for Carcinogens" (J. Ashby and F.J. de Serres, eds), pp. 21–32. Progress in Mutation Research, Vol. 1. Elsevier, New York.
Purchase, I.F.H., Farrar, D.G. and Whitaker, I. (1987). *ATLA* **14**, 184–242.
Rhodes, C., Pemberton, M.A., Scott, R.C. and Oliver, G.J.A. (1986). *Human Toxicol.* **5**, 409–410.

29

The Present Position of *In Vitro* Testing: European Development

T. SMYRNIOTIS

Commission of the European Communities, Directorate General XI, 200 rue de la Loi, 1049 Brussels, Belgium

As we all know, the European Communities' main instrument on animal protection, Directive 86/609/EEC on the protection of animals used for experimental and other scientific purposes, came into force in November 1989. The Commision accepts that animal use in experimentation is at present necessary for the protection of human and animal health and that of the environment as well as for scientific research. The Directive aims to limit the number of animals used by, for instance, the avoidance of duplicate testing, and the mutual recognition of procedure in order to safeguard their welfare to the maximum. Other Community instruments already make reference to the welfare of animals used for experimentation – in fields including animal nutrition, chemicals, cosmetics, food additives, medicines, pesticides and toxicology – and the Commission's current programmes for environmental research and biotechnology aim at the reduction or replacement of animal tests specified in Community regulations, and the development of *in vitro* testing for toxicity and biological activity.

The Commission has a commitment to the goals not only of the internal market and environmental protection in its widest sense, but also to the public in Europe, where there is a need to respond to legitimate concerns

IN VITRO METHODS IN TOXICOLOGY
ISBN 0-12-388175-7

while seeking to avoid extremist positions of all kinds. In recent years, society in Western Europe has demonstrated increasing disquiet with regard to the use of live animals for experimental purposes. This disquiet has stimulated a reappraisal of the rationale underlying human society's use of other species for the experimentation. It is also quite clear that the current trend towards stricter controls is only the first step in the process. The challenge has been laid down to those responsible for the use of animals, principally regulators, industry and scientists, to find alternatives to animal tests.

For regulators concerned with the safety testing of new products prior to registration and/or marketing, the essential requirements for any alternative test method, or test battery, are that they should ensure the same level of protection for man and the environment as the test or tests the alternative is designed to replace. While opportunities currently exist for modifying some test procedures in order to reduce both the numbers of animals used and the degree of suffering to which they are subjected, there are at present very few *in vitro* methods which have been developed to the point where they could be acceptable as part of a regulatory testing scheme. Regulatory bodies should continue to fund research into alternative methods and, where appropriate, provide a mechanism for the evaluation and validation of such methods. The Commission has recently outlined its position with respect to these issues in the Report (COM/88/243) submitted in conformity with Article 23 of the animal experimentation Directive.

In the majority of cases, references to animal testing in Community legislation take the form of guidelines, or notes for guidance, concerning necessary toxicological data which should accompany an application for the placing on the market, or the use, of certain products or ingredients. In some instances such guidelines, or notes for guidance, form part of the text of the legislation itself, as is the case for pharmaceuticals, whereas for other product areas they have been drawn up by one of the Communities' Scientific Advisory Committees. Guidelines or notes for guidance often allow sufficient flexibility so that alternative methods can be used as and when they become available.

I would like now to comment briefly on the problems in the field of industrial chemicals. The 1967 Council Directive on dangerous chemicals (67/548/EEC), as amended for the sixth time by Directive 79/831/EEC, concerns the classification, packaging and labelling of dangerous substances, and requires that before a new substance can be placed on the market a technical dossier must be submitted containing, among other information, toxicological data, including LD_{50} values, and the results of eye and skin irritation tests. The methods which have to be followed in completing these tests are described in detail in Annex V of the Directive, the first part of which was published as a Commission Directive in 1984 (84/449/EEC) and the second part in 1988 (88/133/EEC). Other pieces of Community legislation, existing and proposed, refer to the testing methods required under Directive 67/548/EEC, e.g. additives in animal nutrition, Council Directive 87/153/EEC and the Council Directive concerning dangerous preparations (89/376/EEC).

Directive 67/548/EEC is a central piece of Community legislation which has harmonized chemicals control in the Community. However, it has frequently been criticized for its inflexibility and is often cited as an example of legislation provoking needless animal suffering and testing. In the face of such criticism it has to be pointed out that before its introduction each Community Member State could require different information to be supplied before substances were placed on the market and that this often led to a duplication of animal testing. Now, with the mutual acceptance of data, tests only need to be carried out once according to the prescribed method, and the results are accepted throughout the Community. It is therefore undoubtedly the case that this Directive has brought about a considerable reduction in the total number of animals used for chemicals testing. The Commission is, however, sensitive to its responsibilities to renew the testing requirements of the Directive and an updating procedure has already been initiated.

Annex V of the Directive currently contains some 70 methods for the safety testing of chemicals of which approximately 25 involve the use of vertebrate animals. These methods are constantly being added to and improved and there are groups of national experts in the areas of toxicology, mutagenesis and ecotoxicology who are responsible for the scientific evaluation of new methods or suggested improvements.

Until recently the normal route for the introduction of a new or improved method into the testing package has been as follows: a Member State submits a recommendation to the committee with overall responsibility for the development of testing methods, the Coordinating Committee. This committee and its associated expert sub-groups evaluate the initial proposal and if the method is considered intrinsically valuable, the normal situation is for it to be ring tested throughout the Community. On the basis of the ring test, the method is usually amended and finally adopted for future introduction to the Annex V in all nine languages. This process, proposal stage to publication in the Official Journal, can take up to 5 or 6 years.

In evaluating proposals for new or amended methods, a number of different criteria have been applied.

1) Correspondence to the legal requirements of the Directive (Annex VII, Annex VIII).
2) Intrinsic scientific merit.

3) Repeatability.
4) The utility of the data so derived with respect to classification, labelling and risk assessment.

The latter criterion is often ignored or forgotten, and sometimes regarded as an unnecessary bureaucratic interference in an essentially scientific problem. This is a mistake: the only reason for carrying out safety testing of chemicals in a legislative context is in order to protect man and the environment. This objective is achieved in the case of the EEC Directive on dangerous chemicals by classification, labelling and by risk assessment followed by risk management, i.e. restriction on use. If the data derived from the testing programmes do not lend themselves to this use, then they are virtually useless in a legal context.

In the past, decision-making has been relatively easy. When legislation requiring the systematic safety testing of chemicals was introduced in the 70s, existing methods from classical toxicology were taken off the shelf and were built into the testing schemes; we are talking here about LD_{50}, Draize skin and eye irritation tests, etc. As a result, a whole approach of classification and labelling and risk assessment has been based upon the end points derived from these types of tests.

Over the last 10 years, we have, of course, tried to modify or improve our testing methods, but usually this has involved an adaptation of the existing approach, i.e. carrying out LD_{50} on one sex only, using only one animal in the Draize eye test, etc. But the point is that the end points were the same and they were all immediately compatible with the classification and labelling schemes and the risk assessment models which had been painstakingly developed in the intervening years. The problem is that we cannot ignore this historical perspective. Thousands of chemicals have been classified and labelled using schemes based on LD_{50} and classical Draize tests, etc. and decisions have been taken based upon risk assessments using the same data.

So now, we return to our current problems: the evaluation of alternative testing methods. Our shopping list of criteria for evaluation will remain the same:

1) Correspondence to legal requirements.
2) Scientific merit.
3) Repeatability.
4) Utility of the data so derived with respect to classification, labelling and risk assessment.

But the application of the criteria is now more difficult.

1) As the current legal requirements often specify traditional end points, the legislation must be changed and made more flexible.
2) Intrinsic scientific merit or validity becomes even more pertinent now. Even

a layman can see the direct relevance of classical skin and eye irritation methods to the eventual protection of man and the environment, even though one may argue that results from one species will never entirely predict the response of another. But if it is justifiable to try to predict the potential of a chemical to irritate or damage skin or the eye, how can *in vitro* techniques either individually or as part of a test battery enable a sufficient understanding of the potential effect of a chemical to say with confidence that this substance is or is not a potential danger to the human skin/eye during normal use? The question is an extremely complex one which could easily take up an entire seminar. But this fundamental question of the scientific validation and the appropriate mechanisms and criteria to be applied is one that needs to be resolved at an international level.

3) Repeatability: the problem is the same as for classical methods.

4) Utility of the data from classification and labelling etc. Some scientists say that this is not our problem. That is an abdication of responsibility. To produce a series of alternative test methods for the safety testing of chemicals, methods which are perfect in that they completely satisfy criteria 2 and 3 and yet are completely useless in a regulatory context, are an irresponsible waste of money. In the evaluation of alternative methods it must be demonstrated: (1) how the alternative methods can be used to classify chemicals, i.e. to differentiate and discriminate between the relative potential of chemicals to poison, to irritate, to sensitize etc.; (2) how they can be realistically integrated into models for risk assessment; (3) how classification, labelling and risk assessment based on the new methods relate to the old classification, labelling and risk assessment based upon previous methodologies.

In demonstrating the ability of new methods to satisfy these criteria, scientists should not ignore the fact that administrators using schemes or models for classification and labelling, etc. are faced with over 100 000 existing chemical substances, millions of preparations and, every year, thousands more arriving on the market. It is unreasonable to say, as some toxicologists do, that each substance must be evaluated, case by case, and that only expert judgement is of any value. This is to ignore reality: such systems have to be relatively simple and applicable on a day to day basis by industry and government.

Having said this, the Commission intends to play an active role in coordinating the development and validation of alternative methods. This is in accordance with article 23.1 of the Directive 86/609/EEC on animal experimentation which requires the Commission and the Member States to encourage research into the development and validation of alternative techniques.

On the other hand, paragraph 21 of the Report to the Council, states: "the Commission is aware of the considerable research activities taking place within the Member States, both publicly and privately funded, and proposes that the Commission should be involved in the co-ordination of information exchange on these research activities".

Paragraph 23 of the same Report states "The Commision recognizes that a critical stage in the development of an alternative method is the transition from that of a potentially useful procedure to that of a method accepted as a part of a regulatory testing system. The Commission therefore proposes to provide a framework for the evaluation of alternative test procedures".

On the basis of discussions with representatives of the different Member States it is clear that there are many research initiatives, both publicly and privately funded, which have been launched throughout the Community. While such initiatives are sometimes coordinated at a national level, any coordination at a Community level takes place on a voluntary basis only with information being exchanged frequently after the event. Thus, within the regular meetings of contact points established under Directive 86/609/EEC, a mechanism for information exchange on research activities has been foreseen. However, such information exchange covers only publicly funded initiatives and even in these cases Member States simply provide information on decisions which have already been taken.

Similarly, it is apparent that programmes have been initiated to validate potential alternative methods in some cases involving a duplication of effort and a waste of resources.

It should also be remembered that validation of an alternative test method is an expensive business. To carry out such a validation for one alternative method on a European scale would require the participation of 30–40 laboratories using the same test protocol and applying this to some 40–50 pre-selected test chemicals. It has been estimated that to carry out one test on one chemical would cost in the region of 500 ECU. This gives an approximate cost for the whole validation exercise of between 600 000 and 1 000 000 ECU and there are hundreds of alternative methods waiting to be validated.

The only way the costs of these validation exercises can be controlled is for the participating laboratories to absorb some or all of the costs. As the majority of the participating laboratories are industrial, it is obvious that an extensive programme of validation can only be envisaged with the active support and participation of industry.

In discussions with organizations concerned with alternative testing methods in both Europe and the USA, the barrier of validation is now seen as the single biggest obstacle to the realization of their objectives.

Both the development and the validation of alternative test methods is something that should be coordinated at a European level. Member States, industry and possibly animal welfare groups should be involved in this process; such coordination will avoid a duplication of effort. This is why the Commission services are studying the possibility of establishing a European Centre for Alternative Testing Methods. The objectives and functions of this Centre would be as follows:

1) To coordinate the development activities of alternative procedures within the Community and to act as an information centre with regard to these research activities.

2) To coordinate the validation of alternative testing methods at a Community level. This will involve the standardization of test protocols, the choice of test substances, the organization of double-blind trials and the analysis and evaluation of results.

3) To maintain and manage a data base on alternative testing methods with associated support and user services-help-line, advice service, etc.

4) To act as a conduit for dialogue between regulators, industry and animal welfare groups resulting in the development and validation of test methods which will be accepted internationally.

5) To act as a European focal point for alternative testing methods including as appropriate the organization of conferences, workshops and symposia.

We believe that the establishmment of this Centre will have an enormous impact on the development and acceptance of alternative testing methods.

30

The Position of Academic and Government-Funded Research on *In Vitro* Testing

G. MAHOUY

INSERM, Institut d'Hématologie, Hôpital Saint-Louis-75010, Paris, France

There is no difference in outlook between government-funded and private research with respect to the need to develop and perfect *in vitro* methods. This clearly involves the creation of tests which could enable a reduction in experiments using animals, and, if possible, to replace them. In theory, this would offer only advantages to the researcher, since such *in vitro* methods would make it possible to limit the number of parameters and variables. These tests could also be expected to cost less, though this point still requires confirmation in terms of the costs of infrastructures, reagents and the specialized staff required.

Nevertheless, a certain ambiguity persists concerning the meaning of the word "alternative", and this ambiguity explains in part why this word has become so popular. In the English sense of the term, it suggests that the investigator has the choice between tests of equal performance, some *in vivo* and others *in vitro*, and thus that the questions asked of these models and the results obtained are identical. But we know very well that, while in many cases cell and tissue cultures offer the appropriate solution particularly for the study of molecular and cellular mechanisms, they are unable to take into account the diversity and complexity of the interaction and regulating mechanisms that occur within a complete living

IN VITRO METHODS IN TOXICOLOGY
ISBN 0-12-388175-7

organism. To oppose *in vivo* and *in vitro* methods has no scientific basis. Each of these methods offers a different and complementary manner of approaching a question which has been raised. It is for this reason that the sense of the word "alternative" in French seems to correspond better to reality, since it means "a succession of two things or events which recur in turn" (*Dictionary of the French Language*. Paul-Emile Littré. Encyclopaedia Britannica Inc., Chicago, 1982). In other words, the researcher aware of the advantages, disadvantages and limitations of each method (whole animal, isolated organs, cell cultures) is able to and should move from *in vivo* to *in vitro* and vice versa, according to the complexity of the problems raised and the systems studied. My reason for stressing this point is that I feel that there has been excessive and sometimes inaccurate publicity regarding these problems, raising false hopes among the general public. Therefore, it must be clearly stated that it is highly unlikely that alternative methods could one day totally replace experiments using live animals.

This obviously in no way means that we must not continue to pursue our efforts in the development of *in vitro* tests. Moreover, research at international level with the aim of saving animal lives is impressive. The high quality studies presented at this scientific meeting are an excellent illustration.

A consensus has emerged during this round table in considering that *in vitro* tests should be used routinely in the prescreening of compounds as well as in studying the basic biological mechanisms of toxicity. This point seems particularly positive. A very large number of *in vitro* methods have been suggested for testing toxicity on target organs, reproduction and carcinogenesis. I have noted that some of these methods necessitate large numbers of animals. This would not appear to comply with the aims of the Directive 86/609/EEC which, it should be recalled, are not only to avoid unnecessary suffering but also to reduce to a minimum the number of animals used.

The major problem, and no doubt the one that will be most difficult to resolve, is to demonstrate the reliability of these methods in such a way as to obtain their validation by Health Care Authorities. A very strict approach is required at this stage of research, from both a scientific (interpretation of results) and technical standpoint. It is essential that *in vitro* tests should not be validated prematurely because of various pressures. The consequences could be catastrophic for man but also for animals, since *in vitro* methods would then lose their credibility. Unfortunately, there are precedents. By way of an example, and in a field other than toxicology, we should remember that the safety of a batch of inactivated antipoliomyelitis vaccine was tested on cell cultures in 1955. This batch, which was manufactured by Cutter Laboratories in the USA, was found by this method to be properly inactivated, but caused 250 cases of poliomyelitis among those vaccinated, including five deaths. Subsequent inoculation of monkeys with samples from the same batch showed that the virus had been poorly inactivated. This led to the routine reintroduction of this test in animal experiments considered to be more sensitive than cell cultures. Would it not have been better to have previously ensured the perfect reliability of this *in vitro* method?

What should be the contribution of academic and public research in the development of these *in vitro* tests? It is clear that its role is not to take on the study and selection of methods that would have the best chance for validation. Its purpose is, above all, basic biomedical research. In France, it has two sources of logistical support: research institutions may wholly or in part be responsible for laboratories specializing in the development of these *in vitro* techniques; ministries can also propose and subsidize programmes on specific themes. Thus in 1988 and 1989 the Ministry of Research and Technology undertook to finance two research programmes. The first was devoted to substitute methods in the field of acute toxicity studies and involved the participation of a network of laboratories coordinated by Dr Monique Adolphe on the subject "Improvement in cellular models and development of new methods for evaluation of the toxic signal". The second group, coordinated by Dr André Guillouzo, concerned itself with a multicentric study of acute hepatotoxicity *in vitro*. The aim of these projects was to promote the proposal of standard protocols for the detection of toxicity of new compounds and new products likely to come on to the market. Thus, the contribution of academic and government-funded research is to present new ideas and new technologies, and to test them in cooperation with the pharmaceutical industry.

31

General Discussion

Question 1

C. Roux
Should we use the term "alternative"? Is it not confusing, and would the use of "complementary" not be better?

M. Balls
I think it is too late. This argument was over 10 years ago; the debate is sterile and it is time it was stopped. The Three Rs* definition of alternatives is now widely accepted internationally and we should all agree to use the term alternative. *In vitro* methods can be used as screens, as adjunct or complementary methods alongside animal methods, and as replacements. The word complementary does not apply to prescreens or to replacements, so replacing alternative by complementary would not be an improvement, nor would it reduce confusion.

I. Purchase
I believe that sometimes the word alternative needs qualifying in terms of the purpose for which we want to use it. There are four alternative methods of transport: walking, bicycle, car or plane. If we want to go to

---

* Three Rs = Reduction, Refinement, Replacement.

Geneva we might choose some of them, and the others would be alternatives; if we want to go to New York, different ones might be chosen, and the others would not be alternatives.

G. Mahouy
Prof. Bertrand gave me a definition of alternative in the French language. There are two concepts in the word. It can mean that one method is used, then another, then back to the first one – and so on. Or there is the choice between two methods giving the same results. In the French language at least, alternative should cover the whole field.

M. Balls
In the English language, the word alternative was first used in the last century by the British Prime Minister, William Gladstone, to mean one of a range of choices, not just a direct replacement, one for another. The word alternative in English has a looser meaning; it is not used in a precise way.

Question 2

R. Ulrich
Apart from ourselves and each other, who else do we most need to convince that we have developed and/or can develop alternatives?

M. Balls
I think the people who most need to be convinced are the toxicologists who use animal tests and who are happy to carry on doing so, regulators who think that they can base risk assessment for humans on animal tests, physiologists, pathologists and lawyers. Those who already believe in the potential of alternative tests are politicians, members of the general public and animal welfare advocates.

I think we need increasing debate about both the potential of alternatives and the need for their development. We need honesty at all levels, as Dr Purchase mentioned earlier. The worker who pushes his test based on 10 surfactants as an alternative to the Draize eye test is only doing damage to a field which deserves more serious treatment. We also need more education, so that there is greater realism among toxicologists, the general public and animal welfare advocates.

J. Frazier
There is a difficult situation in terms of the general public, many people not having the scientific background to appreciate the nuances of the

science about which we are talking. These problems are tremendously complex. In terms of education, this is clearly an audience for whom some specific approaches are needed that are designed to explain the complexities of the issues, so that there is not the misconception that one test can replace the whole world of animal toxicology. I do not think a large proportion of the general population understand and appreciate these issues.

This is an audience that needs better education, so that they are able to deal better with the solutions to the problems that will in the long run provide for public safety as well as reduce animal use in toxicological activities.

A. Paine

I would support what has been said. Regulators are working within the framework laid down by the law. I would not say that lawyers are any better scientifically qualified than the general public. It is very important to convince lawyers that alternatives do or do not exist. As far as I understand it, in all product liability law now there is a notion that animal experiments have been done.

M. Balls

I mentioned lawyers for that very reason. Ultimately, it is the courts where decisions are made; for example, if there are claims against companies because of possible damage as a result of exposure to their products.

R. Ulrich

One of the things that we like to do in science, of course, is to focus attention on one question at a time. It is very difficult to answer 50, or sometimes 5, questions all at the same time. The framework of my question was who do we *most* need to convince first. Unfortunately, our biggest constraint is financial. We will not do much good if we continue to diffuse the money and try to convince everybody all at once, all the many isolated groups, that we are trying to do the right thing here. On whom do we really need to target our efforts first, in order to make the money well spent? I do not know if this question can be answered.

F. Zucco

In terms of public information, we also have to stress the role of the press which today plays a big role between the scientific world and public opinion. This requires some thought.

H. van Looy

I believe this question is complicated. What do you want to convince those people about? That there is a potential in and a hope for alternatives? That alternative methods cannot be used today? These are the more important questions.

M. Balls

That is a good point. There is nothing unique about alternatives. Politicians need education in more things than this, as do the general public and ourselves.

M. Bertrand

I think that there are two groups of people who have to be convinced: first, the scientists who, like those of my generation, and after the example of Claude Bernard, are used to working with live animals. They must be shown the potential of *in vitro* tests – and this has been remarkably well presented in the last two days. The other group who have to be convinced include not only journalists, but also animal welfare activists. This is why in Lyon we have set up an ethics committee for the Rhône-Alpes region, which includes members who are responsible for experimentation as well as representatives of the national confederation for animal welfare groups. In this way, we can inform the scientists about the various possibilities offered by *in vitro* methods, help them to choose and explain their experiments, and also "dedramatize" the problem, explaining to the media and to animal welfare groups why research is necessary and thus avoid the violent acts which are regretted by everyone.

Question 3

R. Ulrich

Should serum be used in tissue culture media or should we work to provide serum-free defined media?

M. Balls

During all the 30 years that I have been working in tissue culture, we have been talking about serum. Defined media can be a useful basis for doing more precise work, but the normal physiological state of most cells in the body is to be surrounded by a complex protein-containing solution. That is not foetal calf serum though; there are local factors which alter what is received from the systemic circulation, so that very important micro-environments are produced. I think more work is needed on these micro-environments, as a basis for maintaining differentiated function *in vitro*, also on media and on developing conditions which will provide the kind of cells and tissues in culture that we want to be able to use. This is a huge topic on which we probably should not dwell at length today.

I. Purchase
It seems to me that the artificial environment in which cells are grown *in vitro* is ameliorated only by the introduction of serum. I believe that in the next 20 or 30 years all these various polypeptide and other messaging and nutritional factors which go to support a cell and are found in serum will gradually be identified. There will then be a library of tools which will enable us to create a cell type, to produce a particular result that we want. [*Dr Balls and Dr Ulrich agreed*]

A. Vernadakis
I wonder whether those of us who use brain cultures should use cerebrospinal fluid (CSF) as a substitute. CSF is really closest to the medium with which the cells come in contact. What do colleagues who use brain cultures think about this? Perhaps some company might start collecting CSF from animals.

C. Atterwill
I agree with Dr Vernadakis and the other questioners that we have to produce better media, especially for brain cells, because of the known barrier between the blood and the cells of the brain. If for special tests like EYTEX and SKINTEX, for example, whole lens or skin protein solutions can be developed, why cannot people work on artificial CSF or other solutions for cells in culture?

M. Balls
If people tell us that they use certain growth factors for their cultures, it is important that their papers should not be published unless those factors are available for other workers. Often when we call Sigma and try to obtain something in their catalogue, we are told that it is "not available", presumably because somebody has cornered the whole supply. A certain dishonesty has been involved in the past there, which should not be allowed. It is unprofessional.

I. Purchase
If we were to use CSF either as an *in vitro* culture medium or to contribute to one, it would be very expensive in terms of its requirement for animals.

F. Zucco
A point that antivivisectionists have raised with me concerns serum. Serum comes from animals, so it is a vicious circle.

M. Balls
Most of the serum that is used comes as a by-product of the killing of animals for other purposes, although, of course, horse serum tends to be produced from horses kept for that purpose. It is likely to cause the horses little suffering, and they probably have a good life in between the blood collections to provide serum. Foetal calf serum comes from foetal calves produced when cows are slaughtered for meat. Alternatives are not a way out of all ethical dilemmas.

Question 4

X. Pouradier Duteil
Should we prefer to use primary cell cultures or continuous cell lines?

M.Balls
This is another much debated topic. In the next issue of *Alternatives to Laboratory Animals (ATLA)*, Oliver Flint has written a very provocative article arguing in favour of the use of primary cultures only. I disagree with almost everything he has written, but it will certainly stimulate discussion. In my opinion, any system is appropriate for use, provided that it is used for the purposes for which it is suited and that we are aware of any limitations it may have. This is more or less what Dr Purchase said earlier.

A. Paine
There is not a black and white answer; it depends upon the question we are trying to answer. Many cells obviously do not divide in primary culture, so if we are interested in cell proliferation, it is a waste of time to use them.

M. Balls
Hepatocytes do not divide, but some other primary cultures do.

J. Frazier
I think the issue is one of science that needs to be investigated further. There have recently been some papers about some of the issues involved in comparing primary cultures with cell lines in hepatocytes and probably

in other areas. This is a key question. If somebody could design some nice comparative studies, they would be of significant benefit to answering this particular question in the context of toxicological evaluations.

J.E. Trosko
I agree with what has been said – with one exception. If we understand the question and the limitations, virtually any cell line, primary, transformed or whatever, could be used to answer specific questions. However, there is one question that is fundamental to understanding human carcinogenesis. People are trying to understand it *in vitro* by using human fibroblasts when 80% of human cancers are carcinomas. More importantly, even if we have primary human epithelial cells as a starting point, the people in this field seem to have ignored the statement published by the National Academy of Science in 1975 that not all cells of the body give rise to tumours. In fact, it seems to be stem cells that are responsible. If we are going to ask specific questions, if we want to understand the process of human carcinogenesis *in vitro*, we have to start with the right cells – that is, stem cells – and go forward from there.

Question 5

A. Vernadakis and P. Kramer
Should we use human cells and tissues wherever possible?

M. Balls
Yes, ideally, if we want to predict potential toxicity in man. If we can use human cells *in vitro*, and if we are trying to predict human effects *in vivo*, we then avoid the problem of extrapolation. The species difference problem can be overcome in that way. If, of course, we are trying to use animal data in a validation study or to duplicate animal data, it is more appropriate to use animal cells.

The MEIC scheme, run from Stockholm, has shown that human cell lines sometimes give a better prediction of human toxicity *in vivo* than animal cell lines. One example is digoxin. The people using animal cells in cytotoxicity tests failed to discover the toxicity of digoxin for man, whereas all the human cell lines used in other laboratories picked it up.

I think human hepatocytes are easier to handle than rat hepatocytes. They are more tolerant of the time between obtaining the tissue and isolating the cells. There are possibly also some practical advantages. However, there are ethical problems involved in obtaining human cells, as well as safety and logistical problems. When we get human liver cells, it is always 3 o'clock in the morning on a public holiday, never at 9 o'clock on a Monday morning!

J. Frazier

I think what has been said is correct. The utilization of human cells hopefully solves the problem of the species extrapolation issue, although it clearly does not solve the problem of *in vitro/in vivo* extrapolation, which still has to be dealt with.

In the USA, though, there have been significant efforts to provide human tissues for experimental purposes. The National Disease Research Interchange programme, funded by the Federal Government, has over 120 surgical centres at hospitals around the USA with the specific purpose of obtaining materials for biomedical research. I am not sure whether there is any equivalent organization in the European Community (EC), but the objective of such an organization is to provide human tissues, to maximize their utilization for research purposes.

Efforts are therefore being made to try to solve the problem of human tissue supply. I can only encourage those efforts to go forward.

I. Purchase

Dr Balls said earlier that *in vitro* tests have to be validated to much higher standards than *in vivo* toxicology studies, the argument being that the latter have not been validated in the same way. In fact, the way in which *in vivo* toxicology studies have developed is by taking sensible steps in a stepwise fashion. It seems to me that the argument that has developed about the use of human tissues might be seen in that light. It is a sensible step, but it is a black box – we do not actually know. I would have thought that the *in vitro* toxicologist would want to wait until he had this higher level of scientific proof before he was prepared to do it.

M. Balls

I accept that entirely. When Dr Purchase's reference chemical databank is established, it will be important that he and his colleagues look for human data where they are available. It is true that the quality of human data available at the moment is even more variable than that of animal data, but this does not mean that we should give up.

P. Kramer

There were several major reasons for raising this question, including the following:

1) I perhaps see some problems with primary cells from human tissue, because they are obtained from different people with different histories. This may cause problems in standardizing tests.

2) I would also like to mention the ethical problems which have already been discussed. There are different ethical attitudes in different countries. In Germany, in particular, with our history, it is very difficult to get human tissues, especially for use in industry.

A. Vernadakis

My concern about human cells is in neurotoxicology: how do we test neurotoxicology? We can get liver and parietal cells, but how do we obtain neurons which will be close to the human response?

M. Balls

A great deal is being done with brain slices in animals. There is no reason why we should not have human brain slices – but human brain is not nice material to have around, because of the risk of contracting infectious diseases.

G. Moonen

In response to Dr Vernadakis, I can say that we have designed a method of cultivating adult rat dorsal root ganglion neurons and have applied it to adult humans, taking ganglions from patients operated on for spinal cord tumours. We can obtain 40 cultures from one ganglion and keep them for several months *in vitro*. This opens up the possibility of doing neurotoxicology on adult human neurons *in vitro*.

J. Frazier

I look at the heterogeneity, the polymorphism, in the human populations in two ways. First, it is correct from a statistical point of view that there is variability but, secondly, the positive aspect is that variability is one of the components needed for the risk assessment process. As toxicology is done today with animal testing, very homogeneous populations of animals are used, a set of data is developed from them and extrapolated to the human case by whatever formulae there are for extrapolation for scaling. The safety factors are then thrown in, one of which is for the uncertainty in the extrapolation, and another is for the variability in the human population. The variability is not known, so a factor is used without it having any scientific basis.

If, in fact, human tissues are used for the evaluations, it may take more samples and more analysis, but it will give some measurement of this variability. This can then be used directly in the safety evaluation to justify whether human populations are homogeneous with respect to a response or whether there is a wide diversity, and therefore the safety factor that may be put into the equation can be justified.

J.E. Trosko

I am chief of research on the most studied human population on earth – 120 000 Japanese who have been exposed to the atomic bomb very momentarily, but subsequently for 45 years have been exposed to all kinds of chemicals, in their diet, work-place, drugs and so on. It is a goldmine for toxicologists. No-one is using this information, either retrospectively or prospectively. I invite anyone who wants human toxicological data to come to Hiroshima.

I look at this in a positive sense, that very useful toxicological information is obtained from these kinds of analysis, and that it is not just a statistical problem.

M. Balls

It is very important to make those data available. There are a lot of schemes at the moment for collecting and critically assessing human data. I hope that Dr Trosko's data will be included in that.

B. Bkaily

It is very important that any laboratory that wants to use a human tissue must also do animal testing. Not everybody has access to human tissue, so if the test is not repeated in animals it cannot always be repeated in other laboratories.

Question 6

C. Atterwill

Do early in vivo *studies permit the identification of potential toxicity, or should senior corporate management insist on the use of a battery of screens, in order to reduce the financial impact of the loss of a lead compound later in development?*

Secondly, should the authorities responsible for animal protection laws insist on this approach in order to reduce unnecessary large-scale use of animals?

I. Purchase

The easiest framework within which to answer the first question is the time frame in which we are working. Once a new chemical structure has been invented for, say, an agrochemical (or a pharmaceutical or some other compound) and a patent placed on it, the clock starts ticking. There is a set number of years in which that information can be exploited and the product sold to pay back the investment made in research. Typically, a patent life is about 20 years, and the development stage can take anything from 6 years to 10–14 years. If it takes as long as 10 years, there are only 10 years in which to recoup the costs before somebody else can make the chemical without the investment in the research. That is the important point.

Against that background, it is vitally important for industry to try to get the toxicology done, first, in a way which will not waste chemicals and, secondly, as quickly as possible. Most companies now will do screening tests of various types, *in vivo*, *in vitro* or QSAR, as early as possible, while there are still many different end points, in order to try to screen out those toxicological phenomena.

However, at the moment, it is based not on an empirical list of screening tests but on the skill, experience and knowledge of the toxicologist. He will look at a structure and say that he does not like that sort of chemical, it looks like a carcinogen or a reproductive toxin – and then special testing is done.

We are not yet at the stage, scientifically, when a battery of tests could be put up which would assure us that problems would not be encountered in repeat-dose studies.

C. Atterwill
Dr Purchase mentioned that the predictive value of *in vivo* toxicology tests is extremely good, and that few compounds enter the market and subsequently produce toxic effects which were in the regulatory test battery. In the drug industry, however, quite a number of compounds have entered the market that either have serious adverse reactions reported against them that have been missed in toxicology studies or have to be withdrawn completely from the market for other reasons.

I. Purchase
It is correct that sometimes toxicology tests, whether *in vitro* or *in vivo*, have not predicted those results. Equally, it must be remembered that during its development a pharmaceutical compound has been through clinical studies using a limited number of people and which did not show toxic side effects. Very frequently, we are dealing with a very low incidence effect, 1 in 10000 or something like that. It is conceptually quite difficult to see how such low incidence effects can be picked up by *in vitro*, *in vivo* or clinical studies in man. All those examples that have

been withdrawn after launch were actually submitted to clinical studies in man: if clinical studies have not predicted them, it is asking a lot to expect the laboratory studies to do so.

M. Balls

It is also important for the protection of the work-force, is it not, that there is some early information on which to make that decision?

I. Purchase

Yes, but that early information is derived from relatively few animals. That is not the expensive part of the studies in terms of animals.

J. Frazier

Dr Purchase raised the issue of structure–activity relationships, which have been somewhat neglected at this meeting. This aspect should not be ruled out in terms of its potential. The science that will go into these relationships should also be taken into consideration in the future.

C. Atterwill

I agree with Dr Purchase. More efforts need to be made to harmonize the way in which companies adopt prescreening procedures and the number of compounds that the research chemists are willing to produce to allow some form of rational screening. The more compounds screened by *in vitro* or simple *in vivo* methods, the less the chance that harmful compounds will enter the market later on and the less animals will be used in the developmental regulatory studies.

M. Balls

I think the thought behind Dr Atterwill's second question leads to an answer in the affirmative. In the future, when prescreens are available, it would be quite legitimate for the authorities responsible for animal protection laws to insist that they are used at this early stage.

Question 7

Y. Vandenberghe

What roles can in vitro *methods play in the development of new drugs?*

    1) At which stages can they be useful?
    2) Are they already contributing to a reduction in the use of animals?

3) If used at a very early stage, is there a risk that potentially valuable compounds will be lost?
4) Will in vitro *tests come to be required as part of regulatory toxicology?*

M. Balls

I think that *in vitro* methods are already very useful in pharmacology and have led to a dramatic reduction in the use of animals in screening for pharmacological activity. This leads to a more scientific base to the toxicology approach with drugs, which is now normally based on more information about the compound and its interaction with biological systems.

At any stage of development there is a risk that good compounds will be lost. Judgements are made, and inevitably sometimes, with hindsight, a judgement may be seen as having been wrong.

J. Frazier

The issue of false positives, which is what we mean in talking about throwing out compounds that have value, is an extremely important issue that has to be dealt with. In designing methodologies for these kinds of evaluations, we have to be as sensitive to the issue of false positives as to that of false negatives. If there is either a single method or a group of methods which cumulatively gives a very high false positive rate, the methodology will not be useful from a practical point of view.

It is absolutely certain that *in vitro* tests will come to be required as part of regulatory toxicology – indeed, they already are in genotoxicity testing.

T. Smyrniotis

In the future, of course *in vitro* tests, if properly validated, will be required in regulatory toxicology, provided that they are not more animal-consuming than the *in vivo* tests. We have to be very careful about that.

M.T. van der Venne

In terms of prescreening in the development of new chemicals, we are not talking about regulatory toxicology because, as everybody must be aware, in the Commission of the European Communities we have legislation to control substances that are put on the market. When preliminary research is being done we do not intervene in that.

Differing situations apply to industrial chemicals and to pharmaceuticals. For the former, legislation controls only notification, classification and labelling. The EC 6th Amendment is not intended for risk assessment.

Risk assessment, limitation and banning of chemicals require other legislation and are no longer a question of toxicological aspects.

It is different for pharmaceuticals and pesticides, where it is a matter of registration, and there is a possibility of acceptance or refusal of pharmaceuticals or pesticides: other legislation deals with that aspect.

We are not concerned with prescreening at the developmental level, but it is obvious – and I support what Mr Smyrniotis said – that we want to have these *in vitro* methods. The Commission is open to suggestions and, as Dr Balls knows well, we have already tried to do two pilot studies, one on skin irritation and one on eye irritation. Next month we will try to evaluate our results.

I would stress (as has been said by Dr Purchase and other people) that, before the Commission could consider any alternative *in vitro* methods, they must be reproducible, robust and also, let us say, practical. During this meeting we have heard about wonderful research, but there are very few practical, immediate things that can be done. There is a lot of biotechnology, mutagenicity and other sorts of research being funded by the Commission, and that is where people can introduce their proposals.

M. Balls

I think Dr Purchase is sensitive to the issue of robustness, because of the problems of transferability of cell transformation tests between laboratories. However, the fact is that many of the tests being developed, many of the techniques discussed at this meeting, are very readily transferable between laboratories. This is one of the most impressive things about much of the methodology now being developed. There is a sensitivity in genotoxicology, of which we should be aware and to which we should be sympathetic, but we should not see it as limiting what we can try to do in other areas.

J.R. Claude

What Mrs van der Venne said is exactly the same as the position taken by the World Health Organization experts in February 1990.

Question 8

D. Acosta

In developing in vitro *toxicity tests, should we be more aware of the different requirements of various industries – the chemical, the cosmetics and the pharmaceutical industries?*

M. Balls
I think the background to this question is that much of our general discussion is unsatisfactory, because it does not apply equally to the cosmetics, pesticides and pharmaceutical industries. In the first case, products are designed not to enter the body and to be mild, whereas in the latter two cases the products are designed to interact dynamically and helpfully alter the behaviour of biological systems. There are completely different problems involved; for example, with pesticides, the chemicals are designed to be highly toxic to something, which is a completely different situation from that with cosmetics or drugs.

The answer to the question is both yes and no. In developing potential alternative tests or batteries of tests for irritants, there are a whole set of questions, such as length of exposure, concentration of test material, type of compound and physical form of material, all of which have a big effect on what we are doing.

As a developer of tests, I think it is our job to develop tests with potential. If particular industries are interested in modifying them for their own particular purposes, that is an essential further phase of test development.

I. Purchase
I agree that it depends upon the purpose of the test: it is the same question that is always raised in this field. It has not been brought out in the discussion so far that industry is not interested in toxic chemicals, but in *non-toxic* chemicals. We are not testing for toxicity, but for non-toxicity.

This is very important, because many of the screening tests, like the Ames test, and even *in vitro* irritation and corrosion tests and so on, are designed to test for the presence of irritation. This nearly always means that to confirm that there is not the potential for toxicity, to show the absence of toxicity, a broader base test has to be used.

This is where I think that idea can be linked into what Dr Balls said. New developments in cosmetics usually involve a reformulation of existing products. There is a method of assuring non-toxicity in terms of topical application, in that cosmetics nearly always go through a human volunteer study. This is a different situation from pesticides, where there is not the opportunity to do human volunteer studies. What we are trying to do there is to confirm as best we can that there is absence of toxicity – without exposing people at all.

This affects our thinking about the structure of screening tests if we perceive them in terms of looking for non-toxic chemicals.

M. Balls

It is also being argued in certain quarters in Europe at the moment that, even in the case of ingredients for cosmetics, full toxicity profiles are needed, including testing to toxic levels in these tests. I understand exactly what Dr Purchase has said, but there are other pressures. Some people believe that we need to know at what levels chemicals are toxic in order to know at what levels they are not.

J. Frazier

I take slight issue with Dr Purchase, but not very much. The issue is not whether something is toxic or non-toxic, because we are not really showing non-toxicity. If that was all we had to decide it would be simple: we would say everything is toxic – and not use anything. In fact, everything *is* toxic. We have good examples of this; for example, there was an article in our newspapers not long ago about a documented case of a baby killed by sodium chloride poisoning because the mother put so much salt in the baby's food.

What we are trying to do is to find the appropriate conditions of use, such that adverse effects are not expected in the populations which become exposed. Within that context, there is a whole spectrum of issues that have to be dealt with in terms of risk assessment and so on.

D. Acosta

I do not really have an answer to my question and realize that a variety of responses can be made. The public's perception of *in vitro* alternatives or tests has been modified in terms of what the press and the media have said and how certain industries have responded to *in vitro* alternatives. Obviously, the cosmetic industry has had a great deal of pressure because of the Draize test, whereas other industries, such as the chemical and the pharmaceutical industries, have not had that pressure. Are these other industries now beginning to feel the same pressure as the cosmetic industry?

Question 9

C. Atterwill

Support for hepatotoxicity studies has already resulted in a range of very useful methods, which are in use and making very worthwhile contributions. Could not similar batteries of tests be found for other types of toxicity, and should not more effort be put into their development and validation?

M. Balls

I definitely think so, yes.

J. Frazier

I also agree. Perhaps the issue is how to get more support to do that, but there needs to be more such effort.

C. Atterwill

I certainly agree with these answers. I asked the question because *in vitro* hepatic preparations seem to have gained more credibility because they support two camps, if you like: they first gained credibility on the metabolism side, and then the toxicologist accepted them, used and further developed them. This should apply to other areas. Therefore, credibility and financial support for method development should be given to other areas.

J. Frazier

I agree with the concept that some areas need additional work. Our centre at Johns Hopkins has supported certain areas specifically with the purpose of trying to promote additional research in undeveloped areas. For example, we have what we call a programme project in hypersensitivity testing where three specific projects have been supported to try to move that area forward. In Dr Atterwill's own field, there will probably soon be a programme project in neurotoxicity, so perhaps we will get some support into that area as well.

Question 10

N.G. Carmichael

Is it true to say that in vitro *models for neurotoxicity are still at the development/research stage and cannot yet be used for routine screening?*

M. Balls

From what I have heard here, I thought the answer was yes – but there are now schemes which deserve validation. Let us look forward to the outcome.

C. Atterwill

I agree that there are batteries of tests which can now be put together, as I described, and can be validated. I think the models exist for good mechanistic work. Therefore, these should be incorporated wherever possible into testing strategies.

N.G. Carmichael

My question was trying to bring out the point made earlier by Dr Frazier, that we have to be realistic about whether we are talking about research or testing. Because I have a research history in neurotoxicity, I am extremely interested in all these things which Dr Atterwill and others described. As research tools, they can be extremely interesting. I think we have to be very realistic, though, and say that we have heard nothing at this meeting which comes close to being a routine testing tool in neurotoxicity.

A. Paine

The inhibition of neuropathy target esterase by organophosphorus compounds has not been mentioned at this meeting. The UK Home Office is sponsoring a formal validation study based on the inhibition of an essentially semi-purified enzyme.

Question 11

P. Kramer and F. Ballet

The problem of extrapolation from simple to complex systems must be addressed; for example, do cell growth kinetics in vitro *reflect what happens* in vivo?

M. Balls

They may possibly do so, but not necessarily – it depends upon what cells we are talking about – nor, in a sense, do they need to. There is quite a lot of evidence that basic cytotoxicity tests in which interference with cell growth is investigated will reflect in a promising way acute lethal toxicity *in vivo*. It appears that whatever damages cell viability, survival and proliferation can in the case of certain classes of compounds reflect what happens when these compounds are given in acute oral dose tests.

P. Kramer

I raised the question of cell growth kinetics because I see an important relationship between them and the duration of treatment *in vitro*. In the conjunctiva of the eye, for example, there is a kind of a monolayer which is confluent and very slowly growing. If a cell culture of quite fast growing cells is used and treated for a few hours, it is not the same situation as in the eye where there is only a very short exposure.

M. Balls

We have just worked out a simple method which involves using cell monolayers and exposing the cells for 1 min to high concentrations of test materials. We think that is often what happens in the eye – short exposure, high concentration. We can look at things like recovery with this system. There has been a lot of talk here about the intelligent use of the possibilities around us, and I think intelligence is something we all have to feed into what we are trying to do. I agree entirely that a 3-day cell growth assay is not necessarily a very good way of trying to find an alternative to the Draize eye test.

F. Ballet

The problem of extrapolation from simple to complex systems is very important, and was addressed earlier by Dr Trosko. It is important to consider it further. When *in vitro* models are extrapolated to *in vivo* models, we are, of course, extrapolating from a simple situation to a complex one. There are a lot of difficulties in so doing, which we usually try to overcome by multiplying the number of simple tests. However, we know that the complex system is not the algebraic sum of simple systems, not a minus, plus, plus, and so on.

For example, there are very different cell types in the liver: hepatocytes, Kupffer cells, endothelial cells and so on. If the activity of a compound is tested on these different cell types, we can have, for example, plus on Kupffer cells, minus on endothelial cells, and plus on hepatocytes, but we do not know the final response. This is very important in this kind of problem.

M. Balls

I think we can all agree with that. However, the more complex the system becomes if it is not human, the greater is the problem of relevance to humans. The more molecular, subcellular, the more universal the phenomenon being studied, the more likely it is to be relevant.

A.P.A.H. Woolley

Do we need to look into the use of invertebrate whole-animal models as a replacement for vertebrate whole-animal models?

M. Balls

I think that is a terrible idea. The problems of species differences and extrapolation from non-human to human would be immeasurably worse if *Drosophila*, earthworms or sea urchins were used – although, as in the case of the *Limulus* for pyrogens, there might be some specific instances where there is a good reason for doing exactly that. We heard from Dr Atterwill about the use of the leech neuron, which is also promising as part of a battery approach.

A.P.A.H. Woolley

Dr Balls' arguments against an alternative model of a complex variety (such as an invertebrate would provide) can equally be applied to *in vitro* models. No matter how hard I try, I cannot convince myself that *in vitro* techniques as we know them at the moment offer a viable alternative.

J.E. Trosko

To me, the Ames assay has been the biggest drawback to our understanding of toxicology that I can imagine. I was trained as a human mammalian geneticist, and Bruce Ames is an excellent first-rate National Academy-quality bacterial geneticist. It turns out that Ames assay positives will not be mutagenic in human cells. Those positives that are mutagenic in the Ames test are not necessarily non-toxic to humans, but can be toxic via mechanisms that have nothing to do with mutagenicity. I even doubt whether positives in the Ames assay are useful for prediction of mutagenicity of those compounds in *Salmonella* in the real world – because *Salmonella* is not normally exposed to an S9 mix!

We have to understand the mechanisms behind what each human disease is to begin with. That is a tall order, and we cannot wait. On the other hand, if we are going to use *in vitro* tests, we must understand their mechanisms – I am not saying we should give them up, because we need practical tests.

I come back to Einstein's point, that the world is complex but it is not complicated. Our view of toxicity is complicated, but this is a reflection of our ignorance; we do not understand the mechanisms of the assays we are using to try to predict toxicology.

P. Beaune

Cells *in vitro* are complex. Much more effort should be put into molecular models, subcellular systems, use of enzymes and so on.

M. Balls

Certainly, the *in vitro* systems we use are not simple. I completely agree with Dr Trosko. We should seek understanding of toxic mechanisms at the cellular and molecular levels, because that would be the basis of the better toxicology of the future.

J. Frazier
In an ideal world in which we understood all the mechanisms of toxicology, toxicity and pathological responses to chemicals, it would presumably be simple to design the testing strategies which would identify those mechanisms. The absence of that complete mechanistic knowledge requires us to take a somewhat more empirical approach to the problem

I have some concerns, along the same lines as Dr Balls, in terms of going to lower animals, because it would introduce unknown variables into the system that would be misleading in terms of toxicological evaluations because of our lack of understanding of mechanisms. Lower animal models for specific mechanistic studies are obviously – and will continue to be – of value because the background work has been done: how that system behaves with respect to that particular component of a biological response has been researched.

Question 12

P. Kramer
Is the labelling of compounds for regulatory purposes already possible on the basis of in vitro *tests alone?*

M. Balls
We have heard that it is possible, particularly in the case of corrosivity to the skin and severe irritancy to the eye. I understand that there are two problems in relation to this. First, some regulatory authorities nevertheless insist that at least one animal is used to confirm skin corrosion or severe eye irritancy. Secondly, some companies do the animal studies anyway, in case a regulatory authority asks for confirmation in animals. I think both these practices are immoral and should be stopped.

Is it true that things can be labelled as corrosive without doing the confirmatory animal test?

I. Purchase
Like all these things, it is not quite so simple, but more complicated. It depends upon the use of the chemical. If we have to notify under the EC 6th Amendment, that is one type of situation. However, if a chemical being tested might be used as an intermediate entirely within a factory and the only people who have to be satisfied are our own professionals, if we feel it is possible to label it at the most serious level as an irritant

or a carcinogen, etc. and control it, there is no need to do the testing. It is a complicated question. I do not have personal experience of this, but I believe that most regulatory authorities still require the animal studies for labelling criteria, and it is not possible to bypass them.

M. Balls

In a meeting on regulatory acceptance, held in Greece last spring, 9 of the 17 people there were from regulatory agencies and they all agreed with the principle that if severe effects could be satisfactorily predicted from *in vitro* studies, that should be enough. Saying something is not an irritant is a completely different question, of course.

T. Smyrniotis

The methodology is very well defined in the European labelling system. For the moment, for skin and eye irritation the methods are well defined.

It is clear that national regulatory authorities could probably accept a statement from the industry saying that tests of a chemical with an *in vitro* method indicate that it is very corrosive and it is proposed to label it as a very corrosive substance. I do not think that in this case the regulatory authority would request an animal test. Our methods are regularly updated, and I think in the near future *in vitro* tests will play an increasingly important role, especially in eye and skin irritation. But again, there is the validation problem – and this is underway.

J.R. Claude

I think we are in an intermediate period, and all types of methodology are not at the same stage. Especially for irritancy, ocular toxicity, and probably (as shown by Dr Cordier) embryotoxicity and teratogenicity, there are possibilities of including *in vitro* tests in the battery of tests.

My proposal to the French agency is that, together with the results of their regulatory studies, the companies should report the results of their non-regulatory studies performed by *in vitro* methods. The expected result would be progressive validation by the accumulation of relevant data by *in vitro* procedures.

We must also bear in mind that the agencies have not only a scientific problem, but also in some cases psychological problems before *in vitro* procedures can be accepted. A progressive, positive attitude about *in vitro* experiments must be taken very early – probably *now*.

M. Balls

I think we all have to try to understand the psychology of regulators.

Question 13

F. Zucco
Should parallel testing in vitro *and in* vivo *be encouraged as a part of the validation process and database development?*

M. Balls
Certainly, yes.

H. van Looy
The Organization for Economic Cooperation and Development (OECD) countries are engaged in a rather important programme, a voluntary programme to fill data gaps on certain existing chemicals that are produced in high volumes. It is indeed strange to learn that there are such high-volume chemicals for which there is no basic information.

In this context, there will certainly be a phase of testing in the near future, which we will know more about later this year. It would be nice to believe that there are good systems that can be used for this purpose and given in parallel to the *in vivo* results that will be presented.

Question 14

F. Goethals
What can be done to promote Dr Cordier's proposal for a combined in vitro/in vivo *approach to teratogenicity and carcinogenicity testing, which could lead to the use of one species instead of two in* in vivo *testing?*

M. Balls
There is a lot of concern about carcinogenicity testing, in particular about the relevance of rodent studies and the need for studies in more than one species.

The case for a scheme such as that suggested by Dr Cordier, including the evidence to support it, should first be put to Dr Cordier's peers in toxicology, and then taken to an appropriate national authority, which could in turn take it to the OECD or the EC, because these bodies already have mechanisms for incorporating into practice such new suggestions after full discussion and consensus agreement.

Many toxicologists already question the need for two species' carcinogenicity testing. As long ago as 1982, the toxicologists on the FRAME Toxicity Committee concluded that, unless there was good scientific reason to the contrary, carcinogenicity testing should be carried out in one species, normally the rat.

With rodent studies in carcinogenicity I think we come up against the whole question of relevance. Experienced toxicologists tell me that they can design a study to show that something is or is not a carcinogen, according to what they want.

I. Purchase

To say toxicologists design studies for a perceived outcome is rather cynical, and I hope Dr Balls does not mean it. Many toxicologists, even those in industry who are paid by industry, have ethical standards which would not allow them to pursue that approach.

M. Balls

I am not personally being critical, but am merely reporting what other toxicologists have said.

T. Smyrniotis

Is there agreement among the scientific community about a battery of *in vitro* tests to replace the second species or is it only an expressed wish for the moment?

M. Balls

First, the need for a second species could be questioned anyway and, secondly, it is very hard to get agreement on anything in the scientific community. Scientists do not readily agree with one another; that is not what they are trained to do.

I. Purchase

The image I have of the way carcinogenicity testing will go is not so much a combination of embryotoxicity and carcinogenicity at the *in vitro* stage, but rather to build on the sort of observations that Ames recently published. Basically, he says that such huge doses of genotoxic, but also fairly non-toxic, compounds are being given in these animal studies that there are tumour responses which, when the mechanism is studied, can often be shown to be due to disturbances in hormone balance and similar secondary effects.

This suggests that with a really good battery of genotoxicity assays, once the non-genotoxicity of a chemical has been established, it may be possible completely to avoid doing a long-term carcinogenicity study, and only do a 1-year study looking for organ toxicity. On the basis of the no-effect levels and safety factors there, it should be possible to determine a safety factor which will not result in indirect carcinogenicity in the long-term studies.

N.G. Carmichael

Another form of alternative toxicology might be called "cerebral" or "paper" toxicology. One of the extremely frustrating things in addressing the philosophy of regulators is that on many occasions, for compounds already adequately tested for carcinogenicity, we cannot convince them that there is no need to re-test them at irrelevantly high doses. At present in the USA under the *Federal Insecticide, Fungicide and Rodenticide Act* legislation, we are obliged to slaughter hundreds of animals completely needlessly, because maximum tolerated doses were not achieved in our existing studies. This is something that could be addressed even before starting to talk about whether two species are necessary.

Question 15

F. Zucco

How do we solve the problem of the provision of enough relevant and reliable in vivo *data for use in the validation of* in vitro *methods without doing* in vivo *studies specifically for that purpose?*

M. Balls

I think we should all support the establishment of the international registry of reference chemicals, which has been proposed by Dr Purchase.

Question 16

D. Acosta

Who is funding, or should be funding, the development of in vitro *toxicity tests? Is it industry, governments or private sources?*

M. Balls

To some extent, it is all three, but in no case is it sufficient. I want to record a specific proposal, put to me by a professor of toxicology in the UK, that industrial companies should be required to spend as much on the development of *in vitro* toxicology as on *in vivo* toxicology, and that governments should be required to give grants for *in vitro* toxicology equal to the cost of the *in vivo* testing required by their regulatory agencies. The result would be a dramatic fall in *in vivo* testing, a dramatic increase in *in vitro* toxicology research, and a rationalization and harmonization of the regulatory guidelines. The citizens would be better protected, animals would be caused less suffering, and we would enter the next century in a much better state than we are now.

D. Acosta

I am an academic scientist and do not have all the facilities of industry or even government laboratories to do a thorough validation test. I have had experience with government and/or agencies providing some funds. However, as Dr Balls has said, it is not sufficient. There has to be a coordinated effort between industry, government and private sources, which I do not see at this point. This is a real problem. Funding has to be available if academic scientists are to participate in this type of study.

J. Frazier

This is obviously a serious issue. The sources of funding for these kinds of activities are limited. There is a significant amount of work at the industrial level which should be recognized, but it is often very hard to identify exactly what is going on.

The academic community in the USA, which, as was pointed out earlier, is the source both of a lot of the ideas and of creative new approaches, has a difficult problem. Our centre probably supports the major component of research activities, and our budget for alternative testing research purposes is $300 000 a year – which is a minimal amount of money. The National Institutes of Health will support it, except that such support is impeded by the problem of the mechanisms required to get research support for our basic science activities. This work is more applied toxicology, but the funding is for basic fundamental research, and that creates a barrier.

It is time to have serious discussion about the appropriate level of suport for these activities. I have thought about it, and my answer is that, if I was given $10 million a year for 5 years, I could solve many of the problems being discussed. If I was given $100 million a year for 5 years, I do not think I would do any better than with the $10 million. There is an optimal level of support. Clearly, we are well below that level, but I would be very concerned about throwing a huge amount of money at a problem without having a very good plan for using it.

This is the time, though, to discuss the issue of the optimal level of support and to try to work out the mechanisms to make it available.

M. Balls

That is absolutely right. We all know what happened to President Nixon's attempt to conquer cancer.

I. Purchase

We work in a type of scientific community in which consensus drives the areas which get support. Unfortunately, although alternative toxicology tests are high on the political and emotional agenda, they are not particularly high in terms of quality of science. Until we get our science right we will not get the funding. The problem is that the political and emotional pressure is pulling through bad science.

R. Ulrich

I might suggest that, at least for the pharmaceutical industry, the way to get financial support is perhaps for the government to consider giving a tax deduction for the money spent on alternative research.

H. Bazin

On funding of alternative research through the EC, we in the Community are trying to develop programmes of research for *in vitro* toxicology. We have about 60–80 million ECU to spend on the animal kingdom sector of biotechnology. This programme will be implemented in 1991.

M. Balls

I value what the Directorate General XII (DG XII) is doing. I have been one of the assessors of research on alternatives being funded. Some very valuable projects are about to begin under the BRIDGE programme. The particular value about research funded by DG XII is that it is international, involving good laboratories in a number of countries. I think that is very helpful in terms of the basic research and test validation processes we are talking about.

Question 17

F. Goethals

Are the regulatory authorities likely to accept the use of human data in the validation of non-animal tests, or will they insist on duplication of what is provided by animal tests?

M. Balls
It should depend upon the quality of the human data which are used in the validation process.

A. Paine
The regulatory authorities will accept human data, especially when exposure levels are precisely known. The problem is that, under many conditions, the exposure levels are not known.

Question 18

A. Guillouzo and D. Acosta
Who should control, coordinate, fund and organize validation schemes? Also, who should review the outcomes of validation schemes and make recommendations for the acceptance of well validated and independently judged acceptable non-animal tests, and how should such a review be conducted?

M. Balls
Coordination, in the sense of encouragement without control, is needed. Information on validation schemes should be made publicly available from the very first moment of planning in order to provide for efficiency and lack of duplication of effort. It is also important that reports should be made at stages during the validation process and the final results published and made available through the peer review literature.

The most important point is that the process should be a permissive one and should not be restrictive. I believe that any well-designed scientifically defensible well-conducted study using well-validated and independently assessed methods should be acceptable as a part of the process which helps both to identify potential toxic hazard and subsequently to contribute to risk assessment and risk management.

I believe that industry associations should be able to run validation schemes, as I think the CTFA is doing in the USA, as should private bodies such as FRAME, academic bodies such as Johns Hopkins University, government agencies, such as the BGA in Germany, and international bodies, such as the EC. We need many high-quality well-conducted validation schemes, and some international process of assessment.

J. Frazier

I think there has to be good discussion at the highest level so that we do not have to face the problems of harmonization all over again with the alternative methods.

J.R. Claude

At the end of this meeting, we must be fair to toxicology. First, the use of animals in toxicological experiments accounts for only approximately 12–15% of the total animal consumption.

Secondly, in terms of animal welfare, toxicological experiments are performed according to Good Laboratory Practice. The role of Good Laboratory Practice for the general quality of life of laboratory animals is also very important: it shows that we are not such criminals as is sometimes stated.

M. Balls

I personally would never use such terms, but I think toxicologists have shown that they are capable of defending themselves.

The consumption of animals for food, for example, is quite irrelevant to their use in toxicity testing. If a child is being beaten by its parents in London, it is quite irrelevant to say it would be worse off if it were starving in some other part of the world. That is a completely separate issue. In my opinion, first, there is no connection between the use of animals for food and their use in toxicity testing and, secondly, it is irrelevant to say that we use 3 million animals in Britain in research and eat 50 million.

T. Smyrniotis

With regard to the validation problem, I think we have to create not only a framework for validation, but also to produce constructive methods to be validated. It is very important to have methods that can be validated rapidly and integrated into the regulatory system.

I would like to say to everybody that, of course, we all understand the importance of formal methods of research, science and so on, but the European Commission at least has a commitment not only to the goals of research, the environment, internal markets and the free circulation of products, but also to the European public and has to respond to their legitimate concerns. If we do not respond satisfactorily and rapidly, I am afraid that decisions will be taken which will not be very favourable to research and science.

For example, I am in close contact with the Inter-Group for Animal Welfare within the European Parliament, a powerful group of 50 or 60

Members of Parliament, who are very concerned about animal welfare. After giving money for years for *in vitro* research, they do not understand why nothing has been changed in the regulations. We are not in a position to keep them quiet.

I do not believe that future decisions will be easy to take, but if progress is not made in the near future I am afraid that we will all be in a very difficult position. When you are thinking about science and fundamental research models, please also think about making progress in the field of alternatives.

J. Frazier

What should come out of this meeting in terms of practical things that can be done? The next step that can be addressed in a practical sense is Dr Purchase's suggestion for a reference chemical bank. If our energies could be focused on trying to achieve that, it would make a significant contribution to advancing the validation process. It is not the final solution, but is certainly a step which I think we recognize requires some scientific input, and it is one that can and should be taken. We have the science and I think the technology to do it.

G. Jolles

I want to express thanks to the members of the Panel, especially to Dr Balls. We have had a very good discussion and Dr Balls has done a wonderful job as Chairman. I also wish to thank all the speakers, and the audience for coming, some from a long way. I think your participation in this meeting was extremely helpful.

Concluding Remarks

Over the last five years, substantial progress has been made in the field of *in vitro* toxicology. Whereas early work seemed to focus merely on simple measurements of cell death or cytotoxicity usually through the use of cell lines, the contributions to this book clearly show that new challenges are emerging.

In vitro systems should provide adequate models if the cell's more complex *in vivo* functions are maintained *in vitro* so that mechanisms of toxicity relevant of those observed in the whole animal can be studied.

New *in vitro* models, using primary cultures, now try to maintain cell or organ-specific functions in order to gain the most relevant information. A wide array of specific end points, such as hormone secretion, metabolic changes, transport mechanisms, gene activation and amplification are commonly employed.

The challenge now is to adapt new discoveries to practical use in toxicity testing. The first area, obviously, is toxicological screening, which provides a rapid and inexpensive means to rank compounds with regard to well-defined toxicological properties and biological potency. The second and more important application is in the study of toxicological mechanisms. Indeed, *in vitro* methods could improve extrapolation to human risk assessment, since they often permit the exact determination of safe and toxic concentrations at the target site.

While the integration of *in vitro* methods into the basic sciences of toxicology and industrial research is progressing rapidly, the involvement

IN VITRO METHODS IN TOXICOLOGY
ISBN 0-12-388175-7

and the acceptance of *in vitro* methods as replacements or alternatives to whole animal toxicity testing has been slow and disappointing. At present there is no doubt about the use of *in vitro* data in *addition* to an integrated safety evalution, but they cannot be considered now or in the foreseeable future as a *substitute* for animal experiments.

Contrary to a prevailing misconception, *in vitro* tests need not replace existing *in vivo* procedures in order to be helpful. The way forward could be a combination of tests in various *in vitro* systems together with animal experiments. Such an integrated approach is still at an early stage of development but could be the key to reducing the use of laboratory animals by eliminating unnecessary testing in the light of knowledge of toxicological mechanisms.

In this context, we are convinced that *in vitro* toxicology will generate better and more scientific toxicology in the near future.

G.J. A.C.

Index